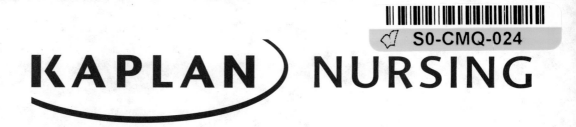

# KAPLAN) NURSING

# THE BASICS

# A COMPREHENSIVE OUTLINE OF NURSING SCHOOL CONTENT

Ninth Edition

**Loretta Aller, PhD, RN**

**Joanne Brown, MSN, MPH, RN**

**Judith A. Burckhardt, PhD, RN**

**Susan Compton, MSN, RN**

**Pamela Gardner, MSN, RN**

**Joseph Ryan Goble, MSN, RN**

**Roberta Harbison, MSN, RN**

**Barbara J. Irwin, MSN, RN**

**Amy Kennedy, MSN, RN**

**Marlene Redemske, MSN, MA, RN**

**Kendra Spaulding, DNP, RN**

Contributing Editors

This book is solely intended for use as preparation for the NCLEX examination. It is not a guide to the clinical treatment of clients. Neither the authors nor the publisher shall be responsible for any harm caused by the use of this book other than for its intended purpose. This book is just a small portion of the Kaplan materials available for you to prepare for the NCLEX examination.

This publication is designed to provide accurate information in regard to the subject matter covered as of its publication date, with the understanding that knowledge and best practice constantly evolve. The publisher is not engaged in rendering medical, legal, accounting, or other professional service. If medical or legal advice or other expert assistance is required, the services of a competent professional should be sought. This publication is not intended for use in clinical practice or the delivery of medical care. To the fullest extent of the law, neither the Publisher nor the Editors assume any liability for any injury and/or damage to persons or property arising out of or related to any use of the material contained in this book.

© 2023 by Kaplan North America, LLC

Published by Kaplan North America, LLC dba Kaplan Publishing
1515 West Cypress Creek Road
Fort Lauderdale, Florida 33309

ISBN: 978-1-5062-8263-3

10 9 8 7 6 5 4 3 2 1

Kaplan Publishing print books are available at special quantity discounts to use for sales promotions, employee premiums, or educational purposes. For more information or to purchase books, please call the Simon & Schuster special sales department at 866-506-1949.

# TABLE OF CONTENTS

**GO ONLINE**

*www.kaptest.com/ nclex/books*

Thinking Exercises, composed of a short case and three questions, are located at the end of chapters 1–16. These exercises provide the reader an opportunity to apply critical thinking and clinical reasoning to arrive at safe clinical judgments. Each question addresses a cognitive skill, identified in parentheses (e.g., recognize cues, analyze cues). The six cognitive skills are derived from the National Council of State Boards of Nursing's Clinical Judgment Measurement Model.

# CHAPTER 1

# HEALTH ASSESSMENT

## Health Promotion

**SECTIONS**

1. Health History

2. Physical Assessment

3. Mental Status Assessment

**CONCEPTS COVERED**

Table 1-1. Normal Vital Signs
Table 1-2. Normal Body Temperature
Table 1-3. Cranial Nerve Assessment

# HEALTH HISTORY

## Health Promotion

## Demographic Data

A. Date

B. Biographical information

C. Client as reliable historian

D. Age, sex, marital status

E. Reason for seeking health care

F. History of present illness/condition

## Past Health History

A. Past health history

1. Medical history

2. Surgical history

3. Medications

4. Communicable diseases

5. Allergies

6. Injuries/accidents

7. Disabilities/handicaps

8. Blood transfusions

9. Childhood illnesses

10. Immunizations

B. Family health history

1. Genogram

2. Familial/genetic diseases

C. Social history

1. Alcohol/tobacco/drug use

2. Travel history

3. Work environment

4. Home environment

5. Hobbies/leisure activities

      6. Stressors

      7. Education

      8. Economic status

      9. Military service

    10. Religion

    11. Culture

    12. Roles/relationships

    13. Sexual history

    14. Patterns of daily living

**D.** Health maintenance

      1. Sleep

      2. Diet

      3. Exercise

      4. Stress management

      5. Safety practices

      6. Patterns of health care practices

      7. Review of systems

# PHYSICAL ASSESSMENT

## Therapeutic Techniques

## Purpose

  **A.** Assess client's current health status

  **B.** Interpret physical data

  **C.** Decide on interventions based on data obtained

## Preparation

  **A.** Gather equipment

    1. Ophthalmoscope

    2. Tuning fork

    3. Cotton swabs

    4. Snellen eye chart

    5. Thermometer

    6. Penlight

    7. Tongue depressor

    8. Ruler/tape measure

    9. Safety pin

    10. Balance scale

    11. Gloves

    12. Nasal speculum

    13. Vaginal speculum

  **B.** Provide for privacy (drape) in quiet, well-lit environment

  **C.** Explain procedure to client

  **D.** Ask client to empty bladder

  **E.** Drape client for privacy

  **F.** Compare findings on one side of body with other side and compare with normal

  **G.** Make use of teaching opportunities (dental care, eye exams, self-exams of breasts or testicles)

  **H.** Use piece of equipment for entire assessment, then return to equipment tray

## Techniques Used In Order Performed, Except for Abdominal Assessment

**A.** General assessment

   1. Inspection

   2. Palpation

   3. Percussion

   4. Auscultation

**B.** Abdominal assessment

   1. Inspection

   2. Auscultation

   3. Percussion

   4. Palpation

**C.** Inspection (visually examined)

   1. Start with first interaction

   2. Provide good lighting

   3. Determine

      a. Size

      b. Shape

      c. Color

      d. Texture

      e. Symmetry

      f. Position

**D.** Palpation (touch)

   1. Warm hands

   2. Approach slowly and proceed systematically

   3. Use fingertips for fine touch (pulses, nodes)

   4. Use dorsum of fingers for temperature

   5. Use palm or ulnar edge of hand for vibration

   6. Start with light palpation, then do deep palpation

   7. Use bimanual palpation (both hands) for deep palpation and to assess movable structure (kidney). Place sensing hand lightly on skin surface, place active hand over sensing hand and apply pressure

   8. Ballottement—push fluid-filled tissue toward palpating hand so object floats against fingertips

   9. Determine

      a. Masses

      b. Pulsation

      c.  Organ size

      d.  Tenderness or pain

      e.  Swelling

      f.  Tissue fullness and elasticity

      g.  Vibration

      h.  Crepitus

      i.  Temperature

      j.  Texture

      k.  Moisture

**E.**  Percussion (tap to produce sound and vibration)

    1.  Types

      a.  Direct—strike body surface with 1 or 2 fingers

      b.  Indirect—strike finger or hand placed over body surface

      c.  Blunt—use reflex hammer to check deep tendon reflexes; use blunt percussion with fist to assess costovertebral angle (CVA) tenderness

    2.  Sounds (produced by direct or indirect percussion)

      a.  Resonance—moderate to loud, low-pitched (clear, hollow) sound of moderate duration; found with air-filled tissue (normal lung)

      b.  Hyperresonance—loud, booming, low-pitched sound of longer duration found with overinflated, air-filled tissue (pulmonary emphysema); normal in child due to thin chest wall

      c.  Tympany—loud, drumlike, high-pitched or musical sound of moderately long duration found with enclosed, air-filled structures (bowel)

      d.  Dull—soft, muffled, moderate to high-pitched sound of short duration; found with dense, fluid-filled tissue (liver)

      e.  Flat—very soft, high-pitched sound of short duration; found with very dense tissue (bone, muscle)

    3.  Determine

      a.  Location, size, density of masses

      b.  Pain in areas up to depth of 3–5 cm (1–2 in)

    4.  Performed after inspection and palpation, except for abdominal assessment; for abdomen, perform inspection, auscultation, percussion, palpation

**F.**  Auscultation (listen to sounds)

    1.  Equipment

      a.  Use diaphragm of stethoscope to listen to high-pitched sounds (lung, bowel, heart); place firmly against skin surface to form tight seal (leave ring)

      b.  Use bell to listen to soft, low-pitched sounds (heart murmurs); place lightly on skin surface

2. Listen over bare skin (not through clothing); moisten body hair to prevent crackling sounds

## Findings

**A.** General survey

1. General appearance

   a. Apparent age

   b. Sex

   c. Racial and ethnic groups

   d. Apparent state of health

   e. Proportionate height and weight

   f. Posture

   g. Gait, movements, range of motion

   h. Suitable clothing

   i. Hygiene

   j. Body and breath odor

   k. Skin color, condition

   l. Presence of assistive device, hearing aid, glasses

2. General behavior

   a. Signs of distress

   b. Level of consciousness, oriented ×3, mood, speech, thought process appropriate

   c. Level of cooperation, eye contact (culture must be considered)

**B.** Vital signs (*see* Table 1-1)

1. Temperature (*see* Table 1-2)

   a. Infants—performed axillary, rectally

   b. Intra-auricular probe allows rapid, noninvasive reading when appropriate

   c. Tympanic membrane sensors—positioning is crucial, ear canal must be straightened

**Table 1-1** Normal Vital Signs

| AGE | NORMAL RESPIRATORY RATE | NORMAL PULSE RATE | NORMAL BLOOD PRESSURE (BP) |
|---|---|---|---|
| Newborn | 30-60 per min | 120-140 beats per minute (bpm)<br><br>May go to 180 when crying | 65/41 mm Hg |
| 1-4 years | 20-30 per min | 70-110 bpm | 85/40-93/50 mm Hg |
| 5-12 years | 16-22 per min | 60-95 bpm | 93/53-106/62 mm Hg |
| Adult | 12-20 per min | 60-100 bpm | Less than 120/80 mm Hg |

Factors influencing respiration: fever, anxiety, medications, disease
Factors influencing BP: disease, medications, anxiety, cardiac output, peripheral resistance, arterial elasticity, blood volume, blood viscosity, age, weight, exercise
Factors influencing pulse rate and rhythm: medications, pathology, exercise, age, sex, temperature, BP, serum electrolytes
Gerontologic considerations: increased systolic blood pressure, possible decrease in diastolic BP, widened pulse pressure

**Table 1-2** Normal Body Temperature

| METHOD USED | FAHRENHEIT | CELSIUS |
|---|---|---|
| Oral | 98.6° | 37° |
| Rectal | 99.6° | 37.6° |
| Axillary | 97.6° | 36.5° |

Factors influencing reading: older adult client (normal temperature may be 95-97°F), faulty thermometer, dehydration, environment, infections

2. Pulse (rate, rhythm)
3. Respirations (rate, pattern, depth)
   a. Adult—costal (chest movement), regular, expiration slower than inspiration, rate 12–20 respirations/min
   b. Neonates—diaphragmatic (abdominal movement), irregular, 30–60 respirations/min
   c. Breathing patterns
      1) Abdominal respirations—breathing accomplished by abdominal muscles and diaphragm; may be used to increase effectiveness of ventilatory process in certain conditions

    2) Apnea—temporary cessation of breathing

    3) Cheyne-Stokes respirations—a repeating period of fast, shallow breathing followed by slow, heavier breathing and seconds of apnea.

    4) Dyspnea—difficult, labored, or painful breathing (considered "normal" at certain times, e.g., after extreme physical exertion)

    5) Hyperpnea—abnormally deep breathing

    6) Hyperventilation—abnormally rapid, deep, and prolonged breathing

        a) Caused by central nervous system disorders, medications that increase sensitivity of respiratory center, or acute anxiety

        b) Produces respiratory alkalosis due to reduction in $CO_2$

    7) Hypoventilation—reduced ventilatory efficiency; produces respiratory acidosis due to elevation in $CO_2$

    8) Kussmaul's respirations (air hunger)—marked increase in depth and rate

    9) Orthopnea—inability to breathe except when trunk is in an upright position

    10) Paradoxical respirations—breathing pattern in which a lung (or portion of a lung) deflates during inspiration (acts opposite to normal)

    11) Periodic breathing—rate, depth, or tidal volume changes markedly from one interval to the next; pattern of change is periodically reproduced

    12) Cyanosis—skin appears blue because of an excessive accumulation of unoxygenated hemoglobin in the blood

    13) Stridor—harsh, high-pitched sound associated with airway obstruction near larynx

    14) Cough

        a) Normal reflex to remove foreign material from the lungs

        b) Normally absent in newborns

4. Blood pressure

    a. Check both arms and compare results (difference 5–10 mm Hg normal)

    b. Pulse pressure is difference between systolic and diastolic readings; normal 30–40 mm Hg

    c. Cover 50% of limb from shoulder to olecranon with cuff; too narrow: abnormally high reading; too wide: abnormally low reading

**C.** Nutrition status

1. Height, weight; ideal body weight, men: 106 lb for first 5 ft, then add 6 lb/in; women: 100 lb for first 5 ft, then add 5 lb/in; add 10% for client with larger frame; subtract 10% for client with small frame

**D.** Skin

1. Check for pallor on buccal mucosa or conjunctivae, cyanosis on nail beds or oral mucosa, jaundice on sclera

2. Scars, bruises, lesions

3. Edema (eyes, sacrum), moisture, hydration

4. Temperature, texture, turgor (pinch skin, tented 3 seconds or less is normal), check over sternum for older adult

**E.** Hair

1. Hirsutism—excess

2. Alopecia—loss or thinning

**F.** Nails (indicates respiratory and nutritional status)

1. Color

2. Shape, contour (normal angle of nail bed $\leq 160°$; clubbing: nail bed angle $\geq 180°$ due to prolonged decreased oxygenation)

3. Texture, thickness

4. Capillary refill—blanch nail beds of fingers or toes and quickly release pressure; color should quickly return to normal ($\leq 3$ seconds)

**G.** Head

1. Size, shape, symmetry

2. Temporal arteries

3. Cranial nerve function (*see* Table 1-3)

**Table 1-3** Cranial Nerve Assessment

| (#) NERVE | FUNCTION | NORMAL FINDINGS | NURSING CONSIDERATIONS |
|---|---|---|---|
| (I) Olfactory | Sense of smell | Able to detect various odors in each nostril | Have client smell a nonirritating substance such as coffee or tobacco with eyes closed<br><br>Test each nostril separately |
| (II) Optic | Sense of vision | Clear (acute) vision near and distant | Snellen eye chart for far vision<br><br>Read newspaper for near vision<br><br>Ophthalmoscopic exam |
| (III) Oculomotor | Pupil constriction, raising of eyelids | Pupils equal in size and equally reactive to light | Observe for symmetry and eye-opening<br><br>Shine penlight into eye as client stares straight ahead<br><br>Eye movements—ask client to watch your finger as you move it toward their face (Examined with CN IV and VI)<br><br>Instruct client to look up, down, inward and laterally. |

*(Continued)*

**Table 1-3** Cranial Nerve Assessment (*Continued*)

| (#) NERVE | FUNCTION | NORMAL FINDINGS | NURSING CONSIDERATIONS |
|---|---|---|---|
| (IV) Trochlear | Downward and inward movement of eyes | Able to move eyes down and inward | (*See* CN III) Examined with CN III and VI (assessment of eye movements) |
| (V) Trigeminal | Motor—jaw movement<br><br>Sensory—sensation on the face and neck | Able to clench and relax jaw<br><br>Able to differentiate between various stimuli touched to the face and neck | Test with pin and wisp of cotton over all three branches (forehead, cheek, jaw on both sides of face)<br><br>Ask client to open jaw, bite down, move jaw laterally against pressure<br><br>Stroke cornea with wisp of cotton |
| (VI) Abducens | Lateral movement of the eyes | Able to move eyes in all directions | (*See* CN III) Examined with CN III and IV (assessment of eye movements) |
| (VII) Facial | Motor—facial muscle movement<br><br>Sensory—taste on the anterior two-thirds of the tongue (sweet and salty) | Able to smile, whistle, wrinkle forehead<br><br>Able to differentiate tastes among various agents | Observe for facial symmetry after asking client to frown, smile, raise eyebrows, close eyelids against resistance, whistle, blow<br><br>Place sweet, sour, bitter, and salty substances on tongue |
| (VIII) Acoustic | Sense of hearing and balance | Hearing intact<br><br>Balance maintained while walking | Test with watch ticking into ear, rubbing fingers together, Rinne, Weber<br><br>Test posture, standing with eyes closed<br><br>Otoscopic exam |
| (IX) Glossopharyngeal | Motor—pharyngeal movement and swallowing<br><br>Sensory—taste on posterior one-third of tongue (sour and bitter) | Gag reflex intact, able to swallow<br><br>Able to taste | Place sweet, sour, bitter, and salty substances on tongue<br><br>Note ability to swallow and manage secretions<br><br>Stimulate pharyngeal wall to elicit gag reflex |

(*Continued*)

**Table 1-3** Cranial Nerve Assessment (*Continued*)

| (#) NERVE | FUNCTION | NORMAL FINDINGS | NURSING CONSIDERATIONS |
|---|---|---|---|
| (X) Vagus | Swallowing and speaking | Able to swallow and speak with a smooth voice | Inspect soft palate—instruct to say "ah"<br><br>Observe uvula for midline position<br><br>Rate quality of voice |
| (XI) Spinal accessory | Motor—flexion and rotation of head; shrugging of shoulders | Able to flex and rotate head; able to shrug shoulders | Inspect and palpate sterno-cleidomastoid and trapezius muscles for size, contour, tone<br><br>Ask client to move head side to side against resistance and shrug shoulders against resistance |
| (XII) Hypoglossal | Motor—tongue movements | Can move tongue side to side and stick it out symmetrically and in midline | Inspect tongue in mouth<br><br>Ask client to stick out tongue and move it quickly side to side<br><br>Observe midline, symmetry, and rhythmic movement |

H. Eyes
1. Ptosis—drooping of upper eyelid
2. Color of sclerae, conjunctivae
3. Pupils—size, shape, equality, reactivity to light and accommodation (PERRLA)
4. Photophobia—light intolerance
5. Nystagmus—abnormal, involuntary, rapid eye movements
6. Strabismus—involuntary drifting of one eye out of alignment with the other eye; "lazy eye"
7. Corneal reflex
8. Visual fields (peripheral vision)
9. Visual acuity—Snellen chart, normal 20/20
10. Ophthalmoscope exam
    a. Red reflex—red glow from light reflected from retina
    b. Fundus
    c. Optic disk (the blind spot)
    d. Macula

11. Gerontologic considerations—sclera yellowish-colored; milky-colored ring around periphery of cornea; decreased corneal reflex; decreased tear secretion; delayed pupil reflex and accommodation; cataracts; presbyopia; increased incidence of "floaters"

**I.** Ears

1. Pull pinna up and back to examine children's ($\geq$3 years of age) and adults' ears

2. Pull pinna down and back to examine infants' and young children's (less than 3 years of age) ears

3. Tympanic membrane—cone of light at 5 o'clock position right ear, 7 o'clock position left ear

4. Weber test—assesses bone conduction; vibrating tuning fork placed in middle of forehead; normal: hear sound equally in ears

5. Rinne test—compares bone conduction with air conduction; vibrating tuning fork placed on mastoid process, when client no longer hears sound, positioned in front of ear canal; normal: should still be able to hear sound; air conduction greater than bone conduction by 2:1 ratio (positive Rinne test)

**J.** Nose and sinuses

1. Septum midline

2. Alignment, color, discharge

3. Palpate and percuss sinuses

**K.** Mouth and pharynx

1. Oral mucosa

2. Teeth (normal: 32)

3. Tongue

4. Hard and soft palate

5. Uvula, midline

6. Tonsils

7. Gag reflex

8. Swallow

9. Taste

**L.** Neck

1. Range of motion of cervical spine

2. Cervical lymph nodes (normal $\leq$1 cm round, soft, mobile) nontender

3. Trachea position

4. Thyroid gland

5. Carotid arteries—check for bruit and thrill

6. Jugular veins

**M.** Thorax and lungs

1. Alignment of spine

2. Anteroposterior to transverse diameter (normal adult 1:2 to 5:7); 1:1 barrel chest

3. Respiratory excursion

4. Respirations

5. Tactile fremitus—vibration produced when client articulates "99"

6. Diaphragmatic excursion—assesses degree and symmetry of diaphragm movement; percuss from areas of resonance to dullness

7. Breath sounds—bilaterally equal

    a. Normal

        1) Vesicular—soft and low-pitched breezy sounds heard over most of peripheral lung fields; inspiration $\geq$ expiration

        2) Bronchovesicular—medium-pitched, moderately loud sounds heard over the mainstem bronchi; inspiration $=$ expiration

        3) Bronchial—loud, coarse, blowing sound heard over the trachea; inspiration $\leq$ expiration

    b. Adventitious (abnormal); caused by fluid or inflammation

        1) Fine crackles—crackling or popping sounds commonly heard on late inspiration; atelectatic crackles clear with coughing

        2) Coarse crackles—harsh, moist popping sounds heard commonly on early inspiration; originate in large bronchus

        3) Sonorous wheeze—low-pitched, coarse snoring sounds commonly heard on expiration

        4) Sibilant wheeze—squeaky sounds heard during inspiration and expiration associated with narrowed airways

        5) Pleural friction rub—grating sound or vibration heard during inspiration and expiration

8. Vocal resonance

    a. Bronchophony—say "99" and hear more clearly than normal; loud transmission of voice sounds caused by consolidation of lung

    b. Egophony—say "E" and hear "A" due to distortion caused by consolidation of lung

    c. Whispered pectoriloquy—hear whispered sounds clearly due to dense consolidation of lung

9. Costovertebral angle percussion—kidneys

**N.** Heart sounds

1. Angle of Louis—manubriosternal junction at second rib

2. Aortic and pulmonic areas—right and left second intercostal spaces alongside sternum

3. Erb's point—third intercostal space just left of sternum

4. Tricuspid area—fourth or fifth intercostal space at lower left of sternal border

5. Mitral area—fifth intercostal space at left midclavicular line (apex of heart)

6. Point of maximal impulse (PMI)

   a. Impulse of the left ventricle felt most strongly

   b. Adult—left fifth intercostal space in the midclavicular line (8–10 cm to the left of the midsternal line)

   c. Infant—lateral to left nipple; heart failure—displaced down and to left

7. S1 and S2

   a. S1 "lub"—closure of tricuspid and mitral valves; dull quality and low pitch; onset of ventricular systole (contraction); louder at apex; use diaphragm

   b. S2 "dub"—closure of aortic and pulmonic valves; snapping quality; onset of diastole (relaxation of atria, then ventricles); loudest at base; use diaphragm

8. Murmurs—abnormal sounds caused by turbulence within a heart valve; turbulence within a blood vessel is called a bruit; three basic factors result in murmurs:

   a. High rate of blood flow through either a normal or abnormal valve

   b. Blood flow through a sclerosed or abnormal valve, or into a dilated heart chamber or vessel

   c. Blood flow regurgitated backward through an incompetent valve or septal defect

9. Pulse deficit—difference between apical and radial rate

10. Jugular veins—normally distend when client lies flat, but are not visible when the client's head is raised 30° to 45°

O. Peripheral vascular system

   1. Pulses

      a. Radial—passes medially across the wrist; felt on radial (or thumb) side of the forearm

      b. Ulnar—passes laterally across the wrist; felt on the ulnar (little finger) side of the wrist

      c. Femoral—passes beneath the inguinal ligament (groin area) into the thigh; felt in groin area

      d. Carotid—pulsations can be felt over medial edge of sternocleidomastoid muscle in neck

      e. Pedal (dorsalis pedis—dorsal artery of the foot)—passes laterally over the foot; felt along top of foot

      f. Posterior tibial—felt on inner side of ankle below medial malleolus

      g. Popliteal—felt in popliteal fossa, the region at the back of the knee

      h. Temporal—felt lateral to eyes

      i. Apical—left at fifth intercostal space at midclavicular line

P. Breasts and axillae

   1. Size, shape, symmetry

   2. Gynecomastia—breast enlargement in males

   3. Nodes—normal: nonpalpable

**Q.** Abdomen

1. Knees flexed to relax muscles and provide for comfort
2. Inspect and auscultate, then percuss and palpate
3. Symmetry, contour (flat, rounded, protuberant, or scaphoid)
4. Umbilicus
5. Bowel sounds; normal high-pitched gurgles heard with the diaphragm of the stethoscope at 5- to 20-s intervals
   a. Hypoactive: less than 3/min
   b. Hyperactive: loud, frequent
6. Aortic, renal, iliac, femoral arteries auscultated with the bell of the stethoscope
7. Peritoneal friction rub—grating sound varies with respirations; inflammation of liver
8. Liver and spleen size
9. Inguinal lymph nodes
10. Rebound tenderness—inflammation of peritoneum
11. Kidneys
12. Abdominal reflexes

**R.** Neurological system

1. Deep tendon reflexes (DTRs)—assess sensory and motor pathways; compare bilaterally; O (absent) through 4+ (hyperactive) scale
2. Cerebellar function—coordination; point-to-point touching, rapid, alternating movements, gait
3. Mental status (cerebral function) (*see* Section 3 of this chapter)
4. Cranial nerve function
5. Motor function
   a. Strength
   b. Tone
6. Sensory function
   a. Touch, tactile localization
   b. Pain
   c. Pressure
   d. Temperature
   e. Vibration
   f. Proprioception (position sense)
   g. Vision
   h. Hearing
   i. Smell
   j. Taste

    **S.** Musculoskeletal system

       1. Muscle tone and strength

       2. Joint movements; crepitus—grating sound abnormal

    **T.** Genitalia

       1. Provide privacy

       2. Use firm, deliberate touch

       3. Male

          a. Penis—foreskin, glans

          b. Hypospadias—meatus located on underside of penile shaft

          c. Epispadias—meatus located on upper side of penile shaft

          d. Scrotum

          e. Inguinal area

       4. Female

          a. Lithotomy position

          b. Cervix

          c. Ovaries

          d. Vaginal canal

    **U.** Anus and rectum

       1. Rectal prolapse—protrusion of rectal mucous membrane through anus

       2. Hemorrhoids—dilated veins

       3. Anal sphincter

       4. Male—prostate gland

       5. Stool—normal color brown; assess for presence of blood

# MENTAL STATUS ASSESSMENT

## Ego Integrity/Self-Concept Intracranial Regulation

Done during interview and neurological assessment

## Data Gathering

**A.** Observation

1. Gait and posture

2. Mode of dress

3. Involuntary movements

4. Voice (consider language and culture)

5. Affect and speech content

6. Logic, judgment, speech patterns

7. Attention, memory, insight

8. Spatial perception, calculation, abstract reasoning, thought processes and content

## General Findings

**A.** Note client's ability to wait patiently

**B.** Posture relaxed, slumped, or stiff

**C.** Body movement—look for control and symmetry

**D.** Abnormal—restlessness, tenseness, pacing, slumped posture, slow gait, poor eye contact (culture must be considered), slow movements or speech, and poor personal hygiene may indicate mental illness

**E.** Communication findings

1. Note client's ability to speak coherently and carry out commands

2. Note client's affect—abnormal findings: blunt, inappropriate, elated, hostile

3. Note presence of aphasia

**F.** Cognitive findings—client should be able to:

1. Demonstrate orientation to time, place, and person

2. Correctly repeat a series of 5 or 6 numbers

3. Give important facts, such as dates or names, and repeat information given in the previous five minutes during exam

4. Make decision(s) based on sound reasoning

5. Demonstrate a realistic awareness of self

6. Copy simple figures and identify familiar sounds

7. Perform simple calculations

8. Give the meaning of a simple figure of speech, as in "a stitch in time saves nine"

9. Give responses that are based in reality and that are logical, goal-oriented, and clear

10. Abnormal findings

   a. Inability to recall immediate or long-term information, recognize objects (agnosia), perform purposeful movements (apraxia), calculate (dyscalculia), describe in abstractions, generalize, apply general principles

   b. Impaired judgment

   c. Unrealistic perceptions of self

   d. Illogical thought processes

   e. Blocking

   f. Flight of ideas

   g. Confabulation (making up answers unrelated to facts)

   h. Echolalia (involuntary repetitions of words spoken by another person)

   i. Delusions of grandeur or persecution

   j. Hallucinations, illusions, and delusions

## Standardized Instrument Screening Tool

A. Mini-Mental State Exam (MMSE)

1. Used to diagnose dementia or delirium

2. Tests orientation, short-term memory and attention, ability to perform calculations, language, and construction

3. Cannot be used if client cannot read, write, or speak English

B. Mental Status Exam

1. Provides a baseline of current cognitive processes

2. Used frequently to assess changes in the client's status

# End-of-Chapter Thinking Exercise

An older adult client is admitted to the medical-surgical unit after being seen in the health care provider's (HCP) office this morning. The client reports no bowel movement or passing gas in five days, no appetite, and constant nausea. Last evening, the client tried to eat some soup and vomited immediately after ingesting. Eighteen months ago, the client was diagnosed with colon cancer after detection on a routine colonoscopy. At that time, the client was treated with a partial colectomy and a course of chemotherapy. The client has been in good health until this week. The client lives in an assisted living facility, is hard of hearing, and ambulates with the assistance of a walker. The nurse prepares to complete the admission physical assessment. The client is alert and oriented to person, place, time, and situation. Vital signs: temperature 98.6°F (37°C), pulse 90 beats/min, respiratory rate 22 breaths/min, BP 154/82 mm Hg, and pain rating of 8/10 in the lower abdomen. The HCP's orders include IV D5 1/2 NS at 75 mL/hr and insertion of a nasogastric (NG) tube to intermittent suction.

1. What factors does the nurse consider when performing an initial physical assessment on this client? (Recognize Cues)

2. What is important to observe when assessing the abdomen of this client? (Analyze Cues)

3. When assessing the client's abdomen, in what order does the nurse perform the techniques of physical assessment? (Take Action)

# Thinking Exercise Explanations

1. What factors does the nurse consider when performing an initial physical assessment on this client? (Recognize Cues)

   - Privacy
   - Quiet environment
   - Adequate lighting
   - Looking directly at the client and talking slowly
   - Explaining the procedure to the client
   - Developing a trusting relationship

   The nurse ensures a safe environment to collect data as well as establishing rapport and communication with the client.

2. What is important to observe when assessing the abdomen of this client? (Analyze Cues)

   - Presence or absence of bowel sounds
   - Presence of abdominal distension
   - Pain, location, quality, pain rating scale

   Because of the diagnosis and signs and symptoms, the nurse expects abnormal findings when assessing the abdomen.

3. When assessing the client's abdomen, in what order does the nurse perform the techniques of physical assessment? (Take Action)

   - Inspection
   - Auscultation
   - Percussion
   - Palpation

   This order allows for accurate assessment of the bowel sounds before touching the abdomen.

# CHAPTER 2

# FUNDAMENTALS OF NURSING

| SECTIONS | CONCEPTS COVERED |
| --- | --- |
| 1. Normal Mobility | Table 2-1. Developmental Stages of the Musculoskeletal System<br>Table 2-2. Joint Movement and Action |
| 2. Altered Functions Related to Immobility | Table 2-3. Adverse Effects of Immobility<br>Table 2-4. Therapeutic Functions of Client Positions<br>Table 2-5. Therapeutic Exercises<br>Table 2-6. Crutch Walking Gaits |
| 3. Safety | Table 2-7. Nursing Management of the Child at Different Developmental Stages |
| 4. Altered Functions Related to Pain | Table 2-8. Types of Pain<br>Table 2-9. Responses to Pain Stimuli<br>Table 2-10. Common Pain Medications |
| 5. Protection from Communicable Diseases | Table 2-11. Recommended Adult Immunizations |
| 6. Maintenance of Skin Integrity | Table 2-12. Therapeutic Baths<br>Table 2-13. Common Skin Medications<br>Table 2-14. General Nursing Measures to Promote Wound Healing<br>Table 2-15. Selected Skin Disorders |
| 7. Perioperative Care | Table 2-16. Fears of Surgery at Different Developmental Stages<br>Table 2-17. Preoperative Teaching Guide<br>Table 2-18. Anesthesia<br>Table 2-19. Premedications and Potential Problems<br>Table 2-20. Potential Complications of Surgery<br>Table 2-21. Surgical Drains |

# NORMAL MOBILITY

## Mobility

## Normal Developmental Structures and Functions— Musculoskeletal System

**A.** Developmental stages and related functions (*see* Table 2-1)

**B.** Joint movement and action (*see* Table 2-2)

**C.** General database

    1. Physical assessment

        a. Body build, height, weight—proportioned within normal limits

        b. Posture, body alignment—erect

        c. Gait, ambulation—smooth

        d. Joints—freely movable

        e. Skin integrity—intact

        f. Muscle tone, elasticity, strength—adequate

    2. History

        g. Psychosocial assessment

            1) Exercise level

            2) Rest and sleep patterns

            3) Sexual activity

            4) Job-related activity

        h. Health history

            1) Pregnancy

            2) Structural or functional defects of the nervous system

            3) Structural or functional defects of the musculoskeletal system

            4) Diagnostic procedures and medical or surgical treatments that require activity restriction

            5) Conditions or treatments that result in pain

            6) Endocrine disorders that affect rest and activity

**Table 2-1** Developmental Stages of the Musculoskeletal System

| AGE | NORMAL FINDINGS |
|---|---|
| 0–1 month (period of involuntary movement) | Full range of motion<br>High degree of muscle tone<br>Moves mostly involuntarily |
| 1–3 months | Turns and raises head and chest when prone<br>Stretches arms<br>Muscles are well flexed |
| 3–6 months | Sits with support<br>Rolls over<br>Shakes objects with two hands<br>Transfers objects from hand to hand |
| 6–9 months | Has erect body posture<br>Sits up<br>Holds a bottle with fingers<br>Feeds self with fingers<br>Grasps with one hand<br>Crawls |
| 9–18 months | Develops lower body control<br>Pulls self up, stands<br>Begins to walk |
| 18 months–4 years | Walks up and down stairs<br>Runs |
| 4–6 years | Hops, skips<br>Dresses self and meets basic needs with direction |
| 6–13 years (period of rapid skeletal growth) | Increases rapidly in height<br>Refines motor skills<br>Likes athletics |
| Adolescent; 13–18 years (period of awkwardness) | Grows taller in spurts with growth of long bones<br>Epiphyses close<br>Reaches maximum height<br>Feels and looks awkward |

*(Continued)*

**Table 2-1** Developmental Stages of the Musculoskeletal System (*Continued*)

| AGE | NORMAL FINDINGS |
|---|---|
| Adult | May begin to develop kyphosis, especially women |
| | Has more fat deposits |
| Older adult | Decreases in height due to bone and cartilage calcifications and kyphosis |
| | Decreasing muscle mass and bulk |
| | Decreasing muscle strength and tone |
| | Decreasing motor activity |
| | Joint stiffness |
| | Decreased range of motion; increased rigidity of neck, shoulders, hips |
| | Slowed reflexes and reaction time |

**Table 2-2** Joint Movement and Action

| MOVEMENT | ACTION |
|---|---|
| Flexion | Decrease angle of joint, e.g., bending elbow |
| Extension | Increase angle of joint, e.g., straightening elbow |
| Hyperextension | Excessively increase angle of joint, e.g., bending the head backward |
| Abduction | Move body part away from midline of body |
| Adduction | Move body part toward midline of body |
| Rotation | Move joint around its central axis |
| Pronation | Turn wrist so that the palm is down |
| Supination | Turn wrist so that the palm is up |
| Dorsiflexion | Point the toes toward the head |
| Plantarflexion | Point the toes away from the head |
| Inversion | Rotate the ankle and sole of foot inward |
| Eversion | Rotate the ankle and sole of foot outward |
| Radial flexion | Rotate the hand inward at the wrist |
| Ulnar flexion | Rotate the hand outward at the wrist |

D. Potential problems

1. Joints—contractures and deformities

2. Body alignment

   a. Poor posture

   b. Lower back pain

   c. Lumbar lordosis—exaggerated concavity in the lumbar region

   d. Kyphosis—exaggerated convexity in the thoracic region

   e. Scoliosis—lateral curvature in a portion of the vertebral column

E. Gerontologic considerations

1. Bones—less dense; less strong; more brittle; decreased mineralization; older adult females have increased osteoclastic bone resorption; osteoporosis incidence higher in women; high incidence of deformity, pain, stiffness, fractures; increased osteoporosis with smoking, decreased calcium intake, alcohol use, physical inactivity

2. Joints—rigid, fragile cartilage; decreased water content in cartilage; decreased intervertebral disk height; limited or painful stiff movement; crepitation with movement

3. Muscles—loss of muscle mass, tone, agility, and strength; slowed reaction time; muscle fatigue; muscle function can be maintained with exercise

## Maintenance and Promotion of Normal Body Structure and Function

A. Rest—basic physiological need

1. Allows body to repair its own damaged cells

2. Enhances removal of waste products from the body

3. Restores tissue to maximum functional ability before another activity is begun

B. Sleep—basic physiological body need, although the purpose and reason for it are unclear; possible theories include:

1. To restore balance among different parts of the central nervous system

2. To mediate stress, anxiety, and tension

3. To help a person cope with daily activities

4. Gerontologic considerations

   a. Older adults do not need more sleep

   b. Hypothalamus changes—decreased stage IV sleep; difficulty getting to sleep, remaining asleep; decreased sleep time; awaken more at night

   c. Contributing factors—depression, heart disease, pain, cognitive dysfunction, sleep apnea, medication

   d. Chronic sleep deprivation—disorientation, increased risk of falls

**C.** Activity and exercise

1. Activity

   a. Maintains muscle tone and posture

   b. Serves as outlet for tension and anxiety

2. Exercise

   a. Maintains joint mobility and function

   b. Promotes muscle strength

   c. Stimulates circulation

   d. Promotes optimum ventilation

   e. Stimulates appetite

   f. Promotes elimination

   g. Enhances metabolic rate

3. Prevents injury

   a. Motor vehicle accidents—use of seat belts and helmets

   b. Job-related accidents—following safety procedures

   c. Contact sports—proper body conditioning and use of protective devices

   d. Aging—rugs should be secure; stairways lit and clear of debris

   e. Pregnancy—bathtub grips; low-heeled shoes

4. Gerontologic concerns

   a. Assess present activity level, medications that may affect activity, range of motion, muscle strength

   b. Include warm-up and cool-down exercises

   c. Maintain hydration and temperature during exercise

   d. Do 30 minutes activity 5 times a week

   e. Swimming, walking, games, exercise programs

# ALTERED FUNCTIONS RELATED TO IMMOBILITY

## Mobility

## Predisposing Factors

A. Musculoskeletal injuries/trauma

B. Congenital defects affecting the musculoskeletal system

C. Diseases of the musculoskeletal system

D. Therapeutic procedures related to the musculoskeletal system

## Adverse Effects of Immobility

(*see* Table 2-3)

**Table 2-3** Adverse Effects of Immobility

| SYSTEM | COMPLICATION | SEQUELAE |
|---|---|---|
| Integumentary | Pressure injury Decreases wound healing | Osteomyelitis |
| | | Tissue maceration |
| | | Infection |
| Musculoskeletal | Osteoporosis | Pathological fractures |
| | Decreased muscle mass strength | Loss of endurance |
| | Atrophy | Deformities |
| | Contractures | Decreased stability |
| Respiratory | Change in lung volume | Decreased lung expansion |
| | Atelectasis | Decreased hemoglobin |
| | Stasis of secretions | Respiratory muscle weakness |
| | | Pneumonia |
| Cardiovascular | Increased cardiac workload | Tachycardia |
| | Thrombus formation | Pulmonary emboli |
| | Orthostatic hypotension | Weakness, faintness, dizziness |

(*Continued*)

**Table 2-3** Adverse Effects of Immobility (*Continued*)

| SYSTEM | COMPLICATION | SEQUELAE |
|---|---|---|
| Metabolic | Decreased basal metabolic rate | Decreased cellular activity |
| | Altered nutrient metabolism | Weight gain |
| | Hypercalcemia | Loss of lean body mass |
| | Altered nutrient metabolism | Negative nitrogen balance |
| | | Anorexia, weight loss, debilitation |
| | | Slow wound healing and tissue growth |
| | Hypercalcemia | Increased diuresis |
| | | Increased excretion of electrolytes |
| Elimination | Constipation | Fecal impaction |
| | Urinary stasis | Urine retention, urinary infections |
| | | Renal calculi |
| Psychosocial | Depression | Insomnia, restlessness |
| | Sensory deprivation | |
| | Confusion | |
| | Increased dependence | |

# Rehabilitation Principles of Mobility

**A.** Positioning

1. Purpose

   a. To prevent contractures

   b. To promote circulation

   c. To promote pulmonary function

   d. To relieve pressure on body parts

   e. To promote pulmonary drainage

2. Common client positions and their corresponding therapeutic functions (*see* Table 2-4)

**B.** Different forms of exercise and their therapeutic functions (*see* Table 2-5)

**C.** Ambulation

1. Use of tilt table

   a. Weight-bearing on long bones to prevent decalcification, resulting in weakening of the bone and renal calculi

   b. Stimulate circulation to lower extremities

   c. Use elastic stockings to prevent postural hypotension

d. Should be done gradually; blood pressure should be checked during the procedure

e. If blood pressure goes down and dizziness, pallor, diaphoresis, tachycardia, or nausea occur, stop procedure

**Table 2-4** Therapeutic Functions of Client Positions

| POSITION | FUNCTION |
|---|---|
| Supine (flat, face up) | Minimizes hip flexion |
| Side | Allows drainage of oral secretions |
| Side with leg bent (Sims) | Allows drainage of oral secretions; decreases abdominal tension |
| Head elevated (Fowler) | Increases venous return; allows maximal lung expansion |
| Head and knees elevated slightly | Increases venous return; relieves pressure on lumbosacral area |
| Elevation of extremity | Increases venous return |
| Flat on back, thighs flexed, legs abducted (lithotomy) | Exposes perineum |
| Prone (flat, face down) | Promotes extension of hip joint |

**Table 2-5** Therapeutic Exercises

| EXERCISE | DESCRIPTION | RATIONALE |
|---|---|---|
| Passive range of motion | Performed by nurse without assistance from client | Retention of joint range of motion; maintenance of circulation |
| Active assistive range of motion | Performed by client with assistance of nurse | Measures motion in the joint |
| Active range of motion | Performed by client without assistance | Maintains joint mobility and increases muscle strength |
| Active resistive range of motion | Performed by client against manual or mechanical resistance | Provision of resistance to increase muscle power; 5-lb bags/weights may be used |
| Isometric exercises | Performed by client; alternate contraction and relaxation of muscle without moving joint | Maintains muscle strength when joint is immobilized |

2. Transfer activities

   a. Definition—to move a client from one surface to another (i.e., from a bed to a stretcher)

   b. Basic guidelines

      1) If client has a stronger and a weaker side, move the client toward the stronger side (easier for client to pull the weak side)

      2) Use the larger muscles of the legs to accomplish a move rather than the smaller muscles of the back

      3) Move client with drawsheet; do not slide a client across a surface

      4) Always have an assistant standing by if there is any possibility of a problem in completing a transfer

3. Technique for sitting client at edge of bed

   a. Place hand under knees and shoulders of client

   b. Instruct client to push elbow into bed; at same time lift shoulders and bring legs over edge of bed, or use one leg to move other leg over edge of bed

4. Technique for assisting client to stand

   a. Place client's feet directly under body; client should wear nonskid slippers

   b. Face client and firmly grasp each side of rib cage

   c. Push one knee against one knee of the client

   d. Rock client forward as client comes to a standing position

   e. Ensure that client's knees are "locked" while standing

   f. Give client enough time to balance while standing

   g. Pivot with client to position and transfer client's weight quickly to chair placed on client's stronger side

5. Use of a transfer board

6. Teaching activities of daily living (ADL)—guidelines

   a. Observe what client can do and allow client to do it

   b. Encourage client to exercise muscles used for activity

   c. Start with gross functional movement before going to finer motions

   d. Extend period of activity as much and as fast as the client can tolerate

   e. There are alternative ways of doing one thing

   f. Give immediate positive feedback after every act of accomplishment

7. Crutch walking

   a. General guidelines

      1) Client should support weight on hand piece, not in axilla—brachial plexus may be damaged, producing "crutch palsy"

      2) Position crutches 8–10 inches to side

      3) Crutches should have rubber tips

   b. Crutch gaits—description and uses (*see* Table 2-6)

**Table 2-6** Crutch Walking Gaits

| GAIT | DESCRIPTION | USES |
|------|-------------|------|
| Four-point | Slow, safe; right crutch, left foot, left crutch, right foot | Use when weight-bearing is allowed for both legs |
| Two-point | Faster, safe; right crutch and left foot advance together; left crutch and right foot advance together | Use when weight-bearing is allowed for both legs; less support than four-point gait |
| Three-point | Faster gait, safe; advance both crutches simultaneously (no weight bearing on affected leg) then advance good leg | Use when weight-bearing is allowed on one leg |
| Swing-to-swing-through | Fast gait but requires more strength and balance; advance both crutches followed by both legs (or one leg is held up) | Use when partial weight-bearing is allowed on both legs; requires coordination |

NOTE: To go up stairs: advance good leg first, followed by crutches and affected leg. To go down stairs: advance crutches with affected leg first, followed by good leg. ("Up with the good, down with the bad.")

# General Nursing Goals and Interventions for Immobility

**A.** Assist with self-care

   1. Assess client's activity level

   2. Encourage motion necessary to improve activity level

   3. Start with simple, gross activity before going to finer motor movements

   4. Increase period of activity as rapidly as client can tolerate

   5. Support client with positive feedback for effort/accomplishments

**B.** Gerontologic considerations

   1. Assess range of motion, ability to perform ADLs, activity level

   2. Good supportive footwear

   3. Walker or cane as needed

   4. Avoid environmental hazards (steps, throw rugs)

   5. Aerobic exercise

   6. Rise slowly from bed or sitting position

**C.** Prevent contracture of muscle

   1. Frequent position change and range of motion exercises

   2. Proper body alignment

      a. Use pillows and trochanter rolls

   3. Balanced diet

**D.** Prevent osteoporosis

   1. Weight-bearing on long bones

   2. Balanced diet

E.   Prevent negative nitrogen balance—give high-protein and easily digestible diet in small, frequent feedings

F.   Prevent constipation

1.   Ambulation as appropriate

2.   Increase fluid intake

3.   Ensure privacy in use of bedpan or commode

4.   Administer stool softeners, e.g., docusate sodium

G.   Prevent urinary stasis

1.   Have client void in normal position, if possible

2.   Increase fluid intake

3.   Low-calcium diet—increase acid-ash residue to acidify urine and prevent formation of calcium stones

4.   Evaluate adequacy of urine output

H.   Prevent pressure injuries

1.   Frequent turning, skin care, keep skin dry

2.   Ambulation as feasible

3.   Use drawsheet when turning to avoid shearing force

4.   Balanced diet with adequate protein, vitamins, and minerals

5.   Use air mattress, flotation pads, elbow and heel pads, sheepskin

6.   Assist with use of Stryker frame or Circolectric bed

7.   Gerontologic considerations

   a.   Increased risk—poor nutritional status and weight loss, vitamin and protein deficiencies, decreased peripheral sensation, moisture

   b.   Identify clients at risk—lower score on Braden scale, weight loss greater than total body weight, serum albumin less than 3.5 g/dL, pressure areas

   c.   Avoid friction during position change, eliminate moisture, move weight-bearing from pressure areas (e.g., heel protectors), include high protein, vitamins, and carbohydrates in diet

I.   Prevent thrombus formation

1.   Leg exercises—flexion, extension of toes and feet for five minutes every hour

2.   Ambulation as appropriate

3.   Frequent change of position

4.   Avoid "gatching" bed or using pillow to support knee flexion for extended periods

5.   Use of antiembolic stockings (TEDs) or elastic hose

**J.** Prevent increase in cardiac workload

1. Use of trapeze to decrease Valsalva maneuver

2. Teach client how to move without holding breath

3. Teach client to rise from bed slowly

4. Increase activity gradually

**K.** Prevent stasis of respiratory secretions

1. Teach client the importance of turning, coughing, and deep breathing

2. Administer postural drainage as appropriate

3. Teach use of incentive spirometer

**L.** Prevent depression and boredom

1. Allow visitors, use of radio, television

2. Schedule occupational therapy

**M.** Usual problems

1. Alterations in comfort

2. Impaired ambulation

3. Inability to perform ADLs

4. Complications of immobility

5. Infection

6. Safety

7. Fatigue

8. Insomnia

# SAFETY

## Growth and Development

## Primary Health Concern of Nursing

**A.** Second level of Maslow's hierarchy of human needs

    1. Besides prevention of injury, includes protection from physical and psychological harm, freedom from pain, and provision of a stable, dependable, orderly, and predictable environment

    2. Nursing has primary responsibility for ensuring the safety of clients in health care facilities and influencing the safety of persons in the home, work, and community environments

**B.** Factors affecting safety

    1. Age/development

        a. Children—accidents constitute leading cause of death in all age groups except infancy (see Table 2-7)

           1) Infants—accidents occur primarily in second half of first year

               a) Mouthing any object that they handle

               b) Unsupervised/unrestrained rolling over, crawling, walking can result in falls and enhance accessibility to small objects, electric cords, poisonous substances, etc.

           2) Toddlers—high incidence of accidents

               a) Increasing curiosity; exploring using all senses (especially taste and touch); learning by trial and error

               b) Increasing gross and fine motor activity, climbing, running, grasping, etc.

               c) Totally uncomprehending and fearless of consequences; increasing negativism as part of autonomy

           3) Preschoolers—continued risk

               a) Increasing imitative behavior

               b) Refining fine and gross motor ability without cognitive ability to foresee potential dangers

4) School-ages—although better muscular control, increased cognitive capacity, and more readiness to respond to rules, there continues to be increased risk of accidents related to identification with "superheroes," increased involvement and competitiveness in sports, and sensitivity to peer pressure

5) Adolescents—high incidence; caused by motor vehicles, physical awkwardness related to growth changes, conflict over dependence/independence; peer orientation and approval seeking; increasing goal orientation and risk-taking behavior; and inner perception of omnipotence and immortality

b. Adults—disregard for safety regulations

c. Older adults—diminished muscular strength and/or coordination, diminished sensory acuity, and impaired balance create special problems

**Table 2-7** Nursing Management of the Child at Different Developmental Stages

| ACTION | RATIONALE |
|---|---|
| **Birth to 6 mo** ||
| Keep sharp and hot objects out of child's reach | Has strong grasp reflex |
| Do not leave unattended; can roll off flat surfaces | Rolls over by about 3 months |
| Administer unpleasant medications slowly via nipple or syringe | Aspirations can easily occur |
| **6 mo to 1 y** ||
| Restrain child adequately | Can resist with entire body, has active cortical control |
| Enlist aid of parent in doing difficult procedures, if possible | Knows parent as source of comfort and security |
| **1 to 3 y** ||
| Administer medications from a cup | Prefers less dependent behavior |
| Expect turbulent temperament; tantrums common | Control environment; be consistent in expectations |
| **3 to 6 y** ||
| Take special care to explain all actions in advance | Illness and procedures are seen as punishment, body mutilation is feared |
| **6 to 13 y** ||
| Provide time for child to handle and play with equipment if possible | Interested in learning; industrious |
| **Adolescent** ||
| Noncompliance is the norm; attempt to impose as few orders as possible | Independence is important to their emotional growth |

2. Awareness of environment, self, and others

   a. Impacts ability to perceive and react to surroundings/circumstances

   b. Factors that may reduce perceptual awareness and ability to perform ADL

      1) Level of consciousness

      2) Neurological function

      3) Sensory perception

   c. Illness-associated signs and symptoms, treatments, anxiety, and degree of weakness/impaired mobility

   d. Hospitalization

   e. Lack of sleep

   f. Medication(s)

3. Ability to communicate—physical impairment, language barrier, illiteracy

4. Environment

   a. Workplace, e.g., hazardous machinery, chemicals, high stress

   b. Residence, e.g., high-crime areas, poorly maintained living conditions

   c. Unfamiliar surroundings in which specific safety information is essential, e.g., hospital

   d. Physical and biological dimensions

      1) Space—defined personal areas sufficient for the purpose (play, chores, hobby), with privacy as appropriate

      2) Lighting—natural/artificial appropriate to function (as above) as well as to provide for day-night cycle; night-lights in bathroom or bedroom

      3) Temperature and humidity—the very young (especially neonate) and very old are particularly vulnerable to extreme variations

      4) Ventilation

         a) Smoking should not be allowed in any confined areas where susceptible individuals may be affected, e.g., any health care facility

         b) Room or central air conditioners should have high-quality filters that are changed frequently

         c) Steps and hallways; handrails

      5) Sound—chronic exposure to loud noises can lead to permanent hearing loss, interfere with work performance, precipitate sleep problems and psychological stress

      6) Physical layout

         a) Neatness and cleanliness—clutter may create hazards

         b) Immediate physical environment at home, work, hospital may have to be adapted to the functional ability of the inhabitant

         c) Steps and hallways; handrails

      e.  Community resources

         1)  Food and water quality

         2)  Waste disposal

         3)  Air quality

         4)  Traffic management

            a)  Child restraint laws

            b)  Advocacy situations, e.g., traffic light for areas of high older adult/children populations, gun laws

**C.** Assessment for individual risk factors at home and in health care facilities

1. History of accidents—if previous incident(s) of accidents, there is increased risk for other mishap(s)

2. Concern for/perception of hazards; cognitive or sensory deficits

3. Evidence of unsafe behaviors—smoking in bed, nonuse of seat belts, storage of toxic substances within reach of children

4. Physical/psychological impediments to safe function—level of alertness, mental status, sensory acuity, mobility limitations

**D.** Plan/Implementation—requires attention to general principles of safety as well as identification of specific hazards/risks and subsequent measures to prevent injury; includes appropriate anticipatory and responsive client education, and prevention of injury by active/passive identification of hazards such as:

1. Orient new client to the immediate environment—call bell/signal, bed controls, location of bathroom, operation of overhead and bed lights, schedule of unit activities

2. Maintain the bed in the lowest position except when care is being provided, side rails in raised position when client is in bed

3. Provide adequate help when ambulating client, especially for the first time

4. Ensure client area is free of clutter—mop up or call housekeeping to remove spills

5. Never leave the client in total darkness—use night-light when room lights are off

6. Always secure call bell/signal within the client's reach

7. Encourage the client to wear shoes when ambulating

8. Use brakes when moving the client in or out of wheelchair, commode, bed

9. Label and report malfunction of any equipment immediately

10. Restrain client only as necessary; restraints used only as long as necessary; padded to prevent undue pressure/constriction; checked every 1–2 h; removed every 2 hours while client is awake; never tied to side rail; health care provider order necessary

11. In case of accident, institute follow-up procedures—document subjective and objective data concerning the incidence of accidents/injury as well as reported/observed use/nonuse of identified safety measures; incident report; fall assessment

12. High environmental temperature—2–3 L fluid/day (precautions when heart failure or renal failure present), wear natural fiber clothing, use tepid or cool baths or showers, fan, or air-conditioning

13. Low environmental temperature—avoid alcohol, keep room temperature greater than 65°F, eat a nutritious, high-protein diet

14. Gerontologic considerations

    a. Risk factors for falls—environment (rugs, clutter, lighting, side rails), medications, sensory deficits, cardiac dysrhythmias, mobility problems, orthostatic hypotension, cognitive impairment, footwear, elimination problems, depression, wandering

    b. Assessment—history of falling, environment, medications, visual acuity, peripheral sensation, muscle strength, range of motion, gait, orthostatic hypotension, cognitive function, heart rate and rhythm, use of assistive devices

    c. Plan/implementation—floor mat or mattress by bed, cleared debris from area, call light within reach, lights in room or bathroom, assistive device within reach, elevated toilet seat, sit on edge of bed before getting up, minimize use of hypnotics and sedatives, wear glasses as needed, wear proper footwear, grab bars in bathroom

# ALTERED FUNCTIONS RELATED TO PAIN

## Sensory Perception

## Characteristics

A. Definition of pain—"whatever the person says it is, and it exists whenever the person says it does"

B. Types (*see* Table 2-8)

    1. Acute—an episode of pain that lasts from a split second to about 6 months; may cause decreased healing, vital sign changes, diaphoresis

    2. Chronic—an episode of pain that lasts for 6 months or longer; may cause depression, weight gain, fatigue, immobility

**Table 2-8** Types of Pain

| SYSTEM | ACUTE PAIN | CHRONIC PAIN |
|---|---|---|
| Musculoskeletal | Disrupts sleep | Fatigue |
| Nutritional | Appetite reduced | Changes in weight |
| Cardiovascular | Fluid intake reduced<br><br>Activation of sympathetic nervous system | Stress-induced changes |
| Psychological | Anxiety present<br><br>Restlessness<br><br>Inability to concentrate | Depression<br><br>Job loss<br><br>Difficulty in concentration<br><br>Problems with interpersonal relationships |
| Digestive | Nausea and vomiting | Constipation, anorexia |
| Immune | | Depresses immune response<br><br>Delays wound healing |

C. Phases of the pain experience (*see* Table 2-9)

 1. Anticipatory (fear, anxiety about impending pain)

 2. Sensation of pain (mild, moderate, severe)

 3. Pain aftermath (weakness, nausea, sweating)

**Table 2-9** Responses to Pain Stimuli

| SYSTEM | CHANGE | RESULT |
|---|---|---|
| Cardiovascular | Increased blood pressure and heart rate lead to increased blood flow to brain and muscles<br><br>Rapid, irregular respiration leads to increased $O_2$ supply to brain and muscles | Enhanced alertness to threats |
| Neurological | Increased papillary diameter leads to increased eye accommodation to light | Visual perception of threat |
| Skin integrity | Increased perspiration | Removal of excess body heat |
| Musculoskeletal | Increased muscle tension or activity leads to neuromuscular responsiveness | Musculoskeletal system ready for rapid motor activity |
| Psychosocial | Aroused apprehension, irritability, and anxiety<br><br>Verbalized pain | Enhanced mental alertness to threat<br><br>Communication of suffering and pleas for help |

D. Factors influencing pain experiences

 1. Cultural factors—individual's responses or reactions to pain are generally dependent on what is expected and accepted in client's culture

 2. Past experiences with pain—past experiences with pain generally make the individual more sensitive to the pain experience

E. Gerontologic considerations—chronic pain affects 50–80% of older population; common types of pain include low back pain, postfracture pain, joint pain; decreased transmission of pain impulse, decreased pressure sensation may influence pain response; client may not use word *pain*, may have decreased ADLs, social interaction, sleep disturbances, and depression due to pain

## Selected Nursing Diagnoses Related to Pain

A. Acute or chronic pain

B. Imbalanced nutrition—less than body requirements

C. Social isolation

D. Activity intolerance

E. Readiness for enhanced comfort

F. Ineffective therapeutic regimen management

# Interventions

**A.** Pain management

1. Allow client to use own words in describing pain experience

2. Use a variety of relief measures

3. Use measures before pain becomes severe

4. Include measures that client believes will be effective

5. Consider the client's ability or willingness to participate in pain relief measures

6. Determine the effectiveness of pain relief measures according to client's response

7. If pain relief measure is ineffective the first time, try it one more time before abandoning the measure

8. Be open-minded about what may relieve the pain

9. Use preventive approach in medication administration

   a. If pain is expected to occur throughout most of a 24-h period, a regular schedule is better than as needed (prn)

   b. Advantages of preventive approach

     1) Usually can take a smaller dose to alleviate mild pain or prevent occurrence of pain

     2) Pain relief is more complete and client spends fewer hours in pain

     3) Helps prevent addiction

   c. Individualized dosage is important because each person may metabolize and absorb medication differently

**B.** Nursing goals and interventions

1. Establish a relationship

   a. Tell client you believe description of pain experience

   b. Listen and allow client to verbalize

2. Establish a 24-hour pain profile

   a. Location and radiation

     1) External

     2) Internal

     3) Both external and internal

     4) Area of body affected

   b. Character and intensity

     1) Acute/chronic

     2) Mild/severe

     3) Allow client to use own words in describing pain

     4) Use same pain scale consistently

       a) Number rating scale (0 to 10)

       b) Visual analogue scale (no pain to unbearable pain)

    c. Onset

      1) Sudden

      2) Insidious

    d. Duration

    e. Precipitating factors/aggravating factors (e.g., What makes pain worse?)

    f. Identify associated manifestations as well as alleviating or aggravating factors for those manifestations

    g. Relieving factors

3. Teach client about pain and its relief

    a. Explain quality and location of impending pain (e.g., before uncomfortable procedure)

    b. Help client learn to use slow, rhythmic breathing to promote relaxation

    c. Explain effects of analgesics and benefits of preventive approach

    d. Demonstrate splinting technique, which helps reduce pain perception

4. Reduce anxiety and fears

    a. Give reassurance; provide information

    b. Offer distraction

    c. Spend time with client

5. Provide comfort measures

    a. Proper positioning

    b. Cool, well-ventilated, quiet room

    c. Patient-controlled analgesia (PCA) pump—a portable device that delivers predetermined dosage of intravenous pain medication (e.g., dose of 1 mg morphine [with a lock-out interval of 5–15 min]); basal rate (e.g., mg/h morphine) and demand dose (varies with medication)

    d. Back rub

    e. Allow for rest

    f. Distraction

    g. Imagery

    h. Relaxation techniques

6. Administer pain medication (*see* Table 2-10)

    a. Use preventive approach

    b. Monitor therapeutic/toxic dose and adverse effects

    c. Heat/cold application as appropriate

    d. Gerontologic considerations—greater risk of adverse reactions and toxicity, greater risk of medication interaction between analgesics and medications (e.g., analgesics, anti-epileptics, and antidepressants); start with lower dose and increase gradually

**Table 2-10** Common Pain Medications

| MEDICATION | ADVERSE EFFECTS | NURSING CONSIDERATIONS |
|---|---|---|
| **Nonopioids** | | |
| Salicylates | Short-term use—GI bleeding, heartburn, occasional nausea <br><br> Prolonged high dosage—salicylism, metabolic acidosis, respiratory alkalosis, dehydration, fluid and electrolyte imbalance, tinnitus | Observe for bleeding gums, bloody or black stools, bruises <br><br> Give with milk, water, or food, or use enteric-coated tablets to minimize gastric distress <br><br> Contraindications—GI disorders, severe anemia, vitamin K deficiency |
| Acetaminophen | Overdosage may be fatal, liver toxicity <br><br> GI adverse effects are not common | Do not exceed recommended dose |
| Nonsteroidal anti-inflammatory drugs (NSAIDs): <br><br> Ibuprofen <br><br> Naproxen <br><br> Ketorolac | Headache, dizziness, epigastric distress <br><br> Peptic ulcer disease <br><br> GI bleeding Prolonged bleeding Renal impairment | Administer with food <br><br> Optimal therapeutic response is seen after two weeks of treatment <br><br> Use cautiously in clients with history of aspirin allergy <br><br> Ketorolac—dosage decreased in clients ≥ 65 years or clients with impaired renal function; duration of treatment ≤ 5 days <br><br> Indomethacin |
| **Opioids** | | |
| Morphine sulfate Fentanyl | Liver damage <br><br> Dizziness, weakness <br><br> Sedation or paradoxical excitement <br><br> Nausea, flushing, and sweating <br><br> Respiratory depression, decreased cough reflex <br><br> Constipation, miosis, hypotension | Give in smallest effective dose <br><br> Observe for development of dependence <br><br> Encourage respiratory exercises <br><br> Use cautiously to prevent respiratory depression <br><br> Monitor vital signs <br><br> Monitor intake and output (I and O), bowel pattern <br><br> Increased constipation in older adults |
| Codeine | Same as morphine <br><br> High doses may cause restlessness and excitement <br><br> Constipation | Less potent and less potential for dependence compared with morphine |

*(Continued)*

**Table 2-10** Common Pain Medications (*Continued*)

| MEDICATION | ADVERSE EFFECTS | NURSING CONSIDERATIONS |
|---|---|---|
| Methadone | Same as morphine | Observe for dependence, respiratory depression<br><br>Encourage fluids and high-bulk foods |
| Hydromorphone | Sedation, hypotension Urine retention | Keep narcotic antagonist (naloxone) available Monitor bowel function |
| **Combinations** | | |
| Oxycodone and acetaminophen | Light-headedness, dizziness, sedation, nausea | Administer with milk after meals |
| Oxycodone and aspirin | Constipation, pruritus<br><br>Increased risk bleeding | |

NOTE: Most narcotic medications exhibit qualitatively the same actions and adverse effects. They differ primarily in potency, onset, and duration of action.

Medications that increase the effects of opioid analgesics include: central nervous system (CNS) depressants (alcohol, barbiturates, sedatives) and phenytoin; other medications with significant interactions include anticholinergics (atropine, antihistamines, some psychiatric medications), antihypertensive medications, metoclopramide.

7. Refer for alternative methods of pain relief
   a. Anesthesia—block pain pathway
   b. Local nerve block
   c. Neurectomy/sympathectomy
   d. Hypnosis
   e. Acupuncture
   f. Biofeedback
   g. Massage
   h. Exercise/yoga
   i. Transcutaneous electrical nerve stimulation (TENS)
   j. Heat/cold application
   k. Distraction
   l. Relaxation
   m. Herbal remedies
   n. Therapeutic touch; consider cultural factors

# PROTECTION FROM COMMUNICABLE DISEASES

## Health Promotion

### Assessment of Communicable Diseases

A. General manifestations

1. Localized infections

   a. Inflammation, redness, warmth, swelling, pain/tenderness, loss of function

   b. Drainage—bloody, serous, cloudy, or purulent

   c. Cellulitis—bacterial skin infection with involvement of connective tissue

2. Generalized infections

   a. Weakness, headache, malaise

   b. Fever, increased pulse, change in blood pressure

B. Diagnostic tests

1. White blood count/leukocytes (WBC)

   a. Neutrophils—increased in most bacterial infections; phagocytosis during acute infection

   b. Eosinophils—increased in allergic reactions

   c. Lymphocytes—increased in chickenpox, mumps, measles, infectious mononucleosis, viral hepatitis; important in immune response

   d. Monocytes—increased in tuberculosis, rickettsial diseases, and convalescent phase of acute infections; immature macrophages

   e. "Shift to left"—increased number immature neutrophils

2. Cultures and antibiotic sensitivity of suspected infectious site

   a. Should be obtained before onset of antibiotic therapy

   b. Specimens must be carefully collected and identified

   c. Preliminary results in 24 hours; final results in 72 hours

3. Highly sensitive C-reactive protein (hsCRP)—marker of inflammation

4. Sedimentation rate

## Analysis of Care

A. Infection control in community

1. International—World Health Organization

2. National Centers for Disease Control

3. Local—public health departments

   a. Food and water control laws

   b. Spraying areas for insect control

   c. Immunizations

      1) Inactivated vaccines

      2) Live attenuated vaccines

B. Infection control in hospital

1. Hospital-acquired infections—nearly 2 million (5%) hospital clients acquire an infection in the hospital

   a. Most common infection—urinary tract infection (UTI)

   b. Most common organism—*Staphylococcus aureus*

2. Prevention of hospital-acquired infections

   a. External environment—handwashing

   b. Internal environment—good nutrition and personal hygiene

   c. Prevention of UTI—strict aseptic technique during instrumentation

   d. Prevention of surgical wound infections—handwashing, surgical asepsis

   e. Prevention of respiratory infections—clean nebulizers

   f. Prevention of bacteremias—excellent sterile technique with intravascular systems

## Plan/Implementation

A. Standard precautions (barrier) used with all clients in all settings

1. Apply to contact with blood, body fluid, nonintact skin, and mucous membranes

2. Handwashing

   a. Done immediately on contact with blood or body fluids

   b. Wash hands before putting on or taking off gloves, between client contacts, between procedures or tasks with same client, or immediately after exposure to blood or bodily fluids

3. Gloves (personal protective equipment)

   a. Use clean, nonsterile gloves when touching blood, body fluids, secretions, excretions, contaminated articles

   b. Put on gloves just before touching mucous membranes or nonintact skin or if gloves torn or heavily soiled

   c. Change gloves between tasks/procedures

   d. Remove gloves promptly after use, before touching items and environmental surfaces

4. Masks, eye protection, face shield (personal protective equipment)

   a. Used to protect mucous membranes of eyes, nose, mouth during procedures and client care activities likely to generate splashes or sprays

5. Gowns (personal protective equipment)

   a. Use clean, nonsterile gowns to protect skin and prevent soiling of clothing during procedures and client care activities likely to generate splashes and sprays—blood, bodily fluids, or excretions

   b. Remove promptly and wash hands after leaving client's environment

6. Environment control

   a. Do not need to use special dishes, glasses, eating utensils; can use either reusable or disposable

   b. Do not recap used sharps or bend, break, or remove used needles

   c. Do not manipulate used needle with two hands; use a one-handed scoop technique

   d. Place used sharps into a puncture-resistant container

   e. Use mouthpieces, resuscitation bags, or other devices for mouth-to-mouth resuscitation

7. Client placement

   a. Private room if client has poor hygiene habits, contaminates the environment, or can't assist in maintaining infection control precautions (e.g., infants, children, altered mental status client)

   b. When cohorting (sharing room), consider the epidemiology and mode of transmission of the infecting organism

8. Transport

   a. Use barriers (e.g., mask, impervious dressings)

   b. Notify personnel of impending arrival and precautions needed

   c. Inform client of ways to assist in prevention of transmission

**B.** Transmission-based precautions—apply to client with documented or suspected infections with highly transmissible or epidemiologically important pathogens; prevent spread of pathogenic organisms

1. Airborne precautions

   a. Used with pathogens smaller than 5 microns that are transmitted by airborne route; droplets or dust particles that remain suspended in the air

   b. Private room with monitored negative air pressure with 6–12 air changes per hour (airborne infection isolation room)

   c. Keep door closed and client in room; susceptible persons should not enter room or should wear N95 HEPA filter

   d. Can cohort or place client with another client with the same organism but no other organism

   e. Place mask on client if being transported

   f. Tuberculosis—wear fit-test respirator mask

      g.  Example of disease in category—measles (rubeola), *Mycobacterium tuberculosis*, chicken pox (varicella), shingles (herpes zoster)

  2.  Droplet precautions

      a.  Used with pathogens transmitted by infectious droplets; droplets larger than 5 microns

      b.  Involves contact of conjunctiva or mucous membranes of nose or mouth; happens during coughing, sneezing, talking, or during procedures such as suctioning or bronchoscopy

      c.  Private room or with client with same infection but no other infection; wear mask if in close contact

      d.  Maintain spatial separation of 3 feet between infected client and visitors or other clients; visitors wear mask if less than 3 feet

      e.  Door may remain open

      f.  Place mask on client if being transported

      g.  Examples of disease in category: diphtheria, Group A *Streptococcus pneumonia*, pneumonia or meningitis caused by *Neisseria meningitidis* or *Haemophilus influenzae* type B, rubella, mumps, pertussis

  3.  Contact precautions

      a.  Needed with client care activities that require physical skin-to-skin contact (e.g., turn clients, bathe clients), or occurs between two clients (e.g., hand contact), or occurs by contact with contaminated inanimate objects in client's environment

      b.  Private room or with client with same infection but no other infection

      c.  Clean, nonsterile gloves for client contact or contact with potentially contaminated areas

      d.  Change gloves after client contact with fecal material or wound drainage

      e.  Remove gloves before leaving client's environment and wash hands with antimicrobial agent

      f.  Wear gown when entering room if clothing will have contact with client or environment surfaces, or if client is incontinent, has diarrhea, an ileostomy, colostomy, or wound drainage

      g.  Remove personal protective equipment (PPE) before leaving room

      h.  Use dedicated equipment or clean and disinfect between clients

      i.  Example of diseases in category: infection caused by multidrug-resistant organisms (e.g., MRSA and vancomycin-resistant organisms), herpes simplex, herpes zoster, *Clostridioides difficile*, respiratory syncytial virus, pediculosis, scabies, excessive wound drainage, fecal incontinence, discharge that suggests increased potential for environmental contamination, rotavirus, hepatitis A (diapered or incontinent clients)

C. Neutropenic precautions—prevent infection among clients with immunosuppression; absolute neutrophil count ≤1000 mm$^3$

1. Assess skin integrity every 8 hours; auscultate breath sounds, presence of cough, sore throat; check temperature every 4 hours; report if greater than 101°F (38°C); monitor complete blood count (CBC) and differential daily

2. Private when possible

3. Thorough hand hygiene before entering client's room

4. Allow no staff with cold or sore throat to care for client

5. No fresh flowers or standing water

6. Clean room daily

7. Low-microbial diet; no fresh salads, unpeeled fruits and vegetables

8. Deep breathe every 4 hours

9. Meticulous body hygiene

10. Inspect IV site; meticulous IV site care

# Immunization Schedules

A. Centers for Disease Control and Prevention (CDC) Recommended Adult Immunization Schedule for ages 19 or older, United States, 2022

https://www.cdc.gov/vaccines/schedules/hcp/imz/adult.html

B. CDC Recommended Adult Immunization Schedule by Medical Condition and Other Indication, United States, 2022

https://www.cdc.gov/vaccines/schedules/hcp/imz/adult-conditions.html

**Table 2-11** Recommended Adult Immunizations

| | RUBELLA | HEPATITIS B (HBV) | POLIOVIRUS (IPV) | VARICELLA | HEPATITIS A | HUMAN PAPILLOMAVIRUS VACCINE (HPV) |
|---|---|---|---|---|---|---|
| **Indications** | Persons (especially women) without proof of vaccine on or after first birthday Health care personnel at risk of exposure to rubella and who have contact with pregnant clients | Persons at risk of exposure to blood or blood-containing body fluids<br><br>Clients and staff at institutions for developmentally disabled<br><br>Hemodialysis clients<br><br>Recipients of clotting factor concentrates<br><br>Household contacts and sex partners of clients with HBV<br><br>Some international travelers<br><br>Injecting drug users<br><br>Men who have sex with men<br><br>Heterosexuals with multiple sex partners or recent STD<br><br>Inmates of long-term correctional facilities<br><br>All unvaccinated adolescents | Travelers to countries where it is epidemic<br><br>Unvaccinated adults whose children receive IPV | Persons without proof of disease or vaccination or who are seronegative<br><br>Susceptible adolescents/adults living in households with children<br><br>Susceptible health care workers<br><br>Susceptible family contacts of immunocompromised persons<br><br>Nonpregnant women of child-bearing age<br><br>International travelers<br><br>High-risk persons: teachers of young children, day care employees, residents and staff in institutional settings, college students, inmates and staff of correctional institutions, military personnel | Travelers to countries with high incidence<br><br>Men who have sex with men<br><br>Injecting and illegal drug users<br><br>Persons with chronic liver disease<br><br>Persons with clotting factor disorders<br><br>Food handlers | Children 11 or 12 years to 26 years (can be given starting at 9 years of age)<br><br>For adults aged 27 through 45 years, public health benefit of HPV vaccination in this age range is minimal |

*(Continued)*

**Table 2-11** Recommended Adult Immunizations (*Continued*)

| | RUBELLA | HEPATITIS B (HBV) | POLIOVIRUS (IPV) | VARICELLA | HEPATITIS A | HUMAN PAPILLOMAVIRUS VACCINE (HPV) |
|---|---|---|---|---|---|---|
| **Schedule** | One dose | Three doses<br><br>Second dose 1-2 months after 1st<br><br>Third 4-6 months after 1st | IPV recommended<br><br>Two doses at 4-8 wk intervals<br><br>Third dose 2-12 months after second<br><br>**OPV no longer recommended in U.S.** | Two doses separated by 4-8 wk | Two doses separated by 6-12 months | Three doses<br><br>Second dose 2 months after 1st<br><br>Third dose 6 months after 2nd |
| **Contraindications** | Allergy to neomycin<br><br>Pregnancy<br><br>Receipt of immune globulin or blood/blood products in previous 3-11 months | Severe allergic reaction to vaccine | Severe allergic reaction after previous dose | Severe allergic reaction to vaccine Immunosuppressive therapy or immunodeficiency (including HIV infection)<br><br>Pregnancy | Severe allergic reaction to vaccine | |
| **Comments** | Check pregnancy status of women<br><br>Should avoid pregnancy for 3 months after vaccination | Precautions:<br><br>Low birth weight infant<br><br>Moderate or severe illness with or without fever | Temperature elevation may be seen for 1-2 weeks Precautions:<br><br>Pregnancy Moderate or severe illness with or without fever | Check pregnancy status of women Should avoid pregnancy for 1 month after vaccination Immune globulin or blood/blood product in previous 11 months<br><br>Moderate or severe illness with or without fever | Swelling and redness at injection site common<br><br>Precaution: pregnancy | HPV vaccination is most effective when given before exposure to any HPV, as in early adolescence |

# [ SECTION 6 ]

# MAINTENANCE OF SKIN INTEGRITY

## Skin Integrity

## Overview

A.  Structure and function of dermal tissue

1.  Structure—largest organ of body

a.  Epidermis—dead squamous cells; no blood supply; outer layer

b.  Dermis—collagen fibers, blood vessels, nerves

c.  Sweat glands

d.  Sebaceous glands

e.  Subcutaneous connective tissue

2.  Functions

a.  Protection against injury

b.  Temperature, water, and electrolyte regulation

B.  Assessment of skin integrity

1.  History of infectious disorders

2.  Potential skin trauma (environmental, occupational) or irritants (dyes)

3.  Seasonal (e.g., dry, low humidity, sun)

4.  Medications (corticosteroids)

5.  Chronic diseases (diabetes)

6.  History of allergic reactions

7.  Inspection

a.  Color—red in inflammation

b.  Temperature—hot with inflammation; cool with decreased perfusion

c.  Elasticity—swollen and painful to movement with inflammation

8.  Skin lesions—describe size, shape, location, color, and distribution

C.  Plan/Implementation

1.  Diagnostic tests

a.  Skin biopsy

b.  Skin culture

2. Nursing interventions

 a. Cleansing baths—remove oils, prevent odor, provide medication (*see* Table 2-12)

 b. Nutrition—deficiencies of nutrients can cause skin disorders, dryness

 c. Promote rest—emotional conditions affect skin

 d. Administer medications (*see* Table 2-13)

 e. Apply dressings

 1) Open wet—antipruritic, vasoconstrictive

 a) Soak nonresidue cloth in tepid solution

 b) Apply for 3–5 min

 c) Reapply repeatedly for 15–20 min

 d) Dry skin

**Table 2-12** Therapeutic Baths

| TYPE | PURPOSE | COMMON USE |
|---|---|---|
| Colloidal, e.g., oatmeal, cornstarch | Antipruritic | Chickenpox |
| Potassium permanganate | Antifungal | Slow-healing ulcers |
| Burow's solution | Antibacterial | Soaks |
| Tar preparations | Antipruritic | Psoriasis |
| Oils | Antipruritic | Moisturizing |

**Table 2-13** Common Skin Medications

| MEDICATION | ADVERSE REACTIONS | NURSING CONSIDERATIONS |
|---|---|---|
| Bacitracin ointment | Nephrotoxicity Ototoxicity | Overgrowth of nonsusceptible organisms can occur |
| Neomycin cream | Nephrotoxicity Ototoxicity | Allergic dermatitis may occur |
| Povidone-iodine solution | Irritation | Do not use around eyes<br>May stain skin<br>Do not use full strength on mucous membranes<br>Allergic dermatitis may occur |
| Silver sulfadiazine cream | Neutropenia Burning | Use cautiously if sensitive to sulfonamides |
| Tolnaftate cream | Irritation | Use small amount of medication Use medication for duration prescribed |
| Nystatin cream | Contact dermatitis | Do not use occlusive dressings |

2) Closed wet—soften keratinized tissue

3) Wet to damp—debride wounds

    f.  Promote wound healing (*see* Table 2-14)

**D.** Evaluation of skin disorders (*see* Table 2-15)

    1.  Performs appropriate skin care

    2.  Adjusts to socialization problems of skin disorders

**Table 2-14** General Nursing Measures to Promote Wound Healing

| MEASURE | RATIONALE |
|---|---|
| Leave dry dressings intact | Prevention of contamination of area |
| Use sterile dressings and technique for open wounds | Prevention of infection |
| Observe for fever, elevated WBC count, swelling, redness of wound; wound culture of drainage | Signs of potential wound infection |
| Elevate extremities | Adequate circulation of WBC, nutrients promote healing |
| Debride or assist with debriding wound if necessary | Debris may also promote increased inflammation |
| Frequent dressing changes if drainage copious | Purulent drainage promotes skin breakdown; moisture promotes bacterial growth |
| Adequate nutrition including protein and vitamin C | Collagen formation requires protein and vitamin C |

**Table 2-15** Selected Skin Disorders

| DISORDER | ASSESSMENT | NURSING CONSIDERATIONS |
|---|---|---|
| Impetigo | Reddish macule becomes honey-colored crusted vesicle, then crust; pruritus<br><br>Caused by *Staphylococcus, Streptococcus* | Skin isolation: careful handwashing; cover draining lesions; discourage touching lesions<br><br>Antibiotics—may be topical ointment and/or by mouth (PO)<br><br>Loosen scabs with Burow's solution compresses; remove gently<br><br>Restraints if necessary; mitts for infants to prevent secondary infection<br><br>Monitor for acute glomerulonephritis (complication of untreated impetigo) |

*(Continued)*

**Table 2-15** Selected Skin Disorders (*Continued*)

| DISORDER | ASSESSMENT | NURSING CONSIDERATIONS |
|---|---|---|
| Herpes simplex type I | Pruritic vesicular groupings on nose, lips, and oral mucous membranes<br><br>Chronically recurrent | Spread by direct contact, handwashing; bland, soft foods; avoid direct contact; administer antivirals (acyclovir, famciclovir, and valacyclovir); topical anesthetics; cold or hot compresses; wash linens and towels in hot water |
| Herpes zoster (shingles) | Vesicular eruption along nerve distribution<br><br>Pain, tenderness, and pruritus over affected region<br><br>Primarily seen on face, thorax, trunk | Caused by reactivation of chickenpox virus (varicella) or decreased immunity<br><br>Analgesics; compresses; oatmeal baths<br><br>Systemic corticosteroids to diminish severity<br><br>Prevent spread—contagious to anyone who has not had chickenpox or who is immunosuppressed; airborne or contact precautions<br><br>Antivirals: famciclovir, valacyclovir, acyclovir |
| Scabies | Minute, reddened, itchy lesions<br><br>Linear burrowing of a mite at finger webs, wrists, elbows, ankles, penis | Reduce itching—topical antipruritic (calamine lotion/topical steroids), permethrin 5% cream or crotamiton 10% cream<br><br>Institute skin precautions to prevent spread<br><br>Scabicide—permethrin or crotamiton lotion; apply lotion (not on face) to cool, dry skin (not after hot shower because of potential for increased absorption); treat all family members (infants upon recommendation of health care provider)<br><br>Repeat in 7 days<br><br>Launder all clothing and linen after above treatment<br><br>The rash and itching may last for 2–3 weeks even though the mite has been destroyed; treat with antipruritic |
| Pediculosis (lice) | Scalp—white eggs (nits) on hair shafts, with itchy scalp<br><br>Body—macules and papules<br><br>Pubis—red macules | Permethrin 1% cream/lotion<br><br>Kills both lice and nits with one application<br><br>May suggest repeating in 7 days—depends on severity |

(*Continued*)

**Table 2-15** Selected Skin Disorders (*Continued*)

| DISORDER | ASSESSMENT | NURSING CONSIDERATIONS |
|---|---|---|
| Tinea | Pedis (athlete's foot)—vesicular eruptions in interdigital webs<br><br>Capitis (ringworm)—breakage and loss of hair; scaly circumscribed red patches on scalp that spread in circular pattern; fluoresces green with Wood's lamp<br><br>Corporis (ringworm of body)—rings of red scaly areas that spread with central clearing | Antifungal—topical ointment, creams, lotions include ketoconazole, miconazole, terbinafine<br><br>Keep areas dry and clean<br><br>Frequent shampooing |
| Psoriasis | Chronic recurrent thick, itchy, erythematous papules/plaques covered with silvery white scales with symmetrical distribution<br><br>Commonly on the scalp, knees, sacrum, elbows, and behind ears<br><br>Elevated sedimentation rate with negative rheumatoid factor | Topical medications: cortisone creams, anthralin, coal tar, moisturizers, creams with vitamins<br><br>Immunosuppressants: methotrexate or cyclosporine<br><br>Biological response modifiers: adalimumab, infliximab, etanercept<br><br>Ultraviolet light (wear goggles to protect eyes)<br><br>Counseling to support/enhance self-image/self-esteem |
| Acne vulgaris | Comedones (blackheads/whiteheads), papules, pustules, cysts occurring most often on the face, neck, shoulders, and back | Good hygiene and nutrition<br><br>PO tetracycline (advise sunscreen with SPF of 15; avoid sun exposure)<br><br>Antibacterial medications—azelaic acid, clindamycin, erythromycin<br><br>Isotretinoin—risk of elevated liver function tests (LFTs), dry skin and fetal damage<br><br>Drying preparations—benzoyl peroxide/vitamin A may cause redness and peeling early in treatment and photosensitivity<br><br>Ultraviolet light and dermabrasion<br><br>Monitor for secondary infection<br><br>Emotional support Isotretinoin (contraindicated with pregnancy) |

(*Continued*)

**Table 2-15** Selected Skin Disorders (*Continued*)

| DISORDER | ASSESSMENT | NURSING CONSIDERATIONS |
|---|---|---|
| Eczema (atopic dermatitis) | Children—rough, dry, erythematous skin lesions that progress to weeping and crusting; distributed on the cheeks, scalp, and extensor surfaces in infants and on flexor surfaces in children<br><br>Adults—hard, dry, flaking, scaling on face, upper chest, and antecubital and popliteal fossa | Onset usually in infancy around 2–3 mo; often outgrown by 2–3 y<br><br>May be precursor of adult asthma or hay fever<br><br>Elimination from diet of common offenders, especially milk, eggs, wheat, citrus fruits, and tomatoes<br><br>Eliminate clothing that is irritating (rough/wool) or that promotes sweating; cotton clothing is best<br><br>Avoid soap and prolonged or hot baths/showers, which tend to be drying; may use warm colloid baths (e.g., cornstarch);<br><br>Emollient lotions to affected areas<br><br>Keep fingernails short and clean; arm restraints/mittens may be necessary<br><br>Topical steroids Antihistamines |

# Effects of Development on Skin Disorders

A. Infant and toddler

    1. Diaper dermatitis—usually on convex areas or folds (often due to *Candida albicans*)

    2. Seborrheic dermatitis (cradle cap)—crusting of infant's scalp due to hyperactive sebaceous glands caused by maternal hormones

        a. Cleanse with shampoo

        b. Oil scalp and remove crusts

B. School-age

    1. Age of communicable diseases

    2. *See* Protection from Communicable Diseases (e.g., tonsillitis)

C. Adolescent

    1. Changes of puberty—sebaceous gland active, eccrine glands functioning, body hair develops

    2. Acne develops

D. Older adults

    1. Assessment—usual changes

        a. Loss of subcutaneous tissue and melanocytes—skin tears more easily; increased risk of ultraviolet damage

        b. Degeneration of collagen and elastic fibers—wrinkling, skin tears more often

     c.  Increased capillary fragility; decreased circulation—increased bruising, decreased wound healing

     d.  Hormonal changes and decreased immune function—dry and more permeable skin

  2.  Intervention—Bathe every day or less often; avoid use of strong, scented, or alcohol-based soaps; avoid bath oil in tubs; keep room humidity at 60%

# Primary Skin Lesions

**A.**  Macule

  1.  Flat and circumscribed

  2.  Nonpalpable

  3.  Smaller than 1 cm

  4.  Example—freckles, flat nevi, petechiae

**B.**  Papule

  1.  Solid elevation

  2.  Palpable

  3.  Less than 1 cm

  4.  Example—wart, mole

**C.**  Nodule

  1.  Elevated solid lesion

  2.  Deep, may extend into dermis

  3.  Greater than 1 cm

  4.  Example—xanthoma, fibroma

**D.**  Wheal

  1.  Localized area of edema

  2.  Elevated and firm, itchy

  3.  Example—mosquito bite, allergic reaction (hive)

**E.**  Vesicle

  1.  Elevation of skin filled with clear fluid

  2.  Less than 1 cm

  3.  Example—blister, herpes simplex, herpes zoster, early chickenpox

**F.**  Pustule

  1.  Elevation of skin filled with pus

  2.  Example—acne, impetigo

**G.**  Ulcer

  1.  Loss of epidermis, dermis, subcutaneous tissue

  2.  Irregular shape, may bleed

  3.  Granulation tissue, slough, necrotic tissue

  4.  Example—pressure sores, chancre

**H.** Atrophy

1. Thinning of skin, may bleed easily

2. Example—aging, disuse syndrome

**I.** Erosion

1. Loss of epidermis; shallow depression

2. Moist with no bleeding; heals without scarring

3. Example—skin trauma

## Dermatological Disorders

**A.** Impetigo—highly contagious superficial streptococcal/staphylococcal infection of outer layers of skin

1. Incubation—1–2 days

2. Assessment—itchy vesicular lesion progressing to thick honey-colored crust most commonly found around the nose and chin (may also be in axillae and on extremities) and spreads peripherally from initial lesion

3. Care

   a. Skin isolation; careful handwashing; cover draining lesions; discourage touching lesions

   b. Antibiotics—may be topical ointment (gentamicin, neomycin) and/or PO; systemic antibiotics if more severe

   c. Loosen scabs with Burow's solution compresses; remove gently

   d. Restraints if necessary; mitts for infants to prevent secondary infection

   e. Monitor for acute glomerulonephritis

**B.** Herpes simplex type I—"fever blisters," "cold sores," canker sores

1. Assessment

   a. Tingling, pruritic, burning vesicular groupings on nose, lips, and oral mucous membranes that usually ulcerate/crust; chronically recurrent; increases with age and immunosuppression

   b. May develop into herpes gingivostomatitis in children with extremely painful lesions in lips, gums, tongue, and hard palate; causes a foul breath odor and difficulty in and refusal to eat/drink; dehydration is of concern

2. Care

   a. Relieve pain—topical anesthetic

   b. Maintain hydration and nutrition—bland, soft, tepid foods and drink; use a straw

   c. Prevent spread—avoid direct contact; maintain scrupulous handwashing; contagious for 3–5 days; wash linens and towels in hot water

   d. Oral antivirals—acyclovir, famciclovir, or valacyclovir

   e. Cold or hot compresses

**C.** Herpes zoster (shingles)—acute viral infection of nervous system caused by reactivation of dormant varicella (chickenpox) virus, may be due to decreased immunity

1. Assessment—several days of unilateral pain, followed by painful, itchy, tender vesicular eruptions along peripheral sensory nerve distribution, primarily on face, thorax, trunk; may reoccur

2. Care

   a. Control pain—analgesics; compresses; oatmeal baths

   b. Systemic corticosteroids to diminish severity

   c. Prevent spread—contagious to anyone who has not had chickenpox or who is immunosuppressed; airborne or contact precautions

   d. Antiviral medications—acyclovir, famciclovir, or valacyclovir

**D.** Scabies—skin disorder caused by mites transmitted via close contact with infested person or clothing/bedding

1. Assessment—intensely itchy (especially at night); red, excoriated, tiny lesions and burrow formation found primarily in the webs of fingers, under the breasts, on groin, knees, and/or elbow surfaces, around the wrists or ankles; not on the face

2. Care

   a. Reduce itching—topical antipruritic (calamine lotion/topical steroids)

   b. Prevent spread

      1) Institute skin precautions

      2) Scabicide—crotamiton lotion or permethrin

         a) Apply lotion (not on face) to cool, dry skin (not after hot shower because of potential for increased absorption); leave on for 8–12 hours then shower off; crotamiton may be applied at bedtime for two or more consecutive nights; risk for neurotoxicity in children

         b) Treat all family members (infants upon recommendation of health care provider)

      3) Launder all clothing and linen after above treatment; dry in hot dryer

      4) The rash and itching may last for 2–3 wk, even though the mite has been destroyed; treat with antipruritic

**E.** Pediculosis—parasitic lice infection spread by close contact and shared clothing, brushes/combs, bedding

1. Assessment

   a. Corporis—white eggs (nits) and lice in clothing; seldom on nonhairy skin of body; intensely itchy, erythematous macules on upper back and areas of tight clothing

   b. Capitis—nits resembling dandruff that are difficult to dislodge, cling to hair shafts in occipital region and over ears; severe itching

   c. Pubis—pubic hair infested with crab-shaped lice, intensely itchy, red macules in hairy regions and abdomen

    2. Care

        a. Avoid transmission—do not share combs, hats, bedding

        b. Permethrin, may repeat if necessary

        c. Launder all clothing as above; soak personal care items in pediculicide

        d. Comb hair with fine-tooth comb to remove nits

**F.** Tinea—fungal infection transmitted via person-to-person contact and animals/soil

    1. Assessment

        a. Pedis (athlete's foot)—vesicular eruptions in interdigital webs

        b. Capitis (ringworm)—breakage and loss of hair; scaly, circumscribed, red patches on scalp that spread in a circular pattern; fluoresces green with Wood's lamp

        c. Corporis (ringworm of body)—rings of red scaly areas that spread with central clearing

    2. Care

        a. Antifungal—topical ointment, creams, lotions

        b. Keep areas dry and clean

        c. Frequent shampooing

**G.** Psoriasis—chronic dermatitis with familial predisposition; often precipitated by stress, trauma, infection

    1. Assessment

        a. Chronic, recurrent, thick, erythematous papules/plaques covered with silvery white scales with symmetrical distribution commonly found on the scalp, knees, sacrum, elbows, and behind ears

        b. May be painful or itchy

        c. Elevated sedimentation rate with negative rheumatoid factor seen with psoriatic arthritis

    2. Care

        a. Topical medications: cortisone creams, anthralin, coal tar, moisturizers, creams with vitamins

        b. Immunosuppressants: methotrexate or cyclosporine

        c. Biological response modifiers: adalimumab, infliximab, etanercept

        d. Ultraviolet light—natural/artificial

        e. Counseling to support/enhance self-image/self-esteem

**H.** Acne vulgaris—chronic skin disorder associated with increased sebum production and inflammation of sebaceous follicles; onset most often at puberty and continues throughout adolescence

1. Assessment—lesions may be comedones (blackheads/whiteheads), papules, pustules, and/or cysts, occurring most often on the face, neck, shoulders, and back

2. Care

   a. Adequate rest, good hygiene and nutrition; eliminate any foods that are associated with increased symptoms

   b. PO tetracycline—advise sunscreen (SPF of at least 15) because of increased sensitivity to sun; do not use in pregnancy/lactation

   c. Drying preparations—benzoyl peroxide/vitamin A acid (may be used concurrently with tetracyclines but not applied at same time); may cause redness and peeling early in treatment; may cause photosensitivity

   d. Isotretinoin—risk of elevated LFTs, dry skin, and depression; teratogenic

   e. Ultraviolet light and surgery may be used for cystic/abscessed lesions (dermabrasion)

   f. Monitor for secondary infections

   g. Emotional support—based on growth and developmental characteristics of adolescence; peer group sessions discussing treatment as part of overall self-image enhancement is often helpful

## [ SECTION 7 ]

# PERIOPERATIVE CARE

## Perioperative Care

A. Assessment

   1. Stress—vasovagal responses

   2. Fears (*see* Table 2-16)

**Table 2-16** Fears of Surgery at Different Developmental Stages

| AGE GROUP | SPECIFIC FEARS | NURSING CONSIDERATIONS |
|---|---|---|
| Toddler | Separation | Teach parents to expect regression, e.g., in toilet training and difficult separations |
| Preschooler | Mutilation | Allow child to play with models of equipment<br>Encourage expression of feelings, e.g., anger |
| School-age | Loss of control | Explain procedures in simple terms<br>Allow choices when possible |
| Adolescence | Loss of independence; being different from peers, e.g., alterations in body image | Involve adolescent in procedures and therapies<br>Expect resistance<br>Express understanding of concerns<br>Point out strengths |
| Older adult | Physical decline<br>Decreased independence<br>Fear of death<br>Fear of long term care facility placement | Assess ability to handle physical and emotional stress<br>Assess cognitive function<br>Explain procedures at level appropriate for client<br>Involve caregivers as appropriate |

**B.** Intervention

1. Teaching (*see* Table 2-17)

   a. Age-appropriate

      1) Toddler—simple directions

      2) Preschool and school-age—allow to play with equipment

      3) Adolescent—expect resistance

   b. Family oriented—have parents reinforce teaching

**Table 2-17** Preoperative Teaching Guide

| Factors for Nurse to Assess Before Teaching |
| --- |
| History of illness |
| Rationale for surgery |
| Nature of surgery—curative or palliative, minor or major, extent of disfigurement, potential alterations, e.g., ostomies |
| Factors related to client's readiness for learning—age, mental status, preexisting knowledge about condition, concerns about condition, family's reaction to need for surgery |
| **Content Areas to Cover During Teaching** |
| Elicit client's concerns, e.g., fears about anesthesia |
| Provide information to clear up misconceptions |
| Explain preoperative procedures, remove jewelry and nail polish |
| Lab tests |
| Skin preparation—cleansing, possibly shaving |
| Enemas if indicated, e.g., before intestinal surgery |
| Rationale for withholding food and fluids, nothing by mouth (NPO) |
| Preoperative medications, IV line |
| Teach postoperative procedures—deep breathing, leg exercises, moving in bed, incentive spirometer (sustained maximal inspiration device), equipment to expect postoperatively |
| Explain importance of reporting pain or discomfort after surgery |
| Explain what will be done to relieve pain, e.g., changing position, medication |
| Provide for growth and development needs of children |

2.  Preparation for surgery (*see* Table 2-18)

    a.  Preoperative Checklist

        1)  Informed consent

        2)  Lab tests, chest x-ray, EKG

        3)  Skin prep

        4)  Bowel prep

        5)  IVs

        6)  NPO

        7)  Preop meds, sedation, antibiotics

        8)  Removal of dentures, jewelry, nail polish

        9)  Nutrition—may need parenteral nutrition (PN) or tube feedings preoperatively

**Table 2-18** Anesthesia

| MEDICATION | ADVERSE EFFECTS | NURSING CONSIDERATIONS |
|---|---|---|
| General anesthesia via inhalation | Respiratory depression, circulatory depression<br><br>Delirium during induction and recovery<br><br>Nausea and vomiting, aspiration during induction, myocardial depression, hepatic toxicity | Check history of sensitization<br><br>Maintain airway<br><br>Protect and orient client<br><br>Monitor vital signs, labs<br><br>Prevent aspiration postop by elevating head of bed, turning head to side (unless contraindicated) |
| Nitrous oxide | Hypotension, postop nausea and vomiting | Monitor vital signs<br><br>Adequate oxygenation is essential, especially during emergence |
| IV thiopental sodium | Respiratory depression, low blood pressure (BP), laryngospasm<br><br>Poor muscle relaxation, hypotension, irritating to skin and subcutaneous tissue | Monitor vital signs, especially airway, breathing<br><br>Straps for operative table, proper positioning<br><br>Protect IV site, check for placement periodically |
| Spinal anesthesia:<br><br>Saddle | Hypotension, headache | Monitor vital signs<br><br>Encourage oral fluids |
| Conduction blocks:<br><br>Epidural<br>Caudal | Hypotension, respiratory depression | Headache not experienced<br><br>Monitor vital signs |

*(Continued)*

**Table 2-18** Anesthesia (*Continued*)

| MEDICATION | ADVERSE EFFECTS | NURSING CONSIDERATIONS |
|---|---|---|
| Local anesthesia | Excitability, toxic reactions such as respiratory difficulties, vasoconstriction if substance contains epinephrine | Monitor client<br><br>Do not use local anesthesia with epinephrine on fingers (circulation is less optimal) |
| Moderate (conscious) sedation:<br><br>Midazolam Diazepam | Respiratory depression, apnea, hypotension, bradycardia | Never leave client alone<br><br>Constantly monitor airway, level of consciousness, pulse oximetry, electrocardiogram (ECG)<br><br>Vital signs every 15–30 min<br><br>Assess client's ability to maintain patent airway and respond to verbal commands |

3. Culturally sensitive perioperative care

   a. Assess primary language spoken

   b. Assess feelings regarding surgery and pain

   c. Determine attitudes about pain management

   d. Determine expectations of the intraoperative and postoperative periods

   e. Evaluate client's support system

   f. Assess feelings about self-care

   g. Use professional interpreters

   h. Use pictures or phrase cards with various languages

   i. Provide printed teaching materials in a variety of languages

4. Complementary and alternative therapies

   a. Supplements should not be taken near the time of surgery; may interact with anesthesia, may affect coagulation parameters

      1) Echinacea

      2) Ephedra (currently removed from the retail market in the United States)

      3) Garlic

      4) Ginkgo

      5) Ginseng

      6) Kava

      7) St. John's wort

   b. Eliminate all dietary supplements (other than multivitamins) at least 2 to 3 weeks before surgery

   c. May resume the supplements with the advice of the health care provider

# Intraoperative Care

A. Assessment
1. Vital signs
2. Aseptic technique
3. Appropriate grounding devices
4. Fluid balance
5. Sponge/instrument count

B. Intervention—monitor effects of anesthesia during post induction (*see* Table 2-19)

**Table 2-19** Premedications and Potential Problems

| MEDICATIONS | ADVERSE EFFECTS | NURSING CONSIDERATIONS |
|---|---|---|
| Morphine | Respiratory depression, gastric irritability | Monitor vital signs, especially respirations; observe for vomiting<br>Side rails elevated to prevent accidents |
| Promethazine hydrochloride (anxiety, antiemetic) | Hypotension | Monitor vital signs |
| Atropine sulfate (to decrease secretions and prevent laryngospasm) | Tachycardia | Monitor vital signs<br>Advise client about dry mouth |

# Postoperative Care

A. Assessment—anesthesia, immobility, and surgery can affect any system in the body and require a full systems assessment (see Table 2-20)

**Table 2-20** Potential Complications of Surgery

| COMPLICATION | ASSESSMENT | NURSING CONSIDERATIONS |
|---|---|---|
| Hemorrhage | Decreased BP, increased pulse, cold, clammy skin | Replace blood volume<br>Monitor vital signs |
| Paralytic ileus | Absent bowel sounds, no flatus or stool | Nasogastric suction<br>IV fluids<br>Decompression tubes |
| Atelectasis and pneumonia | Dyspnea, cyanosis, cough<br>Tachycardia<br>Elevated temperature<br>Pain on affected side | Experienced second day postop<br>Suctioning<br>Postural drainage<br>Antibiotics<br>Cough and turn |

*(Continued)*

**Table 2-20** Potential Complications of Surgery (*Continued*)

| COMPLICATION | ASSESSMENT | NURSING CONSIDERATIONS |
|---|---|---|
| Embolism | Dyspnea, pain, hemoptysis<br><br>Restlessness<br><br>Arterial blood gas (ABG)—low $O_2$, high $CO_2$ | Experienced second day postop<br><br>Oxygen<br><br>Anticoagulants (heparin)<br><br>IV fluids |
| Infection of wound | Elevated WBC and temperature<br><br>Positive cultures | Experienced 3-5 d postop<br><br>Antibiotics, aseptic technique<br><br>Good nutrition |
| Dehiscence | Separation of wound edges | Experienced 5-6 d postop<br><br>Low Fowler position, no coughing<br><br>NPO<br><br>Notify health care provider |
| Evisceration | Bowel erupts through surgical site | Experienced 5-6 d -postop<br><br>Low Fowler position, no coughing<br><br>NPO<br><br>Cover viscera with sterile saline dressing or wax paper (if at home)<br><br>Notify health care provider |
| Psychosis | Inappropriate affect | Therapeutic communication<br><br>Medication |
| Cardiovascular compromise | Decreased BP, increased pulse, cold and clammy skin | Treat cause<br><br>Oxygen<br><br>IV fluids |
| Urinary retention | Unable to void after surgery<br><br>Bladder distention | Experienced 8-12 hours postop<br><br>Catheterize as needed |
| Urinary infection | Foul-smelling urine<br><br>Elevated WBC | Experienced 5-8 days postop<br><br>Antibiotics<br><br>Force fluids |
| Venous thrombo-embolism | Calf pain and/or calf swelling<br><br>Ultrasound | Experienced 6-14 days up to 1 year later<br><br>Anticoagulant therapy |

**B.** Neuropsychosocial

   1. Stimulate client postanesthesia

   2. Monitor level of consciousness

**C.** Cardiovascular

   1. Generally monitor vital signs q 15 min times 4, q 30 min times 2, q 1 hour times 2, then as needed

   2. Monitor I and O

   3. Check potassium level

   4. Monitor central venous pressure (CVP)

**D.** Respiratory

   1. Check breath sounds

   2. Turn, cough, and deep breathe (unless contraindicated; e.g., brain, spinal, eye surgery)

   3. Splint wound

   4. Offer pain medication

   5. Teach incentive spirometer

   6. Get out of bed as soon as possible

**E.** Gastrointestinal

   1. Check bowel sounds in 4 quadrants 5 min each

   2. Keep NPO until bowel sounds present

   3. Provide good mouth care while NPO

   4. Provide antiemetics for nausea and vomiting

   5. Check abdomen for distention

   6. Check for passage of flatus and stool

**F.** Genitourinary

   1. Monitor I and O

   2. Encourage to void

   3. Notify health care provider if unable to void within 8 h

   4. Catheterize, if needed

**G.** Extremities

   1. Check pulses

   2. Assess for color, edema, temperature

   3. Inform client not to cross legs

   4. Keep knee gatch flat

   5. Prohibit pillows behind knee

   6. Apply antiembolic stockings (TED hose) prior to getting out of bed (OOB)

   7. Monitor for calf pain and/or calf swelling

   8. Pneumatic compression device/sequential compression device (SCD)

**H.** Wounds

    1. Dressing

        a. Document amount and character of drainage

        b. Health care provider changes first postop dressing

        c. Aseptic technique

        d. Note presence of drains

    2. Incision

        a. Assess site—edematous, inflamed, excoriated

        b. Assess drainage—serous, serosanguineous, purulent

        c. Note type of sutures

        d. Note if edges are well approximated

        e. Risk of infection 3–5 days postop

        f. Debride wound, if needed, to reduce inflammation

        g. Change dressing frequently to prevent skin breakdown around site and minimize bacterial growth

**I.** Drains—to prevent fluids from accumulating in tissues (*see* Table 2-21)

**Table 2-21** Surgical Drains

| TYPE | DESCRIPTION | NURSING CONSIDERATIONS |
|------|-------------|------------------------|
| Penrose | Simple latex drain | Note location<br><br>Usually not sutured in place but layered in gauze dressing<br><br>Expect drainage on dressing |
| T-tube | Used after gallbladder surgery<br><br>Placed in common bile duct to allow passage of bile | Monitor drainage<br><br>Initially 500–1,000 mL per day<br><br>Usually bloody for first 2 hours<br><br>Keep drainage bag below level of gallbladder<br><br>May be discharged with T-tube in place<br><br>Teach client about care |
| Jackson-Pratt | Portable wound self-suction device with bulb reservoir | Monitor amount and character of drainage<br><br>Notify health care provider if it suddenly increases or becomes bright red |

*(Continued)*

**Table 2-21** Surgical Drains (*Continued*)

| TYPE | DESCRIPTION | NURSING CONSIDERATIONS |
|------|-------------|------------------------|
| Hemovac | Larger portable wound self-suction device with reservoir<br><br>Used after mastectomy | Monitor and record amount and character of drainage<br><br>Notify health care provider if it suddenly increases or becomes bright red<br><br>Empty when full or every 8 h<br><br>Remove plug (maintain sterility), empty contents, place on flat surface, cleanse opening and plug with alcohol sponge, compress evacuator completely to remove air, replace plug, check system for operation |

## End-of-Chapter Thinking Exercise

The nurse cares for an adult client who has just been admitted with stage IV breast cancer. A recent positron emission tomography (PET) scan shows metastasis to the liver and bones. The client was originally diagnosed three years ago and underwent several rounds of chemotherapy. A week ago, the client described having a hard time walking without "stumbling over my own feet" and has had to wear an incontinence pad because she can't seem to get to the bathroom fast enough. The client reports 9/10 pain in the lower back and hips and describes it as "a constant, heavy, dull ache that won't ease up and is worse at night." The client is very thin, with a yellowish skin tone and alopecia noted. Admission vital signs: temperature 97.8°F (36.5°C), pulse 80 beats/min, respiratory rate 16 breaths/min, BP 104/68 mm Hg, peripheral oxygen saturation (SpO$_2$) 95%. The client lives alone and has no family locally. The client's children have encouraged a move out of state to live with them, but the client states, "I'm not ready to give up yet."

1. What factors other than the physical pain influence this client's pain experience? (Recognize Cues)

2. What questions does the nurse ask to assess the physical pain the client is experiencing? (Analyze Cues)

3. What actions does the nurse add to the client's plan of care for pain control? (Take Action)

# Thinking Exercise Explanations

1. What factors other than the physical pain influence this client's pain experience? (Recognize Cues)

   - Past experiences with pain
   - New diagnosis of metastasis
   - Decreased mobility leading to decreased social interactions
   - Increased risk of developing depression

   Chronic pain is multimodal and is a holistic experience for the client. In addition to the physical aspects, the client will need to deal with the advancement of the disease, which can lead to psychosocial changes that may affect the way the client responds to pain. The nurse will need to address all of these to treat the pain effectively.

2. What questions does the nurse ask to assess the physical pain the client is experiencing? (Analyze Cues)

   - Location and radiation
   - Character and intensity
   - Onset
   - Duration
   - Precipitating factors

   Asking questions to obtain the above information will give the nurse a comprehensive record of the client's pain.

3. What actions does the nurse add to the client's plan of care for pain control? (Take Action)

   - Develop a trusting relationship
   - Encourage verbalization about pain, diagnosis, and other issues
   - Establish a pain goal with the client
   - Collaborate with HCP and other team members to establish a medication regimen to control pain
   - Administer medication on a schedule
   - Promote relaxation (deep breathing, guided imagery, listening to music)
   - Ensure frequent position changes

# FLUID AND ELECTROLYTE BALANCE

[ SECTION 1 ]

# FLUID REGULATION

## Fluid and Electrolyte Balance

## Fluid Volume Imbalance

A.  Assessment of fluid volume balance (*see* Table 3-1)

**Table 3-1** Fluid Volume Imbalances

| NURSING PROCESS | DEFICIENT FLUID VOLUME | EXCESS FLUID VOLUME |
|---|---|---|
| Assessment | Thirst (early sign) | No change in temperature |
| | Temperature increases | Pulse increases slightly and is bounding |
| | Rapid and weak pulse | Respirations increase, shortness of breath, dyspnea, fine crackles |
| | Respirations increase | |
| | Poor skin turgor—skin cool, moist | Peripheral edema—bloated appearance, weight increase |
| | Hypotension | Hypertension |
| | Emaciation, weight loss | May have muffled heart sounds |
| | Dry eye sockets, mouth, and mucous membranes | Jugular vein distension |
| | Anxiety, apprehension, exhaustion | Urine specific gravity less than 1.010 |
| | Urine specific gravity greater than 1.030 | Apprehension |
| | | Increased venous pressure |
| | Decreased urine output | Decreased hematocrit, BUN, hemoglobin, Na$^+$, serum osmolality |
| | Increased hemoglobin; hematocrit; Na$^+$ serum osmolality; blood, urea, nitrogen (BUN) | |
| | Headache, lethargy, confusion, disorientation | |

(Continued)

**Table 3-1** Fluid Volume Imbalances (*Continued*)

| NURSING PROCESS | DEFICIENT FLUID VOLUME | EXCESS FLUID VOLUME |
|---|---|---|
| Analysis | Isotonic loss<br><br>Vomiting<br><br>Diarrhea<br><br>GI suction<br><br>Sweating<br><br>Decreased intake<br><br>Hemorrhage<br><br>Third-space shift | Isotonic gain, increase in the interstitial compartment, intravascular compartment, or both<br><br>Congestive heart failure (CHF)<br><br>Renal failure<br><br>Cirrhosis of the liver<br><br>Excessive ingestion of sodium<br><br>Excessive or too rapid intravenous infusion |
| Plan/implementation | Force fluids<br><br>Provide isotonic IV fluids: lactated Ringer's or 0.9% NaCl<br><br>I and O, hourly outputs<br><br>Daily weights (1 liter fluid = 1 kg or 2.2 lb)<br><br>Monitor vital signs<br><br>Check skin turgor<br><br>Assess urine specific gravity | Administer diuretics<br><br>Restrict fluids<br><br>Sodium-restricted diet (average daily diet: 6-15 g $Na^+$)<br><br>Daily weight<br><br>Assess breath sounds<br><br>Check feet/ankle/sacral region for edema<br><br>Semi-Fowler position if dyspneic |

1. Signs and symptoms

2. Diagnostics—central venous pressure (CVP) (right atrial pressure) (*see* Figure 3-1)

   a. Purpose—measurement of effective blood volume and efficiency of cardiac pumping of the right side of the heart; measures pressure in superior vena cava

      1) Indicates ability of right side of heart to manage a fluid load

      2) Guide to fluid replacement

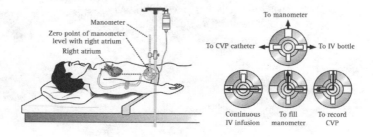

**Figure 3-1.** Central Venous Pressure

    b. Equipment

        1) Central line inserted into superior vena cava

        2) Water manometer with three-way stopcock or transducer

        3) IV fluids

    c. Procedure

        1) Client has catheter in jugular, subclavian, or median antecubital vein

        2) Attach manometer to a three-way stopcock that also connects IV to central catheter inserted into jugular, subclavian, or median cubital vein

        3) Zero on manometer placed at the level of the right atrium at midaxillary line

        4) Measured with client flat in bed

        5) Stopcock opened to the manometer, which allows for filling with IV fluid to level of 18–20 cm

        6) Stopcock turned to allow for fluid in manometer to flow to client

        7) Level of fluid fluctuates with respirations

        8) When level stabilizes, reading is taken at highest level of fluctuation

        9) Return stopcock to proper position and adjust IV flow rate

        10) Normal reading 2–8 mm Hg (3–11 cm of water)

            a) Elevated: greater than 8 mm Hg (11 cm of water) hypervolemia or poor cardiac contractility

            b) Lowered: less than 2 mm Hg (3 cm of water) hypovolemia

        11) Potential complications

            a) Pneumothorax

            b) Air embolism

            c) Infection at insertion site

        12) Nursing management

            a) Dry, sterile dressing

            b) Change dressing, IV fluid bag, manometer, and tubing every 24 h

            c) Instruct client to hold breath (Valsalva maneuver) when tubing changed to prevent air embolism

            d) Check and secure all connections

**B.** Definition of terms (*see* Table 3-1)

    1. Tonicity—concentration of a substance dissolved in water

    2. Isotonic fluids—same concentration as body fluids

    3. Hypertonic solution—solute concentration greater than that of body fluids

    4. Hypotonic solution—solute concentration less than that of body fluids

    5. ECF—extracellular fluid

6. Intake refers to all possible avenues of intake, e.g., oral fluids, food, IV fluids, gavage feedings, irrigations

7. Output refers to all possible avenues of output, e.g., insensible losses, urine, diarrhea, vomitus, sweat, blood, and any drainage

C. Plan/Implementation (*see* Table 3-1)

1. Fluid deficit

   a. Causes

      1) Vomiting

      2) Diarrhea

      3) GI suction

      4) Sweating and warm weather

      5) Decreased intake; increased caffeine and alcohol intake

      6) Hyperthermia

      7) Diuretics

      8) Older adults—decreased total body water; inability to regulate sodium and water balance; decreased thirst perception

   b. Signs and symptoms

      1) Weight loss

      2) Decreased skin turgor

      3) Oliguria

      4) Concentrated urine

      5) Postural hypotension

      6) Weak, rapid pulse

      7) Increased hematocrit, hemoglobin, BUN, $Na^+$, serum osmolality

      8) Hyperthermia—increased pulse, decreased blood pressure, disorientation; treatment is fluid replacement

      9) Older adults—orthostatic hypotension, falls, pressure injuries, constipation, dry oral mucous membranes not reliable, vital signs not reliable in early dehydration

   c. Nursing management (*see* Table 3-2)

      1) Give fluids as appropriate; space fluids over 24 h

      2) Isotonic IV fluids—lactated Ringer's or 0.9% NaCl

      3) I and O, hourly outputs

      4) Daily weights (1 liter fluid = 1 kg or 2.2 lb)

      5) Monitor vital signs and pulse quality

      6) Check skin turgor

      7) Assess urine specific gravity (should be greater than 1.010 but less than 1.030)

**Table 3-2** Intravenous Fluids

| TYPE OF FLUID | IV FLUID | NURSING CONSIDERATIONS FOR IVS |
|---|---|---|
| Isotonic | 0.9% NaCl<br><br>Ringer's solution<br><br>Lactated<br><br>Ringer's 5% dextrose in water* | Main purpose—to maintain or restore fluid and electrolyte balance<br><br>Secondary purpose—to provide a route for medication, nutrition, and blood components<br><br>Type, amount, and sterility of fluid must be carefully checked |
| Hypotonic | 0.45% NaCl | |
| Hypertonic | 10-15% dextrose in water<br><br>3% NaCl<br><br>Sodium bicarbonate 5% | Macrodrip—delivers 10, 12, or 15 drops per milliliter; should be used if rapid administration is needed<br><br>Microdrip—deliver 60 drops per milliliter; should be used when fluid volume needs to be smaller or more controlled, e.g., clients with compromised renal or cardiac status, clients on "keep-open" rates, pediatric clients<br><br>Maintain sterile technique<br><br>Monitor rate of flow; set IV pump properly<br><br>Assess for infiltration—cool skin, swelling, pain<br><br>Assess for phlebitis—redness, pain, heat, swelling<br><br>Change tubing every 72 h, change bottle every 24 h |

*Becomes hypotonic as dextrose is metabolized

2. Fluid overload—isotonic gain

   a. Increase in the interstitial compartment, intravascular compartment, or both

   b. Causes

      1) Heart failure

      2) Renal failure (late phase)

      3) Cirrhosis of the liver

      4) Excessive ingestion of sodium

      5) Excessive or too rapid intravenous infusion

    c.  Signs and symptoms

      1)  Edema

      2)  Distended veins

      3)  Increased blood pressure

      4)  Bounding pulse

      5)  Crackles; increased respiratory rate, shallow respirations

      6)  Decreased hematocrit and BUN—normal: 10–20 mg/dL (3.57–7.14 mmol/L) (adult); slightly higher in older adults

      7)  Weight gain

    d.  Nursing management

      1)  Administration of diuretics

      2)  Restriction of fluids

      3)  Sodium-restricted diet (500 mg to 4 g salt diet)

      4)  I and O

      5)  Daily weight

      6)  Assess breath sounds

      7)  Check for edema feet/ankle/sacral region

      8)  Semi-Fowler position if dyspneic

      9)  Skin care

# [ SECTION 2 ]

# ELECTROLYTE IMBALANCES

## Fluid and Electrolyte Balance

**NOTE: Ranges may vary by resource or facility**

## Potassium Imbalances

Main intracellular ion; involved in cardiac rhythm, nerve transmission (normal level 3.5–5 mEq/L [3.5–5 mmol/L]) (*see* Tables 3-3 and 3-4)

**Table 3-3** Electrolyte(s) Modifiers

| AGENTS | ACTION |
|---|---|
| Alkalinizing | Release bicarbonate ions in stomach and secrete bicarbonate ions in kidneys |
| Calcium salts | Provide calcium for bones, teeth, nerve transmission, muscle contraction, normal blood coagulation, cell membrane strength |
| Hypocalcemic | Decrease blood levels of calcium |
| Hypophosphatemic | Bind phosphates in GI tract, lowering blood levels; neutralize gastric acid, inactivate pepsin |
| Magnesium salts | Provide magnesium for nerve conduction and muscle activity and activate enzyme reactions in carbohydrate metabolism |
| Phosphates | Provide body with phosphorus needed for bone, muscle tissue, metabolism of carbohydrates, fats, proteins, and normal CNS function |
| Potassium exchange resins | Exchange $Na^+$ for $K^+$ in intestines, lowering $K^+$ levels |
| Potassium salts | Provide potassium needed for cell growth and normal functioning of cardiac, skeletal, and smooth muscle |
| Replacement solution | Provide water and $Na^+$ to maintain acid-base and water balance, maintain osmotic pressure |
| Urinary acidifiers | Secrete $H^+$ ions in kidneys, making urine acidic |
| Urinary alkalinizers | Convert to sodium bicarbonate, making the urine alkaline |

**Table 3-4** Electrolytes and Replacement Solutions

| MEDICATION | ADVERSE EFFECTS | NURSING CONSIDERATIONS |
|---|---|---|
| Calcium carbonate<br>Calcium chloride | Dysrhythmias<br>Constipation | Foods containing oxalic acid (rhubarb, spinach), phytic acid (bran, whole cereals), and phosphorus (milk, dairy products) interfere with absorption<br>Monitor EKG<br>Take 1–1.5 hours after meals (pc) if GI upset occurs |
| Magnesium chloride | Weak or absent deep tendon reflexes<br>Hypotension<br>Respiratory paralysis | Respirations should be greater than 16/min before medication given IV<br>Test deep tendon and patellar reflexes before each dose Monitor I and O |
| Potassium chloride<br>Potassium gluconate | Dysrhythmias, cardiac arrest<br>Abdominal pain<br>Respiratory paralysis | Monitor EKG and serum electrolytes<br>Take with or after meals with full glass of water or fruit juice |
| Sodium chloride | Pulmonary edema | Monitor serum electrolytes |

A. Hypokalemia (less than 3.5 mEq/L [3.5 mmol/L])

   1. Causes

      a. Vomiting

      b. Gastric suction

      c. Prolonged diarrhea

      d. Diuretics and steroids

      e. Inadequate intake

   2. Signs and symptoms

      a. Anorexia, nausea, vomiting

      b. Weak peripheral pulses

      c. Muscle weakness, paresthesias; decreased deep tendon reflexes

      d. Impaired urine concentration

      e. Ventricular dysrhythmias

      f. Potential for digitalis toxicity

      g. Shallow respirations

   3. Nursing management

      a. Administration of oral potassium supplements—dilute in juice and give with meals to avoid gastric irritation

    b.  Increase dietary intake—raisins, bananas, apricots, oranges, beans, potatoes, carrots, celery

    c.  IV supplements—20–40 mEq/L usual concentration; cannot give concentration greater than 1 mEq/10 mL into peripheral IV, or without cardiac monitor; do not exceed 20 mEq/hour infusion rate; stop solution immediately if burning occurs

    d.  Assess renal function prior to administration

    e.  Risk for digitalis toxicity

**B.**  Hyperkalemia (greater than 5 mEq/L [5 mmol/L])

  1.  Causes

    a.  Renal failure

    b.  Use of potassium supplements

    c.  Burns

    d.  Crushing injuries

    e.  Severe infection

    f.  Potassium-sparing diuretics

    g.  Angiotensin-converting enzyme (ACE) inhibitors

  2.  Signs and symptoms

    a.  Electrocardiogram (EKG) changes—peaked T waves, wide QRS complexes

    b.  Dysrhythmias, ventricular fibrillation, heart block

    c.  Cardiac arrest

    d.  Muscle twitching and weakness

    e.  Numbness in hands and feet and around mouth

    f.  Nausea

    g.  Diarrhea

  3.  Nursing management

    a.  Restrict dietary potassium and potassium-containing medications or IV solutions

    b.  Sodium polystyrene sulfonate—cation-exchange resin (causes diarrhea)

      1)  Orally—dilute to make more palatable

      2)  Rectally—give in conjunction with sorbitol to avoid fecal impaction

    c.  In emergency situation

      1)  Calcium gluconate given IV

      2)  Sodium bicarbonate given IV

    d.  IV administration of regular insulin and dextrose shifts potassium into the cells

    e.  Peritoneal or hemodialysis

    f.  Diuretics

## Sodium Imbalances

Main extracellular ion; responsible for water balance (normal: 135–145 mEq/L [135-145 mmol/L])

   **A.** Hyponatremia (less than 135 mEq/L [135 mmol/L])

      1. Causes

         a. Vomiting

         b. Diuretics

         c. Excessive administration of dextrose and water IVs

         d. Burns, wound drainage

         e. Excessive water intake

         f. Syndrome of inappropriate antidiuretic hormone secretion (SIADH)

         g. Older adults—kidneys unable to excrete free water

      2. Signs and symptoms

         a. Nausea

         b. Muscle cramps

         c. Confusion

         d. Muscular twitching, coma

         e. Seizures

         f. Headache

         g. Delirium in older adults

      3. Nursing management

         a. Oral administration of sodium-rich foods—beef broth, tomato juice

         b. IV lactated Ringer's or high concentrations of NaCl (0.9%)

         c. Water restriction (safer method)

         d. I and O

         e. Daily weight

   **B.** Hypernatremia (greater than 145 mEq/L [145 mmol/L])

      1. Causes

         a. Hypertonic tube feedings without water supplements

         b. Hyperventilation

         c. Diabetes insipidus

         d. Ingestion of over-the-counter (OTC) medications such as citric acid (1,000 mg), aspirin (325 mg), or sodium bicarbonate

         e. Inhaling large amounts of salt water (near drowning)

         f. Inadequate water ingestion

2. Signs and symptoms

   a. Elevated temperature

   b. Weakness

   c. Disorientation

   d. Irritability and restlessness

   e. Thirst

   f. Dry, swollen tongue

   g. Sticky mucous membranes

   h. Postural hypotension with ↓ ECF

   i. Hypertension with normal or ↑ ECF

   j. Tachycardia

   k. Older adults—mental status changes, coma

3. Nursing management

   a. IV administration of hypotonic solution—0.3% NaCl or 0.45% NaCl; 5% dextrose in water

   b. Offer fluids at regular intervals

   c. Decrease sodium in diet

   d. Daily weight

## Calcium Imbalances

Need for blood clotting, skeletal muscle contraction (normal ionized serum calcium level: 4.6–5.1 mg/dL [1.15–1.27 mmol/L]; normal total serum calcium level: 8.2–10.2 mg/dL [2.05–2.55 mmol/L]); regulated by the parathyroid hormone and vitamin D, which facilitates reabsorption of calcium from bone and enhances reabsorption from the GI tract

**A.** Hypocalcemia (less than 4.6 mg/dL [1.15 mmol/L] for ionized serum calcium or less than 8.2 mg/dL [2.05 mmol/L] for total serum calcium)

1. Causes

   a. Hypoparathyroidism

   b. Pancreatitis

   c. Renal failure

   d. Steroids and loop diuretics

   e. Inadequate intake

   f. Post–thyroid surgery

2. Signs and symptoms

   a. Nervous system becomes increasingly excitable

   b. Tetany

      1) Trousseau sign—inflate BP cuff on upper arm to 20 mm Hg above systolic pressure, carpal spasms within 2–5 min indicate tetany

        2) Chvostek sign—tap facial nerve 2 cm anterior to the earlobe just below the zygomatic arch; twitching of facial muscles indicates tetany

  c. Hyperactive reflexes

  d. Confusion

  e. Paresthesias

  f. Irritability

  g. Seizures

3. Nursing management

  a. Orally—calcium gluconate (less concentrated) or calcium chloride; administer with orange juice to maximize absorption

  b. Parenterally—calcium gluconate

    1) Effect is transitory and additional doses may be necessary

    2) Caution with digitalized clients because both are cardiac depressants

    3) Calcium may cause vessel irritation and should be administered through a long, stable intravenous line

    4) Avoid infiltration because tissue can become necrotic and slough

    5) Administer at a slow rate to avoid high serum concentrations and cardiac depression

    6) Seizure precautions

    7) Maintain airway because laryngeal stridor can occur

    8) Safety needs due to confusion

    9) Increase dietary intake of calcium

    10) Calcium supplements

    11) Regular exercise

    12) Administer phosphate-binding antacids, calcitriol, vitamin D

**B.** Hypercalcemia (greater than 5.1 mg/dL [1.27 mmol/L] for ionized serum calcium or greater than 10.2 mg/dL [2.55 mmol/L] for total serum calcium)

1. Causes

  a. Malignant neoplastic diseases

  b. Hyperparathyroidism

  c. Prolonged immobilization

  d. Excessive intake

  e. Immobility

  f. Excessive intake of calcium carbonate antacids

2. Signs and symptoms

  a. Lack of coordination

  b. Anorexia, nausea, and vomiting

  c. Confusion, decreased level of consciousness

      d.  Personality changes

      e.  Dysrhythmias, heart block, cardiac arrest

  3.  Nursing management

      a.  IV administration of 0.45% NaCl or 0.9% NaCl

      b.  Encourage fluids

      c.  Furosemide

      d.  Calcitonin—decreases calcium level

      e.  Mobilizing the client

      f.  Dietary calcium restriction

      g.  Prevent development of renal calculi

          1)  Increase fluid intake

          2)  Maintain acidic urine

          3)  Prevent urinary tract infection

      h.  Injury prevention

      i.  Limit intake of calcium carbonate antacids

      j.  Surgical intervention may be indicated in hyperparathyroidism (cause of hypercalcemia)

          1)  Preoperatively—directed toward preventing dangerously high serum calcium levels

          2)  Postoperatively

              a)  Observe for signs of hypocalcemia (reverse of preop)

              b)  Due to calcium drop postop, large quantities of calcium salts may be required

              c)  Encourage early ambulation to aid in recalcification of bones

## Magnesium Imbalance

Interdependent with calcium (normal: 1.3–2.1 mEq/L [0.65–1.05 mmol/L])

  **A.**  Hypomagnesemia (less than 1.3 mEq/L [0.65 mmol/L])

    1.  Causes

      a.  Alcoholism

      b.  GI suction

      c.  Diarrhea

      d.  Intestinal fistulas

      e.  Poorly controlled diabetes mellitus

      f.  Malabsorption syndrome

    2.  Signs and symptoms

      a.  Increased neuromuscular irritability

      b.  Tremors

        c.  Tetany

        d.  Hyperactive deep tendon reflexes

        e.  Seizures

        f.  Dysrhythmias especially if hypokalemia present

        g.  Disorientation

        h.  Confusion

    3.  Nursing management

        a.  Increased intake of dietary Mg—green vegetables, nuts, bananas, oranges, peanut butter, chocolate

        b.  Parenteral administration of supplements—magnesium sulfate

            1)  Monitor cardiac rhythm and reflexes to detect depressive effects of magnesium

            2)  Keep self-inflating breathing bag, airways, and oxygen at bedside in case of respiratory emergency

            3)  Calcium preparations may be given to counteract the potential danger of myocardial dysfunction that may result from magnesium intoxication secondary to rapid infusions

        c.  Oral—long-term maintenance with oral magnesium

        d.  IV—assess renal function

        e.  Monitor for digitalis toxicity

        f.  Seizure precautions

        g.  Safety measures for confusion

        h.  Test ability to swallow before PO fluids/food because of dysphagia

**B.**  Hypermagnesemia (greater than 2.1 mEq/L [1.05 mmol/L])—potent vasodilator

    1.  Causes

        a.  Renal failure

        b.  Excessive magnesium administration (antacids, cathartics)

    2.  Signs and symptoms

        a.  Depresses the CNS

        b.  Depresses cardiac impulse transmission

        c.  Cardiac arrest

        d.  Facial flushing

        e.  Muscle weakness

        f.  Absent deep tendon reflexes

        g.  Paralysis

        h.  Shallow respirations

3. Nursing management

   a. Discontinue oral and IV Mg

   b. Emergency

      1) Support ventilation

      2) IV calcium gluconate

   c. Hemodialysis

   d. Monitor reflexes

   e. Teach regarding over-the-counter medications containing Mg (antacids/ some laxatives)

   f. Monitor respiratory status

   g. Monitor cardiac rhythm; have calcium preparations available to antagonize cardiac depressant

[ SECTION 3 ]

# NURSING MEASURES FOR INTRAVENOUS THERAPY

## Fluid and Electrolyte Balance

## Purpose

**A.** Main—to maintain or restore fluid and electrolyte balance

**B.** Secondary—to provide a route for medication, nutrition, and blood components

## Equipment

**A.** Solution

    1. Type, amount, and sterility of fluid must be carefully checked

        a. If sterility is compromised, bacteria will be introduced directly into the bloodstream

        b. Fluid overload is possible

            1) Isotonic

                a) 0.9% NaCl

                b) Ringer's solution

                c) Lactated Ringer's

            2) Hypotonic

                a) 5% dextrose in water (is isotonic but becomes hypotonic when glucose is metabolized)

                b) 0.45% NaCl

            3) Hypertonic

                a) 10–15% dextrose in water

                b) 3% NaCl

                c) Sodium bicarbonate 5%

                d) 5% dextrose in 0.9% saline

**B.** Equipment

    1. Administration set—plays important role in the amount of fluid the client receives

        a. Macrodrip—can deliver 10, 12, or 15 drops per milliliter; should be used if rapid administration is needed

        b. Microdrip—delivers 60 drops per milliliter; should be used when fluid volume needs to be smaller or more controlled, e.g., clients with compromised renal or cardiac status, clients on "keep-open" rates, and pediatric clients

2. Cannula, catheter, wing-tipped needle or intravenous catheter

3. Skin prep, tape, IV, pole, arm board, tourniquet

4. Controller or pump, if indicated

**Table 3-5** Calculations for IV Rate

1) Milliliters per hour:

$$\frac{\text{Total solution}}{\text{Hours to run}} = \text{mL/h}$$

*Example*: 1000 mL in 8 hours

$$\frac{1,000}{8} = 125 \text{ mL/h}$$

2) Drops per minute:

$$\frac{\text{Total volume} \times \text{Drop factor}}{\text{Time in minutes}} = \text{gtts/min}$$

*Example*: 1000 mL in 8 hours, with a drop factor of 15

$$\frac{1,000 \times 15}{8 \times 60} =$$

$$\frac{1,000 \times 1}{8 \times 4} = 31.25 \text{ or } 31 \text{ gtts/min}$$

$$\frac{250}{8} =$$

# Procedure to Begin Intravenous Therapy

**A.** Peripheral IV

1. Location

   a. Condition of vein

   b. Type of fluid/med to be infused

   c. Duration of therapy

   d. Client's age, size, stability

   e. Skill of nurse

2. Insertion of catheter

   a. Explain procedure, check ID

   b. Distend veins by applying tourniquet 4–6″ above site, tap on vessel or have client open and close fist, or hang arm over side of bed

   c. Clean site with povidone-iodine or chlorhexidine antiseptic solution; press applicator against skin and use back-and-forth friction to scrub for at least 30 seconds

   d. Allow to air dry; do not blot skin or "wave" over site to dry

   e. Hold skin taut to stabilize vein

    f.   Insert catheter bevel up at 15–20° (direct method—thrust catheter through skin and vein in one smooth motion; indirect method—first pierce skin, then vessel)

    g.   Watch for flashback of blood in catheter

    h.   Once blood return observed, lessen the angle and advance catheter 1/4″ and then remove tourniquet

    i.   Withdraw needle from catheter; advance catheter up to hub

    j.   Secure catheter

    k.   Attach IV tubing

    l.   Begin IV infusion

    m.   Check for infiltration or hematoma

3.   Complications

    a.   Infiltration—fluid into tissue

       1)  Assessment

          a)  Edema

          b)  Pain

          c)  Coolness in area

          d)  Decrease in flow rate

       2)  Nursing management

          a)  Discontinue IV

          b)  Apply warm compresses to infiltrated site

          c)  Apply sterile dressing

          d)  Elevate arm

          e)  Start IV at new site proximal to infiltrated site if same extremity used; may use different vein distal to infiltrated site (basilic or cephalic)

    b.   Phlebitis—inflammation of vein

       1)  Assessment

          a)  Reddened, warm area around insertion site or on path of vein

          b)  Tenderness

          c)  Swelling

       2)  Nursing management

          a)  Discontinue IV

          b)  Apply warm, moist compresses

          c)  Restart IV at new site

    c.   Thrombophlebitis—inflammation of vein with clot

       1)  Assessment

          a)  Pain at insertion site or above site

          b)  Swelling

          c)  Redness and warmth around insertion site or along path of vein

        d)   Fever

        e)   Leukocytosis

    2)  Nursing management

        a)   Discontinue IV

        b)   Apply warm compress

        c)   Elevate the extremity

        d)   Restart the IV

  d.  Circulatory overload

    1)  Assessment

        a)   Crackles

        b)   Dyspnea

        c)   Confusion

        d)   Seizures

    2)  Nursing care

        a)   Reduce IV rate

        b)   Assess vital signs (VS)

        c)   Assess lab values

        d)   Notify health care provider

  e.  Hematoma

    1)  Assessment

        a)   Ecchymosis

        b)   Immediate swelling at site

        c)   Leakage of blood at site

    2)  Nursing management

        a)   Discontinue IV

        b)   Apply pressure with sterile dressing

        c)   Apply cool compresses (or ice bag) for 24 hours to site, followed by warm compresses

        d)   Restart IV

  f.  Clotting

    1)  Assessment

        a)   Decreased IV flow rate or absent flow rate

        b)   Backflow of blood into IV tubing

    2)  Nursing management

        a)   Discontinue IV

        b)   Do not irrigate or milk the tubing

        c)   Do not increase the IV flow rate or hang the solution higher

d)   Do not aspirate clot from the cannula

e)   Urokinase may be injected into catheter to clear occlusion

# Factors Affecting Flow Rate

A.  Circulatory physiology

1.  Structures

a.  Arteries—originate in the aorta or its branches; transport blood to the systemic circulation

1)  Aorta—assists the flow of blood to the arteries or acts as a reservoir for blood during ejection of the ventricles

2)  Pulmonary artery—originates in the right ventricle and transports unoxygenated blood from the circulation to the lungs to be oxygenated (only artery carrying unoxygenated blood)

b.  Veins—carry unoxygenated blood and body wastes from the systemic circulation to the right atrium by way of the inferior and superior vena cava; valves help to direct the flow of blood toward the heart

c.  Capillaries—small vessels

2.  Circulation

a.  Oxygenated blood leaves left ventricle, travels through aorta and arterioles (smaller branches)

b.  Unoxygenated blood returns to the right side of heart by inferior and superior vena cava

c.  Coronary circulation—circulation to the myocardium

d.  Peripheral circulation—circulation through the periphery (extremities)

3.  Factors regulating circulation

a.  Nervous system—regulates heart rate, influences arteriolar constriction and blood pressure

1)  Neural reflexes are controlled via the vasomotor center in the medulla oblongata; there are four centers:

a)   Vasoconstrictor center—reduces diameter of blood vessels

b)   Vasodilator center—increases diameter of blood vessels

c)   Cardioaccelerator center—increases heart rate

d)   Cardioinhibitory center—decreases heart rate

2)  The four centers are stimulated or inhibited by the following:

a)   Pressoreceptors (baroreceptors)—specialized nerve endings affected by changes in pressure of blood in arteries

b)   Chemoreceptors—located in the aortic arch and carotid bodies; sensitive to oxygen lack, increased blood carbon dioxide, and decreased pH

       c)   Medullary ischemic reflex—produces vasoconstriction of small blood vessels in response to stimulation of the vasoconstrictor center by $CO_2$ excess and diminished oxygen levels

4. Blood pressure—the pressure exerted by the blood against the walls of vessels

   a. Arterial blood pressure (pressure exerted against arterial wall)

     1) Systolic blood pressure—maximum pressure of blood exerted against the arterial wall when the heart is contracting

     2) Diastolic blood pressure—force of blood exerted against the wall of the artery when the heart is at rest

     3) Pulse pressure—difference between diastolic and systolic blood pressure; normal is 30–40 mm Hg

     4) Circulatory factors influencing arterial pressure

       a)   Cardiac output—increase causes increased blood pressure; decrease causes decreased blood pressure

       b)   Peripheral resistance (afterload)—narrowed arterioles increase blood pressure; dilated arterioles decrease blood pressure

       c)   Arterial elasticity—elastic vessels accommodate changes in blood flow; rigid sclerotic vessels cause increases in systolic blood pressure and pulse pressure

       d)   Blood volume (preload)—decreased blood volume (e.g., due to hemorrhage) results in decreased pressure

       e)   Blood viscosity—increased viscosity (e.g., due to overabundance of red blood cells {RBC}) results in high pressure; decreased viscosity (e.g., due to anemia) results in lower pressure

     5) Other factors influencing pressure

       a)   Age—increases with age

       b)   Weight—increases with excess weight

       c)   Emotions—increase with release of epinephrine (caused by strong emotion)

       d)   Exercise—extreme physical activity increases pressure

# Central Venous Access Devices (CVAD) (3 Types)

**A.** Peripherally inserted central catheter (PICC)

  1. Venipuncture performed above or below antecubital fossa into basilic, cephalic, or axillary veins of dominant arm (encourages blood flow and reduces risk of dependent edema)

  2. Tip of catheter is in superior vena cava or brachiocephalic veins

  3. May be single, double, or triple lumen

  4. May stay in place up to weeks or months

  5. Potential complications

      a. Malposition

      b. Dysrhythmias

      c. Nerve or tendon damage

      d. Respiratory distress

      e. Catheter embolism

      f. Thrombophlebitis

6. Nursing management

      a. No blood pressure or phlebotomy affected arm

      b. Change dressing 2–3 times/wk and when wet or nonocclusive

      c. Flush with saline or heparinized saline according to agency policy

**B.** Implanted infusion port

1. Used for long-term home IV therapy

2. Must be surgically placed

3. Long-term use; may remain in place for years

4. End of catheter attached to chamber placed in subcutaneous pocket on client's chest wall or upper arm

5. Use Huber needle to access port; do not use regular beveled needle to access; will "core" diaphragm of port

6. Port must be flushed with heparinized saline when not accessed.

7. Example: port-o-cath

**C.** Tunneled central catheters

1. Increases in size (2 gauges, 2.5 cm in length) 2 hours after insertion, becomes softer

2. Venipuncture 2–3 fingerbreadths above antecubital fossa or 1 fingerbreadth below antecubital fossa into cephalic, basilic, or median cubital vein

3. Long-term use; may remain in place for years

4. Catheter may be single or double lumen; examples: Broviac, Hickman, Groshong

5. Complications

      a. Thrombosis

      b. Phlebitis

      c. Air embolism

      d. Infection

      e. Bleeding

      f. Vascular perforation

6. Nursing management

      a. Change dressing 2–3 times/wk or as prescribed (every 7 days with chlorhexidine patch) and when wet or nonocclusive

      b. Flush with normal saline alone or with normal saline followed by heparinized saline according to agency policy

     c.  Anchor catheter securely

     d.  Avoid chemotherapy or parenteral nutrition

**D.** Nontunneled percutaneous central catheters

  1.  Inserted through subclavian vein; tip in superior vena cava

  2.  Nontunneled central catheters; 7–10 inches long

     a.  Used for short-term IV therapy

     b.  Inserted by health care provider

     c.  Triple-lumen central catheter—distal lumen (16 gauge) used to infuse or draw blood samples; middle lumen (18-gauge) used for parenteral nutrition (PN) infusion; proximal lumen (18-gauge) used to infuse or draw blood and administer medications

  3.  Insertion

     a.  Placed supine in head-low position (dilates vessel and prevents air embolism)

     b.  Client turns head away from site during procedure

     c.  While catheter is being inserted, client performs Valsalva maneuver

     d.  Antibiotic ointment and transparent dressing applied using sterile technique

     e.  Verify position of tip of catheter by x-ray

     f.  Each lumen secured with Luer-Lok cap and labeled to indicate location (proximal, middle, distal)

  4.  Nursing management

     a.  Catheter changed according to agency policy

     b.  Flush with normal saline alone or with normal saline followed by heparinized saline according to agency policy; flushed also after each infusion, specimen withdrawal, medication administration, or when disconnected

     c.  Never use force to flush catheter; if resistance met, notify health care provider

     d.  Dressing changes 2–3 times/wk and as needed (PRN); place in low Fowler position; nurse and client wear masks; alcohol and then iodine swabs or chlorhexidine swabs (agency policy) used to clean site

     e.  Change IV tubing every 72–96 hours according to agency policy

## Blood Transfusions

**A.** Overview

  1.  Purposes

     a.  Restore blood volume following hemorrhage, burns, or injuries to blood vessels

     b.  Combat shock

     c.  Treat severe chronic anemia by increasing the oxygen-carrying capacity of the blood

  2.  Equipment—blood or blood product, normal saline (0.9% NaCl), tubing with filter, 18-gauge needle for venous access (*see* Table 3-6)

**Table 3-6** Blood Components

| PRODUCT | ADVERSE REACTIONS | NURSING CONSIDERATIONS |
|---|---|---|
| Packed red cells | Reactions less common than with whole blood | Companion solution—0.9% NaCl<br><br>Use standard blood filter<br><br>Give over 2–4 hours |
| Platelets | Some febrile reactions | Companion solution—0.9% NaCl<br><br>Nonwettable filter<br><br>Give as quickly as possible, 4 units/hour |
| Plasma | Circulatory overload risk | Administer with straight line set<br><br>Give as quickly as possible (coagulation factors become unstable) |
| Albumin | Circulatory overload risk | Use administration set provided<br><br>25% albumin—give at 1 mL/min<br><br>Give as quickly as possible if client in shock |
| Prothrombin | Hepatitis risk greater than with whole blood<br><br>Allergic/febrile reactions | Use straight line set |
| Factor VIII | Allergic and febrile reactions | Use component drip set or syringe |

3. Procedure
   a. Ask client about any allergies or previous blood reactions (*see* Table 3-7)
   b. Type and crossmatch blood—ensures that the donor's blood and recipient's blood are compatible (*see* Table 3-8)
   c. Check blood for bubbles, dark color, or cloudiness
   d. Change entire IV line for each unit of blood
   e. ID checks by two nurses
      1) Health care provider's order
      2) Hospital ID band name and number
      3) Blood component tag name and number matched to client
      4) Blood type and Rh

**Table 3-7** Blood Transfusion Reactions

| TYPE OF REACTION | CAUSE | SYMPTOMS | NURSING CONSIDERATIONS |
|---|---|---|---|
| Allergic reaction<br><br>Hypersensitivity | Hypersensitivity to antibodies in donor's blood | Occurs immediately or within 24 hours<br><br>Mild—urticaria, itching, flushing<br><br>Anaphylaxis—hypotension, dyspnea, decreased oxygen saturation, flushing | Prevention—premedicate with antihistamines<br><br>Stop the transfusion<br><br>Restart the 0.9% NaCl<br><br>Notify the health care provider<br><br>Supportive care: diphenhydramine, oxygen, corticosteroids |
| Acute intravascular hemolytic reaction | Incompatibility | Occurs within minutes to 24 hours<br><br>Nausea, vomiting, pain in lower back, hypotension, increase in pulse rate, decrease in urinary output, hematuria | Stop the transfusion<br><br>Supportive care—oxygen, diphenhydramine, airway management |
| Febrile nonhemolytic reaction (most common) | Antibodies to donor platelets or leukocytes | Occurs in minutes to hours<br><br>Fever, chills, nausea, headache, flushing, tachycardia, palpitations | Stop the transfusion<br><br>Supportive care<br><br>Aspirin<br><br>Seen with clients after multiple transfusions |
| Sepsis | Contaminated blood products | Occurs within minutes to less than 24 hours<br><br>Tachycardia, hypotension, fever, chills, shock | Stop the transfusion<br><br>Obtain blood culture<br><br>Antibiotics, IV fluids, vasopressors, steroids |
| Circulatory overload | Large volume over short time | Occurs within minutes to hours—dyspnea, crackles, increased respiratory rate, tachycardia | Monitor clients at high risk (older adults, heart disease, children)<br><br>Slow or discontinue transfusion |

**Table 3-8** Blood Group Compatibility

| BLOOD GROUP | CAN ACT AS DONOR TO | CAN RECEIVE BLOOD FROM |
|---|---|---|
| O | O, A, B, AB | O |
| A | A, AB | O, A |
| B | B, AB | O, B |
| AB | AB | O, A, B, AB |

    f.   Check baseline vital signs, including temperature

    g.   Start with normal saline (0.9% NaCl)

    h.   Run blood slowly for first 15 minutes; RN must be present for first 15 minutes

    i.   Stay with client 15–30 min

    j.   Recheck vital signs 15 min after infusion started

    k.   If no untoward effects, increase rate

    l.   Take vital signs every hour until completed, then hourly for 3 hours; licensed practical nurse/licensed vocational nurse (LPN/LVN) may monitor vital signs after first 15 minutes

    m.   Ask client to report itching or flank pain over kidneys

# Burn Management

**A.** Types

    1.   Thermal—contact with hot substance (solids/liquids/gases)

    2.   Chemical—contact with strong acids or strong bases; prolonged contact with almost any chemical

    3.   Electrical—contact with live current; internal damage may be more severe than expected from external injury

    4.   Radiation—exposure to high doses of radioactive material

**B.** Emergency care—on the scene

    1.   Stop the burning process

        a.   Thermal—smother; stop, drop, and roll

        b.   Chemical—remove clothing and flush/irrigate skin/eyes

        c.   Electrical—shut off electrical current or separate person from source with a nonconducting implement

    2.   Ensure airway, breathing, and circulation

    3.   Immediate wound care; keep client warm and dry; wrap in clean, dry sheet/blanket

C. Assessment

  1. Extent of the burn—"Rule of Nines" (*see* Figure 3-2; percentages are used to determine body surface)

  2. Determination of intensity (*see* Table 3-9)

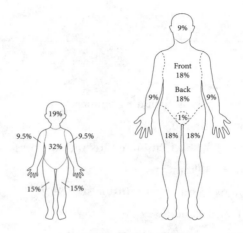

**Figure 3-2.** Child/Adult

**Table 3-9** Classification of Burns

| SUPERFICIAL | SUPERFICIAL PARTIAL-THICKNESS | DEEP PARTIAL-THICKNESS | FULL-THICKNESS | DEEP FULL-THICKNESS |
|---|---|---|---|---|
| Similar to first-degree | Similar to second-degree | Similar to second-degree | Similar to third-degree | Similar to third-degree |
| Skin pink to red<br><br>Painful | Skin pink to red<br><br>Painful | Skin red to white<br><br>Painful | Skin red, white, brown, black<br><br>Pain possible | Skin black<br><br>No pain |
| Epidermis<br><br>Sunburn | Epidermis and dermis<br><br>Scalds, flames | Epidermis and dermis<br><br>Scalds, flames, tar, grease | All skin layers<br><br>Prolonged contact with hot objects | All skin layers, possibly muscles and tendon<br><br>Flames, electricity |
| Heals in 3–5 days | Heals in 2 weeks | Heals in 1 month<br><br>Possible grafting | Heals in weeks to months<br><br>Requires extensive repair | Heals in weeks to months<br><br>Escharotomy<br><br>Grafting |

**D.** Nursing management (*see* Table 3-10)

    1. Fluid replacement

        a. Emergent/resuscitative phase (first 24–48 h)

            1) IV fluids to replace fluid losses; balanced salt solution (lactated Ringer's) to avoid over/under hydration

                a) Rapid for first 8 h

                b) More slowly over remaining 16 h

            2) Plasma to increase blood volume and to increase $O_2$

**Table 3-10** Nursing Care for Burn Client

| GOAL | NURSING CONSIDERATIONS |
|---|---|
| Correct fluid and electrolyte imbalance | First 24–48 hours (emergent/resuscitative phase):<br>• IV fluids balanced salt solution (lactated Ringer's [LR]), plasma<br><br>After calculation of 24-hours replacement—rapid for first 8 hours, more slowly over remaining 16 hours:<br>• 1/2 delivered in first 8 hours, 1/4 over second 8 hours, and 1/4 over third 8 hours<br><br>2–5 d after burn (acute/intermediate phase):<br>• Packed RBCs<br>• Indwelling catheter to monitor hourly output; should be at least 30 mL/hour<br>• Careful administration of IV fluids; check for signs of fluid overload vs. dehydration<br>• Monitor blood pressure; temperature, pulse, respiration (TPR); weight (wt); serum electrolytes |
| Promote healing | Cap, gown, mask, gloves worn by nurse<br><br>Wound care at least once a day<br><br>Debridement (removal of nonviable tissue)—hydrotherapy is used to loosen dead tissue, 30 min maximum<br><br>Escharotomy (incising of leathery covering of dead tissue conducive to bacterial growth)—used to alleviate constriction, minimize infection<br><br>Dressing—careful sterile technique, avoid breaking blisters, wound may be covered or left exposed<br><br>Application of topical antibacterial medications—silver sulfadiazine, mafenide, silver nitrate<br><br>Grafting—biological (human amniotic membrane, cadaver, allograft); autografting when granulation bed is clean and well vascularized<br><br>Tetanus prophylaxis<br><br>Avoid hypothermia and add humidity |

*(Continued)*

**Table 3-10** Nursing Care for Burn Client (*Continued*)

| GOAL | NURSING CONSIDERATIONS |
|---|---|
| Support nutrition | High-caloric, high-carbohydrate, high-protein diet; may require TPN or tube feeding; oral nutrient supplements; vitamins B, C, and iron; H2 histamine blockers and antacids to prevent stress ulcer (Curling's ulcer) |
| | NG tube to prevent gastric distension, early acute gastric dilation, and paralytic ileus associated with burn shock; monitor bowel sounds |
| Control pain | Pain medication (morphine)—given IV at first due to impaired circulation and poor absorption |
| | Monitor VS frequently; analgesic 30 min before wound care |
| Prevent complications of immobility | Prevent contractures—maintain joints in neutral position of extension; shoes to prevent foot drop; splints; active and passive ROM exercises at each dressing change; turn side to side frequently; skin care to prevent breakdown |
| | Stryker frame or Circolectric bed may facilitate change of position |
| | Facial exercises and position that hyperextends neck for burns of face and neck |
| | Consult with physical therapist |
| Support client | Counsel client regarding change in body image |
| | Encourage expression of feelings and demonstrate acceptance of client |
| | Evaluate client's readiness to see scarred areas, especially facial area |
| | Assist client's family to adjust to changed appearance |
| | Consider recommending client for ongoing counseling |
| | Support developmental needs of children, e.g., sick children need limits on behavior |
| | Assist client in coping with immobilization, pain, and isolation |
| | Prepare client for discharge—anticipate readmission for release of contractures/cosmetic surgery; proper use of any correctional orthopedic appliances, pressure garments (used to decrease scarring); how to change dressings |

2. Acute/intermediate phase (2–5 days postburn)
    a. Water and electrolytes to maintain $Na^+$ and $K^+$
    b. Packed RBC to maintain $O_2$ carrying capacity
3. Indwelling catheter to monitor hourly output; should be at least 30 mL/h; weigh daily
4. NG tube to prevent gastric distension, early acute gastric dilation, and paralytic ileus associated with burn shock; monitor bowel sounds; H2 histamine blockers and antacids to prevent a Curling's ulcer

5. Pain medication (morphine)—given IV at first due to impaired circulation and poor absorption from muscles/subcutaneous tissue; monitor VS frequently; analgesic 30 minutes before wound care

6. Tetanus prophylaxis; tetanus immune globulin when history of immunization is questionable

7. Avoidance of hypothermia—warm and humid environment

8. Frequent regular and routine monitoring of VS

9. Clean, safe environment; meticulous hand hygiene; cap, gown, mask, gloves worn by nurse

10. Wound care—early and continuous

    a. Debridement (removal of nonviable tissue)—hydrotherapy is used to loosen dead tissue, 30 minutes maximum; hydrotherapy tank, spray table, tubbing, under as clean conditions as possible (gown, gloves, masks, hat, plastic disposable tub liner)

    b. Escharotomy (incising of leathery covering of dead tissue conducive to bacterial growth)—used to alleviate constriction; minimize infection

    c. Dressing

        1) Wound may be covered or left exposed

        2) Application of topical antibacterial medications

            a) Silver sulfadiazine—closed method; monitor for hypersensitivity, rash, itching, burning sensation in areas other than burn; decreased WBC

            b) Mafenide—open method; monitor acid/base balance and renal function; remove previously applied cream

            c) Silver nitrate—keep dressings wet with solution to avoid overconcentrations; handle carefully, can leave a gray/black stain

    d. Early excision of burn followed by grafting

        1) Biological (human amniotic membrane, cadaver, allograft)

        2) Synthetic

        3) Autografting when granulation bed is clean and well vascularized

11. Diet—high caloric, high carbohydrate, high protein; may require total parenteral nutrition (TPN) or tube feeding at first; oral nutrient supplements; vitamins B and C; iron; possibly zinc (excretion of increased zinc may cause loss of taste)

12. Administration of antacid to prevent stress ulcer (Curling's ulcer)

13. Control of itching—a major problem with healing

14. Psychological counseling

15. Prevent contractures—maintain joints in neutral position of extension; shoes to prevent foot drop; splints; active and passive range of motion (ROM) exercises at each dressing change; turn side to side frequently; skin care to prevent breakdown

16. Assist client in coping with immobilization, pain, and isolation

17. Prepare client for discharge—anticipate readmission for release of contractures/cosmetic surgery; proper use of any correctional orthopedic appliances/pressure garments; how to change dressings

# End-of-Chapter Thinking Exercise

The medical-surgical unit nurse performs an admission assessment on an older adult client. The client lives alone in an apartment in a retirement community. Meals are eaten in a community setting, but the client has not been to meals for several days. The client reports having been sick for the past four days and states, "I can't keep anything down. I've been vomiting and have had diarrhea." The client is in general good health and has a history of hypertension controlled with a daily dose of hydrochlorothiazide (HCTZ). Physical examination reveals dry, cracked lips, dry mucous membranes, and poor skin turgor. The client has not had anything by mouth except ice chips in the last 36 hours. The client voided 50 mL of dark amber urine. The nurse observes weak hand grip strength and decreased deep tendon reflexes (DTR). Vital signs and lab tests are below.

| VITAL SIGN | RESULT |
|---|---|
| Temperature | 99.7°F (37.6°C) |
| Pulse | 115 beats/min, weak and irregular |
| BP | 90/48 mm Hg |
| Respirations | 22 breaths/min |
| SpO$_2$ | 94% |

| LAB TEST | RESULT |
|---|---|
| Sodium | 149 mEq/L (149 mmol/L) |
| Potassium | 2.9 mEq/L (2.9 mmol/L) |
| BUN | 25 mg/dL (8.93 mmol/L) |
| Creatinine | 1.6 mg/dL (141.47 mcmol/L) |

1. What risks for fluid and electrolyte imbalances does the nurse identify? (Recognize Cues)

2. Which findings indicate hypokalemia? (Analyze Cues)

3. Which actions does the nurse implement? (Take Action)

# Thinking Exercise Explanations

1.  What risks for fluid and electrolyte imbalances does the nurse identify? (Recognize Cues)
    - Vomiting
    - Diarrhea
    - Daily diuretic use

    Vomiting and diarrhea lead to volume depletion and increased excretion of potassium. The client's use of a diuretic also causes fluid and potassium losses.

2.  Which findings indicate hypokalemia? (Analyze Cues)
    - Potassium 2.9 mEq/L (2.9 mmol/L); normal: 3.5–5 mEq/L (3.5–5 mmol/L)
    - Weak, irregular pulse
    - Muscle weakness
    - Decreased DTRs

    Because most of the body's potassium is found inside the cell, a disturbance in the extracellular levels can lead to decreased cell membrane excitability, which leads to muscle weakness and cardiac issues. Potassium controls the excitability of cell membranes. Low levels decrease the normal functioning of cardiac, nerve, and muscle tissues.

3.  Which actions does the nurse implement? (Take Action)
    - Notify the HCP of findings
    - Anticipate IV fluid and potassium supplements
    - Monitor vital signs and note any changes
    - Monitor lab values for the return of normal levels

    The client shows signs of dehydration and hypokalemia. The signs and symptoms exhibited indicate an unstable condition, and the nurse needs to notify the HCP for further prescriptions. The nurse will carefully monitor the client's vital signs, lab values, intake and output, and medications for further changes in the client's condition.

# CHAPTER 4

# THE CARDIOVASCULAR SYSTEM

| SECTIONS | CONCEPTS COVERED |
|---|---|
| | Table 4-5. Causes of Heart Failure |
| | Table 4-6. Cardiac Glycoside Medications (Digitalis) |
| | Table 4-7. Diuretic Medication |
| | Figure 4-21. Common Ischemic Pain Pattern |
| | Table 4-8. Selected Cardiac Medications |
| | Figure 4-22. Coronary Artery and Heart |
| | Table 4-9. Antianginal Medication |
| | Table 4-10. Anticoagulant Medications |
| | Table 4-11. Thrombolytic Medications |
| 3. Vascular Alterations: Hypertension | Table 4-12. Antihypertensive Medications |
| 4. Selected Disorders of Tissue Perfusion | Table 4-13. Oxygen Administration |
| | Table 4-14. Emergency Medications for Shock, Cardiac Arrest, and Anaphylaxis |
| 5. Vascular Disorders | |

# THE CARDIOVASCULAR SYSTEM OVERVIEW

## Perfusion

## Anatomy

A. Circulation—functions

   1. Delivers oxygen, nutrients, hormones, and antibodies to organs, tissues, and cells

   2. Removes end products of metabolism from tissue and cells

B. Heart—functions

   1. Pumps oxygenated blood into arterial system to supply capillaries and tissues

   2. Pumps oxygen-poor blood from the venous system through the lungs to be reoxygenated

C. Blood vessels (arteries, capillaries, veins)—function is to carry blood to and from the body's tissues and cells

D. Structure of the heart—cone-shaped, hollow, muscular organ located in the mediastinum (space between lungs in the thoracic cavity) (*see* Figure 4-1)

   1. Base directed toward the body's right side

   2. Apex directed toward the left, resting on the diaphragm

   3. Two-sided double pump

     a. Right side receives deoxygenated blood from the body and pumps it to the lungs

     b. Left side receives oxygenated blood from the lungs and pumps it through the aorta to the body

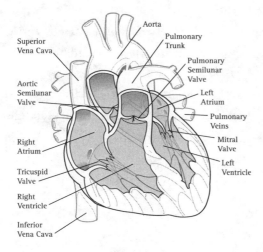

**Figure 4-1.** The Human Heart

4. Pericardium—loose-fitting membrane or fibroserous covering of the heart

5. Cardiac layers

   a. Epicardium—outer layer

   b. Myocardium—middle layer; composed of striated muscle fibers; myocardial fibers stiffen with age

   c. Endocardium—innermost layer; continuous with the blood vessels, lining the heart's cavities and valves

6. Cardiac chambers

   a. Atria (auricles)—two upper "receiving" chambers

      1) Right atrium—receives deoxygenated blood from body via superior and inferior venae cavae and pumps into right ventricle

      2) Left atrium—receives oxygenated blood from lungs and pumps into left ventricle

      3) Interatrial septum separates the atria

      4) Older adults—atrial stretching and distension

   b. Ventricles—two lower "distributing" chambers

      1) Right ventricle—receives blood from right atrium and pumps out to lung via pulmonary artery

      2) Left ventricle (largest, most muscular chamber)—receives oxygenated blood from left atrium and pumps out blood to body

      3) Ventricular septum separates the ventricles

7. Cardiac valves provide for one-way flow of blood

   a. Atrioventricular valves—tricuspid and mitral valves

      1) Tricuspid valve guards opening between right atrium and ventricle (prevents backflow)

      2) Mitral valve guards opening between left atrium and ventricle (prevents backflow)

   b. Semilunar valves—prevent backflow into ventricles

      1) Pulmonary semilunar valve (between pulmonary artery and right ventricle)

      2) Aortic semilunar valve (between aorta and left ventricle)

8. Coronary arteries—disease of these arteries is leading cause of death in the United States (*see* Figure 4-2)

   a. Left coronary arteries—supply the left ventricle, septum, and apex

   b. Right coronary arteries—supply the right ventricle and the sinoatrial (SA) node

   c. Older adults—coronary arteries narrow

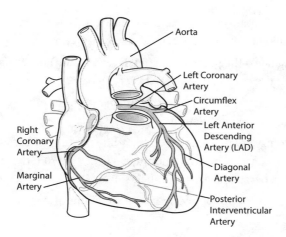

**Figure 4-2.** Coronary Blood Vessels

# Cardiac Function

**A.** Cardiac contraction

   1. Regulation of rate and rhythm—special properties of cardiac muscle

      a. Rhythmicity—rhythm in the formation and conduction of electrical impulses from atria to ventricles

      b. Irritability (excitability)—ability of cardiac muscle cells to respond to stimuli

         1) All or nothing law—irritated muscle responds to stimuli with strongest possible contraction

         2) Adequate oxygen supply, normal neural and hormonal functioning, and balanced diet are essential to maintaining normal function

         3) Medication therapy, infection, lack of oxygen, and disruptions in neural and hormonal balances can increase irritability and result in conduction disturbances

      c. Refractory mechanism—prevents heart muscle from responding to a new stimulus while still in a state of contraction from an earlier stimulus, thereby maintaining rhythm

         1) Absolute refractory period—will not respond to new stimuli of any magnitude

         2) Relative refractory period—muscle begins to be ready for new stimuli; regains irritability

      d. Conductivity—ability of cardiac muscle fibers to transmit electrical impulses

      e. Contractility—shortening of the cardiac muscle fibers in response to a stimulus; occurs rhythmically and is followed by a relaxation period corresponding to the filling and emptying of the cardiac chambers

      f. Automaticity—ability of the heart to beat spontaneously and repetitively without external neurohormonal control; linked to fluid and electrolyte balance rather than to nervous system control

g. Extensibility (expansibility)—ability of heart muscle to expand (stretch) while the chambers fill with blood between muscle contractions

1) Starling law—the greater the stretch (expansion) of cardiac muscle, the more forceful the contraction of the heart

2) Overstretched muscle can result in alterations in filling and decrease forcefulness of contraction

B. Cardiac conduction system—composed of modified cardiac muscle cells able to conduct electrical impulses; controlled by autonomic nervous system (ANS); sympathetic branch increases rate while parasympathetic branch slows rate

1. Sinoatrial node (SA node) or pacemaker—site of impulse initiation 60–100/min (*see* Figure 4-3)

a. Located at junction of superior vena cava and right atrium

b. Regulates heart rate, rhythm, and regularity

c. Other components of conduction pathway have potential to discharge impulses independently; however, the SA node releases impulses more rapidly and therefore assumes control over the process

d. Older adults—decreased number of SA cells; possible decreased heart rate

2. Atrioventricular node (AV node or AV junction)—(*see* Figure 4-3)

a. Located in base of right atrium

b. Receives impulses from SA node and delays them slightly

c. Generates impulses when SA node fails (at a rate of approximately 40–60 beats per minute)

d. Older adults—decreased number of AV node cells

3. Bundle of His (Purkinje system)—continuous with AV node; bundle of His also known as AV bundle

a. Composed of special cardiac muscle fibers that originate in the AV node, then break into left and right bundle branches that extend down the interventricular septum, where they are continuous with Purkinje fibers

b. Relays impulses from AV node to ventricles

c. Purkinje fibers enable electrical impulses responsible for myocardial contraction to spread rapidly over all parts of the ventricles

d. Older adults—decreased number of Purkinje system cells

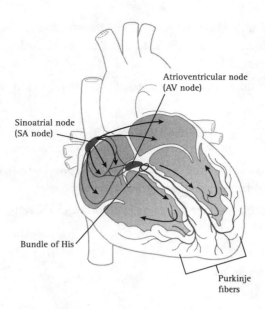

**Figure 4-3.** SA Nodes and AV Nodes

**C.** Cardiac cycle—equivalent to one complete heartbeat

1. Two parts

   a. Systole—contraction of (ejection of blood from) both atria and then both ventricles; initiated by release of impulse by SA node

   b. Diastole—relaxation and filling of both atria and then both ventricles

2. Cardiac output—stroke volume × heart rate

   a. Stroke volume—amount of blood ejected with each beat

   b. Heart rate—number of beats per minute

3. Cardiac output depends upon

   a. Preload

   b. Afterload

   c. Contractility

   d. Age—decreased beta-receptor responsiveness with age; altered autonomic nervous system control

**D.** Cardiac reserve—ability of the heart to adjust to increased demands from stresses such as exercise, excitement, fever, cold, acceleration, deceleration, or disease states; older adults may have significantly decreased cardiac reserve, especially with decreased blood volume, febrile conditions, infections, cardiac dysrhythmias

# Vascular System

**A.** Structure

1. Arteries—originate in the aorta or its branches; transport blood to the systemic circulation

   a. Aorta—assists the flow of blood to the arteries or acts as a reservoir for blood during ejection of the ventricles

    b. Pulmonary artery—originates in the right ventricle and transports deoxygenated blood from the circulation to the lungs to be oxygenated (only artery carrying deoxygenated blood)

  2. Gerontologic considerations—loss of arterial elasticity, blood vessel lumen narrows

  3. Veins

    a. Carry deoxygenated blood and body waste from the systemic circulation to the right atrium by way of the inferior and superior vena cava

    b. Superior vena cava and inferior vena cava—largest veins in the body; bring deoxygenated blood from the upper and lower body to the right atrium

    c. Pulmonary veins—return oxygenated blood from the lungs to the left atrium (only vein carrying oxygenated blood)

  4. Capillaries

    a. Arterioles—smallest arteries

    b. Venules—smallest veins

  5. Layers

    a. Tunica intima—smooth lining of blood vessel

    b. Tunica media—muscle layer

    c. Tunica adventitia—connective tissue binds vessels to adjacent structures

  6. Veins have valves to ensure unidirectional blood flow

**B.** Function (physiology)

  1. Oxygenated blood leaves left ventricle, travels through aorta and arterioles (smaller branches)

  2. Deoxygenated blood returns to the right side of heart by inferior and superior venae cavae

  3. Coronary circulation—circulation to the myocardium

  4. Peripheral circulation—circulation through the periphery (extremities)

    a. Delivers oxygen, nutrients, hormones, and antibodies to organs, tissues, and cells

    b. Removes end products of metabolism from tissues and cells

**C.** Mechanics

  1. Autonomic nervous system—regulates heart rate, influences arteriolar constriction and blood pressure

    a. Neural reflexes are controlled via vasomotor center in the medulla oblongata

    b. Stimulation and inhibition of the circulatory system

      1) Pressoreceptors (baroreceptors)—specialized nerve endings affected by changes in pressure of blood in arteries

      2) Chemoreceptors—located in the aortic arch and carotid bodies; sensitive to lack of oxygen, increased blood $CO_2$, and decreased pH

      3) Medullary ischemic reflex—produces vasoconstriction of small blood vessels in response to stimulation of the vasoconstrictor center by excess $CO_2$ and lack of oxygen

    c. Sympathetic branch ("fight or flight")

       1) Increases blood pressure, heart rate, respiratory rate, blood glucose, and blood flow to the muscles of the legs

       2) Inhibits blood flow to the GI tract

    d. Parasympathetic branch ("rest and relax")

       1) Counterbalances the sympathetic branch to maintain blood pressure, heart rate, and respiratory rate within normal limits

       2) Stimulates blood flow to the GI tract

2. Blood pressure—the pressure exerted by the blood against the walls of vessels

    a. Systolic blood pressure—maximum pressure of blood exerted against the arterial wall when the heart is contracting

    b. Diastolic blood pressure—lowest pressure of blood exerted against the wall of the artery when the heart is at rest

    c. Pulse pressure—difference between systolic and diastolic blood pressure

**D.** Factors affecting cardiovascular performance

1. Cardiac output

    a. Preload—ventricular end-diastolic pressure (VEDP)

       1) Venous return—increased return increases VEDP

       2) End-systolic volume—increased volume increases VEDP

       3) Frank-Starling law of the heart—within a physiologic range of muscle contraction, increased preload will increase cardiac output; excessive preload will decrease cardiac output

    b. Afterload—resistance to ejection of blood from the left ventricle; correlates with aortic systolic pressure; increased afterload increases myocardial oxygen demand

    c. Myocardial contractility—determined by preload, sympathetic nervous stimulation, myocardial oxygen supply

    d. Heart rate—tachycardia or bradycardia decreases cardiac output

# ALTERATIONS IN CARDIAC OUTPUT

## Perfusion, Fluid And Electrolyte Balance

## Cardiopulmonary Arrest

**A.** Assessment—breathless, pulseless, unconscious

**B.** Analysis

1. Failure to institute ventilation within 4–6 minutes will result in cerebral anoxia and brain damage

2. Purpose of cardiopulmonary resuscitation (CPR)—to re-establish $CO_2/O_2$ exchange and adequate circulation so oxygenated blood can be delivered to vital organs

**C.** Plan/implementation

1. Basic life support (BLS)

    a. Recognition

        1) All ages—unresponsive

        2) Adults—no breathing or no normal breathing (e.g., only gasping)

        3) Children and infants—no breathing or only gasping

        4) No pulse palpated within 10 seconds

    b. Activate emergency medical service (EMS) system

    c. CPR sequence: C-A-B

    d. Compression rate—100–120/minute for all populations

    e. Compression depth

        1) Adults—at least 2 inches (5 cm)

        2) Children—at least one-third anterior posterior diameter or about 2 inches (5 cm)

        3) Infants—at least one-third anterior posterior diameter or about 1.5 inches (4 cm)

    f. Chest wall recoil

        1) Allow complete recoil between compressions

        2) HCPs rotate compressors every 2 minutes or sooner if fatigued

    g. Compression interruptions

        1) Minimize interruptions in chest compressions

        2) Attempt to limit interruptions to less than 10 seconds

    h.  Airway

        1)  Head tilt–chin lift

        2)  HCP suspected trauma; jaw thrust

    i.  Compression-to-ventilation ratio (until advance airway placed)

        1)  Adult: 30:2; 1 or 2 rescuers

        2)  Children and infants: 30:2 single rescuer; 15:2 for 2 HCP rescuers

    j.  Ventilations when rescuer untrained or trained and not proficient—compressions only

    k.  Ventilations with advanced airway (HCP)

        1)  1 breath every 6 seconds (10 breaths/minute)

        2)  Avoid excessive ventilation; can cause gastric inflation and subsequent regurgitation and aspiration, increased intrathoracic pressure, decreased venous return to the heart, diminished cardiac output, and reduced blood flow to the brain secondary to cerebral vasoconstriction

        3)  Asynchronous with chest compressions

        4)  Visible chest rise

    l.  Defibrillation

        1)  Attach and use automated external defibrillator (AED) as soon as possible for ventricular fibrillation and pulseless ventricular tachycardia

        2)  Shock energy for defibrillation—initial dose of 120–200 J when using biphasic device; 360 J when using monophasic device

        3)  Resume CPR beginning with compressions immediately after each shock

    m. Continue CPR until one of the following occurs

        1)  Victim responds

        2)  Another qualified person takes over

        3)  Victim is transferred to an emergency department

        4)  Rescuer is physically unable to continue

2.  Advanced cardiac life support (ACLS)

    a.  Medications

        1)  Asystole or pulseless electrical activity (PEA)—epinephrine 1 mg IV or intraosseous (IO) every 3 to 5 minutes

        2)  Ventricular fibrillation or pulseless ventricular tachycardia that is unresponsive to defibrillation; amiodarone 300 mg bolus IV or IO as first dose, 150 mg bolus IV or IO as second dose if indicated, or lidocaine 1–1.5 mg/kg IV or IO as first dose, 0.5–0.75 mg/kg IV or IO as second dose if indicated

    b.  Reversible causes

        1)  Hypovolemia

        2)  Hypoxia

        3)  Hydrogen ion (acidosis)

4) Hypo-/hyperkalemia

5) Hypothermia

6) Tension pneumothorax

7) Tamponade, cardiac

8) Toxins

9) Thrombosis, pulmonary

10) Thrombosis, cardiac

# Disturbances in Cardiac Output

A. Heart disease (see Table 4-1)

**Table 4-1** Cardiac Disorders Classified by Physiological Disturbance

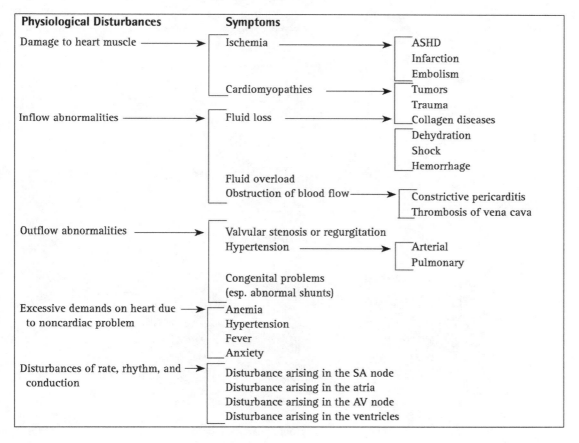

| Physiological Disturbances | Symptoms | |
|---|---|---|
| Damage to heart muscle | Ischemia | ASHD<br>Infarction<br>Embolism |
| | Cardiomyopathies | Tumors<br>Trauma |
| Inflow abnormalities | Fluid loss | Collagen diseases<br>Dehydration<br>Shock<br>Hemorrhage |
| | Fluid overload | |
| | Obstruction of blood flow | Constrictive pericarditis<br>Thrombosis of vena cava |
| Outflow abnormalities | Valvular stenosis or regurgitation | |
| | Hypertension | Arterial<br>Pulmonary |
| | Congenital problems<br>(esp. abnormal shunts) | |
| Excessive demands on heart due to noncardiac problem | Anemia<br>Hypertension<br>Fever<br>Anxiety | |
| Disturbances of rate, rhythm, and conduction | Disturbance arising in the SA node<br>Disturbance arising in the atria<br>Disturbance arising in the AV node<br>Disturbance arising in the ventricles | |

**B.** EKG interpretation (*see* Figures 4-4, 4-5, and 4-6)

1. Determine rate

   a. Count the number of 0.2-s intervals between two R waves, divide by 300

   b. Count the number of R-R intervals in 6 seconds, multiply by 10 (only for regular rhythm)

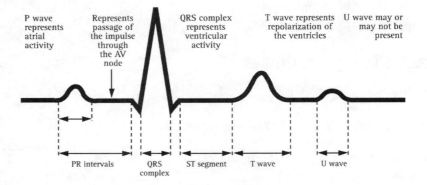

**Figure 4-4.** Components of an EKG

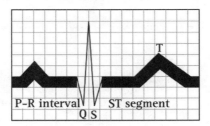

**Figure 4-5.** Components of an EKG

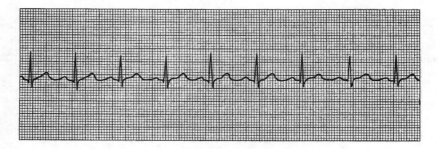

**Figure 4-6.** Rules for Normal Sinus Rhythm

| | |
|---|---|
| Regularity: | The R-R intervals are constant; the rhythm is regular. |
| Rate: | The atrial and ventricular rates are equal; heart rate is between 60 and 100 beats per minute. |
| P wave: | The P waves are uniform. There is one P wave in front of every QRS complex. |
| PRI: | The PR interval (PRI) measures between 0.12 and 0.20 s. |
| QRS: | The QRS complex measures less than 0.12 s. |

2. Determine rhythm

   a. Presence or absence of P wave—SA node originated impulse

   b. Measure P-R interval—normal: 0.12–0.20 s

   c. Measure QRS duration—normal:  less than 0.12 s

   d. Check P wave, QRS complex, ST segment, and T wave

# Rhythm Disturbances (Dysrhythmias)

(*see* Figures 4-7 through 4-18)

**A.** Assessment

   1. Dizziness, syncope

   2. Chest pain, palpitations

   3. Nausea, vomiting

   4. Dyspnea

   5. Abnormal rate—increased, decreased, or irregular

   6. Abnormal heart sounds

**B.** Analysis

   1. Caused by interruption in normal conduction process

   2. Can occur at any point in the normal conduction pathway

   3. Are accompanied by alterations in myocardial tissues, automaticity, regularity, and excitability—these changes can result in hemodynamic alterations affecting the force of contraction and overall cardiac output

   4. Types of dysrhythmias

      a. Sinus dysrhythmias—dysrhythmias originate in the SA node and are conducted along the normal conductive pathways

         1) Tachycardia—sympathetic nervous system increases the automaticity of the SA node

            a) Heart rate is increased above 100 beats per minute

            b) Causes include pain, exercise, hypoxia, pulmonary embolism, hemorrhage, hyperthyroidism, or fever

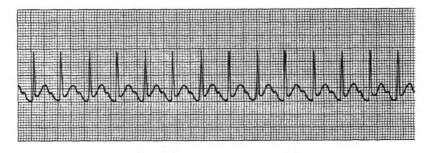

**Figure 4-7.** Rules for Sinus Tachycardia

| | |
|---|---|
| Regularity: | The R-R intervals are constant; the rhythm is regular. |
| Rate: | The atrial and ventricular rates are equal; heart rate is greater than 100 beats per minute (usually between 100 and 160 beats per minute). |
| P wave: | There is a uniform P wave in front of every QRS complex. |
| PRI: | The PR interval measures between 0.12 and 0.20 s; the PRI measurement is constant across the strip. |
| QRS: | The QRS complex measures less than 0.12 s. |

2)  Bradycardia—parasympathetic nervous system (vagal stimulation) causes automaticity of the SA node to be depressed

   a)  Heart rate decreased to below 60 beats per minute

   b)  Causes—myocardial infarction (MI), the Valsalva maneuver, or vomiting; arteriosclerosis in the carotid sinus area; ischemia of SA node; hypothermia; hyperkalemia; depression or medications such as digitalis and propranolol

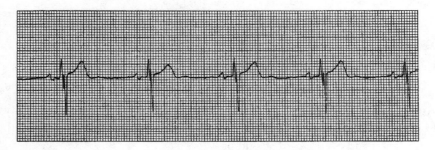

**Figure 4-8.** Rules for Sinus Bradycardia

| | |
|---|---|
| Regularity: | The R-R intervals are constant; the rhythm is regular. |
| Rate: | The atrial and ventricular rates are equal; heart rate is less than 60 beats per minute. |
| P wave: | There is a uniform P wave in front of every QRS complex. |
| PRI: | The PR interval measures between 0.12 and 0.20 s; the PRI measurement is constant across the strip. |
| QRS: | The QRS complex measures less than 0.12 s. |

b.  Atrial dysrhythmias—abnormal electrical activity that results in stimulation outside the SA node but within the atria

   1)  Premature atrial contractions (PAC)

      a)  Ectopic focus within one of the atria when it fires prematurely

      b)  Normal phenomenon in some individuals but may be caused by emotional disturbances, fatigue, tobacco, or caffeine

      c)  May be early sign of abnormal electrical activity associated with organic heart disease

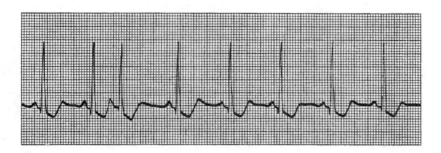

**Figure 4-9.** Rules for Premature Atrial Contractions

| | |
|---|---|
| Regularity: | Because this is a single premature ectopic beat, it will interrupt the regularity of the underlying rhythm. |
| Rate: | The overall heart rate will depend on the rate of the underlying rhythm. |
| P wave: | The P wave of the premature beat will have a different morphology than the P waves of the rest of the strip. The ectopic beat will have a P wave, but it can be flattened, notched, or otherwise unusual. It may be hidden within the T wave of the preceding complex. |
| PRI: | The PRI should measure between 0.12 and 0.20 s but can be prolonged; the PRI of the ectopic beat will probably be different from the PRI measurements of the other complexes. |
| QRS: | The QRS complex measurement will be less than 0.12 s. |

2) Paroxysmal atrial tachycardia (PAT)

a) Rapid rhythmic discharge of impulses originating from an ectopic focus within the atria, followed by a normal ventricular response at a rate of 160–250 beats per minute

b) If prolonged, the period of ventricular filling is shortened, stroke volume is reduced, and cardiac output is diminished, possibly resulting in pump failure, hypotension, and additional dysrhythmias

c) Causes—atrial muscle ischemia, rheumatic heart disease, acute myocardial infarction, psychological factors (e.g., anxiety, stress, emotional trauma), decrease in potassium (leads to cardiac irritability), smoking, caffeine, ingestion of large meals

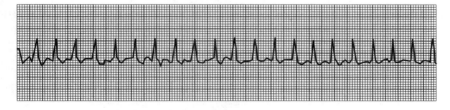

**Figure 4-10.** Rules for Atrial Tachycardia

Regularity: The R-R intervals are constant; the rhythm is regular.

Rate: The atrial and ventricular rates are equal; the heart rate is usually 150–250 beats per minute.

P wave: There is one P wave in front of every QRS complex. The configuration of the P wave will be different from that of sinus P waves; they may be flattened or notched. Because of the rapid rate, the P waves can be hidden in the T waves of the preceding beats.

PRI: The PRI is between 0.12 and 0.20 s and constant across the strip. The PRI may be difficult to measure if the P wave is obscured by the T wave.

QRS: The QRS complex measures less than 0.12 s.

3) Atrial flutter

    a) Arises from an ectopic focus in the atrial wall causing the atrium to contract 250–400 times per minute

    b) AV node blocks most of the impulse, thereby protecting the ventricles from receiving every impulse

    c) Some clients are unaware of this dysrhythmia, whereas others report palpitations or fainting

    d) Causes—stress, hypoxia, medications, or disorders such as chronic heart disease, hypertension

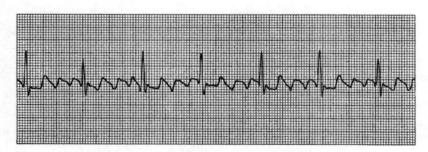

**Figure 4-11.** Rules for Atrial Flutter

Regularity: The atrial rhythm is regular. The ventricular rhythm will be regular if the AV node conducts impulses in a consistent pattern. If the pattern varies, the ventricular rate will be irregular.

Rate: Atrial rate is between 250 and 350 beats per minute. Ventricular rate will depend on the ratio of impulses conducted through to the ventricles.

P wave: When the atria flutter, they produce a series of well-defined P waves. When seen together, these "flutter" waves have a sawtooth appearance.

PRI: Because of the unusual configuration of the P wave (flutter wave) and the proximity of the wave to the QRS complex, it is often impossible to determine a PRI in this dysrhythmia. Therefore, the PRI is not measured in atrial flutter.

QRS: The QRS complex measures less than 0.12 s; measurement can be difficult if one or more flutter waves are concealed within the QRS complex.

4) Atrial fibrillation

a) Most common atrial dysrhythmia arising from several ectopic foci

b) Client presents with a grossly irregular pulse rate

c) Confusion, syncope, and dizziness may occur with severe hypoxia; pump failure may result

d) Causes include chronic lung disease, heart failure, rheumatic heart disease, and hypertension

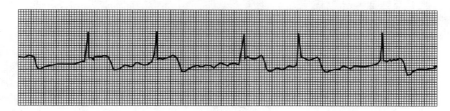

**Figure 4-12.** Rules for Fibrillation

Regularity: The atrial rhythm is unmeasurable; all atrial activity is chaotic. The ventricular rhythm is grossly irregular, having no pattern to its irregularity.

Rate: The atrial rate cannot be measured because it is so chaotic; research indicates that it exceeds 350 beats per minute. The ventricular rate is significantly slower because the AV node blocks most of the impulses. If the ventricular rate is below 100 beats per minute, the rhythm is said to be "controlled"; if it is over 100 beats per minute, it is considered to have a "rapid ventricular response."

P wave: In this dysrhythmia, the atria are not depolarizing in an effective way; instead, they are fibrillating. Thus, no P wave is produced. All atrial activity is depicted as "fibrillatory" waves, or grossly chaotic undulations of the baseline.

PRI: Because no P waves are visible, no PRI can be measured.

QRS: The QRS complex measurement should be less than 0.12 s.

c. Ventricular dysrhythmias—occur when one or more ectopic foci arise within the ventricles

1) Premature ventricular contractions (PVC)

a) One or more ectopic foci stimulate a premature ventricular response

b) May decrease the efficiency of the heart's pumping action

c) Palpitations, a feeling of irregular heartbeat, or a "lump in the throat"

d)   Causes—ischemia due to a myocardial infarction, infection, mechanical damage due to pump failure, deviations in concentrations of electrolytes (e.g., potassium, calcium), nicotine, coffee, tea, alcohol, medications such as digitalis and reserpine, psychogenic factors (stress, anxiety, fatigue), and acute or chronic lung disease

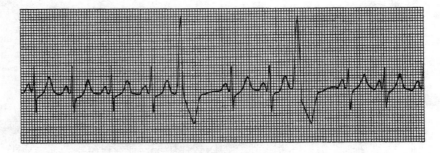

**Figure 4-13.** Rules for Premature Ventricular Contractions

Regularity:   The underlying rhythm can be regular or irregular. The ectopic PVC will interrupt the regularity of the underlying rhythm (unless the PVC is interpolated).

Rate:   The rate will be determined by the underlying rhythm. PVCs are not usually included in the rate determination because they frequently do not produce a pulse.

P wave:   The ectopic PVC is not preceded by a P wave. You may see a coincidental P wave near the PVC, but it is dissociated.

PRI:   Because the ectopic PVC comes from a lower focus, there will be no PRI.

QRS:   The QRS complex will be wide and bizarre, measuring at least 0.12 s. The configuration will differ from the configuration of the underlying QRS complexes. The T wave is frequently in the opposite direction from the QRS complex.

2)   Ventricular tachycardia (VT)

a)   Three or more PVCs occurring in a row

b)   Indicative of severe myocardial irritability

c)   Physical effects include chest pain, dizziness, fainting, occasional collapse

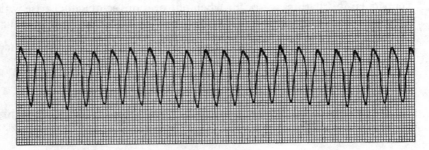

**Figure 4-14.** Rules for Ventricular Tachycardia

| | |
|---|---|
| Regularity: | This rhythm is usually regular, although it can be slightly irregular. |
| Rate: | Atrial rate cannot be determined. The ventricular rate range is 150–250 beats per minute. If the rate is below 150 beats per minute, it is considered a slow VT. If the rate exceeds 250 beats per minute, it's called ventricular flutter. |
| P wave: | None of the QRS complexes will be preceded by P waves. You may see dissociated P waves intermittently across the strip. |
| PRI: | Because the rhythm originates in the ventricles, there will be no PRI. |
| QRS: | The QRS complexes will be wide and bizarre, measuring at least 0.12 s. It is often difficult to differentiate between the QRS and the T wave. |

3) Ventricular fibrillation

    a) Most serious of all dysrhythmias due to potential cardiac standstill; death will occur if not treated

    b) Several ectopic foci within the ventricles are discharged at a very rapid rate

    c) Causes—acute myocardial infarction, hypertension, rheumatic or arteriosclerotic heart disturbances, hypoxia, accidental electrical shock, and hyperkalemia

    d) Unless blood flow is restored by CPR and the dysrhythmia is interrupted (by defibrillation), death will result within 90 s to 5 min

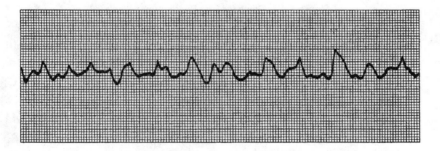

**Figure 4-15.** Rules for Ventricular Fibrillation

| | |
|---|---|
| Regularity: | There are no waves or complexes that can be analyzed to determine regularity. The baseline is totally chaotic. |
| Rate: | The rate cannot be determined because there are no discernible waves or complexes to measure. |
| P wave: | There are no discernible P waves. |
| PRI: | There is no PRI. |
| QRS: | There are no discernible QRS complexes. No cardiac output. Clinical death. |

d. Heart block—delay in the conduction of impulses within the AV system

    1) Bundle branch block (see Figure 4-16)

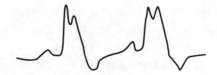

**Figure 4-16.** Bundle Branch Block

a) Right or left branches of the bundle of His are blocked, causing the impulses to change their path of conduction or pass through the myocardial tissue

b) Cause—myocardial ischemia or digitalis toxicity

c) Left bundle branch tends to be more serious and may indicate left-sided heart problems

2) First-degree AV block—AV junction conducts all impulses, but duration of AV conduction is prolonged (see Figure 4.17)

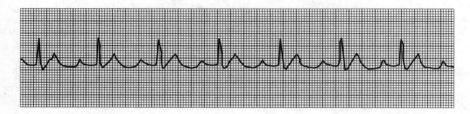

**Figure 4-17.** Rules for First-Degree Heart Block

| | |
|---|---|
| Regularity: | This will depend on the regularity of the underlying rhythm. |
| Rate: | The rate will depend on the rate of the underlying rhythm. |
| P wave: | The P waves will be upright and uniform. Each P wave will be followed by a QRS complex. |
| PRI: | The PRI will be constant across the entire strip, but it will always be greater than 0.20 seconds. |
| QRS: | The QRS complex measurement will be less than 0.12 s. |

3) Second-degree AV block—type I and type II; AV junction conducts only some impulses arising in the atria (see Figures 4-18 and 4-19)

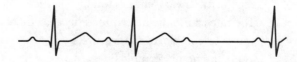

**Figure 4-18.** Second-Degree Heart Block, Type I (Mobitz I, Wenckebach)

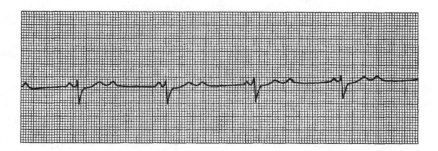

**Figure 4-19.** Second-Degree Heart Block, Type II (Mobitz II)

    a)    Causes—infections, digitalis toxicity, coronary artery disease

    b)    Symptoms—slow heart rate, fainting, decreased blood pressure

| | |
|---|---|
| Regularity: | If the conduction ratio is consistent, the R-R interval will be constant and the rhythm will be regular. If the conduction ratio varies, the R-R will be irregular. |
| Rate: | The atrial rate is usually normal. Because many of the atrial impulses are blocked, the ventricular rate will usually be in the bradycardia range, often one-half, one-third, or one-fourth of the atrial rate. |
| P wave: | P waves are upright and uniform. There are always more P waves than QRS complexes. |
| PRI: | The PRI on conducted beats will be constant across the strip, although it might be longer than a normal PRI measurement. |
| QRS: | The QRS complex measurement will be less than 0.12 s. |

    4)    Third-degree (complete) heart block (see Figure 4-20)

        a)    AV junction blocks all impulses to the ventricles, causing the atria and ventricles to dissociate and beat independently (each with its own pacemaker establishing a rate; ventricular rate is low, 20–40 beats per minute)

        b)    Causes—congenital defects, vascular insufficiency, fibrosis of the myocardial tissue, or myocardial infarction

        c)    Symptoms—palpitations, dizziness, syncope, dyspnea, mental confusion, and cyanosis

        d)    If not treated immediately, may lead to death

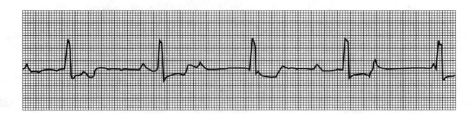

**Figure 4-20.** Rules for Third-Degree Heart Block

Regularity:      Both the atrial and the ventricular foci are firing regularly; thus the P-P intervals and the R-R intervals are regular.

Rate:      The atrial rate will usually be in a normal range. The ventricular rate will be slower. If a junctional focus is controlling the ventricles, the rate will be 40–60 beats per minute. If the focus is ventricular, the rate will be 20–40 beats per minute.

P wave:      The P waves are upright and uniform. There are more P waves than QRS complexes.

PRI:      Because the block at the AV node is complete, none of the atrial impulses is conducted through to the ventricles. There is no PRI. The P waves have no relationship to the QRS complexes. You may occasionally see a P wave superimposed on the QRS complex.

QRS:      If the ventricles are being controlled by a junctional focus, the QRS complex will measure less than 0.12 s. If the focus is ventricular, the QRS will measure 0.12 s or greater.

**C.** Plan/implementation

   1. Vital signs

   2. Cardiac monitor—identify any changes in rhythm and rate

   3. Medications

      a. Antidysrhythmic (*see* Table 4-2)

**Table 4-2** Antidysrhythmic Medication

| MEDICATION | ADVERSE EFFECTS | NURSING CONSIDERATIONS |
|---|---|---|
| **Class IA** | | |
| Quinidine | Hypotension | Monitor blood pressure |
| Procainamide | Heart failure | Monitor for widening of the PR, QRS, or QT intervals |
| Disopyramide | | Toxic effects, has limited use |
| **Class IB** | | |
| Lidocaine | CNS: slurred speech, confusion, drowsiness, confusion, seizures | Monitor for CNS adverse effects |
| | Hypotension and bradycardia | Monitor BP and heart rate and cardiac rhythm |
| **Class IC** | | |
| Flecainide | Bradycardia | Monitor for increasing dysrhythmias |
| Propafenone hydrochloride | Hypotension | Monitor heart rate and blood pressure |
| | Dysrhythmias | Monitor for CNS effects |
| | CNS: anxiety, insomnia, confusion, seizures | |

(Continued)

**Table 4-2** Antidysrhythmic Medication (*Continued*)

| MEDICATION | ADVERSE EFFECTS | NURSING CONSIDERATIONS |
|---|---|---|
| **Class II** | | |
| Beta-blockers:<br><br>Propranolol<br><br>Acebutolol<br><br>Esmolol hydrochloride | Bradycardia and hypotension<br><br>Bronchospasm<br><br>Increase in heart failure<br><br>Fatigue and sleep disturbances | Monitor apical heart rate, cardiac rhythm, and blood pressure<br><br>Assess for shortness of breath and wheezing<br><br>Assess for fatigue, sleep disturbances<br><br>Assess apical heart rate for 1 minute before administration |
| **Class III** | | |
| Amiodarone hydrochloride<br>Ibutilide fumarate | Hypotension<br><br>Bradycardia and atrioventricular block<br><br>Muscle weakness, tremors<br><br>Photosensitivity and photophobia<br><br>Liver toxicity | Continuous monitoring of cardiac rhythm during IV administration<br><br>Monitor QT interval during IV administration<br><br>Monitor heart rate, blood pressure during initiation of therapy<br><br>Instruct client to wear sunglasses and sunscreen |
| **Class IV** | | |
| Calcium channel blockers:<br><br>Verapamil<br><br>Diltiazem hydrochloride | Bradycardia<br><br>Hypotension<br><br>Dizziness and orthostatic hypotension<br><br>Heart failure | Monitor apical heart rate and blood pressure<br><br>Instruct clients about orthostatic precautions<br><br>Instruct clients to report signs of heart failure to health care provider |

4. Provide or assist with emergency treatment

   a. Precordial shock—electric current delivered to the heart through either externally placed paddles (closed chest procedure) or paddles applied directly to myocardium during surgery (open chest procedure); used to halt life-threatening and dangerous dysrhythmias

      1) Defibrillation—paddles placed over right sternal border and over the apex of the heart (*see* Table 4-3)

**Table 4-3** Defibrillation Versus Cardioversion

|  | DEFIBRILLATION | CARDIOVERSION |
|---|---|---|
| Indication | Emergency treatment of ventricular fibrillation | Elective procedure for dysrhythmias such as atrial fibrillation |
| Action | Completely depolarizes all myocardial cells so SA node can re-establish as pacemaker | Same |
| Nursing considerations | Start CPR before defibrillation | Informed consent |
|  | Plug in defibrillator and turn on | Diazepam or midazolam IV |
|  | Turn on monitor and attach leads to client | Digoxin withheld for 48 hours prior to procedure |
|  | Apply gel or paste to paddles (rub paddle surfaces together) | Synchronizer turned on, check at the R wave |
|  | Select electric charge as ordered | Oxygen discontinued |
|  | Paddles placed over right sternal border and over the apex of the heart | Assess airway patency |
|  | Person with paddles calls "all clear" and ensures no one in contact with client | Plug in defibrillator and turn on |
|  | Push discharge button | Turn on monitor and attach leads to client |
|  | Check monitor between shocks for rhythm | Apply gel or paste (rub paddle surfaces together) |
|  | Don't stop to check pulse after shocks, continue CPR, intubate, start IV | Voltage 25–360 joules |
|  | Epinephrine given 1 mg IV push every 3–5 min | Paddles placed over right sternal border and over the apex of the heart |
|  | Sodium bicarbonate given to treat acidosis | Person with paddles calls "all clear" |
|  |  | Push discharge button |
|  |  | Check monitor between shocks for rhythm |
|  |  | After procedure, assess vital signs every 15 min for 1 h, every 30 min for 2 h, then every 4 h |

a) Used in treatment of ventricular fibrillation

b) Completely depolarizes all myocardial cells so SA node can be pacemaker

c) Nursing responsibilities

   i) Start CPR before defibrillation

   ii) Plug in defibrillator and turn on

   iii) Turn on monitor and attach leads to client

   iv) Be sure synchronizer switch is turned off

   v) Apply gel or paste to paddles (rub paddle surfaces together)

   vi) Select electric charge as ordered—360 joules

   vii) Position paddles on chest wall; one to right of sternum just below clavicle, the other to the left of the precordium

   viii) Person with paddles calls "all clear" and checks to ensure no one in contact with client

   ix) Push discharge button

   x) Check carotid pulse

   xi) Sodium bicarbonate given to treat acidosis

2) Cardioversion (*see* Table 4-3)

a) Elective procedure for dysrhythmias such as atrial fibrillation

b) Nursing responsibilities

   i) Informed consent

   ii) Diazepam or midazolam IV

   iii) Voltage 25–360 watts/s

   iv) Digoxin withheld for 48 hours prior to procedure

   v) Synchronizer turned on, check at the R wave

   vi) Oxygen discontinued

   vii) Assess airway patency

   viii) Assess vital signs every 15 min for 1 h, every 30 min for 2 h, then every 4 h

c) Implantable cardioverter-defibrillator available for clients at risk for sudden cardiac death

3) Pacemakers—electronic apparatus used to initiate heartbeat when the SA node is seriously damaged and unable to act as a pacemaker

a) Types of pacemakers (*see* Table 4-4)

**Table 4-4** Pacemakers

| TYPES | ACTION | COMPLICATIONS | NURSING CONSIDERATIONS |
|---|---|---|---|
| Demand (synchronous; noncompetitive) | Functions when heart rate goes below set rate | Dislodgment and migration of endocardial leads | Assess for infection, bleeding |
| Fixed rate (asynchronous; competitive) | Stimulates ventricle at preset constant rate | Wire breakage | Monitor heart rate and rhythm; for preset rate pacemakers, client's rate may vary 5 beats above or below set rate |
| | | Cracking of insulation surrounding wires | |
| Temporary | Used in emergency situations (after MI with heart block, cardiac arrest with bradycardia) Inserted through peripheral vein, tip of catheter is placed at apex of right ventricle | Infection of sites surrounding either pacing wires or pulse generator Interference with pacemaker function by exposure to electromagnetic fields (old microwave ovens, MRI equipment, metal detectors at airports) | Provide emotional support |
| | | | Check pulse daily, report any sudden increase or decrease in rate |
| | | | Carry ID card or wear identification |
| | | | Request hand scanning at security checkpoints at airports |
| Permanent | Lead is passed into right ventricle, or right atrium and right ventricle, and generator is implanted under skin below clavicle or in abdominal wall | | Avoid situations involving electromagnetic fields |
| | | Perforation of myocardium or right ventricle | Periodically check generator |
| | | Abrupt loss of pacing | Take frequent rest periods at home and at work |
| | | | Wear loose clothing over area of pacemaker |
| | | | All electrical equipment used in vicinity of client should be properly grounded |
| | | | Immobilize extremity if temporary electrode pacemaker is used to prevent dislodgment |
| | | | Document model of pacemaker, date and time of insertion, location of pulse generator, stimulation threshold, pacer rate |
| | | | Place cellular phone on side opposite the generator |

        i)     Internal or implantable—stimulating electrodes placed inside the chest wall

        ii)    External—stimulating electrodes placed outside the chest wall

        iii)  Temporary—usually external

        iv)  Permanent—electrode wire inserted percutaneously and threaded through to the ventricle; battery pack is implanted under skin

    b)   Major methods of cardiac pacing

        i)     Rate responsiveness pacemaker—allows faster pacing rates to meet increased bodily demands

        ii)    Demand pacemakers—fire on demand or when necessary to stimulate ventricular contraction; advantageous for clients who are frequently in normal sinus rhythm but suffer periods of bradycardia or syncope

    c)   Technical problems associated with cardiac pacing

        i)     Dislodgment and migration of endocardial leads

        ii)    Wire breakage

        iii)  Cracking of insulation surrounding wires

        iv)  Infection of sites surrounding either pacing wires or pulse generator

        v)    Battery exhaustion

    d)   Nursing responsibilities

        i)     Assess for infection

        ii)    Monitor heart rate and rhythm

        iii)  Provide emotional support

        iv)  Teaching

- Check pulse daily, report any sudden increase or decrease
- Carry ID card
- Request hand scanning at security checkpoints at airports
- Periodic checking of generator
- Take frequent rest periods at home and at work
- Avoid the use of electrocautery devices, ungrounded power tools, large electrical devices

**D.**  Evaluation—client is free from dysrhythmias as evidenced by regular and stable vital signs

# Heart Failure (HF)

Clinical syndrome resulting from structural or functional cardiac disorders that impair the ability of a ventricle to fill or eject blood

**A.**  Assessment—symptoms result from a decrease in cardiac output and involve congestion of either the pulmonary circulatory system, the venous system, or both; almost all manifestations of HF affect tissues and organs that are located away from the heart (e.g., lungs, kidney, brain, liver, and extremities)

1. Left-sided heart failure—develops as a result of left ventricular dysfunction, which causes blood to back up through the left atrium and into the pulmonary veins

   a. Dyspnea—results from pulmonary congestion due to pulmonary engorgement; poor gas exchange because of fluid in the alveoli, resulting in shortness of breath and air hunger

   b. Orthopnea—shortness of breath occurring when the client is in a recumbent position

   c. Paroxysmal nocturnal dyspnea—occurs when client is asleep

   d. Cheyne-Stokes respirations—exact cause in HF unknown; believed they occur as a result of prolonged circulation time between the pulmonary circulation and the central nervous system, which in turn affects the respiratory center

   e. Pleural effusion and pulmonary edema—results from severe pulmonary congestion, causing distended capillaries, which leak fluid into the interstitial and alveolar spaces of the lungs

   f. Cough and cardiac asthma—cough productive of large amounts of frothy, blood-tinged sputum results from edema fluid trapped within the pulmonary tree, irritating the delicate mucosa of the lungs

   g. Decreased renal function, edema, and weight gain—kidney function is adversely affected by the development of HF, resulting in sodium and water retention; sequence of events leading to edema is as follows:

      1) Decreased cardiac output results in decreased arterial pressure in the kidneys, reducing glomerular filtration and output of sodium chloride and water

      2) Reduced circulating blood volume triggers an increase in aldosterone secretion by the adrenal cortex, thereby increasing the rate of reabsorption of sodium by renal tubules

      3) Increased sodium reabsorption results in increased concentration of extracellular fluid

      4) Increased osmotic pressure causes an increase in the release of antidiuretic hormone (ADH) from the neurosecretory cells of the hypothalamus, resulting in increased tubular reabsorption of water

      5) Final result is edema

   h. Cerebral anoxia—develops because of the decrease in cardiac output to the brain, which causes irritability, restlessness, and a shortened attention span

   i. Fatigue and muscular weakness—decreased cardiac output diminishes oxygen to tissues and decreases the speed with which metabolic wastes are swept up into the circulation for excretion, thereby creating profound exhaustion

   j. $S_3$ gallop

   k. B-type natriuretic peptide levels increased

   l. Microalbuminuria

   m. Older adult—may have atypical manifestations (e.g., falls, delirium, chronic cough, weight loss)

2. Right-sided heart failure—develops from a diseased right ventricle that causes backward flow to right atrium and venous circulation; almost always follows left-sided failure due to the stress placed on the right ventricle as it attempts to pump blood against resistance into the congested lungs; venous congestion causes peripheral edema and congestion of organs

   a. Liver enlargement and abdominal pain—as the liver becomes congested with venous blood, it enlarges; stretching of the capsule surrounding the liver causes severe discomfort in the right upper quadrant

   b. Anorexia, nausea, and bloating—secondary to venous congestion of the gastrointestinal tract (anorexia and nausea may also result from digitalis toxicity, a common problem because digitalis is a major medication in treating heart failure)

   c. Dependent edema—early signs of right-sided heart failure include edema of ankles and lower extremities, resulting from venous congestion of kidneys producing compensatory vasoconstriction that decreases renal blood flow, impairing sodium excretion

   d. Coolness of extremities—venous congestion throughout the body reduces peripheral blood flow, often causing coolness of extremities and cyanosis of nail beds

   e. Anxiety and fear—most individuals with heart failure feel anxious and depressed about their condition

   f. Weight gain

3. Advanced heart failure

   a. Weight loss and cachexia—low cardiac output and venous congestion create malnutrition of tissues, although client may appear puffy and bloated due to edema

   b. Shock syndrome—typical clinical picture of shock usually appears during terminal stages of HF

      1) Stupor

      2) Pallor

      3) Rapid, thready pulse

      4) Cold sweats

      5) Restlessness

      6) Profound hypotension

**B.** Etiology

1. Conditions that predispose heart to gradual failure

   a. Inflow of blood to the heart is reduced due to hemorrhage or dehydration

   b. Inflow of blood to the heart is increased due to excessive IV fluids or sodium and water retention

   c. Outflow of blood from the heart is obstructed due to damaged valves and narrowed arteries

   d. The heart muscle is damaged from ischemia or inflammatory processes

   e. The metabolic needs of the body are increased as a result of fever or pregnancy

2. Diseases that lead to heart failure (*see* Table 4-5)

**Table 4-5** Causes of Heart Failure

| DISEASE | PATHOLOGY | RESULTS |
|---|---|---|
| Hypertensive disease | Vessels become narrowed; peripheral resistance increases | Cardiac muscle enlarges beyond its oxygen supply |
| Arteriosclerosis | Degenerative changes in arterial walls cause permanent narrowing of coronary arteries | Cardiac muscle enlarges beyond its oxygen supply |
| Valvular heart disease | Stenosed valves do not open freely; scarring and retraction of valve leaflets result in incomplete closure | Workload increases until heart fails |
| Rheumatic heart disease | Infection causes damage to heart valves, making them incompetent or narrowed | Incompetent valves cause blood to regurgitate backward; workload increases until heart fails |
| Ischemic heart disease | Coronary arteries are sclerosed or thrombosed | Blood supply is insufficient to nourish heart |
| Constrictive pericarditis | Inflamed pericardial sac becomes scarred and constricted, causing obstruction in blood flow | Fibrotic, thickened, and adherent pericardium encases heart, impairing ability of atria and ventricles to stretch during diastolic filling |
| Circulatory overload (IV fluid overload; sodium retention; renal shutdown) | Excessive fluid in circulatory system | Overwhelms heart's ability to pump |
| Pulmonary disease | Damage to arterioles of lungs causes vascular constriction; this increases workload of heart | Right ventricular enlargement and failure |
| Tachydysrhythmias | Decreases ventricular filling time | Decreased cardiac output |

3. Factors that may precipitate heart failure in individuals with diseased hearts
   a. Pregnancy and childbirth
   b. Severe tachycardia or bradycardia
   c. Great mental strain
   d. Sudden elevation of the environmental temperature and humidity
4. Three major mechanisms to compensate for pathological changes in output
   a. Ventricular dilation—increase in the length of muscle fibers, creating an increase in the volume of the heart chambers

1) According to Starling's law, a stretched muscle contracts more forcefully; therefore, dilation causes an increased systolic output within limits

2) This compensatory mechanism is limited because if stretched beyond a certain point, muscle fibers cease to increase contractile power of the heart and because a greatly dilated heart requires more oxygen to meet its metabolic needs, resulting, in time, in hypoxia of the heart muscle

b. Ventricular hypertrophy—increase in diameter of muscle fibers creating a thickening of the walls of the chambers and a corresponding increase in the weight of the heart

1) Generally follows persistent dilation, further increasing the contractile power of muscle fibers

2) Limited compensatory mechanism because, in time, increased muscle mass of heart outgrows coronary blood supply and becomes hypoxic

c. Tachycardia—least effective compensatory mechanism because when heart rate becomes too rapid, the ventricles are unable to fill adequately, with resultant hypotension and shock

5. Cardiac decompensation occurs when the heart is unable to cope with the work demands placed upon it and thus expends most of its reserve

6. Diagnosing heart failure

a. Presence of characteristic symptoms

b. Muffled heart sounds

c. Abnormal heart sounds ($S_3$)

d. Rales (crackles) at the base of the lungs

e. Hazy lung fields and prominent, distended pulmonary veins on x-ray

f. Elevated venous pressure

g. Distended neck veins

h. Prolonged circulation time

i. Reduction in cardiac output

j. Presence of albuminuria

k. Elevated BUN

l. Gerontologic considerations—may see change in grooming habits, change in personality, dizziness or light-headedness, decreased appetite, gait and balance alterations, malaise, chronic cough, nocturia; manifestations are worse during exacerbation of heart failure

7. Complications of heart failure

a. Complications of immobility

b. Acute pulmonary edema—medical emergency that may result in death if not treated immediately; results from fluid from circulation pouring into the alveoli, bronchi, and bronchioles

c. Refractory or intractable heart failure—occurs when diet, medications, and treatments fail to alleviate symptoms

C. Nursing management

1. Medications

a. Cardiac glycosides (*see* Table 4-6)

1) Digitalis (e.g., digoxin)—prescribed for the treatment of heart failure, especially when associated with low cardiac output

a) Actions

i) Direct beneficial effect on myocardial contraction

ii) Increases force of systolic contraction

iii) Increases completeness of ventricular emptying

iv) Increases heart's capacity for work

b) Two categories of dosages

i) Rapid digitalization—aimed at administering the medication rapidly to achieve a detectable effect

ii) Gradual digitalization—client placed on a dose designed to replace the digitalis lost by excretion while maintaining "optimal" cardiac functioning

c) Digitalized state may be maintained even if a maintenance dose is missed

d) Toxicity—the nurse should be aware of and assess for digitalis toxicity; early symptoms include nausea and vomiting followed by anorexia, diarrhea, abdominal pain, confusion, drowsiness, and visual disturbances

e) Dysrhythmias—excessive slowing of pulse (below 60 beats/min)

f) Factors increasing likelihood of toxicity

i) Problems with renal function causing toxic accumulation of digitalis

ii) Depletion of potassium sensitizes the myocardium to digitalis and enhances its effect

iii) Administration of IV calcium presents a danger of digitalis dysrhythmias because digitalis appears to act on the heart by increasing the amount of calcium in the contractile process

g) If toxicity occurs (greater than 2 nanograms/mL)

i) Discontinue the medication and potassium-wasting diuretics

ii) Monitor serum potassium

iii) Administer antidysrhythmic medication as needed: lidocaine

iv) Atropine or electronic pacing for bradycardia or AV block

v) Severe toxicity: Fab body fragments (Digibind) administered

vi) Cholestyramine and activated charcoal orally to suppress absorption

h) Client teaching

i) Understanding of necessity of digitalis, its action, and its adverse effects

ii) Teach how to check pulse rates to detect changes, therefore minimizing risk of toxicity

iii) Notify nurse or health care provider concerning untoward adverse effects

**Table 4-6** Cardiac Glycoside Medications (Digitalis)

| MEDICATION | ADVERSE EFFECTS | NURSING CONSIDERATIONS |
|---|---|---|
| Digoxin | Anorexia<br><br>Nausea<br><br>Bradycardia<br><br>Visual disturbances<br><br>Confusion<br><br>Abdominal pain<br><br>Tachycardia, brady-cardia, heart block<br><br>Anorexia, nausea, vomiting<br><br>Toxicity: Halos around dark objects, blurred vision, halo vision<br><br>Dysrhythmias, heart block | Administer with caution to older adult clients or clients with renal insufficiency<br><br>Monitor renal function and electrolytes<br><br>Instruct clients to eat high-potassium foods<br><br>Take apical pulse for 1 full minute before administering<br><br>Notify health care provider if apical pulse less than 60 (adult), less than 90–110 (infants and young children), less than 70 (older children)<br><br>Rapid digitalization: 0.5–0.75 mg PO, then 0.125 mg–0.375 mg cautiously until adequate effect is noted<br><br>Gradual digitalization: 0.25–0.5 mg PO, may increase dosage every 2 weeks until desired clinical effect achieved<br><br>Digoxin immune fab (Digibind)—used for treatment of life-threatening toxicity<br><br>Maintenance dose: 0.125–0.5 mg IV or PO (average is 0.25 mg)<br><br>Teach client to check pulse rate and discuss adverse effects<br><br>Low $K^+$ increases risk of digitalis toxicity<br><br>Serum therapeutic blood levels 0.5–2 nanograms/mL<br><br>Toxic blood levels ≥2 nanograms/mL<br><br>Instruct client to eat high-potassium foods<br><br>Monitor for digitalis toxicity<br><br>Risk of digitalis toxicity increases if client is hypokalemic |
| **Action** | Increases force of myocardial contraction and slows heart rate by stimulating the vagus nerve and blocking the AV node | |
| **Indications** | Heart failure, dysrhythmias | |
| **Herbal interactions** | Licorice can potentiate action of digoxin by promoting potassium loss<br><br>Hawthorn may increase effects of digoxin<br><br>Ginseng may falsely elevate digoxin levels<br><br>Ma-huang (ephedra) increases risk of digitalis toxicity | |

b. Diuretics (*see* Table 4-7)

    1) Promote physical and mental rest while observing for complications of bedrest

        a) Reduces heart's workload; reduces preload

        b) Promotes diuresis

        c) Reduces work of respiratory muscles (decreases dyspnea)

        d) Reduces tissues' demands for oxygen (lessens circulatory demands)

        e) Decreases venous return (lessens pulmonary congestion and dyspnea) and preload

        f) Lowers blood pressure (diminishes arterial resistance against which heart must pump) and afterload

        g) Lowers heart rate (prolongs the recovery period of cardiac muscle, thereby resulting in a more efficient cardiac contraction)

        h) Promotes comfort and rest (best if taken early to prevent nocturia)

        i) Reduces anxiety

        j) Instruct client to resume activities slowly

**Table 4-7** Diuretic Medication

| MEDICATION | ADVERSE EFFECTS | NURSING CONSIDERATIONS |
|---|---|---|
| **Thiazide Diuretics** | | |
| Hydrochlorothiazide Chlorothiazide | Hypokalemia | Monitor electrolytes, especially potassium |
| | Hyperglycemia | I and O |
| | Blurred vision | Monitor BUN and creatinine |
| | Loss of Na$^+$ | Don't give at bedtime |
| | Dry mouth | Weigh client daily |
| | Hypotension | Encourage potassium-containing foods |
| Potassium sparing:   Spironolactone | Hyperkalemia | Used with other diuretics |
| | Hyponatremia | Give with meals |
| | Hepatic and renal damage | Avoid salt substitutes containing potassium |
| | Tinnitus | Monitor I and O |
| | Rash | |

*(Continued)*

**Table 4-7**  Diuretic Medication (*Continued*)

| MEDICATION | ADVERSE EFFECTS | NURSING CONSIDERATIONS |
|---|---|---|
| Loop diuretics:<br><br>  Furosemide<br><br>  Ethacrynic acid | Hypotension<br><br>Hypokalemia<br><br>Hyperglycemia<br><br>GI upset<br><br>Weakness | Monitor BP, pulse rate, I and O<br><br>Monitor potassium<br><br>Give IV dose over 1–2 minutes → diuresis in 5–10 min<br><br>After PO dose diuresis in about 30 min<br><br>Weigh client daily<br><br>Don't give at bedtime<br><br>Encourage potassium-containing foods |
| Ethacrynic acid<br><br>Bumetanide | Potassium depletion<br><br>Electrolyte imbalance<br><br>Hypovolemia<br><br>Ototoxicity | Supervise ambulation<br><br>Monitor blood pressure and pulse<br><br>Observe for signs of electrolyte imbalance |
| **Osmotic Diuretic** | | |
| Mannitol | Dry mouth<br><br>Thirst | I and O must be measured<br><br>Monitor vital signs<br><br>Monitor for electrolyte imbalance |
| **Other** | | |
| Chlorthalidone | Dizziness<br><br>Aplastic anemia<br><br>Orthostatic hypotension | Acts like a thiazide diuretic<br><br>Acts in 2–3 h, peak 2–6 h, lasts 2–3 days<br><br>Administer in A.M.<br><br>Monitor output, weight, BP, electrolytes<br><br>Increase $K^+$ in diet<br><br>Monitor glucose levels in diabetic clients<br><br>Change position slowly |
| **Action** | Thiazides—inhibits reabsorption of sodium and chloride in distal renal tubule<br><br>Loop—inhibits reabsorption of sodium and chloride in loop of Henle and distal renal tubules<br><br>Potassium sparing—blocks effect of aldosterone on renal tubules, causing loss of sodium and water and retention of potassium<br><br>Osmotic—pulls fluid from tissues due to hypertonic effect | |

(*Continued*)

**Table 4-7** Diuretic Medication (*Continued*)

| MEDICATION | ADVERSE EFFECTS | NURSING CONSIDERATIONS |
|---|---|---|
| **Indications** | Heart failure | |
| | Hypertension | |
| | Renal diseases | |
| | Diabetes insipidus | |
| | Reduction of osteoporosis in postmenopausal women | |
| **Adverse effects** | Dizziness, vertigo | |
| | Dry mouth | |
| | Orthostatic hypotension | |
| | Leukopenia | |
| | Polyuria, nocturia | |
| | Photosensitivity | |
| | Impotence | |
| | Hypokalemia (except for potassium sparing) | |
| | Hyponatremia | |
| **Nursing considerations** | Take with food or milk | |
| | Take in A.M. | |
| | Monitor weight and electrolytes | |
| | Protect skin from the sun | |
| | Diet high in potassium for loop and thiazide diuretics | |
| | Limit potassium intake for potassium-sparing diuretics | |
| | Used as first-line medications for hypertension | |
| **Herbal interactions** | Licorice can promote potassium loss, causing hypokalemia | |
| | Aloe can decrease serum potassium level, causing hypokalemia | |
| | Ginkgo may increase blood pressure when taken with thiazide diuretics | |

    c. Other medications

        1) Angiotensin-converting enzyme inhibitor (ACE) (decreases afterload)

            a) Captopril, enalapril, lisinopril

        2) Angiotensin receptor blockers (ARBs)—decrease afterload

        3) Beta-adrenergic blocking medications—decrease oxygen demand

            a) Carvedilol

4) Vasodilators—nitrates, milrinone; decrease preload and afterload

5) Administer morphine—sedates and decreases afterload

6) Administer human B-type natriuretic peptides—nesiritide; for acute heart failure

2. Diet

   a. Restricted sodium diet

      1) Normal intake—1.5–2.3 g/day

      2) Light in sodium diet—50% less per serving than the usual sodium level

      3) Reduced sodium diet—25% less sodium per serving than the usual sodium level

      4) Low sodium diet—0.14 g/day

      5) Very low sodium diet—0.035 g/day

      6) Sodium-free diet—less than 0.005 g/day

   b. Low calorie, supplemented with vitamins—promotes weight loss, thereby reducing the workload of the heart

   c. Bland, low residue—avoids discomfort from gastric distension and heartburn

   d. Small, frequent feedings to avoid gastric distension, flatulence, and heartburn

3. Record intake and output

4. Weigh daily

5. Good skin care

6. Oxygen therapy

7. Teaching about disease process and medications

# Myocardial Infarction

Formation of localized necrotic areas within the myocardium, usually following the sudden occlusion of a coronary artery and the abrupt cessation of blood and oxygen to the heart muscle

**A.** Assessment—major symptoms vary, depending on whether pain, shock, or pulmonary edema dominates the clinical picture

1. Chest pain—severe, crushing, prolonged; unrelieved by rest or nitroglycerin; often radiating to one or both arms, the neck, and back; caused by accumulation of unoxidized metabolites within ischemic part of myocardium affecting nerve endings (*see* Figure 4-21)

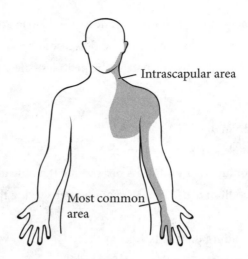

**Figure 4-21.** Common Ischemic Pain Pattern

2. Shock—systolic blood pressure below 80 mm Hg, gray facial color, lethargy, cold diaphoresis, peripheral cyanosis, tachycardia or bradycardia, weak pulse

3. Oliguria—urine output of less than 20 mL/hour as measured by an indwelling urinary catheter, which is indicative of renal hypoxia

4. Low-grade fever—temperature rises to 100–103°F within 24 hours and lasts 3–7 d; accompanied by leukocytosis, elevated sedimentation rate, lactate dehydrogenase (LDH), aspartate aminotransferase (AST), creatine kinase-MB (CK-MB), troponin

    a. Results from destruction of myocardial tissue and accompanying inflammatory process

    b. Fever drops when fibroblasts begin to replace leukocytes and scar tissue starts to form

5. Apprehension—great fear of death;

    a. Severe pain associated with a myocardial infarction can be terrifying

    b. Restlessness results from shock and pain

6. "Indigestion" or "gas pains around the heart," nausea, and vomiting

    a. Client may believe that pain is caused by "indigestion" rather than by heart disease

    b. Nausea and vomiting may result from severe pain or from vasovagal reflexes conducted from the area of damaged myocardium to the gastrointestinal tract

7. Acute pulmonary edema—sense of suffocation, dyspnea, orthopnea, gurgling or bubbling respirations; left ventricle may become severely crippled in pumping action due to infarction, resulting in severe pulmonary congestion accompanied by low cardiac output and shock

8. Dysrhythmias, heart block, asystole

9. Diagnosis

    a. History

    b. EKG changes—ST segment elevation, T wave inversion, Q wave formation

    c. Profound hypotension and shock

d. Lab findings

1) WBC—leukocytosis within 2 d, disappears in 1 wk

2) Erythrocyte sedimentation rate (ESR)—elevated

3) Enzymes

a) Creatinine phosphokinase (CPK), CK-MB isoenzymes—peaks 18–24 h; returns to normal 48–72 h

b) LDH—may remain elevated 5–7 d; peaks 48–72 h; not specific for cardiac damage

c) Myoglobin—begins to rise within 1 h; peaks in 4–6 h; returns to normal in less than 24 h

4) Troponin—peaks in 4–6 hours, remains elevated for up to 2 weeks

**B.** Etiology

1. Predisposing factors—same as for heart failure

2. Causes

a. Complete or near-complete occlusion of a coronary vessel (most common)

b. Decreased blood and oxygen supply to the heart muscle; vasospasm

c. Hypertrophy of the heart muscle from CHF or hypertension

d. Embolism to a coronary artery

3. Selected nursing diagnoses

a. Acute pain

b. Risk for decreased cardiac output

c. Anxiety/fear

d. Deficient knowledge (specify)

**C.** Nursing management

1. Treat acute attack immediately and promptly alleviate symptoms

a. Provide constant supervision, monitoring, expert nursing care

1) Provide thrombolytic therapy—streptokinase or tissue-type plasminogen activator (t-PA) to dissolve thrombus in coronary artery within 6 hours of onset

2) Address client's and family's anxiety

b. Place client in semi-Fowler position—lowers the diaphragm, thereby increasing lung expansion and promoting better ventilation; decreases venous return to the heart, preventing excessive pooling of blood within pulmonary vessels

c. Bedrest to decrease stress on the heart; semi-Fowler position

d. Provide oxygen therapy, if necessary, to help relieve dyspnea, chest pain, shock, cyanosis, and pulmonary edema

e. Monitor vital signs, pain status, lung sounds, level of consciousness, EKG, oxygen saturation

    f.  Monitor I and O

       1)  Intake—fluid intake should be around 2,000 mL daily; too much may precipitate CHF, and too little may precipitate dehydration

       2)  Output—urinary catheter if necessary; oliguria indicates inadequate renal perfusion, and concentrated urine usually indicates dehydration

    g.  Carefully monitor IV infusion—vein should be kept open in case emergency IV medications are necessary

  2.  Administer oxygen

  3.  Medications (*see* Table 4-8)

**Table 4-8** Selected Cardiac Medications

| NAME | ACTION | ADVERSE EFFECTS |
|---|---|---|
| Propranolol | Beta-blocker—blocks sympathetic impulses to heart | Weakness<br>Hypotension<br>Bradycardia<br>Depression<br>Bronchospasm |
| Nifedipine | Calcium channel blocker—reduces workload of left ventricle; coronary vasodilator | Hypotension; dizziness<br>GI distress<br>Liver dysfunction |
| Morphine sulfate | Reduces cardiac workload, preload, and afterload pressures<br>Relieves pain, reduces anxiety | Hypotension<br>Respiratory depression<br>Decreased mental acuity |

  4.  Modify lifestyle

    a.  Stop smoking

    b.  Reduce stress

    c.  Decrease caffeine intake

    d.  Modify intake of calories, sodium, and fat

    e.  Regular physical activity

  5.  Prevent complications and further attacks

    a.  Complications

       1)  Dysrhythmias

       2)  Shock

       3)  CHF

       4)  Rupture of heart muscle

5) Pulmonary embolism

6) Recurrent MI

6. Teaching

   a. Healing not complete for 6–8 weeks

   b. Medication schedule and adverse effects

# Angina Pectoris

Occurs when oxygen supply to the heart is not sufficient, usually due to atherosclerotic changes in the coronary arteries (see Figure 4-22)

**A.** Assessment

1. Pain—may radiate down left arm; associated with stress, exertion, or anxiety

2. Relieved with rest and nitroglycerin

3. Older adults—may not have typical pain

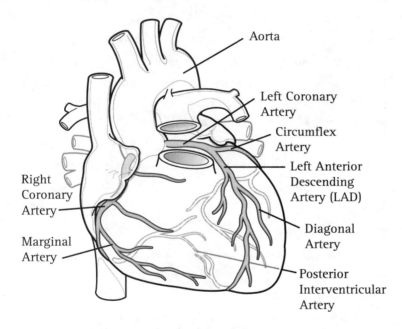

**Figure 4-22.** Coronary Artery and Heart

**B.** Etiology

1. Cause—coronary atherosclerosis

2. Risk factors for coronary artery disease

   a. Nonmodifiable (client has no control)

      1) Increasing age

      2) Family history of coronary heart disease

      3) Men more likely to develop heart disease than are premenopausal women

      4) Race

      b.  Modifiable risk factor (client can exercise control)

         1)  Elevated serum cholesterol

         2)  Cigarette smoking or secondhand exposure

         3)  Hypertension

         4)  Diabetes mellitus

         5)  Physical inactivity

         6)  Obesity

         7)  Depression or chronic stress

         8)  Oral contraceptive use or hormone replacement therapy

         9)  Substance abuse—methamphetamines or cocaine

    3.  Significance—warning sign of ischemia

  **C.**  Nursing management

    1.  Health promotion

      a.  Do not smoke

      b.  Follow balanced diet that limits intake of fat and sodium

      c.  Check blood pressure and cholesterol regularly

      d.  Engage in regular physical activity; goal is reduction of blood pressure and pulse rate upon exertion

    2.  Medications (*see* Tables 4-9 through 4-11)

    3.  Coronary artery bypass surgery

      a.  Indications—to increase blood flow to heart muscle in clients with severe angina

      b.  Saphenous vein is used for graft; as many as five arteries are bypassed

      c.  Preoperative—education and psychological preparation

      d.  Postoperative

         1)  Provide intensive evaluation of organ systems

         2)  Provide chest drainage

         3)  Pain relief

         4)  Be alert to psychological state of disorientation or depression

         5)  Provide activity as tolerated with progress as ordered from foot dangling over side of bed, to sitting in chair, to walking in room by third day

      e.  Provide guidance concerning long-term care and follow-up

      f.  Percutaneous transluminal coronary angioplasty (PTCA)—balloon-tipped catheter is inserted into diseased coronary artery and pressure applied to stenosed artery; possible stent placement

**Table 4-9** Antianginal Medication

| MEDICATION | ADVERSE EFFECTS | NURSING CONSIDERATIONS |
| --- | --- | --- |
| Nitroglycerin | Flushing<br>Hypotension<br>Headache<br>Tachycardia<br>Dizziness<br>Blurred vision | Avoid alcoholic beverages<br>Sublingual dose may be repeated every 5 min for 3 doses<br>Protect medication from light<br>Should wet tablet with saliva and place under tongue<br>Lie down when taking sublingual nitroglycerin<br>Headache most common adverse effect |
| Isosorbide | Headache<br>Orthostatic hypotension | Change position slowly<br>Take between meals<br>Don't discontinue abruptly |
| Beta-blockers:<br>Propranolol<br>Metoprolol<br>Atenolol | Bradycardia<br>Hypotension<br>Bronchoconstriction | Should not be given to clients with known or suspected coronary artery spasms<br>Clients who continue to smoke have reduced effectiveness of therapy<br>Clients with asthma may experience bronchospasms<br>Should be used with caution in clients with diabetes mellitus (may mask signs of hypoglycemia)<br>Should be discontinued gradually to prevent rebound angina |
| Calcium channel blockers:<br>Amlodipine<br>Diltiazem<br>Verapamil | Hypotension | Contraindicated in second- or third-degree heart block, cardiogenic shock, severe bradycardia, heart failure, or hypotension<br>Use cautiously with renal or hepatic impairment<br>Can potentiate the action of digoxin |
| Angiotensin-converting enzyme inhibitors:<br>Captopril | Dry, annoying cough<br>Hypotension<br>Hyperkalemia | Diuretics increase effect<br>Avoid high-potassium foods |

**Table 4-10** Anticoagulant Medications

| MEDICATION | ADVERSE EFFECTS | NURSING CONSIDERATIONS |
|---|---|---|
| **Action: Inhibits Synthesis of Clotting Factors** | | |
| Heparin | Can produce hemorrhage from any body site (10%) | Monitor therapeutic PTT at 1.5–2.5 times the control without signs of hemorrhage |
| | Tissue irritation/pain at injection site | Lower limit of normal 20–25 s; upper limit of normal 32–39 s |
| | Anemia | For IV administration: use infusion pump, peak 5 minutes, duration 2–6 hours |
| | Thrombocytopenia | |
| | Fever | For injection: give deep SQ; never IM (danger of hematoma), onset 20–60 minutes, duration 8–12 hours |
| | Dose dependent on partial thromboplastin time (PTT) | Antidote: protamine sulfate within 30 minutes |
| | | Can be allergenic |
| Low-molecular-weight heparin:<br><br>  Enoxaparin | Bleeding | Less allergenic than heparin |
| | Minimal widespread effect | Must be given deep SQ, never IV or IM |
| | Fixed dose | Does not require lab test monitoring |
| Warfarin | Hemorrhage | Monitor therapeutic prothrombin time (PT) at 1.5–2.5 times the control, or monitor international normalized ratio (INR) |
| | Diarrhea | |
| | Rash | Normal PT 9.5–12 s; normal INR 2–3.5 |
| | Fever | Onset: 36–72 hours, peak 1.5–3 days, duration: 3–5 days |
| | | Antidotes: vitamin K, whole blood, plasma |
| | | Teach measures to avoid venous stasis |
| | | Emphasize importance of regular lab testing |
| | | Client should avoid foods high in vitamin K: many green vegetables, pork, rice, yogurt, cheeses, fish, milk |
| Fondaparinux | Hemorrhage | SQ only |
| | Thrombocytopenia | PT and PTT aren't suitable monitoring tests |

*(Continued)*

**Table 4-10** Anticoagulant Medications (*Continued*)

| MEDICATION | ADVERSE EFFECTS | NURSING CONSIDERATIONS |
|---|---|---|
| \multicolumn{3}{c}{Action: Inhibits Activity of Clotting} |||
| **Dabigatran** | Directly inhibits thrombin<br><br>Used to treat atrial fibrillation<br><br>Increased risk bleeding age greater than 75, kidney disease, gastrointestinal bleeding, use of NSAIDs ||
| **Action** | Note which action each medication uses:<br><br>Heparin blocks conversion of fibrinogen to fibrin<br><br>Warfarin interferes with liver synthesis of vitamin K–dependent clotting factors<br><br>Dabigatran inhibits thrombin ||
| **Indications** | For heparin: prophylaxis and treatment of thromboembolic disorders; in very low doses (10–100 units) to maintain patency of IV catheters (heparin flush)<br><br>For warfarin: management of pulmonary emboli, venous thromboembolism, MI, atrial dysrhythmias, postcardiac valve replacement<br><br>For dipyridamole: as an adjunct to warfarin in postop cardiac valve replacement, as an adjunct to aspirin to reduce the risk of repeat stroke or transient ischemic attacks (TIAs) ||
| **Adverse effects** | Nausea<br><br>Alopecia<br><br>Urticaria<br><br>Hemorrhage<br><br>Bleeding/heparin-induced thrombocytopenia (HIT) ||
| **Nursing considerations** | Check for signs of hemorrhage: bleeding gums, nosebleed, unusual bleeding, black/tarry stools, hematuria, fall in hematocrit or blood pressure, guaiac-positive stools<br><br>Client should avoid IM injections, aspirin (ASA)-containing products, and NSAIDs<br><br>Client should wear medical information tag<br><br>Instruct client to use soft toothbrush, electric razor, to report bleeding gums, petechiae or bruising, epistaxis, black tarry stools<br><br>Monitor platelet counts and signs and symptoms of thrombosis during heparin therapy; if HIT suspected, heparin discontinued and nonheparin anticoagulant (lepirudin) given ||

(*Continued*)

**Table 4-10** Anticoagulant Medications (*Continued*)

| MEDICATION | ADVERSE EFFECTS | NURSING CONSIDERATIONS |
|---|---|---|
| **Herbal interactions** | Garlic, ginger, ginkgo may increase bleeding when taken with warfarin | |
| | Large doses of anise may interfere with anticoagulants | |
| | Ginseng and alfalfa may decrease anticoagulant activity | |
| | Black cohosh increases action of anticoagulant | |
| | Chamomile may interfere with anticoagulants | |
| **Vitamin interaction** | Vitamin C may slightly prolong PT | |
| | Vitamin E will increase warfarin's effect | |

**Table 4-11** Thrombolytic Medications

| MEDICATION | ADVERSE EFFECTS | NURSING CONSIDERATIONS (SPECIFIC) |
|---|---|---|
| Reteplase<br>Alteplase<br>Tissue plasminogen activator | Bleeding | Tissue plasminogen activator is a naturally occurring enzyme<br>Low allergenic risk but high cost |
| Anistreplase<br>Streptokinase | Bleeding | Because streptokinase is made from a bacterium, client can have an allergic reaction. Not used if client had recent *Streptococcus* infection or received streptokinase in past year |
| **Action** | Reteplase and alteplase break down plasminogen into plasmin, which dissolves the fibrin network of a clot | |
| | Anistreplase and streptokinase bind with plasminogen to form a complex that digests fibrin | |
| **Indications** | MIs within the first 6 hours after symptoms, limited arterial thrombosis, thrombotic strokes, occluded shunts | |
| **Nursing considerations (general)** | Check for signs of bleeding; minimize number of punctures for inserting IVs; avoid IM injections; apply pressure at least twice as long as usual after any puncture | |

# VASCULAR ALTERATIONS: HYPERTENSION

## Perfusion

### Hypertension

There are two stages of hypertension, stage 1 and stage 2. Stage 1 hypertension is defined as persistent elevation of the systolic blood pressure between 130–139 mm Hg or the diastolic blood pressure between 80–89 mm Hg. Stage 2 hypertension is defined as a systolic blood pressure of at least 140 mm Hg or a diastolic blood pressure of at least 90 mm Hg.

A. Assessment

1. May be no symptoms

2. Headache, dizziness; facial flushing

3. Anginal pain—insufficient blood flow through coronary arteries to the myocardium

4. Intermittent claudication—decreased adequacy of blood supply to the legs during periods of activity

5. Retinal hemorrhages and exudates—damage to arterioles that supply the retina

6. Severe occipital headaches associated with nausea, vomiting, drowsiness, giddiness, anxiety, and mental impairment due to vessel damage within the brain

7. Polyuria, nocturia, protein, and RBCs in urine, and diminished ability of kidneys to concentrate urine—hardening of arterioles within the kidney (arteriolar nephrosclerosis)

8. Dyspnea upon exertion—left-sided heart failure

9. Edema of the extremities—right-sided heart failure

10. Client's history should include:

   a. Age of onset (all ages, but more common with increasing age)

   b. Family history

   c. History of renal or cardiovascular disease

   d. Recent reports of dyspnea, fatigue, weakness, anginal-type pain, swelling of feet, or nocturia

   e. Sudden gain or loss of weight

   f. Recent severe headaches or drenching sweats

   g. Personality type

   h. Activity level

    i.   Alcohol intake

    j.   Diet, including sodium intake

11.  Physical examination should include

    a.   Blood pressure reading on both arms in supine and erect positions and on one leg: readings should be taken every 1–2 hours over an 8-hour period for 1–2 days (a single blood pressure reading is almost always inaccurate)

    b.   Ophthalmoscopic examination for evidence of vascular changes

    c.   Examination of the heart and aorta by means of auscultation, EKG readings, and aortography

    d.   Palpation of the arteries in the neck, wrists, femoral areas, and feet for evidence of coarctation of the aorta (decreased amplitude of pulses and lower blood pressure in the legs than in the arm)

    e.   Neurological examination for signs of cerebral thrombosis or hemorrhage

    f.   Gerontologic considerations—high incidence of hypertension; parameters the same as for younger adults; increased systolic blood pressure common; treatment goal is less than 139/89 mm Hg or less than 130/80 mm Hg in diabetic clients; consider effects of antihypertensive medications

12.  Laboratory studies—to diagnose type of hypertension present

    a.   Urinalysis and urine cultures to determine the presence of protein, RBCs, pus cells, and casts (all indicative of renal disease)

    b.   Blood count and sedimentation rate

    c.   Serum sodium, potassium, chloride, and carbon dioxide (all indicative of primary aldosteronism)

    d.   Urinary catecholamine metabolites (indicative of pheochromocytoma)

    e.   Urine 17-ketosteroids and blood corticoids (both indicative of Cushing disease)

    f.   Intravenous pyelogram, urine cultures, radioisotope renogram, renal arteriography, intravenous urograms (all tests for renal disease)

    g.   BUN and creatinine

13.  If clinical workup indicates no evidence of coarctation of the aorta, adrenal disease, or primary renal disease, then the condition is diagnosed as essential hypertension

**B.**  Etiology

  1.  Causes

    a.   Risk factors

        1)   Family history of hypertension

        2)   Excessive sodium intake

        3)   Excessive intake of calories

        4)   Physical inactivity

        5)   Excessive alcohol intake

        6)   Low potassium intake

        7)   Age

b. Contributing factors—history of renal or cardiovascular disease; stressful lifestyle

c. Primary (essential or idiopathic)—constitutes 90% of all cases; may be benign (gradual onset and prolonged course) or malignant (abrupt onset and short dramatic course, which is rapidly fatal unless treated)

d. Secondary—develops as a result of another primary disease of the cardiovascular system, renal system, adrenal glands, or neurological system

2. Cycle of hypertensive cardiovascular disease

a. Heart meets increased peripheral resistance (increased afterload)

b. Heart must increase expenditure of energy; increased stretching of muscle fibers

c. Stretching of muscle fibers results in hypertrophy of the heart and increased oxygen demand

d. Hypertrophy of the heart may cause coronary insufficiency and result in MI (the enlarged heart muscle has outgrown its blood supply)

e. If hypertrophied heart maintains cardiac output, left-sided cardiac failure may occur

f. As diastolic pressure rises, the congestion extends back into the entire pulmonary tree

g. Increased pressure of blood in arteries, coupled with arteriosclerotic changes (i.e., in kidneys and brain), can cause blood vessels to rupture, producing hemorrhage

h. Stretching of atrial myocardium may cause atrial fibrillation

3. Complications

a. Renal failure

b. Cerebral vascular accident (CVA)

c. Transient ischemic attacks (TIAs)

d. Retinal hemorrhages

C. Plan/implementation

1. Medications (*see* Table 4-12)

2. Nursing management

a. Provide a restful, quiet hospital environment

b. Provide complete explanations of all procedures and diagnostic studies

c. Listen to the client's fears and worries, and offer reassurance

d. Completely explain dietary restrictions (i.e., salt restriction, low fat)

e. Document client's blood pressure both standing and lying down

f. Encourage weight loss if client is obese

g. Provide moderate salt-restricted diet

h. Plan program of regular physical exercise

i. Encourage changes in job or domestic settings for clients who live or work under considerable stress

**Table 4-12** Antihypertensive Medications

| MEDICATION | ADVERSE EFFECTS | NURSING CONSIDERATIONS |
|---|---|---|
| **Beta-Blockers** | | |
| Atenolol | Bradycardia<br><br>Hypotension<br><br>Bronchospasm | Once-a-day dose increases compliance<br><br>Check apical pulse; if less than 60 bpm, hold medication and call health care provider<br><br>Don't discontinue abruptly<br><br>Masks signs of shock and hypoglycemia |
| Metoprolol | Bradycardia, hypotension<br><br>Heart failure<br><br>Depression | Give with meals<br><br>Teach client to check pulse before each dose; take apical pulse before administration; withhold if pulse is less than 60 bpm |
| Nadolol | Bradycardia, hypotension<br><br>Heart failure | Teach client to check pulse before each dose; check apical pulse before administering<br><br>Withhold if pulse less than 60 bpm<br><br>Don't discontinue abruptly |
| Propranolol | Weakness<br><br>Hypotension<br><br>Bronchospasm<br><br>Bradycardia<br><br>Depression | Blocks sympathetic impulses to heart (beta-blocker)<br><br>Client should take pulse at home before each dose<br><br>Dosage should be reduced gradually before discontinued |
| **Alpha-Blockers** | | |
| Prazosin hydrochloride | Drowsiness, dizziness<br><br>Weakness<br><br>Palpitations<br><br>Nausea | Blocks a mediated vasoconstriction<br><br>Assess for first-dose syncope<br><br>Orthostatic hypotension precautions |
| **Alpha-2 Agonists** | | |
| Methyldopa | Drowsiness, dizziness<br><br>Bradycardia<br><br>Hemolytic anemia<br><br>Fever<br><br>Orthostatic hypotension | Prevent reuptake of norepinephrine<br><br>Monitor CBC<br><br>Monitor liver function<br><br>Take at bedtime to minimize daytime drowsiness<br><br>Change position slowly |

*(Continued)*

**Table 4-12** Anticoagulant Medications (*Continued*)

| MEDICATION | ADVERSE EFFECTS | NURSING CONSIDERATIONS |
|---|---|---|
| Clonidine | Drowsiness, dizziness | Don't discontinue abruptly |
| | Dry mouth, headache Dermatitis | Apply patch to nonhairy area (upper outer arm, anterior chest) |
| | Severe rebound hypertension | Take orthostatic hypotension precautions |
| | | Older adults—high risk of orthostatic hypotension and CNS adverse effects |
| **Thiazide Diuretics** | | |
| Hydrochlorothi-azide | Hypokalemia | Weigh regularly |
| | Dehydration | Monitor for symptoms of hypokalemia |
| | Postural hypotension | Take postural hypotension precautions |
| **Potassium-Sparing Diuretics** | | |
| Spironolactone | Hyperkalemia | Weigh regularly |
| | GI upset | Monitor for symptoms of hyperkalemia |
| **Vasodilators** | | |
| Hydralazine | Headache, palpitations | Dilates arteriolar smooth muscle |
| | Edema | Give with meals |
| | Tachycardia, palpitations | Observe mental status |
| | Lupus erythematosus-like syndrome | Check for weight gain, edema |
| Morphine sulfate | Hypotension | Reduces cardiac workload, preload, and afterload pressures |
| | Respiratory depression | |
| | Decreased mental alertness | Relieves pain, reduces anxiety |
| | Constipation | |
| **Calcium Channel Blockers** | | |
| Nifedipine | Hypotension | Reduces workload of left ventricle (calcium channel blocker) |
| Verapamil | Dizziness | |
| Diltiazem | GI distress | Coronary vasodilator |
| Amlodipine | Liver dysfunction | Monitor blood pressure during dosage adjustments |
| | Jitteriness | Assist client with ambulation at start of therapy |
| | | Nifedipine—high risk of hypotension and constipation in older adults |

(*Continued*)

**Table 4-12** Anticoagulant Medications (*Continued*)

| MEDICATION | ADVERSE EFFECTS | NURSING CONSIDERATIONS |
|---|---|---|
| **ACE Inhibitors** | | |
| Captopril | Dizziness | Blocks conversion of angiotensin I to angiotensin II |
| Enalapril | Orthostatic hypertension | Report swelling of face, light-headedness |
| | Persistent cough | |
| | Hyperkalemia | |
| **Angiotensin II Receptor Blocker (ARB)** | | |
| Losartan | Less likely to cause persistent cough and hyperkalemia than are ACE inhibitors | Prevents binding of angiotensin II with tissue receptor sites |
| | | Maximal effects require 3–6 weeks |
| | | Can be used in combination with a diuretic for better BP control |
| Herbal interactions | Ma-huang (ephedra) decreases effect of antihypertensive medications | |
| | Ephedra increases hypertension when taken with beta-blockers | |
| | Black cohosh increases hypotensive effects of antihypertensives | |
| | Goldenseal counteracts effects of antihypertensives | |

j. Educate client regarding medication therapy

   1) Lie down immediately if faintness, weakness, nausea, or vomiting occurs

   2) Avoid hot baths, excessive amounts of alcohol, and immobility following exercise

   3) Always rise slowly from a lying to a sitting position and from sitting to standing to allow the vascular system to adjust to positional changes

   4) Avoid standing motionless, especially within the first hour or two after receiving medication (standing causes leg vessels to relax, allowing blood to pool within lower extremities)

   5) Use caution when driving an automobile or when operating heavy or dangerous machinery, especially with medications causing sedation

   6) Avoid constipation because it may cause either an increased or irregular absorption of hypotensive medications, which can result in critical hypotensive reactions

   7) Should hypotensive crises occur frequently, wrap legs firmly with elastic bandages when ambulating to promote venous return

   8) Never take a larger dose of medication than prescribed without consulting the health care provider

9) Always take medication on time, and do not skip a dose (noncompliance is common)

10) Never suddenly discontinue a medication without the health care provider's permission to avoid severe rebound hypertensive reaction

11) Always report adverse effects to the health care provider; impotence problems warrant change of therapy

12) Consult with health care provider before taking any prescription or over-the-counter medications

13) Gerontologic considerations

   a) Blood pressure assessment—inflate cuff pressure to level above disappearance of brachial or radial pulse

   b) Assess for orthostatic blood pressure changes; measure blood pressure in supine, sitting, and standing positions

   c) Older adults may not tolerate systolic blood pressure less than 120 mm Hg

   d) Older adults may have significant drop in blood pressure immediately after meals

   e) Polypharmacy—interaction between NSAIDs and antihypertensive medications

## [ SECTION 4 ]

# SELECTED DISORDERS OF TISSUE PERFUSION

## Perfusion

## Selected Disorders of Tissue Perfusion

A.  Shock—sudden reduction of oxygen and nutrients

  1.  Assessment—decreased blood volume causes a reduction in venous return, decreased cardiac output, and a decrease in arterial pressure

    a.  Tachycardia, weak or absent peripheral pulses

    b.  Cyanosis—with severe shock

    c.  Decrease in urinary output ranging from oliguria to anuria, increased urine specific gravity

    d.  Decrease in body temperature and absence of peripheral pulses due to peripheral vasoconstriction

    e.  Anxiety, restlessness, and apprehension due to decreased cerebral tissue perfusion

    f.  Respiration may be shallow and rapid; pulse will be weak and thready

    g.  Decrease in arterial blood pressure

    h.  Dehydration with associated alteration in electrolytes

    i.  Nausea, vomiting

    j.  In advanced shock, signs of pump failure and renal failure will be present

    k.  Cool, clammy skin, decreased capillary refill

    l.  Metabolic acidosis

  2.  Causes

    a.  Types and causes of shock

      1)  Hypovolemic shock—loss of fluid from circulation

        a)  Hemorrhagic shock (external or internal)

        b)  Cutaneous shock, e.g., burns resulting in external fluid loss

        c)  Diabetic ketoacidosis

        d)  Gastrointestinal obstruction, e.g., vomiting and diarrhea

        e)  Diabetes insipidus

        f)  Excessive use of diuretics

        g)  Internal sequestration, e.g., fractures, hemothorax, ascites

      2) Cardiogenic shock—decreased cardiac output

         a) Myocardial infarction

         b) Dysrhythmias

         c) Pump failure

      3) Distributive shock—inadequate vascular tone

         a) Neural-induced loss of vascular tone

            i) Anesthesia

            ii) Pain

            iii) Insulin shock

            iv) Spinal cord injury

         b) Chemical-induced loss of vascular tone

            i) Anaphylaxis

            ii) Toxic shock

            iii) Capillary leak—burns, decreased serum protein levels

  b. Stages of shock—a dynamic condition in which the client's status is constantly changing

      1) Initial stage—cardiac output is insufficient to supply normal nutritional needs of the body's tissues but is not low enough to cause serious symptoms

      2) Compensatory stage—cardiac output is further reduced, but due to compensatory vasoconstriction, blood pressure tends to remain within a normal range

         a) Blood flow to the skin and kidneys decreases

         b) Blood flow to the central nervous system and myocardium tends to be maintained

         c) A decrease occurs in the blood reservoirs

      3) Progressive stage—unfavorable changes become more and more apparent

         a) Falling blood pressure

         b) Increasing vasoconstriction

         c) Increased heart rate

         d) Oliguria

      4) Irreversible stage—no type of therapy can save the client's life

         a) Myocardial depression

         b) Loss of arteriolar tonus

         c) Infused blood tends to remain in the dilated capillary bed

3. Nursing management

  a. Maintain adequate oxygenation (*see* Table 4-13)

  b. Increase tissue perfusion

  c. Maintain systolic BP greater than 90 mm Hg

  d. Treat acidosis

**Table 4-13** Oxygen Administration

| METHOD | OXYGEN DELIVERED | NURSING CONSIDERATIONS |
|---|---|---|
| Nasal cannula or prongs | 23–42% at 1–6 L/min | Assess patency of nostril<br><br>Apply water-soluble jelly to nostrils every 3–4 hours<br><br>Perform good mouth care |
| Face mask | 40–60% at 6–8 L/min (oxygen flow minimum 5 L) | Remove mask every 1–2 hours<br><br>Wash, dry, apply lotion to skin<br><br>Emotional support to decrease feeling of claustrophobia |
| Partial rebreather mask | 50–75% at 8–11 L/min | Adjust oxygen flow to keep reservoir bag two-thirds full during inspiration |
| Nonrebreather mask | 80–100% at 12 L/min | Adjust oxygen flow to keep bag two-thirds full |
| Venturi mask | 24–40% at 4–8 L/min | Provides high humidity and fixed concentrations<br><br>Keep tubing free of kinks |
| Tracheostomy collar or T-piece | 30–100% at 8–10 L/min | Assess for fine mist<br><br>Empty condensation from tubing<br><br>Keep water container full |
| Oxygen hood | 30–100% at 8–10 L/min | Used for infants and young children<br><br>Provides cooled, humid air<br><br>Check $O_2$ concentration with $O_2$ analyzer every 4 hours<br><br>Refill humidity jar with sterile distilled water<br><br>Clean humidity jar daily<br><br>Cover client with light blanket and towel or cap for head<br><br>Change linen frequently<br><br>Monitor client's temperature frequently |

   e. Maintain patent airway

     1) If necessary, ensure ventilation by Ambu bag or ventilator assistance

     2) Provide supplemental oxygen to maintain adequate blood $PO_2$

   f. Indwelling catheter, hourly outputs

   g. Monitor CVP

   h. Monitor vital signs

i. Assess ABGs

j. Keep warm (maintain body temperature)

    1) Heat application is contraindicated because it causes peripheral blood vessels to dilate and draws blood back from vital organs

    2) Hypothermia increases blood viscosity and slows blood flow through the microcirculation

k. Restore fluid volume

    1) Intravenous administration of blood or other appropriate fluids (crystalloids or colloids)

    2) Volume of fluid administered may be pushed until systemic blood pressure, urine volume, and lactate levels return to a relatively normal level or central venous or pulmonary artery pressures, or both, become elevated

l. Medications (*see* Table 4-14)

    1) Antibiotics—when shock is due to an infection (septic shock), antibiotic therapy should be instituted immediately; blood, urine, sputum, and drainage of any kind should be sent for culture

    2) Medications to vasoconstrict and improve myocardial contractility (e.g., dopamine, norepinephrine, phenylephrine, dobutamine, milrinone)

    3) Medications to maintain adequate urine output, e.g., furosemide

    4) Medication to restore blood pressure (adrenergics/sympathomimetics)

    5) Corticosteroids for septic shock

**Table 4-14** Emergency Medications For Shock, Cardiac Arrest, and Anaphylaxis

| MEDICATION | ADVERSE EFFECTS | NURSING CONSIDERATIONS |
|---|---|---|
| Norepinephrine | Headache<br><br>Palpitations<br><br>Nervousness<br><br>Epigastric distress<br><br>Angina, hypertension, tissue necrosis with extravasation | Vasoconstrictor to increase blood pressure and cardiac output<br><br>Reflex bradycardia may occur with rise in BP<br><br>Client should be attended at all times<br><br>Monitor urinary output<br><br>Infuse with dextrose solution, not saline<br><br>Monitor blood pressure<br><br>Protect from light |

*(Continued)*

**Table 4-14** Emergency Medications For Shock, Cardiac Arrest, and Anaphylaxis (*Continued*)

| MEDICATION | ADVERSE EFFECTS | NURSING CONSIDERATIONS |
|---|---|---|
| Dopamine | Increased ocular pressure<br><br>Ectopic beats<br><br>Nausea<br><br>Tachycardia, chest pain, dysrhythmias | Low dose—dilates renal and coronary arteries<br><br>High dose—vasoconstrictor, increases myocardial oxygen consumption<br><br>Headache is an early symptom of medication excess<br><br>Monitor blood pressure, peripheral pulses, urinary output<br><br>Use infusion pump |
| Epinephrine | Nervousness<br><br>Restlessness<br><br>Dizziness<br><br>Local necrosis of skin | Stimulates alpha- and beta-adrenergic receptors<br><br>Monitor BP<br><br>Carefully aspirate syringe before IM and SC doses; inadvertent IV administration can be harmful<br><br>Always check strength:<br>1:100 only for inhalation, 1:1,000 for parenteral administration (SC or IM)<br><br>Ensure adequate hydration |
| Isoproterenol | Headache<br><br>Palpitations<br><br>Tachycardia<br><br>Changes in BP<br><br>Angina, bronchial asthma | Stimulates beta-1 and beta-2 adrenergic receptors<br><br>Used for heart block, ventricular arrhythmias, and bradycardia<br><br>Bronchodilator used for asthma and bronchospasms<br><br>Don't give at bedtime—interrupts sleep patterns<br><br>Monitor BP, pulse |
| Phenylephrine | Palpations<br><br>Tachycardia<br><br>Hypertension<br><br>Dysrhythmia<br><br>Angina<br><br>Tissue necrosis with extravasation | Potent alpha-1 agonist<br><br>Used to treat hypotension |

(*Continued*)

**Table 4-14** Emergency Medications For Shock, Cardiac Arrest, and Anaphylaxis (*Continued*)

| MEDICATION | ADVERSE EFFECTS | NURSING CONSIDERATIONS |
|---|---|---|
| Dobutamine hydrochloride | Hypertension<br><br>PVCs<br><br>Asthmatic episodes<br><br>Headache | Stimulates beta-1 receptors<br><br>Incompatible with alkaline solutions (sodium bicarbonate)<br><br>Administer through central venous catheter or large peripheral vein using an infusion pump<br><br>Don't infuse through line with other meds (incompatible)<br><br>Monitor EKG, BP, I and O, serum potassium |
| Milrinone | Dysrhythmia<br><br>Thrombocytopenia<br><br>Jaundice | Positive inotropic agent<br><br>Smooth muscle relaxant used to treat severe heart failure |
| Sodium nitroprusside | Hypotension | Dilates cardiac veins and arteries<br><br>Decreases preload and afterload<br><br>Increases myocardial perfusion |
| Diphenhydramine HCl | Drowsiness<br><br>Confusion<br><br>Insomnia<br><br>Headache<br><br>Vertigo<br><br>Photosensitivity | Blocks effects of histamine on bronchioles, GI tract, and blood vessels |
| **Actions** | Varies with med | |
| **Indications** | Hypovolemic shock<br><br>Cardiac arrest<br><br>Anaphylaxis | |
| **Adverse effects** | Serious rebound effect may occur<br><br>Balance between underdosing and overdosing | |
| **Nursing considerations** | Monitor vital signs<br><br>Measure urine output<br><br>Assess for extravasation<br><br>Observe extremities for color and perfusion | |

# [ SECTION 5 ]

# VASCULAR DISORDERS

## Perfusion

## Peripheral Vascular Disease

**A.** Assessment

   1. General signs and symptoms

     a. Intermittent claudication—severe pain in calf muscle that occurs with walking and is caused by ischemia and a buildup of lactic acid; pain often described as cramping

       1) Exercise increases metabolic needs of tissues

       2) Damaged arteries are unable to dilate and supply tissues with oxygen

     b. Rest pain (pain in extremities occurring when client is resting)—sudden blockage of a vessel by a thrombus reduces blood supply to tissues and produces ischemic pain; pain relieved by dependent position

     c. Coldness and pallor of extremities during elevation

     d. Dependent rubor—tissues of the extremities are reddish blue in color

       1) Indicative of peripheral vessel damage where vessels remain permanently dilated

       2) Develops after prolonged anoxia or exposure to severe cold

     e. Cyanosis of the tissues—occurs when blood contains too little oxygen

     f. Trophic changes—adverse changes in the skin and nails of the extremities result from prolonged ischemia of tissues (loss of lower extremity hair)

     g. Leg ulcers and cellulitis

       1) Venous stasis is a consequence of venous insufficiency

       2) Venous stasis provides a medium for bacterial growth, which results in ulcerations

     h. Gangrenous changes—death and decay of tissues of the extremities result from severe and prolonged ischemia

**B.** Factors regulating the peripheral vascular system—arteries are contractile in that they can decrease (vasoconstrict) or increase (vasodilate) in response to appropriate stimuli

   1. Arteries have a rich sympathetic nervous system supply

     a. Stimulation causes vasoconstriction

     b. Sympathectomy causes vasodilation

2. Hormonal and chemical control—3 substances within blood help control the caliber of blood vessels

    a. Epinephrine—constricts superficial blood vessels, but in small doses dilates vessels supplying the muscles, brain, and heart

    b. Norepinephrine—constricts all blood vessels, but particularly affects the peripheral vessels

    c. Angiotensin—constricts arteries

3. Local regulatory mechanisms—substances that act locally on blood vessels

    a. Histamine—potent vasodilator of small blood vessels, although may also constrict large arteries

    b. Muscle metabolites—strong vasodilators

    c. Acetylcholine—vasodilator whose action is transient and more apparent in the face and upper limbs than in the lower limbs

    d. Serotonin—substance liberated from platelets that sticks to the injured area of a vessel wall: powerful constrictor of cutaneous arterioles but dilates capillaries

C. Peripheral vascular diseases are characterized by disturbances of blood flow through the peripheral vessels, eventually resulting in damage to tissues of the extremities

1. Adequate blood flow depends on many factors

    a. Efficiency of heart's pumping action

    b. Condition of blood vessels, e.g., patent, dilated, or constricted

    c. Rate of blood flow

    d. Needs of tissues for oxygen and nutrients as well as for removal of waste products

    e. Nervous system activity

    f. Amount of blood flow

## Arterial Peripheral Vascular Disease

Arteries must be capable of dilating and constricting normally

A. Assessment

1. Cool, shiny skin, hair loss

2. Ulcers, gangrene

3. Impaired sensation

4. Intermittent claudication

5. Decreased peripheral pulses

6. Diagnostic tests

    a. Angiography (arteriography)—contrast dye is injected into the arteries, and x-ray films are taken of the vascular tree

        1) May indicate abnormalities of blood flow due to arterial obstruction or narrowing

        2) Magnetic resonance angiography—useful for clients with dye allergy

    b.  Doppler ultrasound—measures velocity of blood flow through a vessel and emits an audible signal

    c.  Duplex imaging—uses Doppler system to map blood throughout artery, and gives anatomic and physiological information about the blood vessels

    d.  Ankle-brachial index (ABI)—divide ankle blood pressure by brachial blood pressure; normal is greater than or equal to 0.9

**B.**  Etiology

    1.  Types of disease

        a.  Arteriosclerosis

        b.  Raynaud disease

        c.  Buerger disease

    2.  Predisposing factors

        a.  Smoking

        b.  Diabetes mellitus

        c.  Hyperlipidemia

        d.  Hypertension

        e.  Obesity

        f.  Sedentary lifestyle

        g.  Age

**C.**  Nursing management

    1.  Check extremities for paleness, coolness, necrosis

    2.  Good foot care

        a.  Use warm water, dry gently and thoroughly

        b.  Use lubricants to keep skin soft

        c.  Wear clean cotton socks

    3.  Do not cross legs

    4.  Regular exercise—promotes collateral circulation

    5.  Stop smoking

    6.  Lose weight

    7.  Interventional radiological procedures

        a.  Percutaneous transluminal angioplasty

        b.  Laser-assisted angioplasty

        c.  Atherectomy catheters

        d.  Intravascular stents

8. Surgical therapy

   a. Arterial bypass with autogenous vein or synthetic graft

   b. Endarterectomy

   c. Patch graft angioplasty

   d. Amputation

9. Medications

   a. Vasodilators

   b. Anticoagulants

   c. Platelet aggregate inhibitors (e.g., aspirin, clopidogrel)

## Venous Peripheral Vascular Disease

Efficiency in returning blood to the heart depends upon competent valves within the veins and adequate pumping action of the muscles surrounding the veins

A. Assessment

   1. Cool, brown skin

   2. Edema

   3. Ulcers

   4. Pain, redness along vein, induration along vein

   5. Normal or decreased pulses

   6. Deep muscle tenderness

   7. Limb may be warmer than opposite limb

   8. Risk for pulmonary embolism

   9. Diagnostic tests

      a. Phlebogram (venogram)

      b. Venous pressure measurements—venous occlusion in one leg causes venous pressure to be higher than in unaffected leg

      c. Venous Doppler evaluation, venous duplex ultrasonography

      d. Lung scan and pulmonary arteriogram

      e. D-dimer test—global marker for coagulation

B. Causes

   1. Thrombophlebitis—inflammation of venous wall with clot formation

   2. Predisposing factors

      a. Venous stasis—conditions causing venous stasis include varicose veins, obesity, surgery, pregnancy, prolonged bedrest, and CHF

      b. Hypercoagulability—may be caused by cancer, blood dyscrasias, decreased fibrinolysis, increased clotting factors or increased blood viscosity, oral contraceptives

      c. Injury to the venous wall—may be caused by IV injections, thromboangiitis obliterans (Buerger disease), fractures and dislocations, chemical injury from sclerosing agents, opaque media for x-ray, certain antibiotics

3. Age-decreased competency of valves; greater incidence of varicose veins; slowed wound healing

C. Nursing management

1. Ambulation and exercise in bed should be encouraged once anticoagulation therapy is started to decrease venous pressure and promote blood flow by the contraction of muscles compressing the veins

2. Elevation of legs above the level of the heart facilitates blood flow by force of gravity, thereby preventing venous stasis and formation of new thrombi; also decreases venous pressure, relieving edema and pain

3. Raise foot of bed rather than using pillows or gatching the bed because these methods often result in elevation of the knee above the foot and interfere with proper flow

4. Apply intermittent or continuous warm, moist packs—to relieve venospasm, produce analgesia, and hasten resolution of inflammation

5. Elastic support hose compresses the superficial veins and, with walking, blood flow in the veins is increased and venous pressure is kept to a minimum

6. Avoid standing and sitting because these increase the hydrostatic pressure in the capillaries, promoting edema

7. Elastic or compression stockings; 6–8 wk

8. Avoid extremes in temperature

9. Monitor peripheral pulses

10. Anticoagulants

11. Thrombolytic therapy—prevents postphlebitis venous insufficiency; risk of bleeding

12. Preventive measures

  a. Passive and active range of motion exercises for clients who are postop, postpartum, or on prolonged bedrest

  b. Early ambulation postop and postpartum

  c. Elastic support hose during and after surgery

  d. Deep breathing exercises postop to promote thoracic pumping action

  e. Avoidance of tight clothing

# Varicose Veins

Dilated veins caused by incompetent valves

A. Predisposing factors

1. Pregnancy

2. Obesity

3. Heart disease

4. Family history

    **B.** Assessment

       1. Pain after prolonged standing

       2. Dilated veins

       3. Feeling of fullness in legs

    **C.** Nursing management

       1. Elevate legs above heart level

       2. Knee-length elastic stockings

       3. Vein ligation

       4. Sclerotherapy—for small or limited number varicosities

       5. Radiofrequency energy—shrinks vein

       6. Endovenous laser treatment

## Chronic Venous Insufficiency

    **A.** Predisposing factors—standing for long periods, constrictive clothing, crossed legs, obesity, age

    **B.** Assessment—venous ulcers

    **C.** Nursing management

       1. Elevate legs while sleeping and 2–3 times per day

       2. Frequent position change

       3. Avoid elastic wraps (uneven pressure)

       4. Compression stockings—replace every 6 months, remove at night, wash with soap every night, do not put into dryer

       5. Wash legs daily with mild soap and water

       6. Used mild moisturizers and creams on legs

       7. Report skin discoloration, swelling, lesions to health care provider

# End-of-Chapter Thinking Exercise

A client is admitted to the hospital for the second time this month. The client lives with an adult child in a 1-story house. The adult child is present and reports the client is having trouble breathing again. "Every morning around 2 o'clock, I awaken to hear gasping. We have tried using three or four pillows, but sleeping in the recliner in the living room is most comfortable and the only way my parent gets any sleep." The client's respiratory rate is 26 and labored. Color is pale, and on auscultation, crackles are heard throughout all lung fields. The client has a wet-sounding productive cough with white sputum. $SpO_2$ 88% on $O_2$ 3 L/min via nasal cannula. The lower extremities show bilateral +3 pitting edema. When asked about diet, the adult child reports they both eat a lot of take-out meals. Last night, they ordered pizza. The client has a history of hypertension and frequent hospitalizations for heart failure. Medications include enalapril 40 mg PO daily and furosemide 80 mg PO daily.

1.  What assessment findings indicate heart failure? (Recognize Clues)

2.  What implementations does the nurse include in the client's plan of care? (Generate Solutions)

3.  Based on the diet information shared by the adult child, what does the nurse include in diet teaching? (Take Action)

# Thinking Exercise Explanations

1. What assessment findings indicate heart failure? (Recognize Clues)

   - Dyspnea
   - Orthopnea
   - Tachypnea
   - Productive cough
   - $SpO_2$ 88%
   - Pitting edema

   The above signs and symptoms indicate decreased cardiac output, increased preload and afterload, and fluid backing up into the pulmonary system from the left side of the heart.

2. What implementations does the nurse include in the client's plan of care? (Generate Solutions)

   - Assess respiratory status every two hours until stable
   - Place in high-Fowler position
   - Encourage coughing and deep breathing
   - Record intake and output
   - Daily weights
   - Assess skin integrity and peripheral edema
   - Administer medications as ordered
   - Report any change in condition to HCP
   - Teach client and family about disease, medications, and diet

   The implementation of the above actions will ensure increased gas exchange and maintain adequate perfusion. Teaching will help to increase compliance with the plan of care while in the home setting.

3. Based on the diet information shared by the adult child, what does the nurse include in diet teaching? (Take Action)

   - Remove foods containing high levels of sodium.

   Heart failure requires sodium restriction. Increased levels of sodium in the diet cause sodium and water to be retained by the kidneys, thereby increasing preload and increasing the workload of the heart.

# [ CHAPTER 5 ]

# THE RESPIRATORY SYSTEM

[ SECTION 1 ]

# THE RESPIRATORY SYSTEM OVERVIEW

## Gas Exchange

## Respiratory System

**A.** Structure

1. Upper respiratory system

   a. Nose—filters, warms, and humidifies inspired air; contains olfactory receptors for sense of smell; older adults have restricted airflow

   b. Sinuses—air-filled cavities provide resonance during speech

   c. Pharynx (throat)—contains adenoids and tonsils; defense mechanisms against infection; gag reflex

   d. Larynx—contains the voice box and epiglottis, which prevents food from entering the trachea; cough reflex

2. Lower respiratory tract

   a. Trachea—smooth, flexible, muscular, tubelike air passage extending from larynx to mainstem bronchi

   b. Mainstem bronchi (right and left)—subdivision of trachea entering lungs

   c. Secondary bronchi—subdivisions of main bronchi branching through each lung field

   d. Bronchioles—smallest subdivisions of bronchi, conducting air from secondary bronchi into alveoli

   e. Alveoli—delicate, thin-walled, minute, hollow chambers within the lungs surrounded by networks of capillaries; contain surfactant that keeps alveoli expanded

3. Thoracic cavity—4 subdivisions

   a. Right pulmonary space—contains right lung

   b. Left pulmonary space—contains left lung

   c. Pericardial space—contains heart and pericardial sac

   d. Mediastinal space—center of thoracic cavity; located between pulmonary spaces; contains esophagus, trachea, great blood vessels, and heart

   e. Gerontologic considerations—loss of elastic recoil; increased residual volume; increased use of accessory muscles

4. Lungs—light, spongy, porous, elastic, cone-shaped organs; inflate with inspiration and deflate (but do not completely collapse) with expiration

   a. Base rests on diaphragm

   b. Apex extends above the first rib

   c. Each lung is divided into lobes—the right has 3 lobes; the left has 2

5. Pleurae—two-layered membrane covering each lung and lining the thoracic cavity

   a. Parietal pleura—lines thoracic cavity within each lung chamber

   b. Visceral (pulmonary) pleura—outer covering of the lung within each chamber

6. Pleural space—space between layers containing thin fluid to prevent friction during respiration

7. Diaphragm—muscular partition separating the thoracic and abdominal cavities

**B.** Function

1. Ventilation—moves air into and out of lungs and along bronchial airways to bring oxygen into the lungs and remove $CO_2$

   a. Inspiration

      1) Contraction of inspiratory muscles

      2) Enlargement of thoracic cage

      3) Reduction in intrapleural and intrapulmonic pressures

      4) Inflow of air until intrapulmonic pressure equals atmospheric pressure

   b. Expiration

      1) Relaxation of inspiratory muscles

      2) Reduction in size of thoracic cage

      3) Increase in intrapleural and intrapulmonic pressures

      4) Outflow of air until intrapulmonic pressure equals atmospheric pressure

      5) Gerontologic considerations–loss of elastic recoil; increased residual volume; increased use of accessory muscles

   c. Normal breath sounds

      1) Bronchial—high-pitched, loud sounds heard over the trachea

      2) Bronchovesicular—medium-pitched, moderately loud sounds heard over the mainstem bronchi

      3) Vesicular—low-pitched, soft sounds heard over the peripheral lung fields

   d. Normal breathing pattern—eupnea

      1) Rate in adult is 12–20 breaths per minute

      2) Smooth with an even respiratory depth

      3) Easy, relaxed; requiring minimal effort

      4) Symmetric chest wall movement

      5) May be abdominal (commonly seen in men) or thoracic (common in women)

2. Effective ventilation—requirements

   a. Patent airway

   b. Elastic, expansive lungs and tracheobronchial tree

   c. Adequate musculoskeletal apparatus of chest wall

**C.** Mechanics of respiration

1. Lungs and circulation act together to convey respiratory gases between atmospheric air and body tissues; respiration regulated by several components

   a. Muscles—diaphragm and intercostal muscles enhance inspiration and expiration

      1) Inspiration—contraction of diaphragm and intercostal muscles, resulting in downward expansion of the thoracic cavity and elevation of the rib cage

      2) Expiration—passive action involving deflation of lungs, relaxation of thoracic musculature, and reduction in the size of the thoracic cavity

      3) Accessory muscles may be used in pathological states or after exercise when additional expansion is needed; abdominal muscles may be used during coughing

   b. Intrapleural pressure—normally negative (below atmospheric pressures)

      1) Inspiration—reduction in intrapleural and intrapulmonic pressures; air enters the lungs until the intrapulmonic and atmospheric pressures equalize

      2) Expiration—increase in intrapleural and intrapulmonic pressures; gases in the pleural cavity are expelled until intrapulmonic and atmospheric pressures equalize

   c. Lung compliance—when lung compliance is lowered, the respiratory effort is increased

   d. Airway resistance—relationship between airflow and pleural pressure

      1) Highest resistance in the nose

      2) Lowest resistance in the bronchioles

      3) Airway problems (e.g., emphysema) increase airway resistance

2. Four "volumes" affected by ventilation

   a. Tidal volume—normal volume of air inspired and expired with each respiration (breath); the tidal volume has two components:

      1) Dead space—air that fills the bronchial tree

      2) Alveolar ventilation—air entering the alveoli

   b. Inspiratory reserve volume—volume of air that can be inspired above the tidal volume

   c. Expiratory reserve volume—amount of air that is expired forcefully at the end normal tidal volume respiration

   d. Residual volume—amount of air present in the lungs after forceful expiration; decreased in older adults

3. Lung capacity—combination of gas volumes within the lung

   a. Inspiratory capacity—tidal volume plus inspiratory reserve volume (amount of air an individual can breathe in from a resting expiratory level)

   b. Functional residual capacity—expiratory reserve volume plus residual volume (amount of air present in the lungs after normal expiration); increased in older adults

   c. Vital capacity—inspiratory reserve volume plus tidal volume plus expiratory reserve volume (maximum amount of air expelled by the lungs after maximum inspiration); decreased in older adults

   d. Total lung capacity—amount of air contained in the lungs on maximum inspiration

4. Changes anywhere in the pulmonary tracheobronchial tree can affect both pulmonary volume and capacity

5. Alveolar ventilation—membrane allows for easy exchange of gases

   a. Diffusing capacity—volume of gas that diffuses through the membranes each minute for a pressure gradient of 1 mm Hg

   b. Perfusion—amount of blood that supplies the lungs

6. Factors regulating $O_2/CO_2$ exchange

   a. Respiratory center—located in the medulla oblongata

      1) Stimulated by the concentration of $CO_2$ in arterial blood; circulating $O_2$ is less significant

         a) Brain chemoreceptors are stimulated primarily by the amount of hydrogen ions and $CO_2$ in the cerebrospinal fluid; excess $CO_2$ and hydrogen ions cause an increase in respiratory rate (loses excess $CO_2$ and restores blood pH balance)

         b) Respiratory acidosis results from a decrease in pulmonary ventilation, causing a high concentration of $CO_2$ in the blood that results in accumulation of carbonic acid and hydrogen ions

         c) Respiratory alkalosis occurs when pulmonary ventilation increases and the number of hydrogen ions decreases

   b. Peripheral chemoreceptors—located in the aortic and carotid bodies

      1) Stimulated when $O_2$ levels drop

      2) Respiratory center responds by stimulating glossopharyngeal, vagus, and phrenic nerve fibers—diaphragm is innervated, and alveolar ventilation and $O_2$ tension are increased

   c. Gerontologic considerations—diminished response of brain stem to arterial oxygen and carbon dioxide changes; slower change in respiratory rate; decreased effectiveness of respiratory and metabolic compensatory mechanisms

# ALTERATIONS IN AIRWAY CLEARANCE AND BREATHING PATTERNS

## Gas Exchange

### Definitions of Breathing Patterns

**A.** Abdominal respirations—breathing accomplished by abdominal muscles and diaphragm; may be used to increase effectiveness of ventilatory process in certain conditions; normal in infants and toddlers

**B.** Apnea—temporary cessation of breathing; may be seen in older adults

**C.** Cheyne-Stokes respirations—breathing followed by slow, heavier breathing and seconds of normal breathing in older adults; seen with brain injury and death

**D.** Dyspnea—difficult, labored, or painful breathing (considered "normal" at certain times, e.g., after extreme physical exertion)

**E.** Hyperpnea—abnormally deep breathing; may be seen with normal, slow, or increased rate; seen with fever, metabolic acidosis

**F.** Hyperventilation—abnormally rapid, deep, and prolonged breathing
   1. Caused by anxiety, pain, diabetic ketoacidosis, brain injury, stroke
   2. Produces respiratory alkalosis due to reduction in $CO_2$ tension

**G.** Hypoventilation—reduced ventilatory efficiency; produces respiratory acidosis due to elevation in $CO_2$ tension; caused by emphysema, pneumonia, pulmonary edema

**H.** Kussmaul respirations (air hunger)—marked increase in depth and rate of breathing; caused by diabetic ketoacidosis or metabolic acidosis

**I.** Orthopnea—inability to breathe except when trunk is in upright position; caused by severe lung or heart disease

**J.** Paradoxical respirations—breathing pattern in which a lung (or portion of a lung) deflates during inspiration (acts opposite to normal); caused by severe lung disease or flail chest

**K.** Periodic breathing—rate, depth, or tidal volume changes markedly from one interval to the next; pattern of change is periodically reproduced

**L.** Agonal respirations—gasping; the last respiratory pattern prior to terminal apnea; seen in cardiac arrest and at end of life

**M.** Adventitious lung sounds—abnormal breath sounds (*see* Table 5-1)

**Table 5-1** Breath Sounds

| ADVENTITIOUS SOUNDS | CHARACTERISTICS | CLINICAL EXAMPLES |
|---|---|---|
| Fine crackles | Popping sounds; heard mostly on late inspiration and not cleared by coughing; originates in the alveoli; sounds like rubbing hair<br><br>May clear with coughing | May be heard in pneumonia, heart failure, chronic bronchitis, and asthma |
| Coarse crackles | Discontinuous popping sounds heard early in inspiration; originate in the large bronchus; sounds are harsh and moist<br><br>May clear with coughing | May be heard in pneumonia, heart failure, chronic bronchitis, and asthma |
| Sibilant wheeze | High-pitched, musical sounds similar to a squeak<br><br>Heard more commonly on expiration, but may be heard on inspiration<br><br>Auscultated over small airways<br><br>Does not clear with coughing | Associated with narrowing of the airways, e.g., asthma, bronchospasm |
| Sonorous wheeze | Low-pitched, coarse, loud, moaning/snoring sounds heard primarily on expiration, but may be present on inspiration, arise from large airways<br><br>Coughing may clear | Associated with inflammation or partial obstruction of the trachea or bronchi, such as in bronchitis, sputum, or foreign body |
| Stridor | Harsh, high-pitched sounds heard over the trachea | Associated with upper airway (larynx and trachea) inflammation and partial obstruction |
| Pleural friction rub | A superficial, low-pitched, coarse rubbing or grating sound (sounds like two surfaces rubbing together)<br><br>Heard throughout inspiration and expiration and not cleared by coughing | Heard in individuals with pleurisy (visceral and parietal pleurae are in contact with each other due to inflammation and edema of the surfaces), pulmonary infarction, lung cancer |

# Upper Airway Obstruction

**A.** Emergency

  1. Choking

    a. Assessment

      1) Inability to breathe or speak

      2) Cyanosis

      3) Collapse

      4) Death can occur within 4–5 minutes

    b. Analysis and nursing diagnosis—impaired gas exchange related to inadequate airway clearance

    c. Nursing management—five-and-five

      1) Give 5 back blows between should blade with heel of hand

      2) Give 5 abdominal thrusts (Heimlich maneuver)

      3) Alternate between 5 back blows and 5 thrusts until blockage is dislodged

    d. Evaluation

      1) Respiratory rate returns to normal

      2) Client is able to speak

**B.** Intubation (*see* Figure 5-1 and Table 5-2)

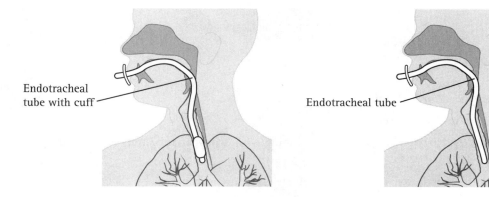

Endotracheal tube with cuff

Endotracheal tube

**Figure 5-1.** Endotracheal Tube

**Table 5-2** Intubation

| METHOD | NURSING CONSIDERATIONS |
|---|---|
| Endotracheal tube—tube passed through the nose or mouth into the trachea | Assess for bilateral breath sounds and bilateral chest excursion<br><br>Mark tube at level it touches mouth or nose<br><br>Secure with tape to stabilize<br><br>Encourage fluids to facilitate removal of secretions |
| Tracheostomy—surgical incision made into trachea via the throat; tube inserted through incision into the trachea | Cuff is used to prevent aspiration and to facilitate mechanical ventilation<br><br>Maintain cuff pressure at 20-25 mm Hg (underinflation could lead to aspiration, whereas overinflation could lead to stenosis and scarring of the trachea)<br><br>Encourage fluids to facilitate removal of secretions<br><br>Sterile suctioning if necessary<br><br>Frequent oral hygiene<br><br>Indications for suctioning tracheostomy<br><br>• Noisy respirations<br>• Restlessness<br>• Increased pulse<br>• Increased respirations<br>• Presence of mucus in airway |

C. Suctioning

1. Assess need for suctioning

2. Wear protective eyewear

3. Hyperoxygenate before and after suctioning—100% oxygen for 3 min, at least 3 deep breaths

4. Explain procedure to client (potentially frightening procedure)

5. Elevate head of bed to semi-Fowler position

6. Lubricate catheter with sterile saline, and insert without applying suction

7. Advance catheter about 16–20 cm; client will begin to cough; do not apply suction

8. Withdraw catheter 1–2 cm, apply suction and withdraw catheter with a rotating motion for no more than 10–15 seconds; wall suction set between 80–120 mm Hg

9. Hyperoxygenate for 1–5 min or until client's baseline heart rate and oxygen saturation are reached

10. Repeat procedure after client has rested, up to 3 total suction passes

11. Endotracheal tube or tracheostomy tube suctioned, then mouth is suctioned; provide mouth care

12. Complications

    a. Hypoxia

    b. Bronchospasm

    c. Tissue trauma

    d. Vagal stimulation

    e. Cardiac dysrhythmias

    f. Infection

D. Tracheostomy care—performed every 8 hours and as needed

    1. Explain procedure

    2. Suction tracheostomy tube

    3. Remove old dressings

    4. Open sterile tracheostomy care kit

    5. Put on sterile gloves

    6. Remove inner cannula (permanent or disposable)

    7. Clean with hydrogen peroxide if permanent inner cannula

    8. Rinse with sterile water, dry

    9. Reinsert into outer cannula

    10. Clean stoma site with hydrogen peroxide and sterile water, then dry

    11. Change ties or Velcro® (hook-and-loop fastener) tracheostomy tube holders as needed; old ties must remain in place until new ties are secured

    12. Apply new sterile dressing; do not cut gauze pads; use precut gauze

    13. Document site of tracheostomy, type/quantity of secretions, client tolerance of procedure

E. Mechanical ventilation

    1. Ventilator used to overcome dangers of respiratory insufficiency

        a. Forces oxygen into lungs to increase the expiration of $CO_2$

        b. Allows well-distributed airflow to the alveoli

        c. Client's breathing efforts and energy expenditure are decreased

        d. Improves the effectiveness of coughing and assists with the expulsion of accumulating secretions

    2. Nursing responsibilities

        a. Prepare client psychologically for use of ventilator

            1) Inadequately prepared clients may panic and defeat the purpose of the ventilator by "fighting" the machine's cycle and breathing ineffectively

            2) Teach client how the apparatus will help, what the client will feel on the machine, how the client can cooperate, and the basic mechanics of the ventilator

    b.  Monitor client's response to the ventilator

        1)  Assess vital signs at least every 2 hours and prn

        2)  Listen to breath sounds (crackles, rhonchi, wheezes, equal breath sounds, decreased or absent breath sounds)

        3)  Respiratory monitoring—pulse oximetry

        4)  Check ABGs, continuous pulse oximetry monitoring

        5)  Provide good oral hygiene at least twice a shift

        6)  Perform nasotracheal suctioning as necessary

        7)  Assess need for suctioning (tracheal/oral/nasal) of 2 hours and perform as necessary

        8)  Check for hypoxia (restlessness, cyanosis, anxiety, tachycardia, increased respiratory rate)

        9)  Check neurological status

      10)  Check chest for bilateral expansion

      11)  Move endotracheal tube to opposite side of mouth every 24 hours to prevent ulcers

      12)  Monitor I and O

    c.  Create alternative methods of communication with client

    d.  Perform and document ventilator checks—care for client first, ventilator second

        1)  Check ventilator settings as ordered by health care provider—tidal volume (TV), respiratory rate, fraction of inspired oxygen ($pO_2$), mode of ventilation, sigh/button cycle

        2)  Check temperature and level of water in humidification system

        3)  Drain condensation from tubing away from client

        4)  Verify that tracheostomy or endotracheal cuff is inflated to ensure tidal volume

        5)  Observe for GI distress

        6)  Document observations/procedures in client care record

**F.**  Oxygen administration (*see* Tables 5-3 and 5-4)

**Table 5-3** Oxygen Administration

| METHOD | OXYGEN DELIVERED | NURSING CONSIDERATIONS |
| --- | --- | --- |
| Nasal cannula or prongs | 23-42% at 1-6 L/min | Assess patency of nostril<br><br>Apply water-soluble jelly to nostrils every 3-4 hours<br><br>Perform good mouth care |
| Face mask | 40-60% at 6-8 L/min (oxygen flow minimum 5 L) | Remove mask every 1-2 hours<br><br>Wash, dry, apply lotion to skin<br><br>Emotional support to decrease feeling of claustrophobia |
| Partial rebreather mask | 50-75% at 8-11 L/min | Adjust oxygen flow to keep reservoir bag two-thirds full during inspiration |
| Nonrebreather mask | 80-100% at 12 L/min | Adjust oxygen flow to keep bag two-thirds full |
| Venturi mask | 24-40% at 4-8 L/min | Provides high humidity and fixed concentrations<br><br>Keep tubing free of kinks |
| Tracheostomy collar or T-piece | 30-100% at 8-10 L/min | Assess for fine mist<br><br>Empty condensation from tubing<br><br>Keep water container full |
| Oxygen hood | 30-100% at 8-10 L/min | Used for neonates<br><br>Provides cooled humid air<br><br>Check $O_2$ concentration with $O_2$ analyzer every 4 hours<br><br>Refill humidity jar with sterile distilled water<br><br>Clean humidity jar daily<br><br>Cover client with light blanket and towel or cap for head<br><br>Change linen frequently<br><br>Monitor client's temperature frequently |

**Table 5-4** Hazards of Oxygen Administration

| COMPLICATION | NURSING CONSIDERATIONS |
|---|---|
| Infection | Change masks, tubing, mouthpieces daily |
| Drying and irritation of mucosa | Administer humidified oxygen |
| Respiratory depression ($CO_2$ narcosis) | Monitor respiratory rates frequently<br><br>Alternate between breathing room air and $O_2$ at prescribed intervals<br><br>Administer mixed $O_2$ (air and $O_2$) rather than pure $O_2$<br><br>Administer minimal concentrations necessary<br><br>Periodically inflate the lungs fully |
| Oxygen toxicity | Premature infants exposed to excessive amounts of $O_2$ for prolonged periods may develop retinopathy of prematurity (ROP); may result in irreversible blindness from vasoconstriction of the retinal blood vessels<br><br>Lungs of clients on respirators (children and adults) are most susceptible to pulmonary damage<br><br>Pulmonary damage includes atelectasis, exudation of protein fluid into alveoli, damage to and proliferation of pulmonary capillaries, and interstitial hemorrhage<br><br>Early symptoms include cough, nasal congestion, sore throat, reduced vital capacity, and substernal discomfort |
| Combustion | Be sure electrical plugs and equipment are properly grounded<br><br>Enforce no-smoking rules<br><br>Do not use oils on the client or on $O_2$ equipment |

# Selected Pulmonary Disorders

**A.** Chronic obstructive pulmonary disease (COPD)—term applied to respiratory disorders that involve persistent obstruction of bronchial airflow

    1. Assessment

        a.  Change in skin color—cyanosis or reddish color

        b.  Weakness

        c.  Use of accessory muscles of breathing

        d.  Weight loss

        e.  Dyspnea

        f.  Changes in posture—day and in sleep

        g.  Cough

        h.  Changes in color, consistency of sputum

        i.  Abnormal ABGs—partial pressure of carbon dioxide ($pCO_2$), $pO_2$

  j. Adventitious breath sounds

  k. Changes in sensorium, memory impairment

2. Etiology—group of conditions associated with obstruction of airflow entering or leaving the lungs, due to genetic and environmental causes (e.g., smoking and air pollution)

  a. Risk factors

   1) Smoking tobacco

   2) Passive tobacco smoke

   3) Occupational exposure

   4) Air pollution, coal, gas, asbestos exposure

   5) Genetic abnormalities—alpha-1 antitrypsin deficiency

   6) Older adults—loss of elastic, alveolar collapse

  b. Asthma—chronic disease with episodic attacks of breathlessness

   1) Precipitating factors

    a) Intrinsic—infection in respiratory tract, sensitivity to aspirin and other NSAIDs

    b) Extrinsic—dust, pollen, food

   2) Secondary factors—stress, fatigue, endocrine changes

   3) Status asthmaticus—acute episode of bronchospasm, not relieved by bronchodilatory therapy

  c. Emphysema—overinflation of alveoli, resulting in destruction of alveolar walls; predisposing factors: smoking, chronic infections, and environmental pollution

  d. Chronic bronchitis—inflammation of bronchi with productive cough; predisposing factors: smoking, infections, environmental pollution

  e. Cystic fibrosis—hereditary dysfunction of exocrine glands, causing production of abnormally thick mucous secretions

   1) Causes—sweat gland dysfunction, respiratory dysfunction, GI dysfunction genetic disease

   2) Diagnostic tests

    a) Sweat chloride analysis—elevated levels of sodium and chloride

    b) GI enzyme evaluation—pancreatic enzyme deficiency

3. Nursing management

  a. Assess airway clearance

  b. Listen to breath sounds

  c. Assess vital signs

  d. Administer oxygen therapy at the lowest concentration to reduce hypoxia, and maintain oxygen levels between 88–92%; monitor response to oxygen therapy

  e. Encourage fluids (6–8 glasses; 3,000 mL/24 h)

  f. Administer medications—bronchodilators, mucolytics, corticosteroids, anticholinergics, leukotriene inhibitors, influenza and pneumococcal vaccines (*see* Table 5-5)

**Table 5-5** Bronchodilators/Mucolytic Medications

| MEDICATION | ADVERSE EFFECTS | NURSING CONSIDERATIONS |
|---|---|---|
| Terbutaline sulfate | Nervousness<br><br>Tremor<br><br>Headache<br><br>Tachycardia<br><br>Palpitations<br><br>Fatigue | Short-acting beta-agonist most useful when about to enter environment or begin activity likely to induce asthma attack<br><br>Pulse and blood pressure should be checked before each dose |
| Ipratropium bromide<br><br>Tiotropium | Nervousness<br><br>Tremor<br><br>Dry mouth<br><br>Palpitations | Cholinergic antagonist<br><br>Don't mix in nebulizer with cromolyn sodium<br><br>Not for acute treatment<br><br>Teach use of metered dose inhaler: inhale, hold breath, exhale slowly |
| Albuterol | Tremors<br><br>Headache<br><br>Hyperactivity<br><br>Tachycardia | Short-acting beta-agonist most useful when about to enter environment or begin activity likely to induce asthma attack<br><br>Monitor for toxicity if using tablets and aerosol<br><br>Teach how to correctly use inhaler |
| Epinephrine | Cerebral hemorrhage<br><br>Hypertension<br><br>Tachycardia | When administered IV, monitor BP, heart rate, EKG<br><br>If used with steroid inhaler, use bronchodilator first, then wait 5 minutes before using steroid inhaler (opens airway for maximum effectiveness) |
| Salmeterol | Headache<br><br>Pharyngitis<br><br>Nervousness<br><br>Tremors | Dry powder preparation<br><br>Not for acute bronchospasm or exacerbations |
| Montelukast sodium<br><br>Zafirlukast<br><br>Zileuton | Headache<br><br>GI distress | Used for prophylactic and maintenance therapy of asthma<br><br>Liver tests may be monitored<br><br>Interacts with theophylline |
| Acetylcysteine | Bronchospasm<br><br>Nausea<br><br>Vomiting | Mucolytic<br><br>Administered by nebulization into face mask or mouthpiece<br><br>Bronchospasm most likely to occur in asthmatics<br><br>Open vials should be refrigerated and used within 90 hours<br><br>Clients should clear airway by coughing prior to aerosol |

g. Chest physiotherapy—to promote removal of secretions with a minimum expenditure of energy and to decrease the need for deep tracheobronchial suctioning

   1) Breathing exercises

      a) Diaphragmatic or abdominal breathing

         i) Client positioned on back with knees bent

         ii) Place hands on abdomen

         iii) Breathe from abdomen and keep chest still

      b) Pursed-lip breathing

         i) Breathe in through nose

         ii) Purse lips and breathe out through mouth

         iii) Exhalation should be twice as long as inspiration

   2) Coughing techniques

      a) Instruct client to lean slightly forward and take several slow, deep breaths through the nose, exhaling slowly through slightly parted or pursed lips

      b) Client should then take another deep breath and cough several times during expiration

      c) Client must be encouraged to cough from deep within the chest and to avoid nonproductive coughing that wastes energy

   3) Postural drainage—uses gravity to facilitate removal of bronchial secretions

      a) Client is placed in a variety of positions to facilitate drainage into larger airways

      b) Secretions may be removed by coughing or suctioning

   4) Percussion and vibration—usually performed during postural drainage to augment the effect of gravity drainage

      a) Percussion—rhythmic striking of chest wall with cupped hands over areas where secretions are retained

      b) Vibration—hand and arm muscles of person doing vibrations are tensed, and a vibrating pressure is applied to the chest as the client exhales

   5) Incentive spirometer—used to maximize inspiration and mobilize secretions

      a) Set incentive spirometer to goal client is to reach or exceed (500 mL often used to start)

      b) Client should do 10 sustained maximal maneuvers per hour and note volume on spirometer

h. Client teaching

   1) Breathing exercises

   2) Methods of improving breathing effectiveness

   3) Stop smoking

   4) Avoid hot/cold air or allergens

        5)  Instructions about infection control

           a)  Avoid close contact with persons who have respiratory infections or the "flu"

           b)  Avoid crowds during times of the year when respiratory infections most commonly occur

           c)  Maintain a high resistance with adequate rest, nourishing diet, avoidance of stress, and avoidance of exposure to temperature extremes, dampness, and drafts

           d)  Practice frequent, thorough oral hygiene

           e)  Advise of prophylactic influenza vaccines

           f)  Instruct to observe sputum for indications of infection

**B.** Restrictive pulmonary disease

    1. Assessment

        a.  Dyspnea

        b.  Pleuritic pain

        c.  Absent or restricted movement on affected side

        d.  Decreased or absent breath sounds

        e.  Cough

        f.  Fever

        g.  Hypotension

        h.  Cyanosis

        i.  Weak, rapid pulse

        j.  Anxiety

    2. Etiology/causes—disorders associated with restrictive pulmonary disease

        a.  Pleural effusion—collection of fluid in pleural space

           1)  Pulmonary congestion so severe that distended capillaries leak fluid into alveolar spaces of the lungs

           2)  Large amounts of fluid can lead to collapse of the lung

           3)  Causes—infection, toxic chemicals, malignancies

        b.  Pneumothorax—collapse of lung due to air in pleural space (*see* Figure 5-2) caused by:

           1)  Thoracentesis—if needle "nicks" lung during procedure

           2)  Thoracic surgery—pleural cavity is entered

           3)  Accidental injury

           4)  Air leak from pulmonary alveoli or erosion of a disease process through the pleura

               a)  Spontaneous—without a known cause; common in tall, thin young men

               b)  Tension—pressure builds up, shifting of heart and great vessels, compromising circulation and respiratory functions

c. Hemothorax—collection of blood in the pleural space (*see* Figure 5-2) caused by:

1) Injury (e.g., pulmonary laceration, puncture by fractured rib)

2) Chest surgery

d. Neoplasms

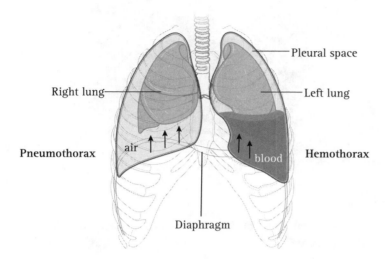

**Figure 5-2.** Pneumothorax and Hemothorax

3. Nursing management

a. Assess vital signs

b. Thoracentesis

c. High Fowler position (head of bed elevated 60–90°)

d. Oxygen therapy

e. Chest tubes (*see* Figures 5-3 and 5-4)

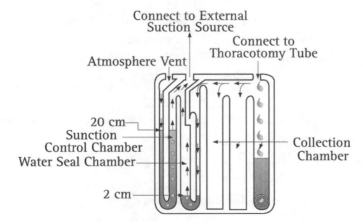

**Figure 5-3.** Water Seal Collection Apparatus

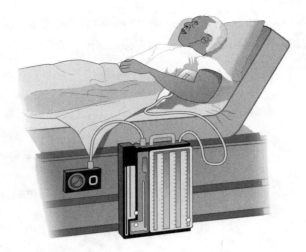

**Figure 5-4.** Pleur-evac

f.  Procedure

1)  Fill water seal chamber with sterile water to the 2-cm level or as required by the manufacturer

2)  If suction is to be used, fill the suction control chamber with sterile water to the 20-cm level or as ordered by the health care provider

3)  Encourage the client to change position frequently

4)  The drainage system must be maintained below the level of insertion

5)  Chest tubes are clamped *only momentarily* to check for air leaks and to change the drainage apparatus

6)  Observe for fluctuations of fluid in the water seal chamber

7)  Gently "milk" tubing in the direction of drainage as needed if agency policy allows

8)  When the health care provider removes the chest tubes, the nurse should instruct the client to do the Valsalva maneuver (forcibly bearing down while holding breath); the chest tube is clamped and quickly removed by the health care provider; an occlusive dressing is applied to the site

g.  Complications

1)  Observe for constant bubbling in the water seal chamber; this indicates a leak in the drainage system

2)  If the chest tube becomes dislodged, apply an occlusive dressing and notify primary health care provider

3)  If the tube becomes disconnected from the drainage system, cut the contaminated tip off the tubing, insert a sterile connector, and reattach to the drainage system; or immerse the end of the chest tube in 2 cm of sterile water until the system can be re-established

h.  Medications

**C.** Infectious pulmonary disorders

   1. Pneumonia

      a. Assessment

         1) Fever, chills

         2) Leukocytosis

         3) Cough productive of rusty-colored sputum, green whitish-yellow sputum (depends on organism)

         4) Dyspnea, accessory muscle use, upright position

         5) Pleuritic pain

         6) Tachycardia, crackles, sonorous wheezes, bronchial breath sounds

         7) Elevated WBC count, sputum culture and sensitivity, blood culture and sensitivity

      b. Etiology

         1) Causes include bacteria, fungi, viruses, parasites, chemical

         2) Inflammatory process that results in edema of lung tissues and extravasation of fluid into alveoli, causing hypoxia

         3) Risk factors

            a) Community-acquired pneumonia

               i) Older adult

               ii) Has not received pneumococcal vaccination

               iii) Has not received yearly flu vaccine

               iv) Chronic illness

               v) Exposed to viral infection or flu

               vi) Smokes or drinks alcohol

            b) Hospital-acquired pneumonia

               i) Older adult

               ii) Chronic lung disease

               iii) Aspiration

               iv) Presence of endotracheal, tracheostomy, or nasogastric tube

               v) Mechanical ventilation

               vi) Decreased level of consciousness

               vii) Immunosuppression (disease or pharmacologic etiology)

            c) Older adults—decreased cough effectiveness; decreased immune response; increased risk with decreased mobility and swallowing disorders

     c.  Nursing management

       1)  Assess vital signs every 4 h

       2)  Cough and breathe deeply every 2 h

       3)  Assess breath sounds and oxygen saturation

       4)  Incentive spirometer—5–10 breaths per hour while awake

       5)  Encourage fluids to 3,000 mL/24 h

       6)  Suctioning as needed

       7)  Oxygen therapy

       8)  Semi-Fowler position/bedrest

       9)  Teaching: fluid intake and stop smoking

      10)  Medications

         a)  Mucolytics

         b)  Expectorants

         c)  Bronchodilators (e.g., beta-2 agonist)—nebulizer or metered dose inhaler (MDI)

         d)  Antibiotics

  2.  Croup syndromes; acute epiglottitis, acute laryngotracheobronchitis, acute laryngitis, respiratory syncytial virus

     a.  Assessment

       1)  Bark-like cough

       2)  Dyspnea

       3)  Inspiratory stridor

       4)  Cyanosis

     b.  Causes

       1)  Viral

       2)  Medical emergency due to narrowed airway in children

     c.  Nursing management

       1)  Care at home

         a)  Steamy shower

         b)  Sudden exposure to cold air

         c)  Sleep with cool humidified air

       2)  Hospitalization required if:

         a)  Increasing respiratory distress

         b)  Hypoxia or depressed sensorium

         c)  High temperature (102°F)

       3)  Nursing care if hospitalized

         a)  Maintain airway

         b)  Mist tent

    c) Monitor heart and respiratory rate

    d) Oxygen with humidification

    e) IV fluids or oral hydration

    f) Medications—antipyretics, antibiotics, bronchodilators

    g) Position in infant seat or prop with pillow

    h) Calm, quiet environment

    i) Cough and deep breathe at least every 2 hours

3. Tuberculosis (TB)

  a. Assessment

    1) Progressive fatigue, nausea, anorexia, weight loss

    2) Irregular menses

    3) Low-grade fevers over a period of time

    4) Night sweats

    5) Irritability

    6) Cough with mucopurulent sputum, occasionally streaked with blood; chest tightness and a dull, aching chest; dyspnea

    7) Diagnostic procedures

      a) Skin testing (*see* Table 5-6)

**Table 5-6** TB Skin Testing

| TEST | NURSING CONSIDERATIONS |
|---|---|
| Mantoux test | Given intradermally in the forearm |
| Purified protein derivative (PPD) | 15 mm or greater induration (hard area under the skin) = significant (positive) reaction for those clients without certain risk factors |
| | Read in 48–72 hours |
| | Positive result does not necessarily mean that active disease is present but indicates exposure to TB or the presence of inactive (dormant) disease |
| | Greater than 5 mm for clients with AIDS = positive reaction |
| | TB infection may still be present in older adults or immunocompromised with induration $\leq$10 mm |
| Multiple puncture test (Tine) | Read test in 48–72 hours |
| | Vesicle formation = positive reaction |
| | Screening test only |
| | Questionable or positive reactions verified by Mantoux test |

        b)    Sputum smear for acid-fast bacilli; induce by respiratory therapy in A.M. and P.M.

        c)    Chest x-ray—routinely performed on all persons with positive purified protein derivative (PPD) to detect old and new lesions; tubercles may be seen in lungs

        d)    Quanti FERON-TB Gold test; results within 24 hours

  b.  Etiology

      1)  Transmitted by airborne release droplet nuclei; bacillus multiplies in bronchi or alveoli, resulting in pneumonitis; may lie dormant for many years and be reactivated in periods of stress; mycobacterium tuberculosis (acid-fast Gram-positive bacillus)

      2)  Risk factors

        a)    Close contact with someone who has active tuberculosis

        b)    Immunocompromised status

        c)    IV drug users

        d)    Persons who live in institutions

        e)    Lower socioeconomic groups

        f)    Immigrants from countries with high prevalence of tuberculosis (Latin America, Southeast Asia, Africa)

      3)  Incidence increasing in immigrant populations, poverty areas, older adults, alcoholics, drug abusers, and persons with AIDS

  c.  Nursing management

      1)  Notification of state health department; evaluation of contacts

      2)  Isoniazid (INH) prophylaxis—not recommended for those individuals greater than 35 years old who are at low risk because of increased risk of associated hepatitis; persons less than 35 get 6–9 month therapy with INH (see Table 5-6)

        a)    Household contacts

        b)    Recent converters

        c)    Persons under age 20 with positive reaction and inactive TB

        d)    Susceptible health care workers

        e)    Newly infected persons

        f)    Significant skin test reactors with abnormal x-ray studies

        g)    Significant skin test reactors up to age 35

      3)  Chemotherapy—to prevent development of resistant strains, two or three medications are usually administered concurrently; frequently a 6- or 9-month regimen of isoniazid and rifampin; ethambutol and streptomycin may be used initially

      4)  Isolation for 2–4 wk (or three negative sputum cultures) after medication therapy is initiated; sent home before this (family already exposed)

5) Teaching

   a) Cover mouth and nose with tissue when coughing, sneezing, laughing; place tissues into plastic bag

   b) Avoid excessive exposure to dust and silicone; wear mask in crowds

   c) Handwashing

   d) Must take full course of medications

   e) Encourage to return to clinic for sputum smears

   f) Good nutrition (increased iron, protein, vitamins B + C)

**Table 5-7** Antitubercular Medications

| MEDICATION | ADVERSE EFFECTS | NURSING CONSIDERATIONS |
|---|---|---|
| **First-Line Medications** | | |
| Isoniazid | Toxic hepatitis<br>Peripheral neuritis<br>Rash<br>Fever | Pyridoxine ($B_6$): 10–50 mg as prophylaxis for neuritis; 50–100 mg as treatment<br>Teach signs of hepatitis<br>Check liver function tests<br>Alcohol increases risk of hepatic complications<br>Therapeutic effects can be expected after 2–3 weeks of therapy<br>Monitor for resolution of symptoms (fever, night sweats, weight loss); hypotension (orthostatic) may occur initially, then resolve; caution client to change position slowly<br>Give before meals<br>Do not combine with Dilantin, causes phenytoin toxicity |
| Ethambutol | Optic neuritis | Use cautiously with renal disease<br>Check visual acuity |
| Rifampin | Toxic hepatitis<br>Fever | Orange urine, tears, saliva<br>Check liver function tests<br>Can take with food |
| Streptomycin | Nephrotoxicity<br>VIII nerve damage | Check creatinine and BUN<br>Audiograms if given long-term |

*(Continued)*

**Table 5-8** Antitubercular Medication (*Continued*)

| MEDICATION | ADVERSE EFFECTS | NURSING CONSIDERATIONS |
|---|---|---|
| **Second-Line Medications** | | |
| Para-aminosalicylic acid | GI disturbances<br><br>Hepatotoxicity | Check for ongoing GI adverse effects |
| Pyrazinamide | Hyperuricemia<br><br>Anemia<br><br>Anorexia | Check liver function tests, uric acid, and hematopoietic studies |
| **Action** | Inhibits cell wall and protein synthesis of *Mycobacterium tuberculosis* | |
| **Indications** | Tuberculosis<br><br>INH—used to prevent disease in person exposed to organism | |
| **Adverse effects** | Toxic hepatitis<br><br>Optic neuritis<br><br>Seizures<br><br>Peripheral neuritis | |
| **Nursing considerations** | Used in combination (2 medications or more)<br><br>Monitor for liver damage and hepatitis<br><br>With active TB, the client should cover mouth and nose when coughing, confine used tissues to plastic bags, and wear a mask with crowds until three sputum cultures are negative (no longer infectious)<br><br>For in-client settings, client is placed under airborne precautions and workers wear an N95 or high-efficiency particulate air (HEPA) respirator until the client is no longer infectious | |

# End-of-Chapter Thinking Exercise

The student nurse is assigned to complete an admission assessment on an older adult client admitted for an exacerbation of COPD. The client is a retired demolition expert and has been a two-pack a day smoker for 40 years. Every year during the winter, the client is admitted to the hospital with a respiratory infection. The client is 5' 9" (175.3 cm), weighs 139 lb (63 kg), and exclaims, "I used to be brawny, but now I'm just scrawny!" Upon assessment, the client has a ruddy facial appearance, a hoarse voice, and cannot complete a sentence without stopping to take a few breaths. Auscultation of the lungs reveals decreased breath sounds throughout and inspiratory wheezes in both upper lobes. The client has a productive cough of thick yellow sputum. The client uses continuous $O_2$ at 2 L/min via nasal cannula, and the $SpO_2$ is 85%. A barrel chest is observed, and the client is using accessory muscles to breathe. Vital signs: Temp 98.6°F (37°C), pulse 103 and regular, respiratory rate 29 and shallow, BP 118/78 mm Hg.

1. The student nurse recognizes that the client has four risk factors for COPD. What are they? (Recognize Cues)

2. Given the respiratory assessment data, what drug classifications does the student nurse expect to see on the Medication Administration Record (MAR)? (Analyze Cues)

3. What does the student nurse include in a teaching plan for this client? (Generate Solutions)

## Thinking Exercise Explanations

1.  The student nurse recognizes that the client has four risk factors for COPD. What are they? (Recognize Cues)

    - Older adult
    - Occupational exposure
    - Smoker
    - Chronic respiratory infections

    These factors cause a decrease in the elasticity of the alveoli and decrease the gas exchange effectiveness of the alveoli over time.

2.  Given the respiratory assessment data, what drug classifications does the student nurse expect to see on the Medication Administration Record (MAR)? (Analyze Cues)

    - Bronchodilators (e.g., albuterol)
    - Mucolytics (e.g., acetylcysteine)
    - Corticosteroids (e.g., prednisone)
    - Leukotriene inhibitors (e.g., montelukast)

    The goal of medication therapy with COPD is to improve breathing patterns, maintain effective airway clearance, and increase oxygen and carbon dioxide exchange in the alveoli.

3.  What does the student nurse include in a teaching plan for this client? (Generate Solutions)

    - Smoking cessation
    - Breathing exercises
    - Prevention techniques for respiratory infections
    - Balance rest and activities
    - Avoid temperature extremes
    - Eat high-calorie, nutrient-dense foods
    - Drink 2–3 L of fluid/24 h

    The above teaching points will enable the client to manage the disease effectively in the home setting, maintaining the optimum quality of life within the limitations of the disease.

## [ CHAPTER 6 ]

# HEMATOLOGICAL AND IMMUNE DISORDERS

**SECTIONS**

**CONCEPTS COVERED**

1. Overview of Hematology

2. Disorders of the Blood

3. The Immune System

# OVERVIEW OF HEMATOLOGY

## Cellular Regulation

### Plasma

A. Albumin—regulates plasma volume; regulates osmotic pressure

B. Serum globulins—transport of lipids, bilirubin; has immune function

C. Fibrinogen—involved in blood coagulation

D. Prothrombin—involved in blood coagulation

E. Plasminogen—involved in blood coagulation

### Cellular Components

A. Produced in bone marrow—hemopoiesis

B. Erythrocytes (RBCs)—transport of oxygen by hemoglobin

C. Leukocytes (WBCs)—protection from infection

D. Thrombocytes (platelets)—involved in coagulation

### Signs and Symptoms of Hematologic Disorders

A. Chronic fatigue and dyspnea—decrease in erythrocytes (e.g., anemias, leukemias, and hemorrhagic disorders) causes a reduction in the oxygen-carrying capacity of the blood

B. Increased susceptibility to infection—decrease in mature circulating leukocytes

C. Gastrointestinal symptoms—anorexia, weight loss, indigestion, sore mouth and tongue

D. Hemorrhage and bleeding into tissues and joints (hemarthrosis) and from mucous membranes— results from either a decrease in the platelet count or absence of one or more clotting factors

E. Bone pain and deformity—result from hyperactivity of bone marrow or from growth of bone tumors (e.g., multiple myeloma)

F. Jaundice—results from rupture and hemolysis of abnormal erythrocytes, as seen in hemolytic anemias and pernicious anemia, causing the release of large amounts of bilirubin into the circulation

G. Enlarged liver and spleen and hyperplasia of bone marrow—caused by either congestion from overproduction of cells (e.g., polycythemia, leukemia) or excessive demands upon these organs to destroy defective cells (e.g., hemolytic anemias)

H. Mental depression—results from the chronicity of most blood diseases and the fatigue and discomfort characteristic of these disorders

I. Protect the client from chills or burns

   1. Due to poor circulation, anemic clients often report feeling cold—offer warm clothing and blankets

   2. Avoid applying heating pads or hot water bottles to clients with anemia because they burn easily

      a. Skin is poorly supplied with blood and oxygen

      b. Client may be unaware of any burning sensation

J. Isolate client from possible sources of infection—severely anemic clients are typically exhausted and debilitated, consequently develop infections easily

# DISORDERS OF THE BLOOD

## Coagulation

## Disorders of the Blood

**A.** Basic physiological disturbances characterizing hematopoietic disorders

   1. Decrease in number of cells (cytopenia)

      a. Decrease in erythrocytes: anemia

      b. Decrease in leukocytes: leukopenia—associated with increased vulnerability to infection

      c. Decrease in thrombocyte or platelet count: thrombocytopenia—associated with increased risk of hemorrhage

**B.** Overproduction of either normal or defective cells

   1. Myeloproliferative diseases—malignant overproduction of cells, takes place within the bone marrow

      a. Polycythemia—abnormal increase in erythrocyte production

      b. Leukemia—increase in manufacture of abnormal, immature leukocytes

      c. Plasma cell myeloma or multiple myeloma—abnormal malignant proliferation of plasma cells

**C.** Lymphoproliferative diseases—cellular overproduction occurs within the lymphatic tissues

   1. Hodgkin lymphoma—malignant proliferation of one form of reticuloendothelial cell within the lymph nodes; lymph nodes contain Reed-Sternberg cells

   2. Non-Hodgkin lymphoma—all lymphoid cancers that do not contain the Reed-Sternberg cell

   3. Leukemia—overproduction of lymphocytes within the lymph nodes

   4. Lymphosarcoma—abnormal proliferation of lymphocytes or lymphoblasts within the lymph nodes

**D.** Defects in coagulation mechanism—caused by depletion or absence of one or more clotting factors

   1. Characterized by persistent bleeding and hemorrhage

   2. Includes the hemophilias, hypoprothrombinemia, and disseminated intravascular coagulation

E.   Disorders of the spleen

   1.   Include enlargement of the spleen (splenomegaly) and splenic rupture (result of accident or trauma)

F.   Causative factors

   1.   Hemorrhage

   2.   Dietary deficiencies

   3.   Malabsorption disorders

   4.   Infection

   5.   Toxicity of medications

   6.   Malignant overproduction of cells

   7.   Increased destruction of cells by an overactive spleen

   8.   Genetic predisposition

   9.   Immunological defects

   10.   Older adults—decreased stem cell function; decreased reticulocyte and platelet production (especially during increased demand)

G.   Abnormalities of erythrocytes

   1.   Two basic pathophysiological developments underlying all erythrocyte disorders

      a.   A deficient number of circulating red blood cells (anemia) due to one or all of the following:

         1)   Insufficient erythrocyte production

         2)   Defective erythrocyte synthesis

         3)   Increased erythrocyte destruction

         4)   Increased erythrocyte loss

      b.   An increased number of circulating red blood cells (polycythemia) due to either:

         1)   A disorder of unknown etiology

         2)   A compensatory mechanism that develops in response to tissue hypoxia (secondary polycythemia); seen with chronic bronchitis

   2.   Types of erythrocyte abnormalities

      a.   Anisocytosis—erythrocytes vary in size from normal

      b.   Poikilocytosis—abnormally shaped erythrocytes, characteristic of any of the anemias with most bizarre shapes seen in the most severe anemias

      c.   Microcyte—abnormally small erythrocytes, characteristic of microcytic anemias (e.g., iron-deficiency anemia, thalassemia major)

      d.   Macrocyte—abnormally large erythrocytes, characterized by microcytic anemias (e.g., pernicious anemia, folic acid deficiency anemia)

      e.   Hypochromic cells—erythrocytes appear pale because of abnormally low hemoglobin content

      f.   Spherocyte—erythrocytes relatively small and round rather than biconcave in shape, characteristic of thalassemia major or hemoglobin C disease

g. Schistocyte—fragmented erythrocytes with extremely bizarre shapes (e.g., triangles, spirals characteristic of hemolytic anemia)

h. Sickle cell—erythrocytes are crescent or sickle shaped due to presence of abnormal hemoglobin (hemoglobin S)

## Iron-Deficiency Anemia

A decrease in the number of erythrocytes or a reduction in hemoglobin

**A.** Iron-deficiency anemia—hemoglobin under 13 g/dL (130 g/L) for males; under 12 g/dL (120 g/L) for females

1. Mild

   a. Asymptomatic at rest

   b. Symptoms usually follow strenuous exertion—palpitations, dyspnea, diaphoresis

2. Moderate

   a. Dyspnea

   b. Palpitations

   c. Diaphoresis

   d. Chronic fatigue

3. Severe

   a. Pale

   b. Exhausted all the time

   c. Severe palpitations

   d. Sensitivity to cold

   e. Loss of appetite

   f. Profound weakness

   g. Dizziness, syncope

   h. Headache

   i. Cardiac complications—CHF, angina pectoris

4. Diagnostic tests

   a. Total erythrocyte count

   b. Hemoglobin and hematocrit (Hct) determination; hemoglobin levels decrease after middle age

   c. Plasma ferritin level

   d. Zinc protoporphyrin/heme (ZnPP/heme) ratio

   e. Transferrin saturation

5. Assessment

   a. Presence of symptoms—fatigue, dizziness, headache, "pins and needles" sensation in fingers and toes

    b. Color of urine and stools over past weeks and months (tarry stools and/or brown, hazy, or smoky urine may indicate internal bleeding)

    c. Adequacy of diet

    d. Tolerance of exercise

    e. Medications taken in recent past (increased risk of gastric irritation)

    f. Recent exposure to poisonous substances or insecticides

    g. Whether client is or has been treated for chronic infections, cancer, renal disease, liver disease, bleeding ulcers, or hemorrhoids

    h. Family history—some blood disorders are hereditary (e.g., hereditary spherocytosis), some are linked with race (e.g., sickle cell anemia), and some with ethnicity (e.g., thalassemia major)

    i. Excessive blood loss, (e.g., bleeding due to trauma or cancer)

    j. Deficiencies and abnormalities of erythrocyte production

    k. Dietary deficiencies

    l. Ingestion or absorption of poisons or medications that suppress the bone marrow

    m. Chronic infections

    n. Genetic abnormalities that result in faulty erythrocyte genesis and/or structure

    o. Excessive destruction of erythrocytes

    p. Gerontologic considerations—iron absorption decreased, iron intake possibly decreased

**B.** Nursing management

  1. Provide specific treatment

    a. Reverse deficiencies, e.g., iron deficiency anemia is cured with iron preparations and diet

    b. Discontinue any damaging medication or chemical agent

    c. In the case of excessive blood loss, identify cause of bleeding, control bleeding, and administer transfusions as ordered and needed

  2. Encourage frequent rest periods—rest is essential to lower the client's oxygen requirements and reduce strain on the heart and lungs

    a. Clients with mild anemia are rarely hospitalized and are fully ambulatory; should be encouraged to rest and nap frequently, especially if the client experiences dizziness or light-headedness

    b. Clients with severe anemia are usually hospitalized and placed on bedrest

  3. Prevent skin breakdown with frequent turning and positioning

    a. Due to reduction in circulating red blood cells, the tissues of the anemic client do not receive adequate amounts of oxygen

    b. Without proper skin care, hypoxic tissues can cause rapid pressure injuries to form

  4. Provide a diet that is high in protein, iron, and vitamins—these substances are essential to normal erythrocyte formation

5. If anorexia is a problem, serve six small, easily digested meals a day instead of three large meals

   a. Avoid hot, spicy foods if the client suffers from a sore mouth or throat

   b. Provide oral hygiene before and after the client eats

   c. Feed the client if too exhausted to feed self

6. Provide good oral hygiene, especially because these clients often suffer from a sore mouth or tongue

   a. Cleanse the teeth before and after meals with a soft-bristled toothbrush or applicator

   b. Encourage client to rinse mouth every two hours with mouthwash that is cool and slightly alkaline

   c. Lubricate lips frequently with mineral oil or petroleum jelly to prevent dryness or cracking

7. Carefully monitor blood transfusions, if indicated—blood transfusions are valuable in the treatment of anemia due to blood loss

8. Provide oxygen therapy, if indicated

   a. Given to clients with severe anemia due to a greatly reduced capacity of the blood to carry oxygen

   b. Supplemental oxygen helps to prevent tissue hypoxia and lessens the work of the heart as it struggles to compensate for the deficiency of oxygen-carrying hemoglobin

9. Protect the client from chills or burns

   a. Due to poor circulation, anemic clients often report feeling cold and being chilled—offer warm clothing and blankets

   b. Avoid applying heating pads or hot water bottles to clients with anemia because they burn easily

      1) Skin is poorly supplied with blood and oxygen, causing tendency to burn

      2) Client may be unaware of any burning sensation

10. Isolate client from possible sources of infection—severely anemic clients are typically exhausted and debilitated, consequently develop infections easily

11. Administer iron supplements

    a. IM or IV iron dextran: IV route preferred; risk of hypersensitivity reaction; IM route may cause skin staining and pain

    b. Oral iron: administer between meals for better absorption; may give with meals if gastric distress occurs; use straw if liquids used; take oral supplements with ascorbic acid to increase absorption

# Thalassemia

A. Etiology

    1. Insufficient production of normal hemoglobin

    2. Autosomal recessive genetic disorder

    3. Affects ethnic groups with origins near the Mediterranean area

    4. Major and minor forms of thalassemia

B. Assessment

    1. General symptoms of anemia

    2. Thalassemia major: hepatomegaly, splenomegaly, jaundice

    3. Growth restriction in children

C. Nursing management

    1. Thalassemia major—blood transfusions and chelation therapy

    2. Splenectomy

    3. Thalassemia minor—generally no treatment as body adapts to reduction of normal hemoglobin

# Megaloblastic Anemias

A. Etiology

    1. Large RBCs; caused by impaired DNA synthesis

    2. Folic acid deficiency, vitamin $B_{12}$ deficiency, medications, inborn errors, erythroleukemia

    3. Common forms—pernicious anemia (megaloblastic) and folic acid deficiency

    4. Pernicious anemia—insidious onset after age 40; high frequency in women

        a. Intrinsic factor no longer secreted by the parietal cells of gastric mucosa

        b. Intrinsic factor necessary for cobalamin ($B_{12}$) absorption

        c. Autoimmune disease; highest incidence in African Americans and in persons of Scandinavian descent

        d. Also occurs with gastrectomy, bowel resection of the ileum, Crohn disease

        e. Older adults—insufficient absorption of vitamin $B_{12}$, decreased vitamin $B_{12}$ intake

B. Assessment

    1. General symptoms of anemia

    2. GI manifestations—sore tongue, anorexia, abdominal pain, nausea, and vomiting

    3. Neuromuscular—paresthesias of hands and feet, ataxia, muscle weakness, impaired thought processes

C. Diagnostic studies

    1. Gastric analysis via NG tube

        a. Pentagastrin injected to stimulate gastric juice secretion, and gastric juice withdrawn via tube

b. Gastric juice with achlorhydria indicates depressed parietal cell function

c. Schilling test—radioactive cobalamin given to client; cobalamin excreted in urine is measured; small amount excreted if client is unable to absorb cobalamin

**D.** Nursing management

1. General anemia precautions

2. Protect client from injury due to decreased sensation to temperature and pain

3. Monthly cobalamin injections or cyanocobalamin nasal spray

4. Evaluate family members for pernicious anemia

5. Client is at higher risk for gastric carcinoma; ongoing evaluation

# Sickle Cell Disease (SCD)

**A.** Etiology

1. Family of genetic disorders caused by mutant sickle cell hemoglobin (HbS)

2. Predominant in African Americans and in people of Mediterranean, Caribbean, South and Central American, Arabian, or East Indian ancestry

3. SCD affects 50,000 Americans; incurable

4. Sickle cell anemia is autosomal recessive genetic disorder

5. Sickle cell trait—25% of hemoglobin in abnormal "S" form; 75% in the normal "A" form

6. Median survival of SCD clients is 40–50 y

**B.** Assessment

1. Hypoxia changes the RBCs containing HbS from biconcave disk to elongated crescent, or sickle cell

2. Sickle cells clog small capillaries, causing more local hypoxia and more sickling

3. Occluded blood vessels → thrombosis

4. Ischemia and necrosis of infarcted tissue

5. Gradual involvement of all body systems

6. Precipitating factors—viral and bacterial infections, high altitudes, emotional/physical stress, surgery, blood loss, dehydration, cold water

7. Children—impairment of growth and development

8. Symptoms of chronic anemia

9. Hand-foot syndrome—bone infarction causing painful swelling of hands and feet; first symptom of SCD

10. Acute sickle cell crisis

a. Tissue hypoxia → tissue death, pain, jaundice

b. Common sites—chest, back, extremities, abdomen

C. Diagnostic studies

1. Hemoglobin (Hgb) level ranges from 7–10 g/dL (70–100 g/L)

2. Peripheral blood smear; sickled cells present

3. Sickle cell preparation

4. Sickling test to determine presence of HbS; determines if trait is present

D. Complications

1. Heart failure

2. Pulmonary infarction

3. Retinal hemorrhage, scarring, detachment, blindness

4. Renal damage

5. Stroke

6. Leg ulcers

7. Osteoporosis and osteosclerosis

8. Priapism

9. Pneumonia

10. Shock

E. Nursing management

1. Acute crisis—$O_2$ therapy, rest, fluids, transfusion therapy for aplastic crisis

2. Pain management—narcotic analgesics; client-controlled analgesia (PCA); morphine or hydromorphone

3. Hydroxyurea; antisickling agent lessens the sickling process, decreases incidence of crises; risk of leukemia and bone marrow depression

4. Preventive care—adequate fluid intake, treatment of infections, antibiotics, folic acid,

5. Client education—avoid high altitudes, extreme temperatures, dehydration; promptly treat infection

## Thrombocytopenia

A. Etiology

1. Reduction in platelets to below 150,000/mm$^3$ (150 × 10$^9$/L)

2. Inherited and acquired disorder

3. May be caused by some foods or medications (chemotherapy or antiseizure medications)

B. Immune thrombocytopenic purpura (ITP)

1. Autoimmune disease seen in children after viral illness; affects adult females between the ages of 20–40

2. Platelets destroyed between 1–3 d instead of 8–10 d

C. Assessment

1. Small, flat, pinpoint red microhemorrhages (petechiae)

2. Numerous petechiae (reddish skin bruise)—purpura; larger lesions—ecchymoses

3. Prolonged bleeding after venipuncture or injection; mucosal bleeding

4. Weakness, fainting, dizziness, tachycardia, abdominal pain, hypotension

D. Diagnostic studies

1. Bleeding time prolonged

2. Activated partial thromboplastin time (aPTT)

3. Prothrombin time (PT)/international normalized ratio (INR)

4. Bone marrow aspiration and biopsy

5. Hgb and Hct decreased

6. Antiplatelet antibodies

E. Nursing management

1. Platelet transfusions (ITP) for platelet counts ≤20,000/mm$^3$ (20 × 10$^9$/L)

2. IV immunoglobulin (ITP)—IV anti-Rho(D), raise platelet count

3. Corticosteroids

4. Plasma infusion to treat thrombotic thrombocytopenic purpura (TTP)

5. Plasmapheresis and plasma exchange (treats TTP)

6. Splenectomy for clients not responsive to medical therapy

7. Danazol—decreases immune response

8. Immunosuppressants, e.g., rituximab, cyclophosphamide, azathioprine

9. Prevent/control hemorrhage

10. Client education

a. Avoid OTC meds that may cause acquired thrombocytopenia

b. Avoid Valsalva maneuver; cough, sneeze, and blow nose gently

c. Avoid any activities that could cause hemorrhage

d. Report development of new petechiae or nosebleed

# Hemophilia

Hereditary bleeding disorder that results from deficiency of or nonfunctioning factor VIII

A. Etiology

1. Hereditary bleeding disorder caused by defective coagulation factor

2. Hemophilia A—factor VIII deficiency; most common

3. Hemophilia B—factor IX deficiency

4. Sex-linked—transmitted to male by female carrier; recessive trait

B. Assessment

1. Spontaneous, easy bruising, subcutaneous hematoma

2. Joint pain with bleeding, hematuria, gingival bleeding, GI bleeding

3. Prolonged internal or external bleeding from mild trauma

4. Pallor, anesthesia from compression caused by hematomas

C. Treatment

1. Transfusions—plasma with factor VIII cryoprecipitate

2. Bedrest

3. Analgesics

D. Diagnostic studies

1. Factor assays—factor VIII, von Willebrand factor (vWF), factor IX

2. Bleeding time

3. Prothrombin time (INR) and thrombin time

4. Platelet count

5. Partial thromboplastin time

E. Nursing management

1. Assess for internal bleeding

2. Analgesics for joint pain, not aspirin

3. Avoid IM injections

4. Stop topical bleeding with pressure or ice

5. Bedrest during bleeding episodes

6. Replacement of deficient clotting factors during acute episodes and prophylactically (cryoprecipitate factor VIII)

7. Client education—prevention of injury; home management; daily oral hygiene

# THE IMMUNE SYSTEM

## Immune Response, Immunity, Infection, Inflammation

### Immune Response

A. Functions of the immune system

   1. Defense—destruction of viruses, fungi, bacteria

   2. Homeostasis—removal of damaged cells

   3. Surveillance—removal of mutated cells

   4. Altered responses—allergic, autoimmune, immunodeficiency disorders, malignancies

B. Types of acquired specific deficiency

   1. Active/natural—contact with antigen (e.g., childhood diseases), develops slowly; protective within weeks; long-term and specific

   2. Active/artificial—immunization with antigen (i.e., immunization with live/killed vaccine, toxoid); protective in a few weeks (lasts several years, booster often needed)

   3. Passive/natural—transplacental and colostrum transfer; temporary (lasts months)

   4. Passive/artificial—injection of serum from immune human or animal (i.e., human gammaglobulin); immediate immunity (lasts several weeks)

C. Gerontologic considerations—total WBC count normal in older adults; may see slight drop in neutrophils; decreased T-cell function; decreased primary and secondary humoral antibody response; higher incidence of malignancies; decreased antibody response to immunizations; higher incidence of infections

## AIDS

Acquired immune deficiency syndrome

A. Etiology—an RNA virus; replicates inside a living cell, transcribes into DNA, which enters cell nuclei, becoming permanent part of genetic structure

   1. Initial infection—viremia

   2. Human immunodeficiency virus (HIV) may remain dormant for 8–10 y

   3. HIV infects human cells with CD4 receptors on the surfaces—lymphocytes, monocytes/macrophages, astrocytes, oligodendrocytes

   4. CD4+ T cells destroyed by HIV

**B.** Assessment

1. HIV—presence of HIV in the blood

2. AIDS—syndrome with CD4/T-cell counts below 200/microL

3. Diagnostic tests

    a. Positive HIV antibody on enzyme-linked immunosorbent assay (ELISA) and confirmed by western blot assay or indirect immunofluorescence assay (IFA)—at least 2-mo window between infection and detection

    b. Viral load testing, $T_4$:$T_8$ ratio, antigen assays

    c. Radioimmunoprecipitation assay (RIPA)

    d. CBC reveals leukopenia with serious lymphopenia, anemia, thrombocytopenia

    e. Home-testing kits on oral secretions

    f. Seroconversion—development of HIV-specific antibodies; flu-like syndrome 1–3 wk after injection

    g. Early disease—CD4+ T-cell count drops below 500–600/microL, oral thrush, headache, aseptic meningitis, peripheral neuropathies, cranial nerve palsy

4. Opportunistic infections

    a. *Pneumocystis jirovecii* pneumonia

        1) Gradually worsening chest tightness and shortness of breath

        2) Persistent, dry, nonproductive cough; crackles

        3) Dyspnea and tachypnea

        4) Low-grade/high fever

        5) Progressive hypoxemia and cyanosis

    b. *Candida albicans* stomatitis or esophagitis

        1) Changes in taste sensation

        2) Difficulty swallowing

        3) Retrosternal pain

        4) White exudate and inflammation of mouth and back of throat

    c. *Cryptococcus neoformans*—severe, debilitating meningitis

        1) Fever, headache, blurred vision

        2) Nausea and vomiting

        3) Stiff neck, mental status changes, seizures

    d. Cytomegalovirus (CMV)—significant factor in morbidity and mortality

        1) Fever, malaise

        2) Weight loss, fatigue

        3) Lymphadenopathy

        4) Retinochoroiditis characterized by inflammation and hemorrhage

        5) Visual impairment

      6) Colitis, encephalitis, pneumonitis

      7) Adrenalitis, hepatitis, disseminated infection

   e. Kaposi sarcoma—most common malignancy

      1) Small, purplish-brown, nonpainful, nonpruritic, palpable lesions occurring on any part of the body

      2) Most commonly seen on the skin

      3) Diagnosed by biopsy

5. AIDS-dementia complex (ADC)

   a. Onset of progressive dementia

6. AIDS (acquired syndrome)—a syndrome distinguished by serious deficits in cellular immune function associated with positive HIV; evidenced clinically by development of opportunistic infections (e.g., *Pneumocystis jirovecii* pneumonia, *Candida albicans,* cytomegalovirus), enteric pathogens, and malignancies (most commonly Kaposi sarcoma)

   a. High-risk groups

      1) Homosexual or bisexual men—especially with multiple partners

      2) Intravenous drug abusers

      3) Hemophiliacs—via contaminated blood products

      4) Blood transfusion recipients prior to 1985

      5) Heterosexual partners of infected persons

      6) Children of infected women, *in utero* or at birth

   b. Transmission—contaminated blood or body fluids, sharing IV drug needles, sexual contact, transplacental, and possibly through breast milk

   c. Time from exposure to symptom manifestation may be prolonged (8–10 y)

**C.** Nursing management

   1. Preventive measures

      a. Avoidance of IV drug use (needle sharing)

      b. Precautions regarding sexual patterns—sex education, condoms, avoid multiple partners

      c. Use of standard precautions—blood/body fluids

   2. Nursing care (*see* Table 6-1)

**Table 6-1** Nursing Care of a Client with Acquired Immune Deficiency Syndrome

| PROBLEM | NURSING CONSIDERATIONS |
|---|---|
| Fatigue | Provide restful environment |
| | Assist with personal care |
| | Monitor tolerance for visitors |
| Pain | Give meds as appropriate |
| | Assess level of pain |
| | Comfort measures |
| | Analgesia |
| Disease susceptibility | Implement infection control precautions |
| | Handwashing or alcohol-based rubs on entering and leaving room |
| | Monitor for oral infections and meningitis |
| | Give antibiotics as ordered |
| | No fresh flowers or plants |
| | Low-bacteria diet |
| Respiratory distress | Monitor vital signs, chest sounds |
| | Give bronchodilators and antibiotics as ordered |
| | Suction and maintain $O_2$ as prescribed |
| | Monitor for symptoms of secondary infections |
| Anxiety, depression | Use tact, sensitivity in gathering personal data |
| | Encourage expression of feelings |
| | Respect client's own limits in ability to discuss problems |
| | Guided imagery |
| Anorexia, diarrhea | Monitor weight |
| | Encourage nutritional supplements |
| | Assess hydration |
| | Give antidiarrheal medication—diphenoxylate |
| | Diet—less roughage, spicy foods |
| | Monitor perineal area for irritation |

a. No effective cure; antiretroviral medications (*see* Table 6-2); highly active antiretroviral therapy (HAART)—combination antiretroviral medications

**Table 6-2** Antiretroviral Medications

| TYPE | MEDICATION NAME |
|---|---|
| Nucleoside reverse transcriptase inhibitors (NRTIs) | Zidovudine |
| | Didanosine |
| | Stavudine |
| | Lamivudine |
| | Combivir (lamivudine and zidovudine combination) |
| Non-nucleoside reverse transcriptase inhibitors (NNRTIs) | Nevirapine |
| | Delavirdine |
| | Efavirenz |
| Protease inhibitors (PIs) | Saquinavir |
| | Indinavir |
| | Ritonavir |
| | Nelfinavir |
| Fusion inhibitors | Enfuvirtide |
| Integrase strand transfer inhibitor | Raltegravir |

b. Treatment specific to the presenting condition
   1) Kaposi sarcoma—local radiation (palliative), single agent/combination chemotherapy
   2) Fungal infections—nystatin swish and swallow, clotrimazole oral solution, amphotericin B with/without flucytosine
   3) Viral infections—acyclovir, ganciclovir
c. Nutrition—high protein and calories; ketoconazole or fluconazole for *Candida* infections
d. Symptomatic relief—comfort measures
e. Maintain confidentiality
f. Provide support
   1) Client and family coping—identify support systems
   2) Minimize social isolation—no isolation precautions are needed to enter room to talk to client, take VS, administer PO medications
   3) Encourage verbalization of feelings

g. Client/family discharge teaching

1) Behaviors to prevent transmission—safe sex, not sharing toothbrushes, razors, and other potentially blood-contaminated objects

2) Measures to prevent infection—good nutrition, hygiene, rest, skin and mouth care, avoid crowds; avoid raw fruits and vegetables, undercooked meat and eggs; use pepper and paprika immediately before eating

## Immune Response

A. Hypersensitivity response

1. Type I: IgE-mediated hypersensitivity reactions—reaction to environmental allergens; rapid

2. Type II: Tissue-specific hypersensitivity reactions—(cytotoxic reactions)—hemolytic anemias, hemolytic blood transfusion reaction

3. Type III: Immune complex reactions—systemic lupus erythematosus, rheumatoid arthritis

4. Type IV: Delayed hypersensitivity reactions—positive PPD, tissue transplant rejection; hypersensitivity reaction delayed or absent in older adults

B. Nursing management

1. Careful health history to determine allergies and triggers

2. Teach avoidance of allergens, triggers

3. Antihistamines, adrenaline, corticosteroids, antipruritic medications, cell-stabilizing medications (cromolyn), immunotherapy

C. Other autoimmune diseases

1. Multiple sclerosis

2. Guillain-Barré syndrome

3. Vasculitis

4. Type 1 diabetes

5. Ulcerative colitis

6. Glomerulonephritis

7. Sjögren syndrome

8. Systemic lupus erythematosus (SLE)

9. Rheumatoid arthritis

10. Graves disease

11. Myasthenia gravis

D. Gerontologic considerations—decreased stem cell function; decreased reticulocyte and platelet production, especially during increased demand (acute or chronic illness)

# Glossary of Terms

1. AIDS (acquired immune deficiency syndrome)—a profound defect in the immune system that strikes previously healthy individuals who have no known cause for the immunosuppression.

2. Antibodies—a collection of protein molecules manufactured by B lymphocytes in response to the presence of specific antigens.

3. Antigens—specific substances that induce the development of an immune response.

4. Contact transmission—direct, indirect, or droplet contact of an infectious agent to a host.

5. Cytomegalovirus (CMV)—one of the herpes-type viruses, commonly found in AIDS clients and also in healthy homosexuals. Recent evidence, based on new genetic engineering techniques, suggests that CMV and the cells of Kaposi sarcoma have many genes in common.

6. Epstein-Barr virus (EBV)—linked with Burkitt lymphoma, a cancer common in children in East Africa, and with nasopharyngeal cancer, a common cancer in China. It is also the cause of infectious mononucleosis, common in adolescents and young adults. EBV is in the herpesvirus family.

7. Hepatitis viruses—occur in several classes. Type A is usually transmitted by the fecal-oral route and causes an illness that is often subclinical in the young and more severe in older adults. Type B causes more severe illness and is associated with liver cancer. Type B can be transmitted by blood transfusions, from mother to newborn, or through saliva, breast milk, or genital secretions. Hepatitis C is transmitted blood to blood. Hepatitis D occurs only with hepatitis B. Hepatitis E is transmitted by fecal contamination of food and water and is not common in the U.S.

8. Herpesviruses—five major types in humans: herpes simplex virus type 1 (HSV-1), 2 (HSV-2), varicella zoster virus (VZV), cytomegalovirus (CMV), and Epstein-Barr virus (EBV). Each type of virus induces a different spectrum of human diseases; e.g., HSV-2 has a strong association with cervical carcinoma; EBV has a strong association with Burkitt lymphoma (prevalent in African children), nasopharyngeal carcinoma (NPC; common in China) and infectious mononucleosis; CMV is associated with Kaposi sarcoma.

9. Immune system—equips an individual to defend against infection. A contemporary definition of the term *immunity* emphasizes the ability to recognize materials or agents as foreign to oneself and to neutralize, eliminate, or metabolize them with or without injury to the host's tissues (see Tables 6-3 and 6-4).

**Table 6-3** Hematopoietic and Immunostimulant Medications

| MEDICATION | INDICATION FOR USE |
| --- | --- |
| Epoetin alfa | Treatment of erythrocytopenia<br><br>Stimulates production of RBC<br><br>Used in chronic renal failure and with clients undergoing anticancer chemotherapy |
| Filgrastim | Treatment of severe neutropenia<br><br>Prevention of infection in clients with cancer chemotherapy–induced neutropenia and in clients undergoing bone marrow transplantation |
| Pegfilgrastim | Prevention of infection in clients with cancer chemotherapy–induced neutropenia |
| Sargramostim | Promotion of bone marrow function after bone marrow transplant |
| Oprelvekin | Prevention of severe thrombocytopenia associated with anticancer chemotherapy |

**Table 6-4** Immunosuppressant Medications

| MEDICATION | INDICATIONS FOR USE |
| --- | --- |
| Azathioprine | Prevent renal transplant rejection<br><br>Treat severe rheumatoid arthritis not responsive to other treatments |
| Cyclosporine | Prevent rejection of solid organ (heart, kidney, liver) transplants<br><br>Prevent graft-versus-host disease in bone marrow transplant |
| Tacrolimus | Prevent liver, kidney, and heart transplant rejection |
| Etanercept | Rheumatoid arthritis treatment (acts to reduce the immune response resulting in inflammation and pain) |
| Infliximab | Treatment of Crohn disease (inflammatory bowel disease thought to have autoimmune origins)<br><br>Treatment of rheumatoid arthritis |
| Methotrexate | Treatment of severe rheumatoid arthritis unresponsive to other treatments |
| Prednisone Prednisolone | Autoimmune disease |
| Basiliximab | After transplant surgery |

10. Incubation period—the time between infection by a disease-causing organism and the onset of overt symptoms of the disease.

11. Infection—presence in the body of a pathogen.

12. Interferon—a protein substance thought to be produced or released by cells after viral infection or by other stimuli.

13. Lymphadenopathy—an abnormal condition of the lymph nodes and glands in which the nodes enlarge, grow and swell, and become palpable.

14. Lymph nodes—oval structures distributed throughout the body; through them pass the lymphocytes. When enlarged, the lymph nodes become palpable, a useful diagnostic sign of infection. Lymph nodes function as a filter of foreign material and also aid in the circulation of lymphocytes.

15. Lymphocytes—originate in the bone marrow, pass through the bloodstream, and enter other organs (such as the thymus or the gut), where they become modified to T or B lymphocytes.

16. Macrophages—cells found in the bloodstream as part of the body's immune system. These cells act by surrounding a foreign particle, virus, or bacterial cell and destroying it—literally "eating" it; T lymphocytes "present" antigen to macrophages. There is evidence that macrophages activate lymphocytes as well by producing factors that affect lymphocyte function.

17. Opportunistic infections—various infectious organisms, mostly viruses, fungi, and parasites, that take the "opportunity" to infect a host whose immune system is deficient and thus cannot fend off the disease caused by the agent; *Candida albicans*, *Pneumocystis jirovecii* pneumonia (PCP), toxoplasmosis, and histoplasmosis are examples.

18. Pathogen—microorganism or substance that is capable of producing diseases.

19. *Pneumocystis jirovecii* pneumonia (PCP)—a form of pneumonia caused by a protozoan parasite. It usually does not cause an infection in a host with an intact immune system.

20. Retroviruses—viruses that are known to cause cancer in animals. Recently, genes from these viruses have been found to be very similar to oncogenes or so-called cancer genes found in human and other cells.

21. Slow virus infections—a group of infections caused by viruses. The incubation periods are very long, and the clinical expressions of disease are relatively slow in progression.

22. Spleen—has both nonimmunologic and immunologic functions. It removes worn-out cells from the circulatory system and is a "graveyard" for red blood cells, reintroducing iron from hemoglobin after red cell death. Like the lymph nodes, the spleen produces lymphocytes and is important early in life. Removal of the spleen has been shown to be associated with overwhelming bacterial infections in infants, children, and young adults.

23. $T_4$:$T_8$ ratio (T-helper to T-suppressor ratio)—$T_4$ is a way of quantifying T-helper cells and $T_8$ is for quantifying T-suppressor cells. In many immunosuppressed states, the ratio of $T_4$:$T_8$ is less than 1:6; in normal states, the ratio is above 1:6.

24. T-helper cells—one of the subpopulations of T lymphocytes that aid in the cytotoxic or killing function of T lymphocytes. In AIDS clients, there is a lowering in the number of T-helper cells and an inverted ratio of helper:suppressor T cells.

25. Thymus—responsible for the development of lymphocytes. The name *T lymphocytes* shows that these lymphocytes are thymus derived.

26. T lymphocytes—arise in the bone marrow and differentiate or mature in the thymus gland. The mature T cell has cytotoxic properties and can destroy "target" cells. To aid in this killing function, there are T-helper cells. A second subpopulation of T cells is the T-suppressor cells, which have the opposite effect.

27. Varicella zoster virus (VZV)—the causative agent for both varicella (chickenpox) and herpes zoster.

# End-of-Chapter Thinking Exercise

The clinic nurse telephones a client who missed an appointment to be seen for follow-up and blood work in the clinic yesterday. The client has been HIV positive but symptom-free with normal CD4+ levels and low viral load for three years. The client reports not feeling well. Upon questioning, the client admits to a fever with chills and night sweats as well as a headache and "feeling like I've been run over by a truck." The nurse schedules a visit for the client to be seen by the nurse practitioner later that day. Lab work results and vital signs are listed below.

| LAB TEST | RESULT |
|---|---|
| Hemoglobin | 13 g/dL (130 g/L) |
| Hematocrit | 42% (0.42) |
| WBC | 2,600/mm$^3$ (2.6 $\times$ 10$^9$/L) |
| Platelets | 140,000/mm$^3$ (140 $\times$ 10$^9$/L) |
| CD4+ | 150 cells/microL |
| HIV viral load | 70,000 copies/mL |

| VITAL SIGN | RESULT |
|---|---|
| Temperature | 102°F (38.8°C) |
| Pulse | 120 beats/min and regular |
| BP | 134/82 mm Hg |
| Respiratory rate | 24 breaths/min |
| SpO$_2$ | 93% (room air) |

The client reports difficulty swallowing and states, "I haven't been eating because it hurts to swallow and everything just tastes funny." The tongue and oral mucous membranes are red with cottage cheese–like white patches over the surface. The client is diagnosed with AIDS and begins combination antiretroviral therapy (cART). The clinic nurse is assigned to teach the client about appropriate self-management.

1. What assessment data lead the nurse to think the client has an opportunistic fungal infection? (Analyze Cues)

2. What information will the nurse include when teaching the client about combination antiretroviral therapy (cART)? (Generate Solutions)

3. Prevention of infection is a priority action in self-management for the client with AIDS. What information will the nurse include when teaching the client about infection prevention? (Generate Solutions)

## Thinking Exercise Explanations

1. What assessment data lead the nurse to think the client has an opportunistic fungal infection? (Analyze Cues)

   - Pain and difficulty swallowing
   - Taste alteration
   - Inflammation of tongue and mucous membranes
   - Cottage cheese–like white patches

   The above signs indicate *Candida albicans*, an opportunistic fungal infection. The reduced functioning of the immune system with AIDS promotes an overgrowth of the fungus.

2. What information will the nurse include when teaching the client about combination antiretroviral therapy (cART)? (Generate Solutions)

   - Be diligent to take the medications exactly as prescribed and not to miss doses
   - Inform client of GI distress as side effect
   - Notify HCP of paresthesias, new-onset muscle pain, or severe abdominal cramping

   cART medications do not kill the HIV virus but decrease the replication of the virus. A constant blood level of the medication is necessary to inhibit replication. Knowing expected adverse effects increases compliance and decreases anxiety when they appear. The HCP needs to be informed of signs of adverse effects of the medication to prevent toxicity.

3. Prevention of infection is a priority action in self-management for the client with AIDS. What information will the nurse include when teaching the client about infection prevention? (Generate Solutions)

   - Avoid crowds
   - Do not share personal toilet articles (toothbrush, razor, toothpaste)
   - Bathe daily using an antimicrobial soap
   - Use strict handwashing technique
   - Avoid eating salads, raw fruits and vegetables, and undercooked meat or eggs
   - Do not drink liquids that have been standing for longer than 1 hour
   - Do not reuse a cup or glass without washing it first
   - Do not change pet litter boxes
   - Maintain a well-balanced diet

   Because of decreased immunity, the client with AIDS is greatly at risk for any kind of infection. Diligence to prevent exposure to microorganisms is crucial in avoiding complications and hospitalizations.

# CHAPTER 7

# THE GASTROINTESTINAL SYSTEM

# CONCEPTS BASIC TO NUTRITION

## Nutrition

## Summary of Digestion

    **A.** Digestive system (*see* Figure 7-1)

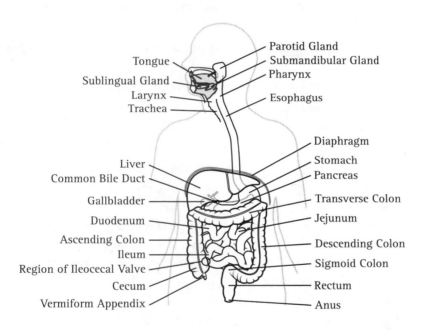

**Figure 7-1.** The Digestive System

1. Alimentary canal—consists of oral cavity, pharynx, esophagus, stomach, small intestine, large intestine, rectum; some nutrients are actively absorbed (requiring energy), and some are passively absorbed; older adults—loss of teeth and enamel; increased risk of cavities; increased risk of periodontal disease

2. Secretory glands—glands such as gastric glands line the stomach; others, such as the pancreas and liver, lie outside the stomach and secrete substances via ducts to the intestinal tract; decreased bicarbonate, mucus, and intrinsic factor in older adults

3. Sphincters

   a. Esophageal—between esophagus and stomach; dilation of lower esophagus in older adults; increased risk of gastroesophageal reflux disease (GERD)

   b. Pyloric—between stomach and small intestine

   c. Ileocecal—between small intestine and large intestine

   d. Anal—controls passage of fluids and fecal material

**B.** Digestive processes

1. Mechanical—food is broken down by teeth, tongue, and peristaltic contractions of stomach and small intestine; sphincters, such as the pyloric sphincter between the stomach and duodenum, control the rate of passage of food through the alimentary canal

2. Chemical

   a. Salivary glands—produce saliva, which lubricates food and begins starch digestion

   b. Esophagus—conducts food to stomach via peristaltic waves; decreased motility in older adults

   c. Stomach—gastric glands produce hydrochloric acid and the enzymes pepsin and rennin

      1) Pepsin—digests proteins into shorter polypeptides

      2) Rennin—curdles milk, which delays its passage through the stomach; enzyme is primarily found in mammalian infants

      3) Intrinsic factor—increased absorption of vitamin $B_{12}$; decreased in older adults

   d. Liver—produces bile, which is stored in the gallbladder before release into the small intestine; bile emulsifies fats into smaller components that are easier to absorb; decreased size in older adults

   e. Pancreas—produces enzymes such as lipase (for fat digestion), amylase (for starch digestion), and trypsin and chymotrypsin (for protein digestion); older adults have pancreatic atrophy and fibrosis, decreased production of proteolytic enzymes

   f. Small intestine—the secretory cells in the walls of the intestine produce lipase (for fat digestion), aminopeptidases (for polypeptide digestion), and disaccharidases (for maltose, sucrose, and lactose digestion); absorption is facilitated by outpocketings in the intestinal wall, called villi, that increase the surface area; decreased absorption of proteins, fats, minerals, vitamins, and carbohydrates in older adults

      1) Duodenum—10–12 in long in adult; upper part of small intestine

      2) Jejunum—8 ft long in adult; middle portion of small intestine

      3) Ileum—11 ft long in adult; lower portion of small intestine

   g. Large intestine—site of water resorption; slowed peristalsis in older adults; risk for decreased fiber intake, immobility and medications may contribute

   h. Rectum—transient storage of feces prior to elimination through the anus

**C.** Gastrointestinal hormones

1. Gastrin

   a. Secreted in response to mechanical distension

   b. Inhibited by acid

   c. Stimulates production of gastric acid and pepsin

   d. Increases gut motility

2. Cholecystokinin

   a. Secreted by cells in the duodenum and jejunum

   b. Secreted in response to presence of the digested fat and protein

   c. Causes the gallbladder to contract, forcing bile into the duodenum for fat absorption

3. Secretin

   a. Produced by the duodenum

   b. Secreted in response to the presence of free fatty acids in the intestine

   c. Stimulates the production of pancreatic juice

4. Enterogastrone

   a. Hormone of the small intestine

   b. Secreted in response to the presence of acid in the duodenum

   c. Inhibits the secretion of gastric acid

**D.** Properties of the gastric mucosa

1. Turnover of gastric mucosa—cells replaced every 3 d; cells continually desquamate into the lumen; decreased new cell formation in older adults

2. Permeability of gastric mucosa—unaffected by osmotic gradients, unlike the remainder of the GI tract; pure water is not absorbed, nor is water lost to the lumen if hypertonic solutions are drunk; the duodenum is highly permeable; all fluids are brought to isotonicity

3. Gastric mucosal barrier—impermeable to (and therefore not digested by) secreted acid

   a. Possible causes of barrier breakdown

      1) Salicylates—aspirin and salicylic acid

      2) Ethanol

      3) Bile acids regurgitated from the duodenum

      4) Injuries or infections

      5) Decreased bicarbonate and mucous in older adults

   b. Consequences of barrier breakdown—acid reaches the mucosa, leading to mucosal injury and bleeding or ulcers

      1) Acid stimulates increased motility of the stomach by direct stimulation of intrinsic plexus; the strong contractions cause pain

      2) Acid penetrating the mucosa permits histamine release, leading to edema of the mucosa as the interstitial spaces fill with fluid

E.  Rate and quantity of gastric secretion

1.  Rate of acid secretion rises to a maximum in the second half hour after eating

2.  Total amount of acid secreted is proportional to the amount of protein ingested

3.  Gerontologic considerations–gastric atrophy and decreased intrinsic factor production; increased risk of vitamin $B_{12}$ deficiency

F.  Malfunctions involving gastric secretion

1.  Loss of gastric juice (e.g., vomiting) leads to metabolic alkalosis—for each $H^+$ lost, one $HCO_3^-$ is retained

2.  Mucosal atrophy (may involve autoimmunity to parietal cells)—no acid or pepsinogen secretion; possible lack of intrinsic factor for $B_{12}$ absorption in the terminal ileum; pernicious anemia develops after approximately three years

G.  Mechanics of gastric digestion

1.  Reception of food—vagally mediated relaxation of the stomach occurs as food distends the esophagus, resulting in little increase in pressure

2.  Mixing of chyme—peristaltic waves over the antrum (moving toward the pyloric sphincter) mix food and gastric secretions thoroughly

3.  Vomiting—forceful expulsion of stomach contents

4.  Gerontologic considerations—decreased gastric motility, volume, blood flow; stomach distension and feeling of fullness may contribute to appetite loss and weight loss

## Sociocultural Influences on Nutritional Intake

*Note: not every member of a culture chooses to follow all of its traditions.

A.  Orthodox Jewish

1.  Dietary laws based on biblical and rabbinical regulations

2.  Laws pertain to selection, preparation, and service of food

3.  Laws

a.  Milk/milk products never eaten at same meal as meat (milk may not be taken until 6 h after eating meat)

b.  Two meals contain dairy products, and one meal contains meat

c.  Separate utensils are used for meat and milk dishes

d.  Meat must be kosher (drained of blood)

e.  Prohibited foods

1)  Pork

2)  Diseased animals or animals who die a natural death

3)  Birds of prey

4)  Fish without fins or scales (shellfish—oysters, crab, shrimp, lobster)

**B.** Muslim

1. Dietary laws based on Islamic teachings in Quran

2. Laws

    a. Fermented fruits and vegetables prohibited

    b. Pork prohibited

    c. Alcohol prohibited

    d. Foods with special value: figs, olives, dates, honey, milk, buttermilk

    e. Humane slaughter of animals for meat

3. 30-day period of daylight fasting required during Ramadan

**C.** South American

1. Basic foods: dried beans, chili peppers, corn

2. Small amounts of meat and eggs

**D.** Puerto Rican

1. Starchy vegetables and fruits (plantains and green bananas)

2. Large amounts of rice and beans

3. Coffee main beverage

**E.** Native American

1. Food has religious and social significance

2. Diet includes meat, bread (tortillas, blue corn bread), eggs, vegetables (corn, potatoes, green beans, tomatoes), fruit

3. Frying common method of food preparation

**F.** African American

1. Minimal milk, eggs, whole grains in diet

2. Leafy greens (turnips, collards, and mustard), fruit

3. High in meat consumption, pork common

**G.** Cajun

1. Foods are strong flavored and spicy

2. Frequently contains seafood (crawfish)

3. Food preparation starts with a roux made from heated oil and flour; vegetables and seafood added

**H.** Chinese

1. Freshest food available cooked at a high temperature in a wok with a small amount of fat and liquid

2. Meat in small amounts

3. Eggs and soybean products used for protein

I. Japanese

1. Rice is basic food

2. Soy sauce is used for seasoning

3. Tea is main beverage

4. Seafood frequently used (sometimes raw fish—sushi)

J. Southeast Asian

1. Rice is basic food, eaten in separate rice bowl

2. Soups

3. Fresh fruits and vegetables frequently part of diet

4. Stir-frying in wok is common method of food preparation

K. Italian

1. Bread and pasta are basic foods

2. Cheese frequently used in cooking

3. Food seasoned with spices, wine, garlic, herbs, olive oil

L. Greek

1. Bread is served with every meal

2. Cheese (feta) is used for cooking

3. Lamb and fish frequent

4. Eggs in main dish but not a breakfast food

5. Fruit for dessert

# Basic Concepts of Nutritional Science

A. Five axioms of food adequacy

1. No single food can provide all that is needed for growth and development

2. The storage and handling of food affect its nutritional value

3. All nutritional requirements for a well-balanced diet can be met by food

4. Nutrients required by humans are similar for all people, but amount varies by activity, age, and size

5. No one food substance operates alone in metabolism

B. Carbohydrates

1. Functions

   a. Provide energy, 4 kcal/g

   b. Regulate some aspects of protein metabolism

2. Classification

   a. Monosaccharides

      1) Simplest form of carbohydrate

      2) Glucose, fructose, and galactose

    b.  Disaccharides

        1)  Double sugars made up of two monosaccharides

        2)  Sucrose, lactose, and maltose

    c.  Polysaccharides—complex carbohydrates made up of more than two monosaccharides

    d.  Fiber—multiple polysaccharides plus nondigestible substances, such as wheat bran and cereals

**C.**  Fats

    1.  Function—storage form of energy; 9 kcal/g

    2.  Classifications

        a.  Simple lipids—triglycerides; main form of fat in diet

        b.  Compound lipids—phospholipids, glycolipids, and lipoproteins; combinations of fat with other compounds

        c.  Derived lipids—digestive products of fats

            1)  Glycerol—water-soluble base of triglycerides, metabolically available to form glucose

            2)  Steroids—fat-related substances that contain sterols, bile acids, sex hormones, hormones of the adrenal cortex, and vitamin D

            3)  Fatty acids—key refined forms of fat

                a)  Saturated—primarily from animal sources; mostly solids at room temperature

                b)  Polyunsaturated—mostly from plant sources; liquids at room temperature

                c)  Essential—needed in diet; body does not manufacture it

                d)  Nonessential—not needed in diet; body manufactures it

**D.**  Proteins

    1.  Function—to build tissue; 4 kcal/g; contains amino acids

    2.  Classifications

        a.  Essential amino acids—structural units of protein that body cannot manufacture

        b.  Nonessential amino acids—structural units of protein that body can manufacture

        c.  Polypeptides—long chains of amino acids

**E.**  Vitamins

    1.  Classification

        a.  Fat soluble—vitamins A, D, E, and K

        b.  Water soluble—vitamin C and B complex

    2.  Characteristics

        a.  Not a carbohydrate, fat, protein, or mineral

        b.  Not manufactured by the body; a necessary dietary substance

    3.  Fat-soluble vitamins

a. Vitamin A

1) Source

a) Derived from beta-carotene

b) Carotene-containing foods are most important: liver, butter, milk, cheese, and egg yolk; yellow, orange, and some green vegetables (yellow and orange colors are due in large part to carotene content)

2) Deficiency symptoms (hypovitaminosis A)

a) Eyes: night blindness, corneal desiccation and ulceration, xerophthalmia

b) Bronchorespiratory epithelium changes from mucous secretion to keratinization

c) Keratinization and xerosis of the skin

d) Genitourinary calculi

e) Sweat gland atrophy

f) Increased cerebrospinal fluid pressure and pseudotumor cerebri

g) Impaired smell and taste secondary to keratinization

h) Defective remodeling of bone

i) Degeneration of testes and gonadal resorption

j) Deficiency enhances carcinogenicity in lab animals

3) Toxicity (hypervitaminosis A)

a) Acute toxicity

i) CNS—lethargy, headache, and papilledema

ii) Skin—dry and pruritic skin, desquamation, and erythema

iii) GI—fatty liver, hepatic cirrhosis, and portal hypertension

iv) Myalgia—gingivitis and cheilosis

v) Tender hyperostoses

vi) Hypercalcemia, hypoprothrombinemia

b) Pharmacokinetics

i) Well absorbed from GI tract

ii) Absorption mediated by a protein carrier—retinol carrier protein

iii) Mostly stored in liver

4) Therapeutic uses of vitamin A

a) Used to treat deficiency symptoms in cases of true deficiency, protein malnutrition (kwashiorkor), or malabsorptive syndromes (steatorrhea, hepatic cirrhosis, postgastrectomy)

b) Dermatologic disease

i) Acne vulgaris

ii) Psoriasis

iii) Ichthyosis

   b. Vitamin D

      1) Source

         a) Primary—sunlight's irradiation of body cholesterol

         b) Secondary—fish oils, fortified dairy products

      2) Deficiency symptoms

         a) Rickets

            i) Uncalcified areas of bone are softened

            ii) Causes deformities of bones from physiological and gravitational stresses on soft sections of bone

         b) Growth restriction and weakness in infants and children

      3) Toxicity symptoms

         a) Hypercalcemia—weakness, vomiting, diarrhea, electrocardiographic changes

         b) Demineralization of bones

         c) Renal calculi and metastatic calcifications of soft tissues

      4) Pharmacokinetics—necessary for absorption of calcium and phosphorus

   c. Vitamin E

      1) Chemically functions most clearly as an antioxidant

      2) The most important lipid-soluble antioxidant in the cell

      3) Reduces harmful free radicals to harmless metabolites

      4) Deficiency symptoms

         a) Loss of deep tendon reflexes

         b) Changes in balance and coordination

         c) Muscle weakness, visual disturbances

      5) Pharmacokinetics—absorbed predominantly via lymphatics

   d. Vitamin K

      1) Source

         a) Chloroplasts of most plant species

         b) Synthesized by many intestinal bacteria

      2) Physiological function

         a) Functions as an essential cofactor for calcium binding in the clotting cascade

         b) Gamma carboxylation occurs in synthesis of prothrombin, proconvertin, Stuart factor, and plasma thromboplastin component or Christmas factor; also called factors II, VII, IX, and X, respectively

      3) Deficiency symptoms—bleeding tendency

      4) Toxicity

         a) Acute intravenous vitamin K toxicity causes chest pain, flushing, and occasionally death

         b) Large parenteral doses may cause anemia, hepatic and renal damage, and hemolysis, particularly in clients with glucose-6-phosphate deficiency

      5) Pharmacokinetics—most commonly given intramuscularly and absorbed via lymphatics

      6) Therapeutic uses

         a) Given for inadequate intake, e.g., hypoprothrombinemia of the newborn

         b) Given for inadequate absorption, e.g., biliary obstruction or malabsorption syndromes

         c) Given for inadequate utilization, e.g., chronic liver disease

4. Water-soluble vitamins—general characteristics

  a. Thiamin (B$_1$)

    1) Sources—quantities in common foods are less than for vitamins A or C

      a) Beef, liver, whole grains, legumes are good sources

      b) Eggs, fish are fair sources

    2) Deficiency symptoms—beriberi

      a) Gastrointestinal—indigestion, appetite loss

      b) Nervous system—nerve irritation and deadening sensations

      c) Cardiovascular—cardiac failure, edema

    3) Toxicity—shock

    4) Therapeutic uses

      a) During times of high energy requirements such as after surgery

      b) During pregnancy and lactation

      c) During growth spurts

      d) In chronic alcoholism

  b. Riboflavin (B$_2$)

    1) Sources

      a) Milk is most important source

      b) Organ meats

      c) Enriched foods

    2) Deficiency symptoms—tissue inflammation

      a) Wound aggravation—poor healing

      b) Glossitis of the tongue

      c) Cheilosis of the mouth

    3) Toxicity—not common

4) Therapeutic uses

    a) After surgery, trauma, and burns

    b) Growth periods

c. Niacin

  1) Sources

    a) Meat

    b) Peanuts, beans

  2) Deficiency symptoms—pellagra

    a) Weakness

    b) Lassitude

    c) Loss of appetite

  3) Toxicity

    a) Vasodilation

    b) Flushing

  4) Therapeutic uses

    a) Surgery, trauma, burns

    b) Hypermetabolic states

d. Pyridoxine ($B_6$)

  1) Sources—widespread in foods

    a) Yeast, liver, and kidney are good sources

    b) Egg yolks are fair sources

  2) Deficiency symptoms—not common

    a) Anemia—hypochromic

    b) CNS disturbances—seizures

  3) Toxicity—peripheral neuropathy

  4) Therapeutic uses

    a) Need greater in high-protein diets and during isoniazid (INH) therapy

    b) Greater requirement during oral contraceptive use and early pregnancy

e. Folic acid and cyanocobalamin ($B_{12}$)

  1) Sources—liver and kidney are best

  2) Deficiency symptoms—anemias

    a) Folic acid—megaloblastic anemia (large, immature red blood cells)

    b) $B_{12}$—pernicious anemia (intrinsic factor needed for intestinal absorption of $B_{12}$)

  3) Toxicity—not common

    4) Therapeutic uses

     a) Intestinal sprue

     b) Mixed anemias

  f. Vitamin C

    1) Sources—citrus fruit and tomatoes

    2) Deficiency symptoms—scurvy

     a) Sore gums

     b) Hemorrhages

     c) Anemia

    3) Toxicity—oxalate hypersensitivity

    4) Therapeutic uses

     a) Postsurgical healing

     b) Fevers and infections

     c) Stress

     d) Growth

**F.** Minerals

 1. Classification

  a. Major minerals—Ca, Mg, Na, K, P, S, Cl (present in relatively large amounts)

  b. Trace minerals—Fe, Cu, I, Mn, Co, Zn, Mo (present in small amounts)

 2. Characteristics

  a. Regulates activities of many enzymes

  b. Varying amounts required; e.g., calcium is 2% of body weight, whereas iron is only 3 g in whole body

  c. Maintains acid-base balance and osmotic pressure

  d. Facilitates membrane transfer of essential nutrients; maintains nerve and muscle irritability

 3. Summary of major minerals (*see* Table 7-1)

**G.** Nursing management

 1. General diet

 2. My Food Plate—recommendations by the U.S. Department of Agriculture for servings of daily food for Americans (*see* Figure 7-2 and Table 7-2)

  a. To reduce all-cause mortality, older adults should consume oral protein and energy supplements

**Table 7-1** Minerals

| MINERAL | PRIMARY FUNCTION(S) | PRIMARY SOURCE(S) | DEFICIENCY SYMPTOM(S) |
|---|---|---|---|
| Calcium | Bone formation<br>Muscle contraction<br>Thrombus formation | Milk products<br>Green leafy vegetables<br>Eggs | Rickets<br>Porous bones<br>Tetany |
| Phosphorus | Bone formation<br>Cell permeability | Milk, eggs<br>Nuts | Rickets |
| Fluoride | Dental health | Water supply | Dental caries |
| Iodine | Thyroid hormone synthesis | Seafood Iodized salt | Goiter |
| Sodium | Osmotic pressure<br>Acid-base balance<br>Nerve irritability | Table salt<br>Canned vegetables<br>Milk, cured meats<br>Processed foods | Fluid and electrolyte imbalance |
| Potassium | Water balance in cells<br>Protein synthesis<br>Heart contractility | Grains, meats<br>Vegetables | Dysrhythmias<br>Fluid and electrolyte imbalance |
| Iron | Hemoglobin synthesis | Liver, oysters<br>Leafy vegetables<br>Apricots | Anemia<br>Lethargy |

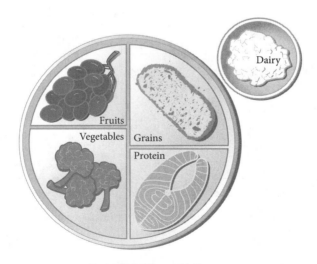

**Figure 7-2.** ChooseMyPlate.gov

**Table 7-2** My Food Plate

| GROUP | FOOD EXAMPLES | RECOMMENDED DAILY INTAKE |
|---|---|---|
| Grains | Bread, cereals, cooked cereals, popcorn, pasta, rice, tortillas<br><br>Half of all grains should be whole grains | Children—3–5 ounce equivalents<br>Teens—5–7 ounce equivalents<br>Young adults—6–8 ounce equivalents<br>Adults—6–7 ounce equivalents<br>Older adults—5–6 ounce equivalents |
| Vegetables | Dark-green vegetables (broccoli, spinach, greens, leafy vegetables), orange vegetables (carrots, pumpkin, sweet potatoes), dried beans and peas (split peas, pinto, kidney, black, soy [tofu]), starchy vegetables (corn, peas, white potatoes) | Children—1–1.5 cups<br>Teens—2–3 cups<br>Young adults—2.5–3 cups<br>Adults—2.5–3 cups<br>Older adults—2–2.5 cups |
| Fruits | Apples, bananas, strawberries, blueberries, oranges, melons, dried fruits, fruit juices | Children—1–1.5 cups<br>Teens—1.5–2 cups<br>Young adults—2 cups<br>Adults—1.5–2 cups<br>Older adults—1.5–2 cups |
| Oils | Nuts, butter, margarine, cooking oils, salad dressings | Children—3–4 teaspoons<br>Teens—5–6 teaspoons<br>Young adults—6–7 teaspoons<br>Adults—5–6 teaspoons<br>Older adults—5–6 teaspoons |
| Milk | Milk, yogurt, cheese, puddings | Children—2 cups<br>Teens—3 cups<br>Young adults—3 cups<br>Adults—3 cups<br>Older adults—3 cups |
| Meat and beans | Meat, poultry, fish, dry beans, eggs, peanut butter, nuts, seeds | Children—2–4 ounce equivalents<br>Teens—5–6 ounce equivalents<br>Young adults—5.5–6.5 ounce equivalents<br>Adults—5–6 ounce equivalents<br>Older adults—5–5.5 ounce equivalents |

3. General guidelines for herbal and dietary supplements

   a. Supplements do not compensate for an inadequate diet

   b. Recommended daily amounts (RDA) should not be exceeded due to the potential for toxicity

   c. Multivitamin-mineral products recommended for certain sex or age groups contain different amounts of some minerals

   d. Iron supplements beyond those contained in multivitamin-mineral combinations are intended for short-term or special-need (e.g., pregnancy) use and should not be taken for longer periods of time due to the potential for toxicity

   e. Most adolescent and adult females should consume 1,000–1,300 mg calcium daily

   f. Supplementing with selenium as an antioxidant and zinc to prevent colds and promote wound healing is not proven

4. Common therapeutic diets (*see* Table 7-3)

**Table 7-3** Common Therapeutic Diets

| CLEAR LIQUID DIET | FULL LIQUID DIET | LOW-FAT, CHOLESTEROL-RESTRICTED DIET |
|---|---|---|
| Sample meal items:<br><br>Gelatin dessert, ice pop, tea with lemon, ginger ale, bouillon, fruit juice without pulp | Sample meal items:<br><br>Milkshakes, soups, custard; all clear liquids | Sample meal items:<br><br>Fruit, vegetables, cereals, lean meat |
| Common medical problems:<br><br>Postoperative; acute vomiting or diarrhea | Common medical problems:<br><br>GI upset (diet progression after surgery) | Common medical problems:<br><br>Atherosclerosis |
| Purpose:<br><br>To maintain fluid balance | Purpose:<br><br>Nutrition without chewing | Purpose:<br><br>To reduce calories from fat and minimize cholesterol intake |
| Not allowed:<br><br>Fruit juices with pulp, milk | Not allowed:<br><br>Jam, fruit, solid foods, nuts | Not allowed:<br><br>Marbled meats, avocados, milk, bacon, egg yolks, butter |

*(Continued)*

**Table 7-3** Common Therapeutic Diets (*Continued*)

| SODIUM-RESTRICTED DIET | HIGH-ROUGHAGE, HIGH-FIBER DIET | LOW-RESIDUE DIET |
|---|---|---|
| Sample meal items:<br><br>Cold baked chicken, lettuce with sliced tomatoes, applesauce | Sample meal items:<br><br>Cracked wheat bread, minestrone soup, apple, brussels sprouts | Sample meal items:<br><br>Roast lamb, buttered rice, sponge cake, "white" processed foods |
| Common medical problems:<br><br>Heart failure, hypertension, cirrhosis | Common medical problems:<br><br>Constipation, large bowel disorders | Common medical problems:<br><br>Temporary GI/elimination problems (e.g., lower bowel surgery) |
| Purpose:<br><br>To lower body water and promote excretion | Purpose:<br><br>To maximize bulk in stools | Purpose:<br><br>To minimize intestinal activity |
| Not allowed:<br><br>Preserved meats, cheese, fried foods, cottage cheese, canned foods, added salt | Not allowed:<br><br>White bread, pies and cakes from white flour, "white" processed foods | Not allowed:<br><br>Whole wheat, corn, bran |
| HIGH-PROTEIN DIET | KIDNEY DIET | LOW-PHENYLALANINE DIET |
| Sample meal items:<br><br>30 grams powdered skim milk and 1 egg in 100 mL water *or* roast beef sandwich and skim milk | Sample meal items:<br><br>Unsalted vegetables, white rice, canned fruits, sweets | Sample meal items:<br><br>Fats, fruits, jams, low-phenylalanine milk |
| Common medical problems:<br><br>Burns, infection, hyperthyroidism | Common medical problems:<br><br>Chronic renal failure | Common medical problems:<br><br>Phenylketonuria (PKU) |
| Purpose:<br><br>To re-establish anabolism to raise albumin levels | Purpose:<br><br>To keep protein, potassium, and sodium low | Purpose:<br><br>Low-protein diet to prevent brain damage from imbalance of amino acids |
| Not allowed:<br><br>Soft drinks, "junk" food | Not allowed:<br><br>Beans, cereals, citrus fruits | Not allowed:<br><br>Meat, eggs, beans, bread |

5. Herbals used to lower cholesterol

a. Flax or flax seed

1) Decreases the absorption of other medications

b. Garlic

1) Increases the effects of anticoagulants

2) Increases the hypoglycemic effects of insulin

c. Green tea

1) Produces a stimulant effect when the tea contains caffeine

d. Soy

# Nutritional Assessment

**A.** Clinical signs of nutritional status (*see* Table 7-4)

**Table 7-4** Physical Signs of Adequate Nutritional Status

| BODY AREA | NORMAL APPEARANCE |
|---|---|
| Hair | Shiny, firm, intact scalp without areas of pigmentation |
| Teeth | Evenly spaced, straight, no cavities, shiny |
| Tongue | Deep red in color |
| Gums | Firm, without redness, even colored |
| Skin | Smooth, moist, even shading |
| Nails | Firm, without ridges |
| Extremities | Full range of motion |
| Abdomen | Flat, nontender |
| Legs | Good color |
| Skeleton | No malformations |
| Weight | Normal for height |
| Posture | Erect |
| Muscles | Firm |
| GI | Good appetite and digestion |
| Vitality | Good endurance, good sleep pattern |

**B.** Health factors

1. Weight—recent gain or loss of 10% is significant

2. Medications—use of antacids, laxatives, diuretics, digitalis, oral contraceptives

3. Illness—cancer, radiation therapy, surgery, GI disease, endocrine disorders, heart disease

# Nutritional Parameters

**A.** Caloric requirement—a calorie is a measurement unit of energy; person's height and weight, as well as level of activity, determine energy need; average adult requires anywhere from 1,500–3,000 kcal/d

**B.** Fluid requirement—average fluid requirement for normal healthy adult is approximately 1,800–2,500 mL/d

**C.** Nutrient requirements

1. Carbohydrates—first substance utilized for energy production in starvation; only source of energy production for the brain

2. Fats—second source of energy production utilized by the body in starvation; its waste products are ketone bodies, which can create an acidic environment in the blood

3. Proteins—last energy source utilized in starvation; depletion of protein leads to muscle wasting as well as loss of pressure in the vascular space; low albumin level in the blood indicates protein malnutrition

**D.** Diagnostic tests

1. Blood (*see* Table 7-5)

2. Urine

   a. Urinalysis—an elevated level of ketone bodies indicates altered fat metabolism

      1) Schilling test—diagnoses vitamin $B_{12}$ deficiency (pernicious anemia); radioactive vitamin $B_{12}$ is administered to the client; low value excreted in urine indicates pernicious anemia (normal is greater than 10% of dose excreted in 24 h)

3. Gastric aspirate

   a. pH—measures acid/alkaline range; generally overly acidic environment can lead to ulcerative activity; gastric pH of 1–4 indicates proper placement of NG tube

   b. Guaiac—tests for presence of blood in aspirate; normally, blood absent

4. Stool

   a. Fecal occult blood test (FOBT)—tests for presence of blood; normally, blood absent

   b. Quantitative analysis—reviewed for color, consistency, and amount

   c. Tested for presence of *Clostridioides difficile* infection

**Table 7-5** Blood Tests

| BLOOD TEST | CONVENTIONAL VALUES* | SI VALUES* |
|---|---|---|
| Serum albumin | 3.5–5 g/dL | 35–50 g/L |
| Prealbumin | 19.5–35.8 mg/dL | 195–358 mg/L |
| Lymphocyte count | 20–40% of total white cells | 0.2–0.4 of total white cells |
| Hemoglobin: | | |
| Male | 13–18 g/dL | 130–180 g/L |
| Female | 12–16 g/dL | 120–160 g/L |
| Children (3–12 years) | 11–12.5 g/dL | 110–125 g/L |
| Hematocrit: | | |
| Male | 42–52% | 0.42–0.52 |
| Female | 35–47% | 0.35–0.47 |
| Children (3–12 years) | 35–45% | 0.35–0.45 |
| Glucose tolerance test | 1 hour—190 mg/100 mL | 1 hour—10.5 mmol//L |
| | 2 hours—140 mg/mL | 2 hours—7.7 mmol/L |
| | 3 hours—125 mg/mL | 3 hours—6.9 mmol/L |
| Total cholesterol | 150–200 mg/dL | 3.9–5.2 mmol/L |
| Low-density lipoproteins (LDL), mg/100 mL | Less than 160 (no coronary artery disease [CAD] and less than 2 risk factors)<br><br>Less than 130 (no CAD and 2 or more risk factors)<br><br>Less than 100 if CAD present | Less than 160 (no CAD and less than 2 risk factors)<br><br>Less than 130 (no CAD 2 or more risk factors)<br><br>Less than 100 if CAD present |

*Ranges May Vary by Resource and Facility

5. Special procedures
   a. Upper GI series (barium swallow)
      1) Definition—ingestion of barium sulfate to determine patency and size of esophagus, size and condition of gastric walls, patency of pyloric valve, and rate of passage to small bowel or into small bowel
      2) Preparation
         a) Maintain NPO after midnight; avoid opioids and anticholinergic medications
         b) Inform client that stool will be light colored after procedure
      3) Posttest—encourage fluids and/or laxative to prevent constipation

    b.  Endoscopy

       1)  Definition—visualization of esophagus and/or stomach and/or duodenum by means of a lighted, flexible fiber-optic tube introduced through the mouth to the stomach or from rectum through intestines to determine presence of ulcerations or tumors or to obtain tissue or fluid samples

       2)  Preparation

          a)  Verify that informed consent from client has been obtained

          b)  Maintain NPO before procedure (at least 8 h)

          c)  Teach client about numbness in throat due to local anesthetic applied to posterior pharynx by spray or gargle; conscious sedation used

       3)  Postprocedure nursing care

          a)  Maintain NPO until gag reflex returns

          b)  Observe for vomiting of blood, respiratory distress, aspiration

          c)  Inform client to expect sore throat for 3–4 days after procedure

    c.  Gastric analysis

       1)  Definition—aspiration of gastric contents to evaluate for presence of abnormal constituents such as blood, abnormal bacteria, abnormal pH, or malignant cells

       2)  Preparation—client must be NPO before test; NG tube is passed; contents aspirated and sent for evaluation

       3)  Pentagastrin is sometimes used to stimulate hydrochloric acid secretion

    d.  Lower GI series (barium enema)

       1)  Definition—instillation of barium into colon via rectum for fluoroscopy x-rays to view tumors, polyps, strictures, ulcerations, inflammation, or obstructions of colon

       2)  Preparation

          a)  Low-residue diet for 1–2 days

          b)  Clear liquid diet and laxative evening before test

          c)  Cleansing enemas until clear morning of test

       3)  Postprocedure nursing care

          a)  Cleansing enemas after exam to remove barium and prevent impaction; laxatives administered

          b)  X-rays may be repeated after all barium is expelled

**E.**  Nursing management

  1.  Weight for height tables—ideal body weight at specific heights

  2.  Exchange lists

    a.  Six classifications; client is given number of allowances

    b.  Foods on each list nearly equal in carbohydrates, protein, fat, and calories

  3.  Evaluation methods—24-h food recall or 3-d food diary

# Alternative Techniques

A. Enteral nutrition—liquid delivered to stomach, distal duodenum, or proximal jejunum via a nasogastric, percutaneous endoscopic gastrostomy (PEG) or percutaneous endoscopic jejunostomy (PEJ) tube (*see* Table 7-6)

**Table 7-6** Conditions Requiring Enteral Feeding

| CONDITION | CAUSE |
|---|---|
| Preoperative need for nutritional support | Inadequate intake preoperatively, resulting in poor nutritional state |
| Gastrointestinal problems | Fistula, short-bowel syndrome, Crohn disease, ulcerative colitis, nonspecific maldigestion or malabsorption |
| Oncology therapy | Radiation, chemotherapy |
| Alcoholism, chronic depression, eating disorders | Chronic illness, psychiatric, or neurologic disorder |
| Head and neck disorders or surgery | Disease or trauma |

1. Definition—providing nourishment via a tube due to inability of GI tract use
2. Basic principles
    a. Tube must be in proper position before infusion of food or aspiration into lungs can result
    b. Feeding must be administered at room or body temperature at a controlled rate or diarrhea may result
3. Nursing management of tube feeding
    a. Insert tube through the nose to the stomach
        1) X-ray verification most reliable method
        2) Auscultation of sound when air instilled into tube does not indicate placement in stomach
        3) Aspirate gastric or duodenal contents for pH testing
            a) pH 0–4 indicates gastric placement
            b) pH greater than or equal to 6 indicates placement in lungs or intestines
        4) Observe color—gastric aspirate usually cloudy and green but may also be off-white, tan, bloody, or brown
    b. Aspirate for gastric contents; if more than 50–100 mL residual, hold feeding
    c. Control rate of feeding administration—use enteral pump or count drops in gravity administration
    d. Flush tube with water or normal saline after feeding and before and after medications are administered through the tube
4. Complications of enteral feeding (*see* Table 7-7)

**Table 7-7** Complications of Enteral Feedings

| COMPLICATION | NURSING CONSIDERATIONS |
|---|---|
| Mechanical tube displacement | Replace tube |
| Aspiration | Elevate head of bed |
| | Check residual before feeding for intermittent |
| | Check residual every 4 hours for continuous |
| | If excess residual present, stop for 1 hour and recheck residual |
| Gastrointestinal cramping, vomiting, diarrhea | Decrease feeding rate |
| | Change formula |
| | Administer at room temperature |
| Metabolic hyperglycemia | Monitor glucose, serum osmolality |
| | Administer insulin if needed |
| | Reduce infusion rate |
| Dehydration | Flush tube with water or normal saline according to hospital policy |
| Formula-medication interactions | Check compatibility |
| | Flush tubing prior to and after medication |

**B.** Parenteral nutrition (PN) (*see* Figure 7-3)

1. Definition—liquid concentrate of hypertonic glucose, amino acids, electrolytes, vitamins, and minerals; given to selected clients to provide nutrition when enteral feeding is not possible or desirable

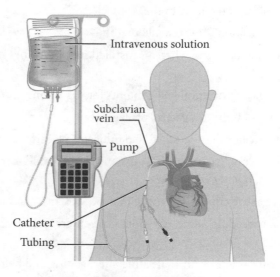

Intravenous solution

Subclavian vein

Pump

Catheter

Tubing

**Figure 7-3.** Parenteral Nutrition

2. Basic principles

   a. Concentrated solution must be infused in large vessel; rapid dilution is mandatory to prevent complications of high osmolarity

   b. Client must be carefully monitored for signs of complications; infection and hyperglycemia are common; fluid volume overload possible

3. Nursing management

   a. Do not infuse solution until placement of tube is verified as correct by x-ray

   b. Use aseptic technique when changing dressing or handling infusion bottle; use filter

   c. Infuse solution by pump at constant rate to prevent abrupt change in infusion rate

      1) Increased rate results in hyperosmolar state

      2) Slowed rate results in "rebound" hypoglycemia due to delayed pancreatic reaction to change in insulin requirements

4. Types of solutions

   a. PN—amino acid-dextrose formulas; 2–3 L of solution given over 24 h; 500 mL of 10% fat emulsions (Intralipid) given with PN over 6 h 1–3 times/wk; fine bacterial filter used

   b. TNA (total nutrient admixture)—amino acid-dextrose-lipid, "3-in-1" formula; 1 L solution given over 24 h

   c. Lipids—provide fatty acids

5. Methods of administration

   a. Peripheral—used for peripheral parenteral nutrition to supplement oral intake; should not administer dextrose concentrations above 10% due to irritation of vessel walls; usually used for less than 2 wk

   b. Central—catheter inserted into subclavian vein

      1) Peripherally inserted central catheter (PICC)—catheter threaded through basilic or cephalic vein to superior vena cava; dextrose solution greater than or equal to 10%; duration less than or equal to 4 wk

      2) Percutaneous central catheter through subclavian vein

      3) Triple-lumen central catheter often used; distal lumen (16-gauge) used to infuse or draw blood samples, middle lumen (18-gauge) used for PN infusion, proximal lumen (18-gauge) used to infuse or draw blood and administer medications; duration less than or equal to 4 wk

      4) If single-lumen catheter used, cannot use to administer medications (may be incompatible) or give blood (RBCs coat catheter lumen); medications and blood must be given through peripheral IV line, not piggybacked to the PN IV line

   c. Tunneled central catheters/access devices

      1) Right atrial catheters—Hickman, Broviac, and Groshong

      2) Subcutaneous port—Huber needle used to access port through skin

6. Nursing management

   a. Initial rate of infusion (50 mL/h) and gradually increased (100–125 mL/h) as client's fluid and electrolyte tolerance permits

   b. Infuse solution by pump at constant rate to prevent abrupt change in infusion rate

      1) Increased rate results in hyperosmolar state (headache, nausea, fever, chills, malaise)

      2) Slowed rate results in "rebound" hypoglycemia caused by delayed pancreatic reaction to change in insulin requirements; do not discontinue suddenly

   c. Client must be carefully monitored for signs of complications; infection and hyperglycemia are common (*see* Table 7-8)

   d. Change IV tubing and filter every 24 h

   e. Keep solutions refrigerated until needed; allow to warm to room temperature before use

   f. If new solution unavailable, use 10% dextrose and water solution until available

**Table 7-8** Complications of Parenteral Nutrition

| COMPLICATION | NURSING CONSIDERATIONS |
|---|---|
| Infection/sepsis | Maintain closed intravenous systems with filter |
| | No blood drawn or medications given through PN line |
| | Dry, sterile, occlusive dressing applied to site |
| Pneumothorax because of line placement | PN to be started only after chest x-ray validates correct placement |
| | Monitor breath sounds and for presence of shortness of breath |
| Hyperglycemia | Monitor glucose level and serum osmolality |
| Hyperosmolar coma | Administer insulin according to sliding scale insulin |
| Hypoglycemia | Hang 10% dextrose solution if PN discontinued suddenly |
| Fluid overload | Monitor breath sounds, weight, and peripheral perfusion |
| | Do not "catch up" if PN behind |
| Air embolism | Monitor for respiratory distress |
| | Valsalva maneuver during tubing and cap change |

7. Monitor daily weight, glucose, temperatures, I and O; check BUN, electrolytes (calcium, magnesium) three times a week; check CBC, platelets, prothrombin time, liver function studies (aspartate aminotransferase [AST], alanine aminotransferase [ALT]), prealbumin and serum albumin once per week

8. Do not increase flow rate if PN behind scheduled administration time

9. Discontinuation

   a. Gradually tapered to allow client to adjust to decreased levels of glucose

   b. After discontinuation, isotonic glucose solution administered to prevent rebound hypoglycemia (weakness, faintness, diaphoresis, shakiness, confusion, tachycardia)

# ALTERATIONS IN METABOLISM

## Metabolism, Elimination

## Alterations In Metabolism

A. Alterations in protein metabolism (*see* Table 7-9)

**Table 7-9** Alterations in Protein Metabolism

| DISORDER | ASSESSMENT | NURSING CONSIDERATIONS |
|---|---|---|
| Phenylketonuria (PKU)—inborn error of phenylalanine utilization | High blood phenylalanine that leads to intellectual delay | Specially prepared milk substitutes for infants (Lofenalac)<br><br>Low-protein diet for children (no meat, dairy products, eggs, NutraSweet) |
| Gout—inborn error of purine metabolism | High uric acid level that leads to progressive joint deterioration | Low-purine diet (no fish or organ meats) |
| Celiac disease (sprue)—inborn error of wheat and rye metabolism | Intestinal malabsorption that leads to malnutrition Diarrhea<br><br>Failure to thrive | Gluten-free diet (no wheat, rye, barley)<br><br>*Pure oats are gluten free; however, oats may become contaminated with gluten if processed in the same facility as wheat, rye, barley |
| Kidney failure | Increased protein and albumin losses in urine leads to protein deficiency | High-calorie, low-protein diet, as allowed by kidney function |
| Protein allergy | Diarrhea that leads to malnutrition and water loss | Change dietary protein source |

B. Alterations in fat metabolism (*see* Table 7-10)

**Table 7-10** Alterations in Fat Metabolism

| DISORDER | ASSESSMENT | NURSING CONSIDERATIONS |
|---|---|---|
| Hepatobiliary disease | Decreased bile leads to fat malabsorption | Low-fat, high-protein diet<br>Vitamins |
| Cystic fibrosis | Absence of pancreatic enzymes leads to malabsorption of fat (and fat-soluble vitamins), weight loss Infection and lung disease lead to increased need for calories and protein | Pancreatic enzyme replacement (pancrelipase) before or with meals High-protein diet High-calorie diet in advanced stages |
| Atherosclerosis (thickening and hardening of the arteries) | Associated with high blood cholesterol and triglyceride levels | Low-saturated-fat diet Cholesterol-lowering medications given before meals |

# Impaired Absorption of Nutrients

A. Infections of the GI tract

    1. Assessment

        a. Definition—acute illness caused by ingested food or water contaminated by toxins or parasites

        b. Signs and symptoms

            1) Headache

            2) Abdominal discomfort, anorexia

            3) Watery diarrhea, nausea, vomiting

            4) Low-grade fever

        c. Predisposing conditions—ingestion of contaminated food/liquid

    2. Types of infection (*see* Table 7-11)

    3. Nursing management

        a. Prevention

            1) Good sanitation

            2) Good hygiene measures (e.g., handwashing)

            3) Proper food preparation (e.g., thorough cooking); heat canned foods 10–20 min; inspect cans for gas bubbles

            4) Proper food storage

b. Treatment

1) Maintain fluid and electrolytes; oral rehydration preferred (infants 1–3 tsp every 10–15 min)

2) Monitor vital signs

3) Medication: antibiotics, antispasmodics as ordered

4) Maintain respiratory status—botulism can require tracheostomy, respiratory support

**Table 7-11** Common Infections of the Gastrointestinal Tract

| PARASITE OR BACTERIUM | SOURCE | NURSING CONSIDERATIONS |
|---|---|---|
| Enterotoxigenic *Escherichia coli* | Undercooked beef | Causes rapid, severe dehydration<br><br>Cook beef until meat no longer pink and juices run clear |
| *Salmonella* | Poultry, eggs | Causes gastroenteritis, systemic infection |
| *Campylobacter* | Poultry, beef, pork | Cook and store food at appropriate temperatures |
| *Giardia lamblia* | Protozoan, contaminated water | Treated with metronidazole, good personal hygiene |
| *Shigella* | Fecal contamination | Affects pediatric population, antimicrobial therapy |
| *Clostridioides difficile* | Fecal contamination | Greater risk in older adults<br><br>Often preceded by antibiotic therapy |

**B.** Vomiting

1. Characteristics—color, amount, quality, odor

2. Predisposing factors

   a. Health history—medication adverse effects, GI tract and neurological conditions

   b. Emotional factors—stress can precipitate vomiting

3. Diagnostic Studies

   a. Gastroscopy—direct visualization of gastric mucosa through a lighted endoscope

   b. Barium swallow radiologic study—client swallows a radiopaque liquid

4. Nursing management

   a. Antiemetics—medications that relieve vomiting (*see* Table 7-12)

   b. Replace lost fluids and electrolytes; oral rehydration preferred

   c. Control odors

**Table 7-12** Selected Antiemetic Medications

| MEDICATION | ADVERSE EFFECTS | NURSING CONSIDERATIONS |
|---|---|---|
| Prochlorperazine | Drowsiness<br><br>Orthostatic hypotension<br><br>Diplopia, photosensitivity | Check CBC and liver function with prolonged use |
| Ondansetron | Headache, sedation<br><br>Diarrhea, constipation<br><br>Transient elevations in liver enzymes | New class of antiemetics—serotonin receptor antagonist Administer 30 min prior to chemotherapy |
| Metoclopramide | Restlessness, anxiety, drowsiness<br><br>Extrapyramidal symptoms<br><br>Dystonic reactions | Monitor BP<br><br>Avoid activities requiring mental alertness<br><br>Take before meals<br><br>Used with tube feeding to decrease residual and risk of aspiration<br><br>Administer 30 min prior to chemotherapy |
| Meclizine | Drowsiness, dry mouth<br><br>Blurred vision<br><br>Excitation, restlessness | Contraindicated with glaucoma<br><br>Avoid activities requiring mental alertness |
| Dimenhydrinate | Drowsiness<br><br>Palpitations, hypotension<br><br>Blurred vision | Avoid activities requiring mental alertness |
| Promethazine | Drowsiness<br><br>Dizziness<br><br>Constipation<br><br>Urinary retention<br><br>Dry mouth | Administer PO, IM, rectal suppository<br><br>Report excessive sedation<br><br>Avoid alcohol, other CNS depressants |
| Ginger | Minor heartburn | May increase risk of bleeding if taken with anticoagulants, antiplatelet, or thrombolytic medications Instruct to stop medication if easy bruising or other signs of bleeding noted; report to health care provider |

# SELECTED DISORDERS

## Metabolism, Elimination, Client Education

### Hiatal Hernia

A. Definition—opening in diaphragm through which the esophagus passes becomes enlarged and part of the upper stomach comes up into the lower portion of the thorax

B. Etiology

   1. Structural—weakening of diaphragm

   2. Increased abdominal pressure—obesity, pregnancy, heavy lifting

   3. Gerontologic considerations—weakened diaphragm, kyphosis, medications (calcium channel blockers, nitrates)

C. Clinical manifestations

   1. Often no symptoms

   2. Feeling of fullness in chest with pain when lying down

   3. Client reports chest pain, heartburn, belching, dysphagia

D. Treatment

   1. Antacids (with limitations)

   2. H₂ receptor blockers (e.g., cimetidine, ranitidine)

   3. Cryoprotective medications (e.g., sucralfate)

   4. Proton pump inhibitors (e.g., omeprazole)

   5. Surgery to tighten cardiac sphincter (valvuloplasty or antireflux procedure)

E. Dietary

   1. Small, frequent meals; avoid caffeine, chocolate, alcohol, fatty foods, NSAIDs

F. Nursing management: client teaching—do not lie down for at least 1 hour after meals; elevate head of bed when sleeping

### Gastritis

A. Definition—inflammation of stomach, which may be acute or chronic

B. Clinical manifestations—uncomfortable feeling in abdomen, headache, anorexia, nausea, vomiting (possibly bloody), hiccuping

   **C.** Causes—*Helicobacter pylori*, NSAIDs, alcohol, radiation therapy, atrophic gastritis in older adults

   **D.** Nursing management

      1. Nothing by mouth, slowly progressing to bland diet

      2. Antacids often relieve pain

      3. Referral to appropriate agency if alcohol abuse is verified

      4. Medications—$H_2$ receptor blockers, proton pump inhibitors, cryoprotective medications, antibiotics

## Peptic Ulcer Disease

   **A.** Definition—excavation formed in the mucosal wall, caused by erosion that may extend to muscle layers or through the muscle to the peritoneum (*see* Table 7-13)

   **B.** Assessment—sites (*see* Figure 7-4)

   **C.** Risk factors

      1. *H. pylori* infection

      2. Acute responses to medical or surgical stressors

      3. Psychological stress

      4. Gerontologic considerations—increased use of NSAIDs

**Table 7-13** Duodenal Versus Gastric Ulcer

| | CHRONIC DUODENAL ULCER | CHRONIC GASTRIC ULCER |
|---|---|---|
| Age | 30–60 years | 50 years and older |
| Sex | Male to female ratio of 3:1 | Male to female ratio of 1:1 |
| Risk factors | Blood group type O, COPD, chronic renal failure, alcohol, smoking, cirrhosis, stress | Gastritis, alcohol, smoking, NSAIDs, stress |
| Gastric secretion | Hypersecretion | Normal to hyposecretion |
| Pain | 2–3 hours after meal; nighttime, often in early sleeping hours<br><br>Food intake relieves pain<br><br>Older adults—pain may not be first symptom | 0.1–1 hour after meal or when fasting<br><br>Relieved by vomiting<br><br>Ingestion of food does not help<br><br>Older adults—pain may not be first symptom |
| Vomiting | Rare | Frequent |
| Hemorrhage | Less likely | More likely |
| Malignancy | Rare | Occasionally |

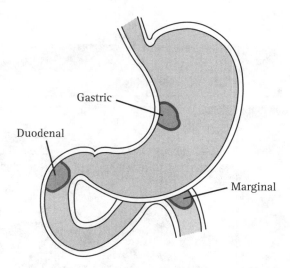

**Figure 7-4.** Sites for Ulcers

**D.** Nursing management—nonsurgical

1. Diet

   a. Avoid oversecretion and hypermotility in the gastrointestinal tract

   b. Eat three meals per day; small, frequent feedings not necessary if taking antacids or histamine blocker

   c. Avoid coffee, alcohol, highly seasoned foods, milk and cream, extremes in food temperature

2. Reduce stress

3. Medications (*see* Table 7-14)

   a. Antacids: administer 1 h before or after meals; antacids decrease absorption of other medications

   b. Histamine receptor site antagonist (e.g., cimetidine, ranitidine); administer with meals

   c. Sucralfate; give 1 hour before meals

   d. Proton pump inhibitors

   e. Antibiotic therapy for *H. pylori* (e.g., metronidazole, tetracycline)

**Table 7-14** GI Medications

| MEDICATION | ADVERSE EFFECTS | NURSING CONSIDERATIONS |
|---|---|---|
| **Antacids** | | |
| Aluminum hydroxide gel Calcium carbonate<br><br>Aluminum hydroxide and magnesium trisilicate | Constipation that may lead to impaction<br><br>Phosphate depletion (aluminum-only products) | Monitor bowel pattern<br><br>Compounds contain sodium; check if client is on sodium-restricted diet<br><br>Aluminum and magnesium antacid compounds interfere with tetracycline absorption<br><br>Calcium compounds can cause hypercalcemia and hypersecretion of gastric acid, causing acid rebound<br><br>Encourage fluids<br><br>Monitor for signs of phosphate deficiency—malaise, weakness, tremors, bone pain<br><br>Shake well |
| Magnesium hydroxide | None at normal dose<br><br>Excessive dose can produce nausea, vomiting, and diarrhea | Store at room temperature with tight lid to prevent absorption of $CO_2$<br><br>Prolonged and frequent use of cathartic dose can lead to dependence<br><br>Administer with caution to clients with renal disease |
| Magnesium trisilicate in combination with aluminum hydroxide | (See aluminum hydroxide gel and magnesium hydroxide, above) | (See aluminum hydroxide gel and magnesium hydroxide, above)<br><br>Careful use advised for kidney dysfunction |
| Aluminum hydroxide and magnesium hydroxide combined | Slight laxative effect | Encourage fluid intake |
| **Cytoprotective** | | |
| Sucralfate | Constipation<br><br>Dizziness | Take medication 1 h before each meal<br><br>Should not be taken with antacids or $H_2$ blockers |

(Continued)

**Table 7-14** GI Medications (*Continued*)

| MEDICATION | ADVERSE EFFECTS | NURSING CONSIDERATIONS |
|---|---|---|
| **H₂ Antagonists** | | |
| Cimetidine<br><br>Ranitidine<br><br>Famotidine | Diarrhea<br><br>Confusion and dizziness (esp. in older adults with large doses)<br><br>Headache | Bedtime dose suppresses nocturnal acid production<br><br>Compliance may increase with single-dose regimen<br><br>Avoid antacids within 1 hour of dose<br><br>Dysrhythmias<br><br>Cimetidine—high risk of confusion in older adults |
| **Proton Pump Inhibitors** | | |
| Omeprazole<br><br>Lansoprazole<br><br>Rabeprazole<br><br>Esomeprazole<br><br>Pantoprazole | Dizziness<br><br>Diarrhea | Typically administered 30–60 minutes before breakfast<br><br>Do not crush sustained-release capsule; contents may be sprinkled on food or instilled with fluid in NG tube |
| **Anti-Ulcer** | | |
| Sucralfate | Nausea<br><br>Vomiting<br><br>Decreased absorption of some medication | Shake well before pouring<br><br>Give on an empty stomach<br><br>Give 1–2 hours before meals |
| **Prostaglandin Analogs** | | |
| Misoprostol | Abdominal pain Diarrhea (13%) Miscarriage | Notify health care provider if diarrhea more than 1 week or severe abdominal pain or black, tarry stools |
| **Nursing considerations** | Other medications may be prescribed, including antacids (time administration to avoid canceling med effect) and antimicrobials to eradicate *H. pylori* infections<br><br>Client should avoid smoking, alcohol, aspirin (ASA), and caffeine, all of which increase stomach acid | |

    4. Complications

      a. Perforation

      b. Hemorrhage

      c. Periodontitis

**E.** Surgical intervention (*see* Figure 7-5)

    1. Diagnostic work—upper GI series, endoscopy, CT scan, esophagogastroduodenoscopy (EGD)

    2. Minimally invasive surgery by laparoscopy

    3. Gastrectomy—removal of stomach and attachment to upper portion of duodenum

    4. Pyloroplasty

    5. Vagotomy—cutting the vagus nerve (decreases HCl secretion)

    6. Billroth I—partial removal (distal one-third to one-half) of stomach, anastomosis with duodenum

    7. Billroth II—removal of distal segment of stomach and antrum, anastomosis with jejunum

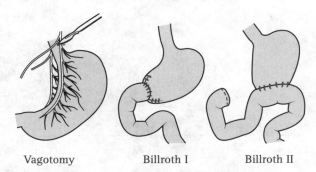

Vagotomy      Billroth I      Billroth II

**Figure 7-5.** Common Surgeries for Ulcers

**F.** Nursing management—surgical

    1. Postoperative

      a. Assess vital signs

      b. Inspect dressings

      c. Observe nasogastric drainage for volume and blood

      d. Provide gastric decompression as ordered

        1) Levin tube—single lumen at low suction

        2) Salem sump—double lumen for drainage

          a) Prevent irritation to nostril

          b) Lubricate tube around nares with water soluble jelly

          c) Control excessive nasal secretions

2. $B_{12}$ via parenteral route (required for life)

3. Encourage deep breathing

4. Observe for peristalsis

   a. Listen for bowel sounds

   b. Record passage of flatus or stool

5. Teach preventive measures for "dumping syndrome" (rapid passage of food to stomach, causing diaphoresis, diarrhea, hypotension); usually occurs 10–15 minutes after eating

   a. Restrict fluids with meals

   b. Avoid stress after eating

   c. Eat smaller, frequent meals

   d. Lie down after eating

# Pyloric Stenosis in Adults

**A.** Definition—in adults, narrowing or obstruction of the pyloric sphincter caused by scarring from healing ulcers

**B.** Assessment

1. Vomiting

2. Epigastric fullness

3. Anorexia

4. Weight loss

5. Constipation

**C.** Surgical intervention

1. Pyloroplasty—incision through circular muscles of the pylorus

2. Vagotomy and gastroenterostomy—establishes gastric drainage, involves severing of vagus nerve

**D.** Nursing management

1. Perioperative

   a. Correct fluid and electrolyte abnormalities—alkalosis, hypokalemia

   b. Gastric decompression or small frequent feedings

2. Postoperative

   a. Observe for signs of dumping syndrome, gastritis, and esophagitis (adults)

   b. Check incision; provide fluids

# ACCESSORY ORGANS OF DIGESTION (LIVER, GALLBLADDER, PANCREAS)

## Metabolism, Nutrition, Elimination

### Overview of Accessory Organs

A.  Liver (*see* Figure 7-6)

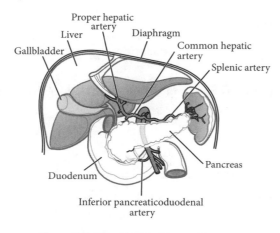

**Figure 7-6.** Liver, Gallbladder, and Pancreas

1.  Anatomy

    a.  Gland located in right upper quadrant of abdomen below diaphragm

    b.  Arterial blood brought to liver by hepatic artery

    c.  Filtered blood returns to body via hepatic vein

    d.  Blood from the stomach, spleen, pancreas, and intestine is brought to liver for filtration via the portal vein

    e.  Older adults—decreased liver size

2.  Functions

    a.  Manufacture and secrete bile

        1)  Bilirubin—from hemoglobin released by red blood cells at end of their life cycle

        2)  Bile salts

        3)  Cholesterol

        4)  Color—greenish or brownish yellow

        5)  Bile aids in digestion and leaves liver via channels that form the hepatic duct

          b.  Manufacture of fibrinogen and prothrombin

          c.  Manufacture of heparin

          d.  Aids in destruction of aging red blood cells

          e.  Manufacture of vitamin A

          f.  Storage of vitamins A, B, D, iron, copper

          g.  Metabolism of carbohydrates, fats, proteins

          h.  Manufacture of immunoglobulins

          i.  Metabolism of medications, alcohol, and hormones

          j.  Regulation of blood volume by storing up to 400 mL of blood

          k.  Older adults—decreased enzymatic reactions; decreased metabolism of medications and hormones

**B.** Biliary tract

    1.  Common bile duct

          a.  Anatomy—composed of cystic duct from the gallbladder and hepatic duct from the liver; leads to duodenum

          b.  Function—transports bile from liver and gallbladder to duodenum when food is present in small intestine

    2.  Cystic duct

          a.  Anatomy—leads from gallbladder to the common bile duct

          b.  Function—passageway for bile to and from gallbladder

             1)  When duodenum is empty, sphincter closes, causing bile from the liver to flow through the cystic duct into the gallbladder

             2)  During digestion, sphincter opens as the gallbladder contracts, forcing bile through the cystic duct to the common bile duct into the duodenum

    3.  Gallbladder (*see* Figure 7-6)

          a.  Anatomy—sac located under the right side of liver

          b.  Function—storage and concentration of bile; stimulated to contract by cholecystokinin (a hormone secreted by the small intestine in response to the presence of fat)

**C.** Pancreas (*see* Figure 7-6)

    1.  Anatomy

          a.  Gland located behind stomach on left side of abdomen

          b.  Composed of lobes, lobules, and ducts

          c.  Pancreatic duct joins with the common bile duct at the duodenum

          d.  Contains the islets of Langerhans—specialized cells that produce insulin and glucagon

    2.  Functions—digestive and exocrine gland functions

          a.  Manufacture and release (via pancreatic duct) of pancreatic enzymes to aid digestion

             1)  Amylase—helps break down carbohydrates

             2)  Lipase—helps break down fats

             3)  Trypsin—helps break down protein

    b.  Production and release of insulin and glucagon directly into the bloodstream

        1)  Alpha cells synthesize glucagon

        2)  Beta cells synthesize insulin

# Diagnostic Testing

**A.**  Liver function studies

    1.  Liver function test—over 70% of the parenchyma of the liver may be damaged before liver function tests become abnormal (*see* Table 7-15)

**B.**  Radiographic

    1.  Abdominal x-rays—show enlargement or displacement of organs

    2.  Cholangiogram—x-ray permitting visualization of bile ducts after IV injection of dye

    3.  Liver scan—scanning of liver with radioisotope-sensitive device after IV injection of radioisotopes; detects cysts or masses in the liver

**C.**  Ultrasound

**D.**  Liver biopsy

    1.  Client preparation

        a.  Obtain vital signs and weight

        b.  Done at bedside—client in supine position or lateral with upper arms elevated

        c.  Empty bladder prior to procedure to avoid accidental perforation

        d.  Administer vitamin K IM to decrease chance of hemorrhage; check clotting time

        e.  NPO morning of procedure (6 h before)

        f.  Sedative administration just prior to procedure; teach client about holding breath for 5–10 s during procedure

    2.  Nursing management

        a.  Check vital signs frequently for hemorrhage and/or infection; weigh client

        b.  Assess dressing and insertion site

        c.  Report elevated temperature and/or abdominal pain to health care provider

**E.**  Paracentesis

    1.  Needle aspiration of abnormal fluid accumulated in abdominal cavity (ascites) for analysis or as therapeutic measure

    2.  Client preparation

        a.  Obtain vital signs and weight

        b.  Done at bedside—client typically placed in supine position with HOB slightly elevated

        c.  Empty bladder prior to procedure to avoid accidental perforation

    3.  Nursing management

        a.  Check vital signs frequently for hemorrhage and/or infection; weigh client

        b.  Assess dressing and insertion site

        c.  Report elevated temperature and/or abdominal pain to health care provider

        d.  Maintain bedrest according to agency policy

**Table 7-15** Liver Function Tests

| TEST | PURPOSE | PREPARATION/TESTING CONVENTIONAL UNITS (SI UNITS) | POSTTEST NURSING CARE |
|---|---|---|---|
| Pigment studies | Parameters of hepatic ability to conjugate and excrete bilirubin<br><br>Abnormal in liver and gallbladder disorders, e.g., with jaundice<br><br>Direct bilirubin increases in obstruction | Fast 4 h<br><br>Normal:<br>Serum bilirubin, direct 0.1–0.4 mg/dL (1.7–3.7 mcmol/L)<br>Serum bilirubin, total 0.3–1 mg/dL (5–17 mcmol/L)<br>Urine bilirubin, total 0 | Over 70% of the parenchyma of the liver may be damaged before liver function tests become abnormal |
| Protein studies:<br>Serum albumin | Proteins are produced by the liver<br><br>Levels may diminish in hepatic disease<br><br>Severely decreased serum albumin results in generalized edema | Normal:<br><br>3.5–5.5 g/dL  (35–55 g/L) | None |
| Coagulation studies:<br>Prothrombin time (PT) or international normalized ratio (INR)<br><br>Partial thromboplastin time (PTT) | May be prolonged in hepatic disease<br><br>In liver disease, PTT prolonged due to lack of vitamin K | Normal:<br><br>PT 9–12 seconds<br>PTT 20–39 seconds | Put specimen in ice<br><br>Apply pressure to site for 5 min (15 min if on anticoagulants) |
| Liver enzymes | With damaged liver cells, enzymes are released into bloodstream | Normal:<br><br>AST 10–40 units/L<br>ALT 7–56 units/L<br>LDH less than 176 units/L | None |
| Blood ammonia (arterial) | Liver converts ammonia to urea<br><br>With liver disease, ammonia levels rise | Normal:<br><br>15–45 mcg/dL (11–32 mcmol/L) | None |
| Abdominal x-ray | To determine gross liver size | None | None |
| Liver/spleen scan | To demonstrate size, shape of liver; visualize scar tissue, cysts, or tumors; radioactive isotope injected intravenously | Client is not a source of radioactivity | None |

| TEST | PURPOSE | PREPARATION/TESTING CONVENTIONAL UNITS (SI UNITS) | POSTTEST NURSING CARE |
|---|---|---|---|
| Cholecystogram and cholangiography (percutaneous, surgical, or magnetic resonance) | For gallbladder and bile duct visualization; radiopaque material injected directly into biliary tree; determines filling of hepatic and biliary ducts | Question client about seafood (iodine) allergy<br><br>Fat-free dinner evening before exam<br><br>Ingestion of dye in tablet form<br><br>(Telepaque tablets—check history of allergies to iodine) evening before<br><br>NPO after dye ingestion<br><br>X-rays followed by ingestion of high-fat meal followed by further x-rays | None |
| Celiac axis arteriography | For liver and pancreas visualization; uses contrast medium of organic iodine | Question client about seafood (iodine) allergy prior to radiopaque dye administration; anaphylaxis possible | None |
| Splenoportogram (splenic portal venography) | To determine adequacy of portal blood flow; uses contrast medium of organic iodine | Question client about seafood (iodine) allergy prior to radiopaque dye administration; anaphylaxis possible | None |
| Liver biopsy | Sampling of tissue by percutaneous needle aspiration | Administer vitamin K IM to decrease chance of hemorrhage<br><br>Informed consent<br><br>NPO morning of exam (6 h)<br><br>Sedative administration just before exam<br><br>Ask client to hold breath for 5–10 seconds during insertion<br><br>Performed at bedside, supine position, lateral with upper arms elevated | Position on right side for 1–2 h and gradually elevate head of bed (HOB), 30° 1st 2 h, 45° 2nd 2 h<br><br>Maintain bedrest for 24 h<br><br>Frequently check vital signs to detect hemorrhage and shock; check clotting time, platelets, hematocrit<br><br>Expect mild local pain radiating to right shoulder<br><br>Note reports of severe abdominal pain immediately— may be indication of perforation of bile duct and peritonitis |
| Bilirubin | Detect presence of bilirubin due to hemolytic or liver disease | Total bilirubin 0.3–1 mg/dL (5–17 mcmol/L)<br><br>Direct (conjugated) bilirubin 0.1–0.4 mg/dL (1.7–3.7 mcmol/L)<br><br>Indirect (unconjugated) bilirubin 0.1–0.4 mg/dL (3.4–11.2 mcmol/L) | None |

# Selected Disorders of the Digestive Accessory Organs

A. Liver disorders

1. Cirrhosis

   a. Definition—group of chronic diseases in which liver tissue is gradually replaced by scar tissue; results in gradual loss of liver function

   b. Assessment

      1) Alcoholic cirrhosis—result of alcoholism and poor nutrition

      2) Biliary cirrhosis—result of chronic biliary obstruction and infection

      3) Postnecrotic cirrhosis—result of a previous viral hepatitis

      4) Older adults—hepatitis C, obesity, chronic alcohol use

      5) Complications

         a) Portal hypertension—elevated blood pressure throughout entire portal venous system

         b) Esophageal varices

            i) Dilated tortuous veins usually found in the submucosa of the lower esophagus

            ii) Hemorrhage from rupture leading cause of death in clients with cirrhosis

            iii) Ascites

            iv) Bleeding disorders

   c. Surgical intervention—cirrhosis/bleeding esophageal varices

      1) Shunts to relieve portal hypertension—last resort intervention for portal hypertension and esophageal varices

         a) Portacaval—blood diverted from portal circulation to vena cava

         b) Splenorenal—blood diverted from splenic vein to left renal artery

         c) Transjugular intrahepatic portosystemic shunt (TIPS)

      2) Liver transplant

      3) TIPS—for clients who have not responded to any other nonsurgical management

   d. Surgical/nonsurgical intervention—bleeding esophageal varices

      1) Insertion of Sengstaken-Blakemore tube with three openings (*see* Figure 7-7)

         a) Gastric balloon—inflation lumen

         b) Esophageal balloon—inflation lumen

         c) Gastric aspiration lumen

      2) Minnesota tube

         a) Similar to Sengstaken-Blakemore tube but has four lumens

         b) Fourth lumen allows for aspiration of secretions that collect above the esophageal balloon

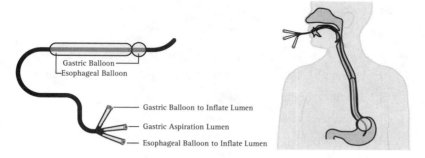

**Figure 7-7.** Sengstaken-Blakemore Tube

3) Injection sclerotherapy—endoscopic injection of a chemical into the esophagus; causes varices to become fibrotic

4) Endoscopic variceal ligation

5) Administration of desmopressin acetate—temporarily lowers portal pressure

6) Shunting procedure—TIPS

e. History

1) Digestive disturbances

a) Indigestion

b) Flatulence

c) Anorexia

d) Nausea and vomiting

2) Circulatory

a) Esophageal varices

b) Hematemesis

c) Hemorrhage

d) Ascites

e) Hemorrhoids

f) Increased bleeding tendencies

g) Edema in extremities

3) Biliary

a) Jaundice

b) Pruritus

c) Dark urine

d) Clay-colored stools

4) Hepatorenal failure

5) Hepatic failure

    f. Nursing management

      1) Provide appropriate nutrition

        a) Early stages—high protein, high carbohydrates

        b) Advanced stages—fiber, protein, fat, and sodium restrictions

        c) Small, frequent feedings

        d) Fluid restriction

        e) No alcohol

      2) Maintain skin integrity

        a) Avoid strong soaps

        b) Alleviate dry, itching skin

      3) Promote rest

      4) Reduce exposure to infection

      5) Reduce ascites

        a) Sodium/fluid restrictions

        b) Medications—diuretics

        c) Paracentesis

      6) Monitor fluid/electrolyte balance

      7) Lactulose—decreases serum ammonia levels

2. Jaundice

    a. Definition—condition in which all tissues, including skin and sclera, are yellow or greenish yellow because of an increased concentration of bilirubin in the blood

    b. Causes

      1) Hemolytic (prehepatic)—caused by destruction of great number of blood cells, causing a high concentration of bilirubin, exceeding the liver's ability to excrete it

        a) Hemolytic transfusion reactions

        b) Autoimmune hemolytic anemia

        c) Erythroblastosis fetalis

      2) Intrahepatic—due to inability of normal amounts of bilirubin to be excreted by a diseased liver

        a) Cirrhosis

        b) Hepatitis

      3) Obstructive (posthepatic)—due to intrahepatic or extrahepatic obstruction interfering with bile flow

        a) Cholelithiasis

        b) Tumors

        c) Adverse effect of medications—e.g., phenothiazine derivative, sulfonamides

    c.  History and assessment

        1)  Yellowish or greenish yellow discoloration of skin and sclera

        2)  Dark-colored urine

        3)  Clay-colored stools

        4)  Pruritus

    d.  Nursing management

        1)  Treatment of underlying cause

        2)  Relief of pruritus

            a)  Medications—e.g., antihistamines, topical steroids

            b)  Diversionary activities

            c)  Corn starch, baking soda, oatmeal bath

            d)  Keep nails trimmed and clean

3.  Hepatitis (*see* Table 7-16)

    a.  Assessment

        1)  Fatigue

        2)  Jaundice (icterus), yellow sclera

        3)  Anorexia, right upper quadrant (RUQ) pain and tenderness, malaise

        4)  Clay-colored stools, tea-colored urine

        5)  Pruritus—accumulation of bile salts under the skin

        6)  Liver function studies; elevated ALT, AST, alkaline phosphatase (ALP)

        7)  Prolonged PT

        8)  Percutaneous liver biopsy

        9)  Antibodies to specific virus; (e.g., anti–hepatitis A [anti-HAV])

    b.  Nursing management

        1)  Frequent rest periods

        2)  Appropriate transmission-based precautions

            a)  HAV—enteric precautions

            b)  Hepatitis B (HBV), hepatitis C (HCV)—blood and body fluids precautions

        3)  Diet low in fat, high in calories, carbohydrates, and protein; no alcoholic beverages

        4)  For pruritus—calamine; short, clean nails; antihistamines

        5)  Medications

            a)  Vitamin K

            b)  Antiviral medications—interferon and lamivudine

            c)  After exposure to hepatitis B vaccine

**Table 7-16** Classifications of Hepatitis

| TYPE | HIGH RISK GROUP | INCUBATION | TRANSMISSION | NURSING CONSIDERATIONS |
|---|---|---|---|---|
| Hepatitis A (HAV) | Young children<br><br>Institutions for custodial care<br><br>International travelers to developing countries | 15–50 days | Common in fall, early winter<br><br>Fecal-oral<br><br>Shellfish from contaminated water<br><br>Poor sanitation<br><br>Contaminated food handlers<br><br>Oral-anal sexual activity | Survives on hands<br><br>Diagnostic tests—Cultured in stool and detected in serum before onset of disease<br><br>Prevention—improved sanitation; hepatitis A vaccine<br><br>Treated with gamma globulin early postexposure<br><br>No preparation of food |
| Hepatitis B (HBV) | Immigrants from areas of HBV endemicity<br><br>Drug addicts<br><br>Fetuses from infected mothers<br><br>Homosexually active men<br><br>Clients on dialysis<br><br>Male prisoners<br><br>Transfusion recipients<br><br>Health care workers | 28–160 days | Blood and body fluids<br><br>Parenteral drug abuse<br><br>Sexual contact Hemodialysis<br><br>Accidental contaminated needle exposure<br><br>Maternal-fetal route | Diagnostic tests—antibodies to hepatitis B surface antigen, antibodies to hepatitis B core antigen, antibodies to hepatitis B e antigen<br><br>Treatment—hepatitis B vaccine (Heptavax-B, Recombivax HB), hepatitis B immune globulin (HBIg) postexposure, interferon alpha-2b, lamivudine<br><br>Chronic carriers—frequent, potential for chronicity 5–10%<br><br>Complications—cirrhosis, liver cancer |
| Hepatitis C (HCV) | Persons receiving frequent blood transfusions<br><br>International travelers<br><br>Hemophilia clients | 15–160 days | Contact with blood and body fluids<br><br>IV drug users | May be asymptomatic<br><br>Complications—cirrhosis, liver cancer<br><br>Great potential for chronicity |

*(Continued)*

**Table 7-16** Classifications of Hepatitis (*Continued*)

| TYPE | HIGH RISK GROUP | INCUBATION | TRANSMISSION | NURSING CONSIDERATIONS |
|---|---|---|---|---|
| Delta or hepatitis D (HDV) | Drug addicts<br><br>Concurrent HBV infection | 28–160 days | Coinfects with hepatitis B<br><br>Close personal contact<br><br>Parenteral transmission | Diagnostic test—hepatitis D antigen (HD Ag) in serum |
| Hepatitis E | Persons living in underdeveloped countries | 28–35 days | Oral-fecal<br><br>Contaminated water | Resembles hepatitis A<br><br>Does not become chronic<br><br>Usually seen in young adults<br><br>Seen in travelers from Asia, Africa, Mexico |
| Toxic hepatitis | Older adults (increased use of prescription and over-the-counter medications, decreased liver metabolism)<br><br>Medication-induced (INH, diuretics, tetracycline, carbon tetrachloride acetaminophen) Ethyl alcohol | | Noninfectious inflammation of liver | Removal of causative substance<br><br>Check level of consciousness<br><br>Encourage fluids |

6) Teach client and family

    a) Avoid alcohol and potentially hepatotoxic prescription/OTC medications (particularly acetaminophen and sedatives)

    b) Balance rest and activity periods

    c) Techniques to prevent spread

    d) Cannot give blood donation

    e) Instruct to note and report recurrence of signs and symptoms

    **B.** Biliary disorders

      1. Cholecystitis

        a. Definition—inflammation of gallbladder

        b. Causes—bacterial invasion via blood, lymph, or bile ducts

        c. Risk factors

          1) Cholelithiasis

          2) Obesity

          3) Sedentary lifestyle

          4) Women affected more than men

          5) Highest incidence age 50–60 y

        d. Assessment

          1) Intolerance to fatty foods

          2) Indigestion

          3) Nausea, vomiting, flatulence

          4) Severe pain in upper right quadrant of abdomen radiating to back and right shoulder

          5) Elevated temperature

          6) Leukocytosis

          7) Dark urine, clay-colored stools

        e. Nursing management

          1) Antibiotics

          2) NPO until acute symptoms subside

          3) Gastric decompression

          4) Analgesics

          5) Weight-reduction diet if needed

          6) Avoidance of fatty, fried foods

      2. Laparoscopic cholecystectomy

        a. Laparoscope attached to a video camera visualizes the gallbladder through a small, 10-mm puncture at the umbilicus

        b. A laser is used to dissect the gallbladder away from the liver bed

        c. Laparoscopic forceps extract the gallbladder through puncture site

      3. Surgical management of the client with biliary disease

        a. Types of surgery

          1) Cholecystectomy—removal of gallbladder; a Penrose drain may be inserted through the incision to promote drainage into dressings

          2) Cholecystostomy—opening of gallbladder to remove stones, bile, or pus (decompression); a tube (cholecystostomy tube) is sutured into the gallbladder for drainage

3) Choledochostomy—opening into the common bile duct to remove obstructing stones; a drainage tube (T-tube) is inserted into the duct and connected to drainage

4) Extracorporeal shock wave lithotripsy—shock wave therapy to destroy stones in the biliary system

  a) Strong analgesics and sedation used before procedure

  b) Treatment followed with oral dissolution therapy

b. Preoperative care

1) Routine preop care

2) Nutritional supplements of glucose and protein hydrolysates to aid in wound healing and prevent liver damage

3) NG tube insertion before surgery

c. Postoperative care

1) Routine postop care to prevent respiratory, circulatory, and fluid electrolyte complications

2) Promotion of drainage from cholecystostomy or T-tube until normal bile flow is reestablished

  a) Semi-Fowler position

  b) Prevent kinking or twisting of tubes

  c) Position drainage bottle as ordered (usually kept on bed at or below level as gallbladder)

  d) Observe and record amount and character of drainage (expect 500–1,000 mL/d at first)

3) Check orders regarding clamping of T-tube before/after meals

4) Check orders regarding fluid replacement of drainage

5) Provide low-fat, high-carbohydrate, high-protein diet

6) Note color changes of skin, sclera, and stool as indicators of improved bile flow after T-tube removal

  a) Jaundice should lessen

  b) Stool should slowly progress from light to dark color

7) Protect skin around incision from drainage and leakage

  a) Apply coat of zinc oxide or petroleum jelly

  b) Change dressing frequently

  c) If drainage amount remains large, record finding (may indicate fistula)

8) Provide pain medication as needed

  a) Position frequently for comfort

  b) Evaluate pain intensity; may indicate other problems, e.g., infection, urinary retention, gas in intestines

9) Monitor signs for $K^+$ and $Na^+$ alterations; check serum electrolytes

4. Cholelithiasis

   a. Definition—presence of stones in the gallbladder; cholesterol stones or pigment stones

   b. Causes—an increased concentration and precipitation of bile substances (cholesterol, bile acids, bile pigments)

      1) Metabolic factors—an increased serum cholesterol

         a) Obesity

         b) Pregnancy

         c) Diabetes

         d) Hypothyroidism

      2) Biliary stasis

      3) Biliary system inflammation and cirrhosis of liver

   c. Assessment

      1) Belching immediately following a meal; flatulence

      2) Indigestion following rich, fatty foods

      3) Severe right upper quadrant abdominal pain radiating to back and right shoulder (biliary colic); rebound tenderness

      4) Nausea and vomiting

      5) Biliary colic—severe pain, tachycardia, diaphoresis

   d. Nursing management

      1) Relief of pain—analgesics; meperidine avoided

      2) Anticholinergics—dicyclomine

      3) Control of nausea and vomiting

      4) Gastric decompression

      5) Monitor for dehydration

5. Biliary carcinoma

   a. Risk factors—chronic cholelithiasis

   b. Cause—unknown

   c. Signs and symptoms

      1) Jaundice (advanced disease)

      2) Same as cholelithiasis

   d. Management—cholecystectomy, radiation therapy, chemotherapy

6. Biliary atresia

   a. Definition—congenital absence of bile ducts

   b. Cause—unknown

   c. Assessment

      1) Jaundice of progressive intensity starting at age 2–3 wk

      2) Dark urine

3) Clay-colored stools

4) Decreased nutritional fat absorption

5) Vitamin A, D, E, K (fat-soluble) deficiencies

6) Low prothrombin level and easy bleeding

7) Lethargy and slow movement

d. Nursing management

1) Reconstructive surgery to create pathway for bile flow into intestines

2) Poor prognosis—only small percentage of infants can tolerate the surgery

**C.** Pancreatic disorders

1. Acute pancreatitis

a. Definition—inflammatory condition of the pancreas in which pancreatic function can be restored

b. Etiology

1) Possible factors: tumors, cysts, abscesses, penetrating ulcers, infections, medication toxicities, heredity, neurogenic and emotional factors, alcoholism, trauma to abdomen

2) Theory—"autodigestion" of the pancreas by its own enzymes

c. Assessment

1) Nausea and vomiting; vomiting does not relieve pain or nausea; may occur after heavy meal or alcohol ingestion

2) Fluid/electrolyte imbalance

3) Abdominal and back pain major symptom; pain increased after meals and is unrelieved with antacids

4) Fever

5) Jaundice

6) Hyperglycemia

7) Weight loss

8) Ascites

9) Increased serum amylase and lipase, elevated urine amylase, decreased serum calcium, elevated bilirubin

d. Nursing management

1) NPO

2) Gastric decompression

3) Antacids and proton pump inhibitors

4) Analgesics (meperidine contraindicated)

5) Treating fluid/electrolyte imbalance

6) Monitor for signs of infection

7) Monitor for shock, renal failure

        8)    Monitor for hyperglycemia

        9)    PN

     10)    Long-term treatment includes avoidance of alcohol; low-fat, bland diet; and small, frequent meals

2. Chronic pancreatitis

   a. Definition—chronic fibrosis of the pancreas with obstruction of pancreatic ducts and destruction of pancreatic secreting cells

   b. Causes and risk factors

      1)    Develops after repeated episodes of alcohol-induced acute pancreatitis

      2)    Associated with chronic obstruction of bile duct

   c. Assessment

      1)    Severe upper abdominal and back pain difficult to relieve; pain flares up

      2)    Nausea and vomiting

      3)    Jaundice

      4)    Dark urine

      5)    Fever

      6)    Diarrhea and steatorrhea

      7)    Weight loss and muscle wasting

      8)    Diabetes mellitus (polyuria, polydipsia, polyphagia)

   d. Nursing management

      1)    Analgesics—opioid and nonopioid analgesics

      2)    Medications to decrease gastric acid—$H_2$ receptor blockers, proton pump inhibitors, or octreotide

      3)    Bland, low-fat diet

      4)    Six small feedings daily—increased caloric intake

      5)    Treatment of exocrine insufficiency—medications containing amylase, lipase, and trypsin to aid digestion, e.g., pancrelipase

      6)    Monitor signs and symptoms of diabetes mellitus; possible oral hypoglycemics or insulin

      7)    Avoid alcohol

3. Pancreatic cancer

   a. Assessment

      1)    Pain is absent in early stages

      2)    Pain (abdominal: vague, dull)

      3)    Anorexia and fatigue

      4)    Weight loss

      5)    Nausea, vomiting, flatulence

      6)    Jaundice (initial sign, but disease may be advanced)

7) Clay-colored stools

8) Dark urine; frothy urine

9) GI bleeding

10) Ascites

b. Nursing management

1) High-calorie, bland, low-fat diet

2) Avoid alcohol

3) Anticholinergics

4) Chemotherapy—combination of medications

5) Radiation therapy (external beam or radioactive iodine implantation)

6) Stent placement for obstruction

7) Surgery (Whipple procedure)—removal of head of pancreas, distal portion of common bile duct, the duodenum, and part of the stomach or minimally invasive surgery via laparoscopy

8) Postop nursing management

a) Monitor for peritonitis, hemorrhage, thrombophlebitis, diabetes or hypoglycemia

b) Monitor for intestinal obstruction, paralytic (adynamic) ileus

c) Monitor for shock, pancreatitis, hepatic failure

# SECTION 5

# THE LOWER INTESTINAL TRACT

## Nutrition, Elimination

## Assessment of Elimination Function

A. Anatomy

  1. Cecum—first portion; pouch-like structure in lower right quadrant; receives chyme from ileum

  2. Colon

    a. Ascending colon—up right side of abdomen

    b. Transverse colon—across abdomen

    c. Descending colon—down left side of abdomen

    d. Sigmoid colon—lower portion of descending colon; contains feces ready for excretion, empties into rectum

    e. Rectum—end portion of large intestine; 7 in long; usually empty except during and immediately before defecation; decreased rectal sensation in older adults

    f. Anal canal—1 in long; has internal and external sphincter

B. Process

  1. Waste products are moved along GI tract by muscular contractions called peristalsis

  2. Peristalsis is stimulated by presence of bulk in intestine

  3. Consistency of stool affected by length of time in large intestine and amount of water reabsorbed

  4. Anatomical process

    a. Reflex action

      1) Internal anal sphincter is under autonomic nervous system control

      2) When rectum is full, parasympathetic nerves are stimulated, causing internal anal sphincter to relax

    b. Voluntary action—external anal sphincter is under cerebral cortex control

# Diagnostic Tests

**A.** Diagnostic tests of stool—test for presence of fat, pus, pathogens, parasites, occult blood

**B.** Endoscopy—direct visualization via hollow tube with illuminated fiberoptic scope

    1. Proctosigmoidoscopy (sigmoidoscopy)

        a. Definition—visualization of sigmoid colon or rectum and anal canal

        b. Client preparation

            1) Laxative night before exam and enema or suppository morning of procedure

            2) Clear liquid diet 12–24 h before exam (per health care provider order); clear liquids restricted 2-4 h before procedure

        c. Postoperative nursing care—allow client to rest; observe for hemorrhage, perforation; some flatulence and gas pain expected

    2. Colonoscopy

        a. Definition—visualization of entire large intestine to assess for cancer, polyps, strictures, ulcers

        b. Client preparation

            1) Clear liquid diet 12–24 h before exam (per health care provider order); clear liquids restricted 2-4 h before procedure

            2) Cathartic in evening, evening before exam

            3) Enema evening before exam (electrolyte-balanced solution may be given to induce diarrhea)

            4) Enema or suppositories may be required

        c. Nursing management

            1) Allow rest

            2) Observe for passage of blood and abdominal pain—signs of perforation; instruct client to report immediately

**C.** Barium enema—instillation of barium (radiopaque substance) into colon via rectum for fluoroscopy x-rays

    1. Purpose—viewing tumors, polyps, strictures, ulcerations, inflammation, or obstructions of colon

    2. Client preparation to clear large intestine of most fecal material

        a. Liquid diet and laxative night before exam

        b. Enema on morning of exam

    3. Nursing management

        a. Cleansing enemas or laxative to remove barium to prevent impaction

        b. X-rays may be repeated after all barium is expelled

        c. Instruct client that white-colored stools are expected

# Nursing Implications

**A.** Promotion of normal elimination

   1. Teach client to respond to urge to defecate

   2. Provide facilities, privacy, and sufficient time

   3. Fluids—encourage adequate intake; 8 or more glasses of fluid daily

   4. Encourage consumption of fiber—fruits, vegetables, grains

   5. Activity—encourage exercise and ambulation to maintain muscle tone

   6. Emotional state—teach client that stress affects autonomic nervous system, which controls peristalsis

**B.** Nutritional alterations

   1. Encourage high-fiber diet

      a. Fruits and vegetables

      b. Bran

      c. Whole-wheat flours and cereals

   2. Diet must be of adequate quantity of food to provide stimulus for peristalsis

**C.** Decompression of the intestinal tract

   1. Definition—removal of air and fluids from intestines via tube inserted through nose or mouth and attached to suction

   2. Purpose

      a. Drain fluids and gas due to obstruction

      b. Deflate bowel before or after intestinal surgery

      c. Drain fluids and gas due to paralytic ileus

   3. Types

      a. Salem sump, Levin and Anderson tubes (NG)

         1) Attached to low suction

         2) Levin to low intermittent suction

      b. Miller-Abbott tube—for obstruction of small intestine

         1) Double-lumen nasointestinal (NI) tube—one lumen leads to balloon; other lumen has openings all along tube for drainage

            a) When irrigating, be sure to use lumen marked "suction"

            b) The balloon is inflated with mercury after tube is inserted; clamp the lumen to the balloon and label with "Do Not Touch"

      c. Cantor tube (NI)

         1) Single lumen

         2) Sealed, mercury-filled rubber bag/balloon tip; used to decompress or stent small intestine

    4. Insertion of NI tubes

      a. Mechanical passage into stomach same as NG tube

      b. Passage of tube along intestines is aided by gravity, weight of mercury, and peristalsis

      c. After tube is in stomach, have client lie on right side, then on back (in Fowler position), and then on left side to use gravity to position tube

      d. Position of tube is ascertained by x-ray—do not tape tube to face but coil loosely on bed

      e. Position of tube and absence of telescoping of bowel from weight of tube is ascertained daily by x-ray

    5. Nursing management

      a. Measure drainage q shift

      b. Maintain liquid diet

      c. Irrigate as ordered—if unable to aspirate returns, record fluid instilled to be subtracted from total drainage output

      d. General care of client with NG tube

      e. Report signs of return of peristalsis, e.g., bowel sounds, flatus

**D.** Bowel surgery

    1. Overview—purposes of bowel surgery

      a. Removal of diseased portion of bowel

      b. Creation of an outlet for passage of stool when there is an obstruction or need for bowel rest

    2. Assessment

      a. Resection and anastomosis (also called partial or hemicolectomy)—diseased portion of bowel is removed and remaining ends are joined together

      b. Temporary cecostomy—opening into cecum (lower right quadrant of abdomen); catheter is inserted into bowel to provide temporary outlet for feces

      c. Abdominoperineal resection

        1) Abdominal incision through which the proximal end of the sigmoid colon is brought out to provide permanent colostomy

        2) Perineal incision through which the anus, the rectum, and the distal portion of the sigmoid are removed

      d. Intestinal ostomies for fecal diversion (*see* Figure 7-8)

        1) Sigmoid colostomy—characteristics

          a) Proximal portion of sigmoid colon brought out through abdominal wall to form stoma

          b) Distal portion of colon is removed

          c) Stoma is located in the lower left quadrant

          d) Feces are formed

          e) Permanent colostomy—usually done for cancer of the rectum

    f) Drainage may be regulated by irrigation, and ostomy appliance may eventually not be needed

2) Transverse loop colostomy

    a) Loop is created by bringing a section of transverse colon out through an abdominal incision

    b) Support ring is slid under the protruding bowel section to prevent the bowel from sliding back into the abdomen

    c) Anterior wall of the bowel loop is cut open while the posterior wall remains intact

    d) Single stoma with a proximal opening leading to the ascending colon and a distal opening leading to the descending colon

    e) Stoma is located in the upper abdomen

    f) Feces are soft

    g) Temporary colostomy—divert feces from injured or diseased section of bowel

    h) Skin breakdown may be a problem

    i) When healing has occurred, the anterior wall of the bowel loop is sutured, and the bowel section is reinserted into the abdomen

3) Transverse double-barrel colostomy—usually temporary

    a) Same as single barrel, with two distinct stomas on the abdomen

    b) May be permanent colostomy if the distal portion of the colon is later removed

4) Ascending colostomy

    a) Portion of the ascending colon is brought out to abdomen to form stoma

    b) Stoma location is right upper quadrant

    c) All portions of the colon distal to the stoma are removed

    d) Permanent colostomy

    e) Feces are liquid to soft

    f) Skin breakdown is common

5) Ileostomy

    a) Portion of the ileum brought to abdomen to create stoma

    b) All portions of the large intestine are removed

    c) Permanent ostomy; pouch must be worn at all times

    d) Usually done for ulcerative colitis or Crohn disease

    e) Stoma is located in the right lower quadrant

    f) Drainage is liquid or semiliquid

    g) Skin breakdown and fluid/electrolyte imbalance occur easily

h) Continent ileostomy (Kock pouch)—intra-abdominal reservoir with valve formed in distal ileum; pouch is reservoir for fecal material and cleaned at regular intervals by catheter insertion

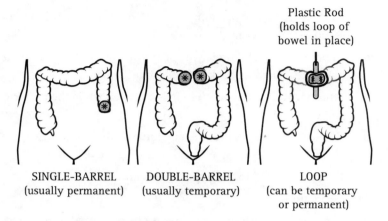

**Figure 7-8.** Types of Colostomies

3. Preop nursing management

a. Psychological support and explanations

b. Medications—antibiotics before surgery

c. Diet—high calorie, high protein, high carbohydrates, low residue week before; full liquid diet 24–48 hours before; NPO after midnight

d. Elimination—laxatives, enemas evening before and morning of surgery

e. Activity—assist prn; client will be weakened from extensive prep procedures

f. Monitor for fluid/electrolyte imbalance

g. Place tube prior to surgery—NG or intestinal

h. Have enterostomal health care provider see client for optimum placement of stoma

4. Postop nursing management

a. NG or intestinal decompression until peristalsis returns—maintain NPO status

b. Clear liquids progressing to solid, low-residue diet for 6–8 weeks

c. Monitor I and O and fluid/electrolyte balance

d. Observe and record condition of stoma

1) First few days appears beefy red and swollen

2) Gradually, swelling recedes and color is pink or red

3) Notify health care provider immediately if stoma is dark blue, blackish, or purple—indicates insufficient blood supply

e. Observe and record description of any drainage from stoma (*see* Figure 7-9)

1) Usually just mucus or serosanguineous fluid for first 1–2 d

2) Fecal drainage begins 3–6 days postop

f. Care of peristomal skin, emptying and changing appliance, irrigation (unless ascending cholecystostomy or ileostomy)

g. Promote positive adjustment to ostomy

1) Encourage client to look at stoma

2) Encourage early participation in ostomy care

3) Reinforce positive aspects of colostomy

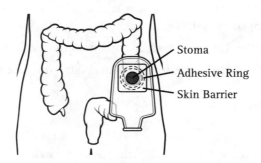

**Figure 7-9.** Colostomy Appliance

5. Nursing management

a. Skin care

1) Influencing factors

a) Composition, quantity, consistency of drainage

b) Medications

c) Location of stoma

d) Frequency in removal of appliance adhesive

2) Principles of skin protection

a) Use skin sealant under all tapes

b) Use skin barrier to protect skin immediately surrounding the stoma

c) Cleanse skin gently and pat dry; do not rub

d) Change appliance immediately when seal breaks; use pouch deodorants

b. Colostomy irrigations for sigmoid colostomy

1) Purpose—to stimulate emptying of colon at scheduled times

2) Usually begins 5–7 d postop

3) If distal loop of transverse colostomy is irrigated, mucus may be seen in drainage from rectum or through stoma

4) Ileostomies and ascending colostomies are not irrigated—drainage is liquid

5) 500–1,000 mL of tepid water used for solution

6) Special irrigating sleeve and cone are used

7) Insert catheter 8 cm

8) Hang irrigating container at shoulder height

9) Stop procedure if client reports cramps or if water is forcefully returning around cone or catheter

        10)    Time required for return flow varies from 15–45 min

        11)    When possible, client should be sitting upright on toilet for procedure

  c.  Diet

      1)  Usually not restricted after first 6 wk with colostomy

      2)  Ileostomy clients remain on low-residue diet—avoid foods that cause diarrhea or constipation in the client

  d.  Activity—optimal recovery within 3 mo; no restrictions

  e.  Sexuality—no physical interference with ability, conception, pregnancy, or delivery

# Selected Bowel Disorders

**A.**  Constipation

  1.  Definition—passage of dry, hard, difficult-to-evacuate stools

  2.  Causes

    a.  Paralytic ileus (absence of peristalsis) resulting from trauma to intestinal nerve endings during abdominal surgery

    b.  Atrophy or decreased muscle strength—part of aging process or overuse of laxatives

    c.  Decreased level of activity and exercise, causing decreased muscle strength and tone

    d.  Inadequate or poor choices of food intake

    e.  Older adults—medications (opiates), decreased intake of fluids and fiber, decreased activity level

  3.  Nursing management

    a.  Administration of laxatives (*see* Table 7-17)

    b.  Administration of enemas

      1)  Types

        a)  Oil retention—softens feces

        b)  Soapsuds—irritates colon, causing reflex evacuation, volume expander

        c)  Tap water—softens feces, stimulating evacuation

      2)  Procedure

        a)  Position on left side

        b)  Use tepid solution

        c)  Hold irrigation set no more than 18 in above rectum

        d)  Insert tube no more than 4 in

        e)  Ask client to retain fluid for 5–10 minutes

        f)  Do not administer in presence of abdominal pain, nausea, vomiting, or suspected appendicitis

**Table 7-17** Laxatives and Stool Softener Medications

| MEDICATION | ADVERSE EFFECTS | NURSING CONSIDERATIONS |
|---|---|---|
| **Stimulant** | | |
| Bisacodyl | Mild cramps, rash, nausea, diarrhea | Tablets should not be taken with milk or antacids (cause dissolution of enteric coating and loss of cathartic action) |
| | | Can cause gastric irritation Effects in 6–12 h |
| **Lubricant** | | |
| Mineral oil | Pruritus, anorexia, nausea | Administer in upright position |
| | | Prolonged use can cause fat-soluble vitamin malabsorption |
| | | Softens stool |
| **Emollient** | | |
| Docusate | Few adverse effects | Contraindicated in atonic bowel, nausea, vomiting, GI pain |
| | Abdominal cramps | Softens stool |
| | | Effects in 1–3 d |
| **Osmotic** | | |
| Magnesium hydroxide | Hypermagnesemia, dehydration | Na$^+$ salts can exacerbate heart failure |
| Polyethylene glycol and electrolytes | Nausea and bloating | Large-volume product—allow time to consume it safely |
| **Bulk Forming** | | |
| Psyllium hydro-philic mucilloid | Obstruction of GI tract | Take with a full glass of water; do not take dry |
| | | Report abdominal distension or unusual amount of flatulence |
| **Action** | Bulk forming—absorbs water into stool mass, making stool bulky, thus stimulating peristalsis | |
| | Lubricants—coat surface of stool and soften fecal mass, allowing for easier passage | |
| | Osmotic agents and saline laxatives—draw water from plasma by osmosis, increasing bulk of fecal mass, thus promoting peristalsis | |
| | Stimulants—stimulate peristalsis when they come in contact with intestinal mucosa | |
| | Stool softeners—soften fecal mass | |
| **Indications** | Constipation | |
| | Preparation for procedures or surgery | |
| **Adverse effects** | Diarrhea | |
| | Dependence | |
| **Nursing considerations** | Contraindicated for clients with abdominal pain, nausea and vomiting, fever (acute abdomen) | |
| | Chronic use may cause hypokalemia | |

       c.  Provide client education regarding promotion of normal elimination

          1)  Sit or squat during defecation

          2)  Gastrocolic reflex—try to have bowel movement after meals or after warm drink

          3)  Avoid routine use of laxatives or enemas

          4)  Gerontologic considerations—assess medication use, determine fluid and fiber intake, encourage increased fluid and fiber intake (bran, fruits, vegetables, nuts), avoid routine laxative and enema use

**B.** Diarrhea

  1.  Definition—passage of an increased number of loose stools

  2.  Causes

       a.  Systemic diseases—e.g., uremia, hyperthyroidism

       b.  Conditions causing parasympathetic nervous system stimulation—e.g., prolonged stress

       c.  Dietary changes in infants

       d.  Conditions directly affecting the GI tract, e.g., food allergies, poisoning, or abuse of cathartics

  3.  Nursing management

       a.  Perineal care—prevention of skin breakdown around anus

       b.  Prevent dehydration and electrolyte imbalance, especially in infants and older adults

       c.  Prevent metabolic acidosis, especially in infants

       d.  Administration of antidiarrheal medications (*see* Table 7-18)

**C.** Malabsorption syndrome

  1.  Definition—group of conditions caused by inadequate absorption of nutrients from the small intestine, resulting in abnormal digestion

  2.  Causes

       a.  Tropical sprue

       b.  Gastric resection/bowel resection

       c.  Antibiotics

       d.  Massive bowel resection

       e.  Parasitic infections

       f.  Overgrowth of bacteria in small intestine

       g.  Radiation injury to mucosa of small intestine

       h.  Enteritis

**Table 7-18** Antidiarrheal Medications

| MEDICATION | ADVERSE EFFECTS | NURSING CONSIDERATIONS |
|---|---|---|
| Bismuth subsa-licylate | Darkening of stools and tongue<br><br>Constipation | Give 2 h before or 3 h after other meds to prevent impaired absorption<br><br>Encourage fluids<br><br>Take after each loose stool until diarrhea controlled<br><br>Notify health care provider if diarrhea not controlled in 48 h<br><br>Absorbs irritants and soothes intestinal muscle<br><br>Do not administer for more than 2 d in presence of fever or in client less than 3 y of age<br><br>Monitor for salicylate toxicity<br><br>Use cautiously if already taking aspirin<br><br>Avoid use before x-rays (is radiopaque) |
| Diphenoxylate hydrochloride and atropine sulfate | Sedation<br><br>Dizziness<br><br>Tachycardia<br><br>Dry mouth<br><br>Paralytic ileus | Onset 45–60 min<br><br>Monitor fluid and electrolytes<br><br>Increases intestinal tone and decreases peristalsis<br><br>May potentiate action of barbiturates, depressants |
| Opium alkaloids<br><br>Loperamide | Narcotic dependence, nausea<br><br>Drowsiness<br><br>Constipation | Acts on smooth muscle to increase tone<br><br>Administer with glass of water<br><br>Discontinue as soon as stools are controlled<br><br>Monitor children closely for CNS effects |
| **Action** | Absorbs water, gas, toxins, irritants, and nutrients in bowel; slow peristalsis; increases tone of smooth muscles and sphincters | |
| **Indications** | Diarrhea | |
| **Adverse effects** | Constipation, fecal impaction; anticholinergic effects | |
| **Nursing considerations** | Not used with abdominal pain of unknown origin; monitor for urinary retention | |

    3. Assessment

        a. Steatorrhea—excessive fat in stool

        b. Light yellow to gray, greasy, soft stool

        c. Weight loss, anemia, fatigue

        d. Anorexia

        e. Vitamin deficiency

    4. Nursing management

        a. Nutritional support

            1) Enteral feedings

            2) Total parenteral nutrition (PN)

        b. Skin care

        c. Observe for vitamin and mineral deficiencies

        d. Monitor for pulse irregularities, edema

**D.** Adult celiac disease (nontropical sprue)

    1. Definition—an intolerance to gluten, a protein found in wheat and rye flour

    2. Causes

        a. Hypersensitivity response

        b. Hereditary tendency

        c. History of childhood celiac disease

    3. Assessment

        a. Same as malabsorption syndrome

        b. Onset usually age 30–60

    4. Nursing management

        a. Gluten-free diet

        b. Substitute cornmeal and rice for wheat, rye, oats, barley

**E.** Appendicitis (inflammation of appendix)

    1. Cause—occlusion of lumen of appendix from infection, strictures, or fecal masses

    2. Assessment

        a. Abdominal pain in right lower quadrant (McBurney's point)

        b. Anorexia

        c. Nausea and vomiting

        d. Diarrhea or constipation

        e. Rigid abdomen, muscle guarding

        f. Increased temperature

        g. Leukocytosis (WBC 15,000–20,000 cells/$\mu$L)

        h. Highest incidence 10–30 y of age

3. Nursing management

   a. No heating pads, enemas, or laxatives preop

   b. Maintain NPO status until blood count reports received

   c. No analgesics until cause of pain is determined

   d. Ice bag to abdomen to alleviate pain

   e. Observe for signs and symptoms of peritonitis

   f. Sudden absence of pain can indicate appendix has ruptured

4. Surgical removal of appendix (appendectomy)

F. Peritonitis (inflammation of peritoneal membrane covering abdominal organs)

1. Causes

   a. Ruptured appendix

   b. Perforated ulcer

   c. Bowel perforation

   d. Pelvic inflammatory disease (PID)

   e. Bladder perforation

   f. Traumatic rupture of liver or spleen

2. Assessment

   a. Severe abdominal pain

   b. Abdominal rigidity; decreased bowel sounds

   c. Nausea

   d. Vomiting

   e. Increased temperature

   f. Leukocytosis

   g. Shock: weakness, pallor, diaphoresis

   h. Paralytic ileus

   i. Symptoms may be masked in older adults or those receiving corticosteroids

3. Nursing management

   a. Antibiotics and intravenous fluids, as ordered

   b. Gastric decompression; monitor NG drainage

   c. NPO

   d. Re-establish fluid/electrolyte balance; monitor serum electrolyte levels

4. Surgery to alleviate cause—closure of abnormal opening into abdomen and drainage of fluid

G. Meckel diverticulum—a congenital sac or pouch in the ileum

1. Assessment

   a. Usually asymptomatic: may cause problems in childhood

   b. Signs and symptoms of appendicitis if diverticulum becomes inflamed from infection

2. Nursing management

    a. Antibiotics

    b. Rest

    c. Warm application to abdomen

    d. Antispasmodics

3. Surgical (if symptomatic)—removal of the diverticulum

**H.** Ileitis (acute Crohn disease)

1. Definition—inflammatory condition of intestine

2. Assessment—same as appendicitis

3. Nursing management

    a. Nutrition—high-protein, high-calorie, low-fat, and low-fiber diet

    b. Medications—antibiotics, antidiarrheals

    c. Management of client with diarrhea

**I.** Crohn disease—regional enteritis, ileitis, or enterocolitis (*see* Table 7-19)

1. Definition—inflammatory condition of any area of large or small intestine, usually ileum and ascending colon

2. Assessment—characterized by exacerbations and remissions

    a. Severe abdominal pain and cramping in lower-right quadrant of abdomen

    b. Chronic diarrhea

    c. Mucus, pus, fat in stools

    d. Fatigue

    e. Increased temperature

    f. Decreased weight

    g. Highest incidence ages 20–30 and 50–80 y

    h. Diagnostic tests—upper GI series, barium enema, colonoscopy

3. Nursing management

    a. Diet—high protein, high calorie, low fat, and low fiber; PN used for bowel rest

    b. Medications—analgesics, anticholinergics, antibiotics, corticosteroids, immune modulators, salicylate containing compounds

    c. Maintenance of fluid/electrolyte balance

4. Surgical intervention—hemicolectomy or ileostomy

**Table 7-19** Crohn Disease Versus Ulcerative Colitis

| | CROHN DISEASE REGIONAL ENTERITIS | ULCERATIVE COLITIS |
|---|---|---|
| **Assessment** | | |
| Usual age of onset | 20-30 and 50-80 years | Young adult to middle age (30-50) |
| Fatty stool (steatorrhea) | Frequent | Absent |
| Malignancy results | Rare | 10-15% |
| Rectal bleeding | Occasional: mucus, pus, fat in stool | Common; blood, pus, mucus in stool |
| Abdominal pain | After meals | Predefecation |
| Diarrhea | Diarrhea rare; 5-6 unformed stools per day | 10-20 liquid stools per day; often bloody |
| Nutritional deficit, weight loss, anemia, dehydration | Common | Common |
| Fever | Present | Present |
| Anal abscess | Common | Common |
| Fistula and anorectal fissure fistula | Common | Rare |
| **Diagnosis** | | |
| Level of involvement | Ileum, right colon | Rectum, left colon |
| Inflammation | Noncontinuous segment | Continuous segment |
| Course of disease | Prolonged, variable | Remissions and relapses |
| | Complications—bowel abscess, fistula formation, intestinal obstruction | Complications—hemorrhage, abscess formation, arthritis, uveitis |
| Nursing considerations | High-protein, high-calorie, low-fat, and low-fiber diet | |
| | May require PN to rest bowel | |
| | Analgesics, anticholinergics, sulfonamides, corticosteroids, antidiarrheals, and antiperistaltics | |
| | Maintain fluid/electrolyte balance | |
| | Monitor electrolytes | |
| | Promote rest, relieve anxiety | |
| | Ileostomy in severe cases | |

J. Ulcerative colitis (*see* Table 7-19)

1. Definition—inflammatory condition of the colon characterized by eroded areas of the mucous membrane and tissues beneath it

2. Assessment

   a. Diarrhea—10–20 stools per day

   b. Blood, pus, mucus in stool; pain

   c. Fecal incontinence

   d. Dehydration

   e. Weight loss

   f. Weakness, cachexia

   g. Metabolic acidosis

   h. Exacerbations and remissions

   i. Highest incidence age 30–50 y

   j. High correlation to personality traits of perfectionism, rigidity, dependence, insecurity

3. Nursing management

   a. Management of client with diarrhea

   b. Reduce inflammation—steroids

   c. Maintain nutrition—low-residue, high-protein, high-calorie diet

   d. Maintain fluid/electrolyte balance; monitor electrolyte levels

   e. Promote rest and relieve anxiety

4. Surgical intervention—ileostomy

K. Diverticular disease

1. Definition—infection, inflammation, or obstruction of diverticula (sacs or pouches in the intestinal wall), causing the client to become symptomatic

2. Assessment

   a. Colicky pain in left-lower quadrant of abdomen; pain described as cramping

   b. Fever, increased WBC

   c. Constipation, diarrhea, vomiting; constipation may alternate with diarrhea

   d. Decreased bowel sounds

3. Nursing management

   a. Analgesics

   b. Anticholinergics

   c. Antibiotics—broad-spectrum

   d. No laxatives or enemas

   e. Clear liquid diet or NPO to rest bowel

     f.  High-fiber diet; there are no evidence-based studies to suggest the avoidance of nuts, seeds, or popcorn; certain clients may have food triggers (that trigger an attack), so these foods should be avoided

  4.  Surgical intervention—colon resection with or without colostomy

**L.**  Intestinal obstruction

  1.  Types

     a.  Mechanical—physical blockage of passage through intestines

       1)  Strangulated hernia

       2)  Tumors

       3)  Adhesions

       4)  Fecal impaction

       5)  Strictures

          a)  Radiation

          b)  Congenital

       6)  Intussusception (telescoping of bowel within itself)

       7)  Volvulus—twisting of bowel

     b.  Nonmechanical (paralytic ileus)—no mechanical blockage, absence of peristalsis

       1)  Abdominal trauma/surgery

       2)  Spinal injuries

       3)  Peritonitis

       4)  Wound dehiscence (breakdown)

  2.  Assessment

     a.  High-pitched bowel sound above area of obstruction, decreased or absent bowel sounds below the area of obstruction

     b.  Abdominal pain and distension; pain often described as "colicky"

     c.  Obstipation (absence of stools or gas)

     d.  Nausea and vomiting

  3.  Nursing management

     a.  NG or intestinal decompression

     b.  NPO

     c.  Fluid/electrolyte replacement; monitor electrolyte levels

     d.  Assist with ADL

     e.  Good oral and skin care

     f.  Fowler position to facilitate breathing

     g.  Measure abdominal girth

     h.  Analgesics

**M.** Abdominal hernias

1. Definition—protrusion of an organ through the wall of the cavity in which it is normally contained

2. Types

    a. Inguinal—protrusion of intestine through abdominal ring into inguinal canal

    b. Femoral—protrusion of intestine into femoral canal

    c. Umbilical—protrusion of intestine through umbilical ring

    d. Ventral or incisional—protrusion through site of an old surgical incision

    e. Reducible—the protruding structure can be replaced by manipulation into the abdominal cavity

    f. Irreducible—the protruding structure cannot be replaced by manipulation

    g. Incarcerated—intestinal flow is completely obstructed

    h. Strangulated—blood flow to the intestines, as well as intestinal flow, is completely obstructed

3. Assessment

    a. Lump at site of hernia

    b. Lump may disappear in reclining position and reappear on standing/coughing

    c. Strangulated hernia—severe abdominal pain, nausea and vomiting, distension, intestinal obstruction

4. Nursing management—herniorrhaphy

    a. Preop nursing management

       1) Assess respiratory system for potential causes of increased intra-abdominal pressure—may cause interference with postop healing

       2) Surgery is postponed until respiratory conditions are controlled

    b. Postop nursing management

       1) Relieve urinary retention

       2) Prevent paroxysmal coughing

       3) Provide scrotal support

       4) Provide ice packs for swollen scrotum

       5) Advise no pulling, pushing, heavy lifting for 6 wk

       6) Inform client that sexual function is not affected

       7) Instruct client that ecchymosis will fade in a few days

# End-of-Chapter Thinking Exercise

An adult client was seen in the health care provider's (HCP) office reporting fatigue, rectal bleeding, and abdominal cramping followed by diarrhea 10 times a day. The symptoms have been increasing in intensity for the past two weeks. The client reports almost constant nausea and has not eaten any solid food for the last week. The client states, "I've been sipping broth and an electrolyte solution because that's all I can tolerate." Weight is 100 lb (45.36 kg), height 5′ 6″ (167.6 cm), with a calculated BMI of 16.1. Hemoglobin is 9 g/dL (90 g/L), hematocrit 31% (0.31), WBC count 14,000/mm³ (14 × 10⁹/L). The client is admitted to the medical-surgical unit for bowel rest and total parenteral nutrition (TPN). When the nurse receives report, the TPN is infusing at 50 mL/hr through a left arm peripherally inserted central catheter (PICC). There is a new prescription to increase the rate of the TPN to 100 mL/hr. Two hours later, the unlicensed assistive personnel (UAP) reports to the nurse that the client's demeanor seems "different" since admission. The client is in bed with the door closed saying, "I'm so sleepy this morning, I'm going back to bed." Upon assessment, the nurse learns the client has a headache and can't watch TV because of "seeing double." The nurse notices the client has voided 300 mL in the last two hours.

1.  When caring for a client receiving TPN, the nurse observes for what complications that can result from TPN? (Recognize Cues)

2.  Which complication is likely present based on the assessment findings? (Prioritize Hypothesis)

3.  What nursing implementations need to be incorporated into the plan of care to prevent infection? (Generate Solutions)

# Thinking Exercise Explanations

1.  When caring for a client receiving TPN, the nurse observes for what complications that can result from TPN? (Recognize Cues)

    - Infection
    - Hyperglycemia
    - Fluid overload or depletion

    There is an increased risk of both localized infection at the catheter site and catheter-related bloodstream infection due to the high dextrose concentration of TPN. Hyperglycemia can occur due to high concentrations of glucose after a malnourished state as well as osmotic diuresis and subsequent fluid depletion. Fluid overload can occur with too rapid administration of the solution.

2.  Which complication is likely present based on the assessment findings? (Prioritize Hypothesis)

    - Hyperglycemia

    The assessed signs and symptoms are most consistent with osmotic diuresis secondary to hyperglycemia from the rate increase.

3.  What nursing implementations need to be incorporated into the plan of care to prevent infection? (Generate Solutions)

    - Strict adherence to aseptic technique
    - Replace transparent dressings every 7 days or according to institutional policy
    - Replace PICC dressing if it becomes loose, damp, or visibly soiled
    - Assess catheter site every 4 hours for redness, swelling, and tenderness
    - Monitor temperature every 4 hours
    - Monitor WBC count daily
    - Change IV tubing and filter once daily
    - Maintain line only for TPN administration

    The nurse needs to be aware of the importance of reducing the risk of infection with both a centrally placed catheter and because of the high dextrose concentration of the parenteral nutrition solution. This is the ideal medium for bacterial and fungal growth, and strict aseptic technique must be employed at all times.

# [ CHAPTER 8 ]

# THE ENDOCRINE SYSTEM

# THE ENDOCRINE SYSTEM OVERVIEW

## Metabolism, Cellular Regulation

## Overview

A. Chemical communication and coordination system that enables reproductive growth and development and also regulation of energy

  1. Maintains internal homeostasis of body

  2. Coordinates responses to external and internal environmental changes

B. Composed of glands/glandular tissue

  1. Secrete, store, and synthesize chemical messengers (hormones) that travel to target cells throughout the body

  2. Include: hypothalamus, pituitary, thyroid, parathyroids, adrenals, pancreas, ovaries, testes, pineal, and thymus

  3. Major hormones are amines, peptides, and steroids

  4. Important functions include reproduction, stress response, electrolyte balance, energy metabolism, growth, maturation, and aging (*see* Table 8-1)

**Table 8.1** Important Functions of the Endocrine System

| GLAND/HORMONE | TARGET TISSUE | FUNCTION |
|---|---|---|
| Thyroid:<br><br>Thyroxine ($T_4$)<br>Triiodothyronine ($T_3$)<br>Calcitonin | All body tissues<br><br>Bones | Regulation of metabolic rate of all cells and processes of cell growth, tissue differentiation<br><br>Regulates calcium and phosphorus blood levels |
| Parathyroids:<br><br>Parathyroid hormone (PTH) | Bones, intestines, kidneys | Regulates calcium and phosphorus blood levels (bone demineralization and intestinal absorption) |
| Adrenal medulla:<br><br>Epinephrine<br>Norepinephrine | Sympathetic effectors | Enhances and prolongs effects of sympathetic nervous system<br><br>Response to stress |

*(Continued)*

**Table 8.1** Important Functions of the Endocrine System (*Continued*)

| GLAND/HORMONE | TARGET TISSUE | FUNCTION |
|---|---|---|
| Adrenal cortex: | All body tissues | Metabolism; stress response |
| Corticosteroids | Sex organs | Masculinization |
| Androgens | Kidneys | Growth and sexual activity in women |
| Estrogen | | Regulates sodium/potassium balance, water balance |
| Mineralocorticoids | | |
| Pancreas: | General | Promotes movement of glucose out of blood into cells |
| Islets of Langerhans | Pancreas | |
| Insulin (beta cells) | | Promotes movement of glucose from storage into blood |
| Glucagon (alpha cells) | | |
| Somatostatin | | Inhibits insulin and glucagon secretion |
| Women—ovaries: | Reproductive system | Development of secondary sex characteristics, oogenesis, preparation of uterus for fertilization and fetal development; bone growth |
| Estrogen | Breasts | |
| Progesterone | | Maintains lining of uterus necessary for successful pregnancy |
| Men—testes | Reproductive system | Stimulates development of secondary sexual characteristics, spermatogenesis |

# [ SECTION 2 ]

# ENDOCRINE DISORDERS

## Metabolism, Client Education: Providing

## Diabetes Mellitus

A. Overview—diabetes mellitus is defined as a genetically heterogeneous group of disorders characterized by glucose intolerance (*see* Table 8-2)

**Table 8.2** Alterations in Glucose Metabolism

| TYPE | NURSING CONSIDERATIONS |
|------|------------------------|
| Type 1 diabetes | Acute onset before age 30 |
| | Insulin-producing pancreatic beta cells destroyed by autoimmune process |
| | Requires lifelong insulin injections |
| | Ketosis prone |
| Type 2 diabetes | Usually older than 30 and obese |
| | Decreased sensitivity to insulin (insulin resistance) or decreased insulin production |
| | Ketosis rare |
| | Treated with diet and exercise |
| | Supplemented with oral hypoglycemic medications |
| | insulin may be used |
| Others:<br><br>Gestational diabetes<br>Impaired fasting<br>glucose | Onset during pregnancy, second or third trimester |
| | High-risk pregnancy |
| | Fasting plasma glucose of $\geq$100 mg/dL ($\geq$ 5.6 mmol/L) and less than 126 mg/dL (less than 7 mmol/L); risk factor for future diabetes risk |

B. Risk factors for type 2 diabetes

1. Parents or siblings with diabetes

2. Obesity (20% or more above ideal body weight)

3. African American, Hispanic, Native American, or Asian American

4. Older than 45 years

    5. Previously impaired glucose tolerance

    6. Hypertension

**C.** Diagnostic tests

    1. Blood glucose monitoring—presence of sugar in the urine is a sign of diabetes that calls for an immediate blood glucose test; normal range in fasting blood is 70–99 mg/dL (3.89–5.49 mmol/L); older adults may normally have higher glucose levels

    2. Oral glucose tolerance test—blood samples are drawn at 1-, 2-, and 3-h intervals after glucose ingestion

        a. Fasting glucose greater than 125 mg/dL (6.9 mmol/L) and 2-h glucose greater than 190 mg/dL (5 mmol/L) on two occasions are diagnostic of diabetes; may see increased fasting glucose in older adults

        b. Preparation—usually NPO after midnight (10–12-h fast); client sometimes ingests high-carbohydrate diet for 3 d preceding test

        c. Fasting blood sample taken

        d. Glucose load (about 75 g/300 mL of flavored beverage) is given

        e. Specimens are drawn at 1, 2, and 3 h after glucose ingestion

    3. Urine ketones indicate that diabetic control has deteriorated; body has started to break down stored fat for energy

    4. Special considerations—medications, illness, and stress will affect testing

    5. Glycosylated hemoglobin (HbA1c)—blood sample can be taken without fasting

        a. Measures control over last 3 months; not affected by carbohydrate intake or exercise

        b. Normal is 4–6%

**D.** Nursing management

    1. Dietary management

        a. Provide all essential food constituents—lower lipid levels if elevated

        b. Achieve and maintain ideal weight

        c. Meet energy needs

        d. Achieve normal range glucose levels

        e. Review food exchange method of meal and snack planning with client/family; foods on list in specified amounts contain equal number of calories and grams of protein, fat, and carbohydrate

    2. Proper management of insulin regimen—insulin is secreted by beta cells of the islets of Langerhans and works to lower blood glucose by facilitating uptake and the utilization of glucose by muscle and fat cells and by decreasing the release of glucose from the liver; injection sites must be rotated (*see* Table 8-3)

**Table 8.3** Antidiabetic Medications: Insulin

| INSULIN TYPES | ONSET OF ACTION; (MIN) | PEAK ACTION | DURATION OF ACTION | TIME OF ADVERSE REACTION | CHARACTERISTICS |
|---|---|---|---|---|---|
| **Rapid Acting** | | | | | |
| Lispro | 15–30 | 0.5–1.5 h | 3–5 h | Midmorning: trembling, weakness | Client should eat within 5–15 min after injection; also used in insulin pumps |
| Aspart | 15–30 | 1–3 h | 3–5 h | | |
| Glulisine | 10–15 | 1–1.5 h | 3–5 h | | |
| **Short Acting** | | | | | |
| Regular | 30–60 min | 1–5 h | 6–10 h | Midmorning, midafternoon: weakness, fatigue | Clear solution; given 20–30 min before meal; can be used alone or with other insulins |
| **Intermediate Acting** | | | | | |
| Neutral protamine hagedorn (NPH) | 1–2 h | 4–12 h | 16 h | Early evening: weakness, fatigue | White and cloudy solution; can be given after meals |
| **Very Long Acting** | | | | | |
| Glargine Insulin detemir | 3–4 h | Continuous (no peak) | 24 h | | Maintains blood glucose levels regardless of meals; cannot be mixed with other insulins; given at bedtime |
| **Action** | Reduces blood glucose levels by increasing glucose transport across cell membranes; enhances conversion of glucose to glycogen | | | | |
| **Indications** | Type 1 diabetes; type 2 diabetes not responding to oral hypoglycemic medications; gestational diabetes not responding to diet | | | | |
| **Adverse effects** | Hypoglycemia | | | | |
| **Nursing considerations** | Teach client to rotate sites to prevent lipohypertrophy, fibrofatty masses at injection sites; do not inject into these masses | | | | |
| | Only regular insulin can be given IV; all can be given SQ | | | | |
| **Herbal interactions** | Bee pollen, glucosamine may increase blood glucose | | | | |
| | Basil, bay leaf, chromium, echinacea, garlic, ginseng may decrease blood glucose | | | | |
| | Ginkgo biloba might interfere with the management of diabetes mellitus; if taking ginkgo, closely monitor blood glucose levels | | | | |

3. Oral hypoglycemic medications appear to work by improving both tissue responsiveness to insulin and/or the ability of the pancreatic cells to secrete insulin (*see* Table 8-4)

4. Hypoglycemia prevention and early detection

    a. Signs and symptoms of hypoglycemia (insulin reaction)

        1) Irritability, confusion, tremors, blurring of vision, coma, seizures

        2) Hypotension, tachycardia

        3) Skin cool and clammy, diaphoresis

    b. Treatment of hypoglycemia

        1) If conscious and able to swallow—15 g of quick acting carbohydrate; liquids containing glucose or commercially prepared glucose tablets ideal

        2) If unable to safely swallow or unconscious—glucagon IM, dextrose 50% (D50W) IV

    c. Signs and symptoms of hyperglycemia/diabetic ketoacidosis (DKA)

        1) Headache, drowsiness, stupor, coma

        2) Hypotension, tachycardia

        3) Skin warm and dry, dry mucous membranes, elevated temperature

        4) Polyuria progressing to oliguria, polydipsia, polyphagia

        5) Kussmaul respirations (rapid and deep)

        6) Fruity odor to breath

    d. Treatment of hyperglycemia (DKA)

        1) Normal saline or 0.45% NaCl (DKA)

        2) Regular insulin

        3) Potassium as soon as urine output is satisfactory (DKA)

        4) Determine and address cause

        5) Client education

        6) Exercise regimen

**Table 8.4** Oral Hypoglycemic Medications

| MEDICATION | ADVERSE EFFECTS | NURSING CONSIDERATIONS |
|---|---|---|
| **ORAL** | | |
| **Sulfonylureas** | | |
| Glimepiride<br>Glipizide<br>Glyburide | GI symptoms and dermatologic reactions | Only used if some pancreas beta cell function<br>Stimulates release of insulin from pancreas<br>Many medications can potentiate or interfere with actions<br>Take with food if GI upset occurs |
| **Biguanides** | | |
| Metformin | Nausea<br>Diarrhea<br>Abdominal discomfort | No effect on pancreatic beta cells; decreases glucose production by liver<br>Not given if renal impairment<br>Can cause lactic acidosis<br>Avoid alcohol<br>Do not give with alpha-glucosidase inhibitors |
| **Alpha-Glucosidase Inhibitors** | | |
| Acarbose<br>Miglitol | Abdominal discomfort<br>Diarrhea<br>Flatulence | Delays digestion of carbohydrates<br>Must be taken immediately before a meal<br>Can be taken alone or with other medications |
| **Thiazolidinediones** | | |
| Rosiglitazone<br>Pioglitazone | Infection<br>Headache<br>Pain<br>Rare cases of liver failure | Decreases insulin resistance and inhibits gluconeogenesis<br>Regularly scheduled liver function studies<br>Can cause resumption of ovulation in perimenopause |
| **Glitinides** | | |
| Repaglinide | Hypoglycemia<br>GI disturbances<br>Upper respiratory tract infections (URIs)<br>Back pain<br>Headache | Increases pancreatic insulin release<br>Medication should not be taken if meal skipped |

*(Continued)*

**Table 8.4** Oral Hypoglycemic Medications (*Continued*)

| MEDICATION | ADVERSE EFFECTS | NURSING CONSIDERATIONS |
|---|---|---|
| **Gliptins** | | |
| Linagliptin | URIs | Enhances action of incretin hormones |
| Sitagliptin | Hypoglycemia | |
| **INJECTED** | | |
| **Incretin Mimetics** | | |
| Exenatide | GI upset | Interacts with many medications |
| | Hypoglycemia | Administer 1 hour before meals |
| | Pancreatitis | |
| **Amylin Mimetics** | | |
| Pramlintide | Hypoglycemia | Delays gastric emptying |
| | Nausea | Suppresses glucagon secretion |
| | Injection site reaction | |
| **Indications** | Type 2 diabetes | |
| **Nursing considerations** | Monitor serum glucose levels | |
| | Avoid alcohol | |
| | Teaching for disease: dietary control, symptoms of hypoglycemia and hyperglycemia | |
| | Good skin care | |
| **Herbal interactions** | Bee pollen, ginkgo biloba, glucosamine may increase blood glucose | |
| | Basil, bay leaf, chromium, echinacea, garlic, ginseng may decrease blood glucose | |

# Acromegaly

A. Definition—hypersecretion of growth hormone; often caused by pituitary adenoma

B. Assessment (*see* Table 8-5)

   1. Enlarged flat bones and terminal portions of long bones; lower jaw and forehead protrude

   2. Poor coordination

   3. Muscle weakness and atrophy

   4. Lethargy

   5. Arthralgias and arthritis

   6. Changes in visual fields

   7. Deep voice and enlarged tongue

   8. Emotional instability

   9. Sexual abnormalities

**Table 8.5** Pituitary Disorders

| | HYPOPITUITARISM (DWARFISM) | ACROMEGALY |
|---|---|---|
| Assessment | Height below normal, body proportions normal, bone/tooth development retarded, sexual maturity delayed, skin fine, features delicate | Body size enlarged, coordination poor, flat bones enlarged, sexual abnormalities, deep voice, skin thick and soft, visual field changes |
| Diagnosis | Hyposecretion of growth hormone, occurs before maturity | Hypersecretion of growth hormone occurs after maturity |
| | Etiology unclear, predisposition: pituitary tumors, idiopathic hyperplasia | Etiology: unclear |
| | Treatment: hormone replacement (human growth hormone, thyroid growth hormone, testosterone) | Diagnosis: growth hormone measured in blood plasma |
| | Complication: diabetes | Treatment: external irradiation of tumor, atrium-90 implant transnasally, hypophysectomy (removal of pituitary or portion of it with hormone replacement) |
| Potential nursing diagnosis | Self-esteem disturbance | Body image disturbance |
| | Risk for sexual dysfunction | Nutrition altered |
| | | Chronic pain |
| | | Risk for sexual dysfunction |
| Plan/ implementation | Monitor growth and development | Monitor blood glucose level |
| | Provide emotional support | Provide emotional support |
| | Assess body image | Provide safety due to poor coordination and vision |
| | Refer for psychological counseling as needed | Administer dopamine agonists, somatostatin analogs, growth hormone receptor blockers |
| | Monitor medications | Provide care during radiation therapy |
| | Hormone replacement therapy | Provide posthypophysectomy care: |
| | Thyroid hormone replacement | Elevate head |
| | Testosterone therapy | Check neurological status and nasal drainage |
| | Human chorionic gonadotropin (hCG) injections | Monitor BP frequently |
| | | Observe for hormonal deficiencies (thyroid, glucocorticoid) |
| | | Observe for hypoglycemia |
| | | Monitor intake and output |
| | | Provide cortisone replacement before and after surgery |
| | | Avoid coughing Avoid brushing teeth for 2 weeks |

10. Hypertension and heart failure

11. Impaired glucose tolerance and diabetes mellitus

C. Diagnosis—growth hormone measured in blood plasma, MRI, increased insulin-like growth factor 1 (IGF-1) levels

D. Nursing management

1. Monitor blood glucose level

2. Provide emotional support

3. Administer medications—dopamine agonists (e.g., cabergoline), growth receptor antagonists (e.g., pegvisomant), somatostatin analogues (e.g., octreotide)

4. Monitor for adverse effects of radiation therapy

5. Surgery best approach to cure: hypophysectomy (transsphenoidal)

   a. Monitor neurologic status and vision

   b. "Mustache" dressing under nose

   c. Instruct client to report postnasal drip

   d. Monitor for halo sign—clear drainage surrounded by yellow or slight serosanguineous drainage (indicates CSF leak)

   e. Instruct client to avoid coughing, sneezing, blowing nose, bending forward (increases intracranial pressure) and to avoid brushing teeth for 2 weeks

   f. Monitor for meningitis—photophobia, neck stiffness, headache

   g. Administer hormonal replacement as needed—gonadal hormones, cortisol and thyroid

# Hypopituitarism

A. Definition—hyposecretion of growth hormone

B. Assessment (*see* Table 8-5)

1. Height is below normal

2. Proportion of weight to height is normal

3. Bone and tooth development are retarded

4. Sexual maturity is delayed

5. Features are delicate

C. Diagnosis—growth hormone measured in blood plasma; decreased in hypopituitarism

D. Nursing management

1. Monitor growth and development

2. Provide emotional support

3. Assess body image

4. Refer for psychological counseling as needed

5. Monitor medications

   a. Hormone replacement therapy

   b. Thyroid hormone replacement

   c. Testosterone therapy (males)

# Diabetes Insipidus

A. Definition—deficiency of antidiuretic hormone (ADH)

B. Assessment (*see* Table 8-6)

1. Excessive urine output, dilute urine

2. Severe dehydration, hypotension, tachycardia, decreased pedal pulse strength

3. Excessive thirst

4. Anorexia

5. Weight loss

6. Mental status changes—irritability, decreased alertness, lethargy, possible coma

7. Poor skin turgor, dry mucous membranes

**Table 8.6** ADH Disorders

|  | **DIABETES INSIPIDUS (DECREASED ADH)** | **SYNDROME OF INAPPROPRIATE ANTIDIURETIC HORMONE SECRETION—SIADH (INCREASED ADH)** |
|---|---|---|
| Assessment | Excessive urine output | Anorexia, nausea, vomiting |
|  | Chronic, severe dehydration | Lethargy |
|  | Excessive thirst | Headaches |
|  | Anorexia, weight loss | Change in level of consciousness (LOC) |
|  | Weakness | Decreased deep tendon reflexes |
|  | Constipation | Tachycardia |
|  |  | Increased circulating blood volume |
|  |  | Decreased urinary output |
| Diagnosis | Head trauma | Small-cell carcinoma of lung |
|  | Brain tumor | Pneumonia positive-pressure ventilation |
|  | Meningitis Encephalitis | Brain tumors |
|  | Deficiency of ADH | Head trauma |
|  | Diagnosis tests: | Stroke |
|  | Low urine specific gravity | Meningitis |
|  | Urinary osmolality below plasma level High serum sodium | Encephalitis |
|  |  | Feedback mechanism that regulates ADH does not function properly; ADH is released even when plasma hypo-osmolality is present |
|  |  | Diagnostic tests—serum sodium decreased, plasma osmolality decreased, increased urine specific gravity |

(*Continued*)

**Table 8.6** ADH Disorders (*Continued*)

| | DIABETES INSIPIDUS (DECREASED ADH) | SYNDROME OF INAPPROPRIATE ANTIDIURETIC HORMONE SECRETION—SIADH (INCREASED ADH) |
|---|---|---|
| Nursing considerations | Record intake and output<br><br>Monitor urine specific gravity, skin condition, weight, blood pressure, pulse, temperature<br><br>Administer desmopressin acetate | Restrict water intake (500–600 mL/24 h)<br><br>Administer diuretics to promote excretion of water<br><br>Hypertonic saline (3% NaCl) IV<br><br>Administer demeclocycline<br><br>Weigh daily<br><br>I and O<br><br>Monitor serum $Na^+$ levels<br><br>Assess LOC |

C. Diagnostic tests

    1. Low urine specific gravity (normal for adult 1.010–1.030)

    2. Clinical manifestations—especially frequent urination

    3. Urinary osmolality below plasma level

    4. Increased hemoglobin, hematocrit, BUN

D. Nursing management

    1. Monitor fluids and electrolytes

        a. Record intake and output

        b. Urine specific gravity

        c. Skin condition

        d. Weight

        e. Blood pressure, pulse, temperature

    2. Administer prescribed medications (hormone replacement)—observe for expected therapeutic effects

        a. Desmopressin acetate (DDAVP) nasal spray

        b. Desmopressin by subcutaneous or intravascular injection (*see* Table 8-7)

**Table 8.7** Diabetes Insipidus Medications

| MEDICATION | ADVERSE EFFECTS | NURSING CONSIDERATIONS |
|---|---|---|
| Desmopressin:<br><br>    Nasal spray<br>    SQ<br>    IV | Excess—smooth muscle contraction, especially arterioles and capillaries<br><br>Water intoxication<br><br>Other—hypersensitivity, hypertension, nausea | Antidiuretic hormone<br><br>Increases water retention by kidney<br><br>Used to treat diabetes insipidus |

3. Prevent constipation—laxatives and stool softeners

4. Provide skin care

5. Client teaching

    a. How to measure intake and output and also signs of early dehydration

    b. Expected responses from medications, e.g., decreased thirst and urination

    c. Lifelong replacement may be needed

# Pheochromocytoma

**A.** Definition—hypersecretion of catecholamines (epinephrine and norepinephrine) due to secreting tumors of the adrenal medulla; tumor can also occur anywhere, from neck to pelvis along course of sympathetic nerve chain; caused by tumor in adrenal medulla

**B.** Assessment

1. Intermittent hypertension lasting several minutes to several hours; episodes precipitated by increased abdominal pressure (Valsalva maneuver, abdominal palpation)

2. Increased heart rate; palpitations during hypertensive episodes

3. Nausea and vomiting; weight loss

4. Hyperglycemia, glucosuria, polyuria

5. Diaphoresis, pallor

6. Tremor, nervousness during hypertensive episodes

7. Pounding headache during hypertensive episodes

8. Weakness during hypertensive episodes

9. Visual disturbances during hypertensive episodes

10. Pain during hypertensive episodes

**C.** Diagnostic tests

1. Histamine test, provocative test—causes rise in blood pressure (rarely done)

    a. Normally causes drop in blood pressure, but in this disease, a rise occurs

    b. Given subcutaneously if blood pressure not higher than 170/110 mm Hg

    c. If blood pressure over 170/110 mm Hg, phentolamine test done

2. Phentolamine test (rarely done)

    a. At least 3 days prior to test, should not receive any sedatives, antihypertensives (especially reserpine), or narcotics—may cause false-positive reactions

    b. Phentolamine given IV—adrenergic blocking agent neutralizes epinephrine and causes drop in blood pressure

    c. Decrease in blood pressure of at least 35 mm Hg systolic and 25 mm Hg diastolic within 3–5 minutes considered positive for tumor

    d. Drop in blood pressure lasts 10 min

    e. Vasopressors should be readily available

3. Urinary vanillylmandelic acid (VMA) test

    a. 24-h urine for VMA—breakdown product of catecholamine metabolism

    b. Normal results: 1–5 mg; positive for tumor if significantly higher

    c. Foods affecting VMA excretion excluded 3 d before test:

        1) Coffee

        2) Tea

        3) Bananas

        4) Vanilla

        5) Chocolate

    d. All medications discontinued during test

    e. Urine collected on ice or refrigeration and preservative needed

4. Clonidine suppression test—clonidine levels not decreased

**D.** Nursing management

1. Promote comfort

    a. Avoid physical and emotional stress

    b. Monitor blood pressure in sitting and lying positions

    c. Frequent bathing but avoid chilling

    d. Administer analgesics for pain, sedatives and tranquilizers for rest and relaxation

2. Provide appropriate nutrition

    a. Increase calorie, vitamin, and mineral intake because of increased metabolic demand (compatible with hyperglycemia and weight loss)

    b. Avoid coffee, tea, cola, and other stimulating foods, foods containing tyramine

3. Limit activity

4. Administer adrenergic blocking medications (e.g., phenoxybenzamine)

5. Administer hydralazine for hypertensive crisis

6. Promote safety

    a. Assist with self-care

    b. Eliminate unnecessary equipment and material from client's immediate vicinity

    c. Recruit help and assistance of significant other

    d. Allow time to verbalize concerns to decrease nervousness and tremors

7. Provide postsurgical care—adrenalectomy or medullectomy

# Addison Disease (Adrenal Insufficiency)

**A.** Definition—adrenocortical hypofunction due to insufficient secretion from adrenal cortex

**B.** Assessment (see Table 8-8)

1. Fatigue and weakness
2. Dehydration
3. Alopecia
4. "Tan" skin
5. Depression
6. Emaciation, weight loss
7. Immune deficiency
8. Fluid and electrolyte imbalance
9. Pathological fractures

**Table 8.8** Adrenal Disorders

| | ADDISON DISEASE | CUSHING SYNDROME |
|---|---|---|
| Assessment | Fatigue, weakness, dehydration, ↓ BP, hyperpigmentation, ↓resistance to stress, alopecia<br><br>Weight loss, pathological fractures<br><br>Depression, lethargy, emotional liability | Fatigue, weakness, osteoporosis, muscle wasting, cramps, edema, ↑ BP, purple skin striations, hirsutism, emaciation, depression, decreased resistance to infection, moon face, buffalo hump, obesity (trunk), mood swings, masculinization in females, blood glucose imbalance |
| Diagnosis | Hyposecretion of adrenal hormones (mineralocorticoids, glucocorticoids, androgens)<br><br>Pathophysiology:<br>　↓ Na$^+$ dehydration<br>　↓ Blood volume + shock<br>　↑ K$^+$ metabolic acidosis + Arrhythmias<br>　↓ Blood glucose + insulin shock<br><br>Diagnostic tests:<br>　CT and MRI<br>　Hyperkalemia and hyponatremia<br>　↓ Plasma cortisol<br>　↓ Urinary 17-hydroxycorticosteroids and 17-ketosteroids<br>　ACTH stimulation test<br><br>Treatment:<br>　Hormone replacement | Hypersecretion of adrenal hormones (mineralocorticoids, glucocorticoids, androgens)<br><br>Pathophysiology:<br>　↑ Na$^+$ + ↑ blood volume + ↑ BP<br>　↓ K$^+$ + metabolic alkalosis + shock<br>　↑ Blood glucose + ketoacidosis<br><br>Diagnostic tests:<br>　Skull films<br>　Blood glucose analysis<br>　Hypokalemia and hypernatremia<br>　↑ Plasma cortisol level<br>　↑ Urinary 17-hydroxycorticosteroids and 17-ketosteroids<br><br>Treatment:<br>　Hypophysectomy, adrenalectomy |

335

**C.** Diagnostic tests

1. Skull films, CT, MRI

2. Hyperkalemia and hyponatremia

3. Plasma cortisol decreased

4. Urinary 17-hydroxycorticosteroids and 17-ketosteroids decreased

5. ACTH stimulation test

**D.** Nursing management

1. Teach appropriate diet—high protein, high carbohydrate, high sodium, low potassium

2. Provide emotional support

3. Prevent complications

   a. Wear MedicAlert bracelet

   b. Protect from infection

   c. Monitor for hypoglycemia, hyponatremia

4. Avoid factors that precipitate Addisonian crisis (adrenal crisis)

   a. Physical stress

   b. Psychological stress

   c. Inadequate steroid replacement

5. Assist with treatment of Addisonian crisis (precipitated by physical or emotional stress, sudden withdrawal of hormones)

   a. Observe for clinical manifestations

      1) Nausea and vomiting

      2) Abdominal pain

      3) Fever

      4) Extreme weakness

      5) Severe hypoglycemia, hyperkalemia, and dehydration (develop rapidly)

      6) Blood pressure falls, leading to shock and coma; death results if not promptly treated

   b. Provide treatment and nursing care (see Tables 8-9 and 8-10)

      1) Administer hydrocortisone or dexamethasone (*see* Table 8-11)

      2) Carefully monitor IV infusion of 0.9% NaCl or D5W/NaCl

      3) Administer IV glucose, glucagon

      4) Administer insulin with dextrose in normal saline; administer potassium binding and excreting resin (e.g., sodium polystyrene sulfonate)

      5) Monitor vital signs, ECG, serum potassium, serum glucose

      6) Assist with 24-h urine collection for 17-hydroxycorticosteroids; refrigeration of urine during collection is necessary

   c. Administer hormonal replacement—may be lifelong

**Table 8.9** Glucocorticoid Medications

| MEDICATION | ADVERSE EFFECTS: | NURSING CONSIDERATIONS |
|---|---|---|
| Short acting:<br><br>    Cortisone acetate<br>    Hydrocortisone<br><br>Intermediate acting:<br><br>    Methylprednisolone<br>    Prednisone<br><br>Long acting:<br><br>    Betamethasone<br>    Dexamethasone | Increases susceptibility to infection<br><br>May mask symptoms of infection<br><br>Edema, changes in appetite<br><br>Euphoria, insomnia<br><br>Delayed wound healing<br><br>Hypokalemia, hypocalcemia<br><br>Hyperglycemia<br><br>Osteoporosis, fractures<br><br>Peptic ulcer, gastric hemorrhage<br><br>Psychosis | Prevents/suppresses cell-mediated immune reactors<br><br>Used for adrenal insufficiency<br><br>Overdose produces Cushing syndrome<br><br>Abrupt withdrawal of medication may cause headache, nausea and vomiting, and papilledema (Addisonian crisis)<br><br>Give single dose before 9 A.M.<br><br>Give multiple doses at evenly spaced intervals<br><br>Infection may produce few symptoms due to anti-inflammatory action<br><br>Stress (surgery, illness, psychic) may lead to increased need for steroids<br><br>Nightmares are often the first indication of the onset of steroid psychosis<br><br>Check weight, BP, electrolytes, I and O, weight<br><br>Use cautiously with history of TB (may reactivate disease)<br><br>May decrease effects of oral hypoglycemics, insulin, diuretics, $K^+$ supplements<br><br>Assess children for growth restriction<br><br>Protect from pathological fractures<br><br>Administer with antacids<br><br>Do not stop abruptly<br><br>Methylprednisolone succinate also used for arthritis, asthma, allergic reactions, cerebral edema<br><br>Dexamethasone also used for allergic disorders, cerebral edema, asthmatic attack, shock |
| **Action** | Stimulates formation of glucose (gluconeogenesis) and decreases use of glucose by body cells; increases formation and storage of fat in muscle tissue; alters normal immune response | |

*(Continued)*

**Table 8.9** Glucocorticoid Medications (*Continued*)

| MEDICATION | ADVERSE EFFECTS: | NURSING CONSIDERATIONS |
|---|---|---|
| **Indications** | Addison disease | |
| | Crohn disease | |
| | COPD | |
| | Lupus erythematosus | |
| | Leukemias, lymphomas, myelomas | |
| | Head trauma, tumors to prevent/treat cerebral edema | |
| **Adverse effects** | Psychoses, depression | |
| | Weight gain | |
| | Hypokalemia, hypocalcemia | |
| | Stunted growth in children | |
| | Petechiae | |
| | Buffalo hump | |
| **Nursing considerations** | Monitor fluid and electrolyte balance | |
| | Don't discontinue abruptly | |
| | Monitor for signs of infection | |
| **Herbal interactions** | Henna, celery seed, juniper may decrease serum potassium; when taken with corticosteroids, may increase hypoglycemia | |
| | Ginseng taken with corticosteroids may cause insomnia | |
| | Echinacea may counteract effects of corticosteroids | |
| | Licorice potentiates effect of corticosteroids | |

**Table 8.10** Mineralocorticoid Medications

| MEDICATION | ADVERSE EFFECTS | NURSING CONSIDERATIONS |
|---|---|---|
| Fludrocortisone acetate | Hypertension, edema due to sodium retention | Give PO dose with food |
| | Muscle weakness and dysrhythmia due to hypokalemia | Check BP, electrolytes, I and O, weight |
| | | Give low-sodium, high-protein, high-potassium diet |
| | | May decrease effects of oral hypoglycemics, insulin, diuretics, $K^+$ supplements |

(*Continued*)

**Table 8.10** Mineralocorticoid Medications (*Continued*)

| MEDICATION | ADVERSE EFFECTS | NURSING CONSIDERATIONS |
|---|---|---|
| Action | Increases sodium reabsorption, potassium and hydrogen excretion in the distal convoluted tubules of the nephron | |
| Indications | Adrenal insufficiency | |
| Adverse effects | Sodium and water retention<br><br>Hypokalemia | |
| Nursing considerations | Monitor BP and serum electrolytes<br><br>Daily weight, report sudden weight gain to health care provider<br><br>Used with cortisone or hydrocortisone in adrenal insufficiency | |

# Cushing Disease (Cortisol Excess)

A. Definition—increased secretion of cortisol from three main causes

1. Hyperplasia of adrenocortical tissue due to pituitary dysfunction

2. Adrenocortical hyperplasia from a separate neoplasm secreting **adrenocorticotrophic** hormone (ACTH)

3. Primary adrenocortical hyperplasia from an adrenal tumor

B. Assessment (see Table 8-8)

1. Muscle wasting

2. Weakness

3. Osteoporosis

4. Edema

5. Purple striations on skin

6. Truncal obesity

7. Mood swings

8. Poor resistance to infections

9. Blood glucose imbalance

10. Hypertension

11. Buffalo hump

C. Diagnostic tests

1. Skull films, CT, MRI

2. Blood glucose analysis

3. Hypokalemia and hypernatremia

4. Plasma cortisol level increased

5. Urinary 17-hydroxycorticosteroids and 17-ketosteroid levels increased

**D.** Nursing management

1. Provide emotional support—assure the client that most physical changes are reversible with treatment

2. Teach appropriate diet—high protein, low carbohydrate, low sodium, high potassium, low calorie; fluid restriction

3. Prevent complications

   a. Use careful technique to prevent infection

   b. Assist with ambulation

   c. Eliminate environmental hazards for pathological fractures

   d. Observe for hyperactivity and GI bleeding, fluid volume overload

4. Administer aminoglutethimide or metyrapone to decrease cortisol production

5. Provide postadrenalectomy care

   a. Flank incision—painful breathing, so encourage coughing and deep breathing

   b. Hormone imbalance likely

      1) Monitor for shock

      2) Monitor for hypertension

      3) Administer cortisol as ordered

   c. Monitor urine output

   d. Anticipate slow recovery from anesthesia in obese client

   e. Anticipate slow wound healing

   f. Monitor glucose level

   g. Ensure client safety to decrease risk of fractures

   h. Teach low-sodium, high-potassium diet

   i. Provide long-term hormone therapy because of cortical and mineralocorticoid deficiency

      1) Given in schedule to mimic diurnal rhythm, with two-thirds dosage in early morning and one-third dosage in late afternoon

      2) Dose should meet needs of stress

6. Avoid factors that precipitate Addisonian crisis

   a. Physical stress

   b. Psychological stress

   c. Inadequate steroid replacement

7. Observe for clinical manifestations of Addisonian crisis

   a. Nausea and vomiting

   b. Abdominal pain

   c. Fever

   d. Extreme weakness

e. Severe hypoglycemia and dehydration develop rapidly

f. Blood pressure falls, leading to shock and coma; death results if not promptly treated

8. Treatment of Addisonian crisis

a. Monitor hydrocortisone therapy (*see* Table 8-11)

b. Carefully monitor IV infusion of NaCl

c. Administer vasopressors

d. Ensure absolute rest

e. Monitor vital signs

**Table 8.11** Adrenal Disorder Medications

| MEDICATION | ADVERSE EFFECTS | NURSING CONSIDERATIONS |
|---|---|---|
| Cortisone acetate<br>Hydrocortisone<br>Prednisone | Hyperglycemia, gastric and duodenal ulcers, muscle wasting, fluid retention, $K^+$ excretion, striae, acne, hirsutism, hypopigmentation, cataracts, osteoporosis<br><br>Centripetal fat buildup, moon face, buffalo hump<br><br>Adverse effects occur after prolonged therapy | Overdosage produces<br>Cushing syndrome<br>Abrupt withdrawal of medication may cause headache, nausea and vomiting, and papilledema<br>Give oral replacement preparation two-thirds in A.M., one-third in P.M.<br>Monitor labs, BP, physical exam<br>Infection may produce few symptoms due to anti-inflammatory action<br>Stress (surgery, illness, psychic) may lead to increased need for steroids<br>Nightmares are often the first indication of the onset of steroid psychosis |
| Dexamethasone | Euphoria, insomnia<br><br>Peptic ulcer, delayed wound healing | Effects of local injections persist for approximately 24 h<br>Check weight, BP, electrolytes<br>Check for depression<br>Give PO dose with food |

# Hypothyroidism (Myxedema)

**A.** Definition—insufficient secretion of thyroid hormone

**B.** Assessment (*see* Table 8-12)

1. Early hypothyroidism—cold intolerance, lethargy, tiredness, slightly decreased temperature, constipation, weight gain

2. Myxedema—periorbital and peripheral edema, thick speech, hoarseness, alopecia, bradycardia

C. Nursing management

1. Provide appropriate pacing of activities

    a. Allow client extra time to think, speak, act

    b. Teaching should be done slowly and in simple terms

2. Promote comfort, rest, and sleep

    a. Frequent rest periods between activities

    b. Maintain room temperature at approximately 75°F

    c. Provide client with extra clothing and bedding

3. Maintain skin integrity—restrict use of soaps, apply lanolin or creams to skin

    a. Teach appropriate diet

        1) High protein, low calorie

        2) Small, frequent feedings

    b. Prevent constipation—high-fiber, high-cellulose foods

    c. Increase fluid intake

    d. Cathartics or stool softeners as ordered

4. Provide emotional support to client

    a. Explain to client that symptoms are reversible with treatment

    b. Explain to family that client's behavior is part of the condition and will change when treatment begins

5. Administer medication replacement therapy

    a. Desiccated thyroid hormone

    b. Levothyroxine (Synthroid); dose gradually increased and adjusted

    c. Liothyronine sodium

6. Administer sedatives carefully—risk of respiratory depression

7. Instruct client about causes of myxedema coma (acute illness, surgery, chemotherapy, discontinuation of medication)

## Hyperthyroidism (Graves Disease)

A. Definition—oversecretion of thyroid hormone

B. Assessment (*see* Table 8-12)

1. Increased physical activity

2. Tachycardia

3. Increased sensitivity to heat

4. Fine, soft hair

5. Enlarged thyroid

6. Nervous, jittery, irritable, talkative

7. Exophthalmos

8. Weight loss

 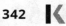

**Table 8.12** Thyroid Disorders

| | MYXEDEMA/HYPOTHYROIDISM | GRAVES DISEASE/ HYPERTHYROIDISM |
|---|---|---|
| Assessment | Diagnostic tests:<br><br>$\downarrow$ basal metabolic rate (BMR)<br>$\downarrow T_3$<br>$\downarrow T_4$<br>$\uparrow$ thyroid-stimulating hormone (TSH)<br><br>Decreased activity level<br><br>Sensitivity to cold<br><br>Potential alteration in skin integrity<br><br>Decreased perception of stimuli<br><br>Obesity, weight gain<br><br>Potential for respiratory difficulty<br><br>Constipation<br><br>Alopecia<br><br>Bradycardia<br><br>Dry skin and hair<br><br>Decreased ability to perspire<br><br>Reproductive problems | Diagnostic tests:<br><br>$\uparrow$ BMR<br>$\uparrow T_3$<br>$\uparrow T_4$<br>High-titer antithyroid antibodies<br>Hyperactivity<br><br>Sensitivity to heat<br><br>Rest and sleep deprivation<br><br>Increased perception of stimuli<br><br>Weight loss<br><br>Potential for respiratory difficulty<br><br>Diarrhea<br><br>Tachycardia<br><br>Exophthalmos<br><br>Frequent mood swings<br><br>Nervous, jittery<br><br>Fine, soft hair |
| Analysis | Hyposecretion of thyroid hormone<br><br>Slowed physical and mental functions | Hypersecretion of thyroid hormone<br><br>Accelerated physical and mental functions |
| Predisposing factors | Inflammation of thyroid Iatrogenic—thyroidectomy, irradiation, overtreatment with antithyroids<br><br>Pituitary deficiencies Iodine deficiency Idiopathic<br><br>Older adults—atrophy, fibrosis | Thyroid-secreting tumors<br><br>Iatrogenic—overtreatment for hypothyroid<br><br>Pituitary hyperactivity<br><br>Severe stress, e.g., pregnancy |
| Treatment and management | Hormone replacement:<br><br>Synthetic thyroxine ($T_4$) levothyroxine | Antithyroid medications (saturated solution of potassium iodide [SSKI], methimazole, propylthiouracil)<br>Irradiation ($^{131}$I)<br><br>Surgery |

*(Continued)*

**Table 8.12** Thyroid Disorder (*Continued*)

| | MYXEDEMA/HYPOTHYROIDISM | GRAVES DISEASE/ HYPERTHYROIDISM |
|---|---|---|
| Potential nursing diagnosis | Disturbed body image | Activity intolerance |
| | Imbalanced nutrition: more than body requirements | Altered body temperature |
| | Activity intolerance Constipation | Social interaction, impaired |
| | Hypothermia | Imbalanced nutrition: less than body requirements |
| | Deficient knowledge | Hyperthermia |
| | Decreased cardiac output | Fatigue |
| | | Risk for impaired tissue integrity |

**C.** Treatment

    1. Antithyroid medications (e.g., propylthiouracil, methimazole)

    2. Irradiation ($^{131}$I PO)—short-term

    3. Thyroidectomy—usually subtotal resection

**D.** Nursing management

    1. Promote comfort, rest, and sleep

       a. Limit activities to quiet ones (e.g., reading, knitting)

       b. Provide for frequent rest

       c. Restrict visitors and control choice of roommates

       d. Keep room cool; advise light, cool clothing

       e. Avoid stimulants (e.g., coffee)

    2. Provide emotional support

       a. Accept behavior

       b. Use calm, unhurried manner when caring for client

       c. Interpret behavior to family

    3. Administer antithyroid medication (*see* Table 8-13)

    4. Provide postthyroidectomy care

       a. Prevent strain on suture line

          1) Low or semi-Fowler position

          2) Support head, neck, and shoulders to prevent flexion or hyperextension; elevate head of bed 30°

          3) Tracheostomy set and suction supplies at bedside

       b. Give fluids as tolerated

**Table 8.13** Hyperthyroidism and Hypothyroidism Medications

| MEDICATION | ADVERSE EFFECTS | NURSING CONSIDERATIONS |
|---|---|---|
| **Hyperthyroidism Medications** | | |
| Carbimazole<br>Methimazole<br>Propylthiouracil | Leukopenia<br>Fever<br>Rash<br>Sore throat<br>Jaundice | Inhibits synthesis of thyroid hormone by thyroid gland<br>Check CBC and hepatic function<br>Report fever, sore throat to health care provider |
| Lugol's iodine solution<br>Potassium iodide | Nausea, vomiting, metallic taste<br>Rash | Iodine preparation<br>Used 2 wk prior to surgery; decreases vascularity, decreases hormone release<br>Only effective for a short period<br>Give after meals<br>Dilute in water, milk, or fruit juice<br>Stains teeth<br>Give through straw |
| Radioactive iodine ($^{131}$I) | Feeling of fullness in neck<br>Metallic taste<br>Leukemia | Destroys thyroid tissue<br>Contraindicated for women of childbearing age<br>Fast overnight before administration<br>Urine, saliva, vomit radioactive 3 d<br>Use full radiation precautions<br>Encourage fluids |
| **Hypothyroidism Medication** | | |
| Levothyroxine | Nervousness, tremors<br>Insomnia<br>Tachycardia, palpitations<br>Dysrhythmias, angina | Tell client to report chest pain, palpitations, sweating, nervousness, shortness of breath to health care provider |

      c.  Check Chvostek and Trousseau signs

        1)  Chvostek sign

           a)  An abnormal spasm of the facial muscles elicited by light tapping on the cheek of a client with hypocalcemia

           b)  Surgical removal of the thyroid gland can damage or remove the parathyroid glands (because they are embedded in the posterior thyroid gland)

           c)  Parathyroidectomy causes hypocalcemia and produces symptoms of tetany, including Chvostek sign

        2)  Trousseau sign

           a)  Involuntary flexion of the wrist caused by inflating a blood pressure cuff above the systolic pressure on the upper arm

           b)  Occurs in clients with hypocalcemia or hypomagnesemia

        3)  Have IV calcium gluconate or calcium chloride available

      d.  Offer throat lozenges, analgesics, cold steam inhalations for sore throat

      e.  Adjust diet to new metabolic needs

  5.  Observe for complications

      a.  Laryngeal nerve injury—detected by hoarseness

      b.  Thyrotoxic crisis (abrupt onset of HF, pulmonary edema, delirium, increased temperature and increased pulse, systolic hypertension, altered clotting, seizures, abdominal pain, diarrhea); treatment—hypothermia blanket, $O_2$, D5W, potassium iodine, propylthiouracil (PTU), digitalis, propranolol, hydrocortisone, acetaminophen

      c.  Hemorrhage; check back of neck and upper chest for bleeding

      d.  Respiratory obstruction

      e.  Tetany (decreased calcium from parathyroid involvement)—check Chvostek and Trousseau signs; have IV calcium gluconate or IV calcium chloride available

## Hypoparathyroidism

**A.**  Decreased secretion of parathyroid hormone; causes low serum calcium levels (hypocalcemia); may be due to neck surgery; possible decreased calcium absorption in older adults

**B.**  Assessment

  1.  Tetany, hyperactive deep tendon reflexes

  2.  Muscular irritability (paresthesias of lips, hands, feet)

  3.  Carpopedal spasm

  4.  Tremor, seizures

  5.  Dysphagia

  6.  Disorientation and confusion

  7.  Laryngeal spasm

  8.  Personality changes

9. Weakness and muscle cramps

10. Tachycardia and dysrhythmias; decreased cardiac output

11. Positive Chvostek sign

12. Positive Trousseau sign

**C.** Diagnostic

1. tests Serum calcium

2. Serum phosphorus

3. X-ray—bones appear dense

4. Sulkowitch test—test urine for calcium

**D.** Nursing management

1. Emergency Rx—calcium chloride, calcium gluconate, calcium gluceptate; infuse slowly to prevent hypotension and cardiac arrest

2. Replacement therapy

   a. Vitamin D—calcitriol, ergocalciferol

   b. Elemental calcium as lactate, gluconate, or carbonate—1.5–3 g/day

3. Observe for tetany

4. Administer appropriate diet—low phosphorus, high calcium (green leafy vegetables, soybeans, tofu)

# Hyperparathyroidism

**A.** Oversecretion of parathyroid hormone; causes elevated serum calcium levels (hypercalcemia); may be due to benign tumor, vitamin D deficiency, long-term kidney disease

**B.** Assessment (*see* Table 8-14)

**C.** Diagnostic tests

1. Serum calcium— greater than or equal to 10 mg/dL

2. Serum phosphorus— less than or equal to 4.5 mg/dL

3. X-ray—bones appear porous

4. Sulkowitch test—calcium in urine

5. Parathyroid hormone levels

6. Dual-energy x-ray absorptiometry (DEXA) scan—bone loss

**Table 8.14** Parathyroid Disorders

| | HYPOPARATHYROIDISM | HYPERPARATHYROIDISM |
|---|---|---|
| Assessment | Tetany<br><br>Muscular irritability (cramps, spasms)<br><br>Carpopedal spasm, clonic convulsions<br><br>Dysphagia<br><br>Paresthesia, laryngeal spasm<br><br>Anxiety, depression, irritability<br><br>Tachycardia<br><br>    + Chvostek sign<br>    + Trousseau sign | Fatigue, muscle weakness<br><br>Cardiac dysrhythmias<br><br>Emotional irritability<br><br>Renal calculi<br><br>Back and joint pain, pathological fractures<br><br>Pancreatitis, peptic ulcer |
| Diagnosis | Decreased secretion of parathyroid hormone<br><br>Iatrogenic—post thyroidectomy<br><br>Hypomagnesemia<br><br>Diagnostic tests:<br><br>    ↓ Serum calcium<br>    ↑ Serum phosphorus<br>    ↓ Parathyroid hormone (PTH)<br><br>X-ray—bones appear dense | Oversecretion of parathyroid hormone<br><br>Benign parathyroid tumor<br><br>Parathyroid carcinoma<br><br>Neck trauma<br><br>Neck radiation<br><br>Diagnostic tests:<br><br>    ↑ Serum calcium<br>    ↓ Serum phosphorus<br>    ↑ Serum parathyroid hormone<br><br>X-ray—bones appear porous |
| Potential nursing diagnosis | Risk for injury<br><br>Deficient knowledge | Risk for injury<br><br>Impaired urinary elimination<br><br>Nutrition—less than body requirements<br><br>Constipation |

*(Continued)*

**Table 8.14** Parathyroid Disorders (*Continued*)

| | HYPOPARATHYROIDISM | HYPERPARATHYROIDISM |
|---|---|---|
| Plan/ implementation | Emergency treatment—calcium chloride or gluconate over 10-15 minutes<br><br>Calcitriol 0.5-2 mg daily for acute hypocalcemia<br><br>Ergocalciferol 50,000-400,000 units daily<br><br>Observe for tetany<br><br>Low-phosphorus, high-calcium diet | Relieve pain<br><br>Prevent formation of renal calculi increase fluid intake<br><br>Offer acid-ash juices (improves solubility of calcium)<br><br>Administer appropriate diet<br><br>Prevent fractures<br><br>Safety precautions<br><br>Monitor potassium levels (counteracts effect of calcium on cardiac muscles)<br><br>Provide postparathyroidectomy care (essentially same as for thyroidectomy)<br><br>IV furosemide and saline promote calcium excretion<br><br>IV phosphorus is used only for rapid lowering of calcium level<br><br>Surgery—parathyroidectomy |

D. Treatment

1. IV furosemide and saline promote calcium excretion
2. IV phosphorus is used only for rapid lowering of calcium level
3. Bisphosphonates (e.g., alendronate) increase bone density and decrease calcium levels
4. Surgery—parathyroidectomy

E. Nursing management

1. Relieve pain
2. Prevent formation of renal calculi: increase fluid intake
3. Offer acid-ash juices (improves solubility of calcium)
4. Administer appropriate diet
5. Prevent fractures
6. Promote body alignment
7. Safety precautions
8. Monitor potassium levels (counteracts effect of calcium on cardiac muscles)
9. Provide postparathyroidectomy care (essentially same as for thyroidectomy)

## End-of-Chapter Thinking Exercise

A middle-aged client diagnosed with hypertension visits the clinic every 3 months for blood pressure monitoring. On a routine visit last week, the client reported increased tiredness and not being able to get through the day without a short nap before dinner. The client was burned while cooking a month ago, and the burn still has not healed. The nurse practitioner (NP) notes the client's medical history includes a father and older brother who have type 2 diabetes. The NP orders lab tests and schedules a return visit in 1 week. At today's visit, the client's weight is 200 lb (90.7 kg) and calculated BMI is 34.3. The NP reviews the following labs with the client: fasting blood glucose 168 mg/dL (9.3 mmol/L), glycosylated hemoglobin (HbA1c) 9%, urinalysis positive for glucose. The client is diagnosed with type 2 diabetes. The nurse instructs the client about diet and exercise requirements, and metformin 500 mg PO daily is ordered.

1. What risk factors are present that show an increased risk for type 2 diabetes? (Recognize Cues)

2. Which assessment findings indicate hyperglycemia? (Analyze Cues)

3. What information is important to include when teaching the client about metformin? (Generate Solutions)

# Thinking Exercise Explanations

1. What risk factors are present that show an increased risk for type 2 diabetes? (Recognize Cues)

   - Age—older than 45
   - Hypertension
   - Familial history
   - Obesity

   Many adults have undiagnosed type 2 diabetes. Insulin resistance is present before a diagnosis is made and increases the risk of accompanying cardiovascular disease. Identifying risk factors and screening for type 2 diabetes is essential in controlling hyperglycemia and decreasing complications of the disease in the future.

2. Which assessment findings indicate hyperglycemia? (Analyze Cues)

   - Elevated fasting blood glucose
   - Elevated glycosylated hemoglobin (HbA1c)
   - Glucose in the urine
   - Delayed wound healing

   A fasting blood glucose reading greater than or equal to 100 mg/dL (5.55 mmol/L) and a glycosylated hemoglobin (HbA1c) greater than 6.5% indicate insulin resistance or decreased insulin secretion. Chronic hyperglycemia is the hallmark sign of diabetes mellitus. When the blood glucose concentration is over 180 mg/dL (9.99 mmol/L), the kidneys begin to excrete glucose in the urine, indirectly demonstrating hyperglycemia. Chronic hyperglycemia causes a lack of elasticity and narrowing of the blood vessels. This in turn decreases the body's ability to adequately deliver oxygen and nutrients to cells, causing a delay in healing.

3. What information is important to include when teaching the client about metformin? (Generate Solutions)

   - Adverse effects of the medication can include GI distress, such as nausea, flatulence, abdominal pain, and diarrhea
   - Avoid alcohol while taking this medication to prevent lactic acidosis
   - Remind the client that the medication needs to be discontinued 48 hours before any testing with contrast medium to prevent kidney damage and lactic acidosis
   - Avoid medication interactions by asking the health care provider before taking any over-the-counter (OTC) medications

[ CHAPTER 9 ]

# THE RENAL AND UROLOGICAL SYSTEMS

# THE URINARY SYSTEM OVERVIEW

## Acid-Base Balance, Fluid and Electrolyte Balance, Elimination

## Overview of the Urinary System

A. Kidneys

1. Anatomy (*see* Figure 9-1)

   a. Bean-shaped, paired organs

   b. Left kidney larger and higher

   c. Positioned adjacent to vertebral column

   d. Two layers—outer cortex, inner medulla

   e. Functional unit—nephron (*see* Figure 9-2)

      1) Glomerulus—removes filtrate from blood

      2) Bowman's capsule—filtrate passes through to tubule

      3) Tubule

         a) Proximal convoluted tubule

         b) Loop of Henle

         c) Distal convoluted tubule

         d) Collecting tubule

   f. Gerontologic concerns—decreased kidney size; decreased tone and elasticity of bladder, ureters, urethra; decreased bladder capacity

2. Physiology

   a. Elimination of waste products

   b. Fluid and electrolyte balance regulator

   c. Production of red blood cells

   d. Hormonal control of blood pressure

   e. Gerontologic concerns—glomerular sclerosis and decreased renal perfusion; decreased ability to concentrate urine

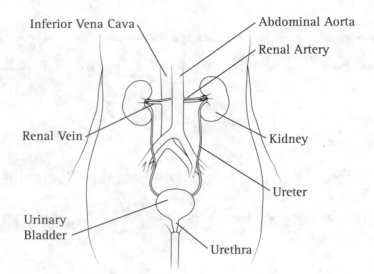

**Figure 9-1.** Urinary System

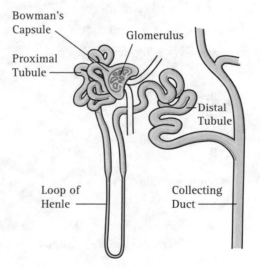

**Figure 9-2.** Nephron

**B.** Ureters

1.  Anatomy—hollow tubes, about 12 inches long

2.  Physiology—propel urine to bladder from kidneys

**C.** Bladder

1.  Hollow, muscular organ

2.  Lies within pelvic cavity

3.  Normal capacity—500 mL

4.  Contracts under voluntary and involuntary control

5.  Nerve supply—parasympathetic and sympathetic

# URINARY FUNCTION

## Acid-Base Balance, Fluid and Electrolyte Balance, Elimination

## Overview of Urinary Function

A. Urine production

1. Glomerular filtration—begins in afferent arteriole, then to glomerular capillaries, then to glomerulus

2. Tubular reabsorption—ultrafiltrate passes through remainder of nephron

B. Characteristics of urine

1. Color—yellow

2. Consistency—clear, transparent

3. Specific gravity—1.010–1.025

4. pH—4.5–8

5. 24-hour production—1,000–2,000 mL

C. Serum changes

1. BUN—normal 10–20 mg/dL (3.6–7.1 mmol/L); greater than 60 yo 8–20 mg/dL (2.8–7.1 mmol/L)

2. Creatinine—normal 0.7–1.4 mg/dL (62–124 mcmol/L)

D. Diagnostic studies of the urinary system (*see* Table 9-1)

E. Promotion of normal urinary function

1. Adults

a. Adequate hydration

b. Activity (maintenance of muscle tone)

c. Regular voiding habits

2. Children

a. Proper toilet training

1) 2.5 to 3.5 years old—bladder reflex control

2) 3 years old—regular voiding habits

3) 4 years old—independent bathroom activity

4) 5 years old (approximate)—nighttime control

b. Enuresis—lack of nighttime bladder control in school-age child

**Table 9-1** Diagnostic Studies of the Urinary System

| TEST | CLIENT PREPARATION AND PROCEDURE | NURSING CONSIDERATIONS |
|---|---|---|
| Urinalysis<br><br>Urine culture | Advise client to save first A.M. urine specimen<br><br>Cleanse external meatus with povidone-iodine or soap and water prior to test | Overnight urine specimen is more concentrated Obtain midstream specimen<br><br>Normal—less than 100,000 colonies/mL |
| Cystometrogram—test of muscle tone | Prepare client for indwelling urinary catheter<br><br>Instillation of saline may cause feeling of pressure in bladder during test<br><br>Client should report bladder sensations during test | Advise client to report any posttest symptoms |
| Creatinine clearance | 24-hour urine collection | Blood drawn for creatinine level at end of urine collection<br><br>Normal—Women: 75–115 mL/min Men: 85–125 mL/min |
| Cystoscopy—direct visualization by cystoscope inserted into bladder | Bowel preparation<br><br>Teach client to deep breathe to decrease discomfort<br><br>NPO if general anesthesia used | Posttest nursing care:<br><br>Monitor character and volume of urine<br><br>Check for abdominal distention, frequency, fever<br><br>Check for bleeding<br><br>Provide antimicrobial prophylaxis |
| Cystourethrogram—x-ray study of bladder and urethra | Explain procedure to client—catheter inserted into urethra, radiopaque dye injected, client voids, x-rays taken during voiding | Posttest nursing care:<br><br>Advise client to report any symptoms |
| Intravenous pyelogram—provides x-ray visualization of kidneys, ureters, and bladder | Bowel preparation<br><br>NPO after midnight<br><br>Check for allergies<br><br>Burning may occur during injection of radiopaque dye into vein<br><br>X-rays are taken at intervals after dye | Postprocedure x-rays usually done<br><br>Client should be alert to signs of dye reaction—edema, itching, wheezing, dyspnea |

*(Continued)*

**Table 9-1** Diagnostic Studies of the Urinary System (*Continued*)

| TEST | CLIENT PREPARATION AND PROCEDURE | NURSING CONSIDERATIONS |
|---|---|---|
| Renal scan—evaluation of kidneys | Radioactive isotope injected IV<br><br>Radioactivity measured by radioactivity counter<br><br>Fluids forced before procedure | No posttest care required |
| Ultrasound—images of renal structures obtained by sound waves | Noninvasive procedure; no preparation; requires full bladder | No preparation or posttest care required |
| Renal biopsy—kidney tissue obtained by needle aspiration for pathological evaluation | X-ray taken prior to procedure<br><br>Skin is marked to indicate lower pole of kidney (fewer blood vessels)<br><br>Position—prone and bent at diaphragm<br><br>Client instructed to hold breath during needle insertion | Posttest nursing care:<br><br>Pressure applied to site for 20 min; check vital signs every 15 min for 1 h<br><br>Pressure dressing applied; position on affected side for 30-60 min<br><br>Client kept flat in bed<br><br>Bedrest for 6-8 h<br><br>Fluid intake 3,000 mL/day<br><br>Observe for hematuria and site bleeding |

# Management of Urinary Retention

A. Clinical manifestations
   1. Voiding at frequent intervals in small amounts
   2. Suprapubic discomfort and bladder distention
   3. Appropriate hydration with no urinary output for more than 6 h
   4. Specific gravity is elevated
B. Causes
   1. Functional—neurogenic bladder
   2. Mechanical—stricture, calculi, trauma
C. Predisposing factors
   1. Bedrest
   2. Tumors
   3. Prostatic hypertrophy
   4. Decreased bladder tone—postoperative, neurological
   5. Bladder or urethral cancer

      6. Postop effects

      7. Calculi

      8. Medications—nephrotoxicity

   **D.** Complications

      1. Rupture of bladder

      2. Infection

      3. Uremia

   **E.** Nursing care

      1. Stimulate voiding, e.g., running water

      2. Pouring tepid water over perineum

      3. Positioning

      4. Catheterization—temporary, may be emergency

   **F.** Surgical Intervention (*see* Table 9-2)

      1. Suprapubic cystostomy—opening into bladder, drainage via catheter through abdominal wall

      2. Surgery for kidney stones

**Table 9-2** Urinary Diversion

| NAME | PROCEDURE | NURSING CONSIDERATIONS |
|---|---|---|
| Nephrostomy | Flank incision and insertion of nephrostomy tube into renal pelvis | Penrose drain<br>Surgical dressing |
| Ureterosigmoidostomy | Ureters detached from bladder and anastomosed to sigmoid colon | Urine and stool are evacuated through anus<br>Encourage voiding via rectum every 2-4 h; no enemas or cathartics<br>Monitor complications—fluid and electrolyte imbalance, pyelonephritis, obstruction |
| Cutaneous ureterostomy | Single- or double-barreled stoma, formed from ureter(s) excised from bladder and brought out through the skin into the abdominal wall | Stoma usually constructed on right side of abdomen below waist<br>Extensive nursing intervention required for alteration in body image |
| Ileal conduit | Portion of terminal ileum is used as a conduit; ureters are replanted into ileal segment; distal end is brought out through skin and forms a stoma | Most common urinary diversion<br>Check for obstruction (occurs at the anastomosis)<br>Postop mucus threads normal |

*(Continued)*

**Table 9-2** Urinary Diversion (*Continued*)

| NAME | PROCEDURE | NURSING CONSIDERATIONS |
|------|-----------|------------------------|
| Kock pouch, continent ileal conduit | Ureters are transplanted to an isolated segment of ileum (pouch) with a one-way valve; urine is drained by a catheter | Urine collects in pouch until drained by catheter<br><br>Valve prevents leakage of urine<br><br>Drainage of urine by catheter is under control of client<br><br>Pouch must be drained at regular intervals |

# Care of Urinary Drainage Systems

**A.** Urinary catheters (*see* Table 9-3)

  1. To facilitate healing of portion of urinary tract

  2. To empty bladder contents, e.g., postoperatively or spinal cord injuries

  3. To promote continence

  4. To facilitate measurement of urine output

**Table 9-3** Urinary Catheters

| TYPE | CHARACTERISTICS | COMMENTS |
|------|-----------------|----------|
| Bladder drainage system | Double lumen with inflatable balloon toward tip | Indwelling for urinary drainage |
| Nephrostomy | Placed on temporary basis | Used as nephrostomy tube—anchored in renal pelvis through flank incision |
| Suprapubic | Placed in bladder via abdominal incision<br><br>Dressing over site | Used in conjunction with urethral drainage |
| Straight | Intermittent | Used for neurogenic bladder; bladder outlet obstruction in men; postop after surgical problems in reproductive organs |

**B.** Procedure for catheterization

  1. Female

   a. Explain procedure to client

   b. Assemble equipment

   c. Client should be placed in dorsal recumbent position or in Sims' position

   d. Drape client with sterile drapes, using sterile technique

e.   Apply sterile gloves

f.   Lubricate catheter tip and place in sterile catheter tray

g.   Separate labia with thumb and forefinger, and wipe from the meatus toward the rectum with sterile cleansing swab and discard

h.   Insert catheter 2–3 in into the urethra; insert catheter an additional inch after urine begins to flow to ensure balloon portion of catheter is in the bladder

i.   Inflate balloon

j.   Gently apply traction to the catheter

k.   Tape drainage tubing to client's thigh

2.   Male

a.   If uncircumcised, retract the foreskin to expose urinary meatus

b.   Cleanse glans and meatus with sterile cleansing swabs in circular motion

c.   Hold penis perpendicular to the body; insert catheter into urethra 6–7 in

d.   Replace the foreskin

e.   Inflate balloon

f.   Gently apply traction to the catheter until resistance is felt, indicating the catheter is at the base of the bladder

g.   Tape drainage tubing to client's thigh

3.   Principles of drainage system care

a.   Catheter should not be disconnected from drainage system except to perform ordered irrigations

b.   Urine samples should be obtained from drainage port with a small-bore needle, using sterile technique; clamp tubing below port

c.   Drainage bags should not be elevated above level of cavity being drained (to prevent reflux)

d.   Avoid kinks in tubing

e.   Avoid removing more than 1,000 mL at one time; if more urine in bladder, clamp after 1,000 mL, wait 15–30 min, and then continue

f.   Coil excess tubing on bed

4.   Catheter irrigation

a.   Purpose—prevent obstruction of flow and catheter

b.   Procedure—urethral catheter irrigation

1)   Use closed system; if frequent irrigation is required, replace single lumen catheter with multilumen catheter

2)   Draw up required solution

3)   Clamp catheter just below port (specimen or irrigation)

4)   Thoroughly clean injection port

5)   Insert syringe into port

6)   Slowly and evenly inject solution into catheter and bladder

      7) Withdraw syringe, cleanse port, remove clamp

      8) Note drainage and document procedure, including resistance to flush, client comfort, drainage returned

  5. Nursing management

    a. Use aseptic technique on insertion

    b. Do not disturb integrity of closed drainage system

    c. Check for kinks

    d. Keep urine collection bag below the level of the urinary bladder

    e. Monitor intake and output; minimum urinary drainage catheter output should be 30 mL/h

    f. Monitor for signs and symptoms of infection (foul-smelling urine with pus, blood, or mucus streaks)

    g. Adhere to special precautions for type of catheter used

      1) Ureterostomy tube—never irrigate

      2) Nephrostomy tube—never clamp

    h. Clamp indwelling catheters intermittently prior to removal to improve bladder tone

**C.** Promotion of normal urinary function

  1. Adequate hydration

  2. Activity (maintenance of muscle tone)

  3. Regular voiding habits

# Incontinence

**A.** Definition—involuntary loss of bladder control due to infection, neurogenic bladder, sphincter weakness, or reduced muscle tone

**B.** Types

  1. Urge incontinence—strong and sudden urge to void; unknown cause

  2. Stress incontinence—occurs with physical exertion such as lifting, sneezing; common in women after childbirth

  3. Overflow incontinence—constant dribbling of urine; diabetic neuropathy, prostatic hyperplasia, uterine prolapse

  4. Reflex incontinence—large amount of urine retained; central nervous system disease (CVA, MS)

**C.** Intervention—short-term; varies according to type

  1. Scheduling, bladder retraining, prompted voiding

  2. Pelvic exercises

  3. Surgical approaches

  4. Condom catheters, incontinence pads

  5. Avoid delay in assisting client to bathroom

## Surgery for Urinary Diversion Following Surgery for Bladder Cancer or Urethral Cancer

(*see* Figure 9-3 and Table 9-2)

A. Ureterosigmoidostomy—ureters are attached to the sigmoid colon to allow drainage into rectum and elimination control by anus; not commonly used

B. Cutaneous ureterostomy—one or both ureters are brought to the skin surface to form a stoma to drain urine

C. Ileal conduit—both ureters are attached to a segment of ileum, which is brought to the surface of the lower abdomen to form a stoma to drain urine; most commonly used urinary diversion

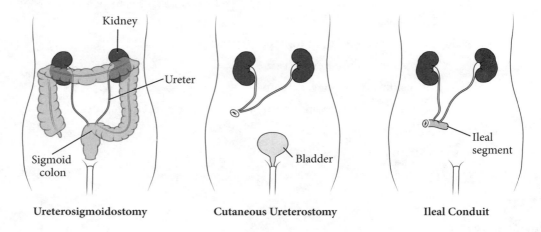

**Figure 9-3.** Types of Urinary Diversions

# SELECTED DISORDERS

## Acid-Base Balance, Fluid and Electrolyte Balance, Elimination

## Selected Disorders of the Urinary System

A. Cystitis

1. Definition—inflammation of the bladder; may be infectious (bacteria, virus, fungal) or noninfectious (irritation)

2. Assessment

   a. Signs and symptoms

      1) Urgency

      2) Frequency

      3) Burning during urination (dysuria)

      4) Cloudy, foul smelling urine

   b. Predisposing factors

      1) Female more prone

      2) Catheterization, instrumentation

      3) Hospital-acquired infections (e.g., *E. coli*)

3. Nursing management

   a. Encourage/increase fluids to 3,000 mL/d

   b. Urine for culture and sensitivity (C and S)

   c. Antibiotic therapy (e.g., trimethoprim/sulfamethoxazole) or antifungals (e.g., ketoconazole)

   d. Urinary antiseptics (e.g., nitrofurantoin)

   e. Bladder analgesics (e.g., phenazopyridine)

   f. Encourage drinking cranberry juice to maintain acid urine

   g. Discourage caffeine, carbonated beverages, tomatoes

   h. Teach females to void following intercourse

   i. Clean properly after defecation (front to back)

**B.** Pyelonephritis—inflammation of the kidney

   1. History

      a. Pregnancy

      b. Urinary obstruction

      c. Metabolic disorder (e.g., diabetes mellitus, hypertension)

      d. Trauma

      e. Tumor

      f. Urinary tract infection

   2. Assessment

      a. Chills

      b. Fever

      c. General malaise

      d. Urinary frequency, dysuria

      e. Flank pain

      f. Costovertebral angle (CVA) tenderness

   3. Nursing management

      a. Serial urine culture—usually caused by *E. coli*

      b. Periodic blood tests

      c. Bedrest during acute phase

      d. Antibiotic therapy, antiseptics, analgesics

      e. Encourage fluid intake 3,000 mL/day

**C.** Urinary tract calculi

   1. Definition—mineral crystallization formed around organic matter

      a. Urolithiasis—urinary stones

      b. Nephrolithiasis—kidney stones

   2. History

      a. UTI, dehydration

      b. Hypercalcemia or increased uric acid

      c. Urinary stasis

      d. Obstruction

   3. Assessment

      a. Pain (renal colic)

         1) Location depends on location of stone

         2) Radiates from flank to abdomen, labia, or scrotum

      b. Nausea, vomiting

      c. Hematuria, WBCs and bacteria in urine

      d. Diaphoresis

e. Low-grade fever and chills

f. Diagnostic tests—intravenous pyelogram (IVP), CT, MRI, cystoscopy, and kidneys, ureters, and bladder (KUB)

4. Nursing management

a. Monitor I and O

b. Force fluids

c. Strain urine and check pH of urine

d. Monitor temperature

e. Pain management—NSAIDs, oxybutynin, propantheline, opioids

f. Diet for prevention depends on identified stone from urinary tract

1) Low in oxalate—spinach, black tea, rhubarb for calcium oxalate stones

2) Low in protein—to prevent cystine stones, calcium phosphate

3) Low in sodium—sodium increases calcium in urine

4) Low in purines to prevent uric acid stones

5. Medical management

a. Lithotripsy

1) Laser lithotripsy and extracorporeal shock wave lithotripsy most common

2) Laser probes or high-energy acoustic shock waves shatter the stones

b. Surgery—stent placement, nephrolithotomy, nephrostomy, retrograde ureteroscopy

D. Hydronephrosis —kidney pelvis dilation, leading to tissue destruction and renal failure

1. Assessment

a. Pain

1) Dull flank

2) Stabbing in flank or abdomen radiating to genitalia

b. Nausea, vomiting

c. Signs and symptoms of UTI

d. Abdominal muscle spasms

2. Nursing management

a. Bedrest

b. Antibiotic therapy

c. Catheterization

d. Force fluids to 3,000 mL/d

e. Urinary diversion

f. Surgical correction

g. Strain all urine

**E.** Benign prostatic hyperplasia (BPH)

1. Definition—prostate gland enlargement

2. History

   a. Retention

   b. Hesitancy, frequency, urgency, dysuria

   c. Nocturia

   d. Hematuria before or after voiding

   e. Urinary stream alterations; dilated ureter

   f. Dribbling

3. Diagnostic tests—BUN, prostate-specific antigen (PSA), ultrasound, biopsy

4. Management

   a. Urinary antiseptics

   b. 5-alpha reductase inhibitor (e.g., finasteride)

   c. Alpha-blocking medications (e.g., tamsulosin)

   d. Saw palmetto or lycopene

   e. Suprapubic cystostomy—to empty bladder

   f. Surgery—three common approaches to prostate gland removal

      1) Transurethral resection of prostate (TURP)

      2) Suprapubic resection (incision through bladder)

      3) Retropubic resection (incision through abdomen)

   g. Postop care of TURP

      1) Assess for shock and hemorrhage—check dressing and drainage: urine may be bright red for 12 h; monitor vital signs

      2) I and O—after catheter removed, expect dribbling and urinary leakage around wound

      3) Avoid long periods of sitting and strenuous activity until danger of bleeding is over

**F.** Nephrosis (nephrotic syndrome)—idiopathic syndrome characterized by proteinuria and hypoalbuminemia

1. Definition

   a. Congenital nephrotic syndrome

   b. Secondary nephrotic syndrome—occurs after known glomerular disease

   c. Idiopathic nephrotic syndrome—most common

2. Assessment

   a. Edema

   b. Pallor

   c. Lethargy

   d. Oliguria

      e.   Dark, frothy urine

      f.   Decreased serum protein, increased serum cholesterol and plasma lipids

  3.  Nursing management

      a.   Steroid and antibiotic therapy; monitor for infection

      b.   Bedrest

      c.   Fluid restriction, I and O

      d.   High-protein, low-sodium, high-caloric diet

**G.**  Acute kidney injury

  1.  Definition—a rapid loss of renal function due to damage to the kidney.

  2.  History

      a.   Prerenal injury

         1)  Circulating volume depletion

         2)  Vascular obstruction

         3)  Vascular resistance

      b.   Intrarenal failure

         1)  Acute tubular necrosis (ATN) from nephrotoxic medications or transfusion reaction

         2)  Trauma

         3)  Glomerulonephritis

         4)  Severe muscle exertion

         5)  Genetic conditions—polycystic kidney disease

      c.   Postrenal failure—obstruction of urine outflow from the kidney; reflux of urine from the bladder back into the kidneys; tumors or renal calculi

  3.  Assessment

      a.   Oliguric phase

         1)  Urinary output 0.5 mL/kg/hr

         2)  Nausea, vomiting

         3)  Irritability

         4)  Drowsiness, confusion, coma

         5)  Restlessness, twitching, seizures

         6)  Increased serum $K^+$, BUN, creatinine

         7)  Increased $Ca^+$, $Na^+$, pH, $CO_2$

         8)  Anemia

         9)  Pulmonary edema, CHF

         10)  Hypertension

         11)  Albuminuria

    b. Diuretic or recovery phase

      1) Urinary output 4–5 L/d

      2) Increased serum BUN

      3) $Na^+$ and $K^+$ loss in urine

      4) Increased mental and physical activity

  4. Nursing management

    a. Oliguric and anuric phases—protein-sparing diet, restrict fluids, observe for hyponatremia and hypokalemia, dialyze as ordered, prevent infection

    b. Diuretic phase—monitor I and O, observe for electrolyte imbalance, provide adequate nutrition, prevent infection

**H.** Chronic kidney disease

  1. Definition—ongoing deterioration of kidney function, resulting in uremia

  2. History

    a. Hypertension

    b. Diabetes mellitus

    c. Lupus erythematosus

    d. Sickle cell disease

    e. Chronic glomerulonephritis

    f. Repeated pyelonephritis

    g. Polycystic kidney disease

    h. Nephrotoxins

  3. Assessment

    a. Anemia

    b. Acidosis

    c. Azotemia

    d. Fluid retention

    e. Urinary output alterations

  4. Nursing management

    a. Antihypertensives

    b. Fluid and sodium restrictions

    c. Adherence to diet

    d. Monitor I and O

    e. Skin care

    f. Dialysis—movement of fluid and particles across a semipermeable membrane (*see* Table 9-4 and Figure 9-4)

**Table 9-4** Hemodialysis and Peritoneal Dialysis

| | HEMODIALYSIS | PERITONEAL DIALYSIS |
|---|---|---|
| Circulatory access | Subclavian catheter<br><br>AV fistula, AV graft | Catheter in peritoneal cavity<br><br>(Tenckhoff, Gore-Tex) |
| Dialysis bath | Electrolyte solution similar to that of normal plasma | Similar to hemodialysis |
| Dialyzer | Artificial kidney machine with semipermeable membrane | Peritoneum is dialyzing membrane |
| Procedure | Blood shunted through dialyzer for 3–5 h, 2–3 times/wk | Weigh client before and after dialysis<br><br>Repeated cycles can be continuous<br><br>Catheter is cleansed and attached to line leading to peritoneal cavity<br><br>Dialysate infused into peritoneal cavity to prescribed volume<br><br>Dialysate is then drained from abdomen after prescribed amount of time |
| Complications | Hemorrhage<br><br>Hepatitis<br><br>Nausea and vomiting<br><br>Disequilibrium syndrome (headache, mental confusion)<br><br>Muscle cramps<br><br>Air embolism<br><br>Sepsis<br><br>Arterial steal syndrome (fistula) | Protein loss<br><br>Peritonitis<br><br>Cloudy outflow, bleeding<br><br>Fever<br><br>Abdominal tenderness, lower-back problems<br><br>Nausea and vomiting<br><br>Exit site infection<br><br>Hypotension and hypovolemia |
| Nursing considerations | Check "thrill" and bruit every 8 h<br><br>Don't use extremity for BP or to obtain blood specimens<br><br>Monitor BP, apical pulse, temperature, respirations, breath sounds, weight<br><br>Monitor for hemorrhage during dialysis and 1 h after procedure | Constipation may cause problems with infusion and outflow; high-fiber diet, stool softener<br><br>If problems with outflow, reposition (supine or low Fowler, client to side)<br><br>Monitor BP, apical pulse, temperature, respirations, breath sounds, weight<br><br>Clean catheter insertion site and apply sterile dressing |

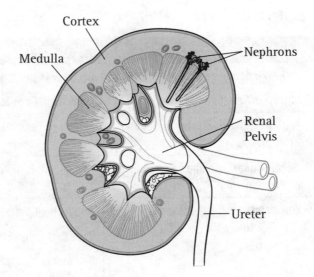

**Figure 9-4.** Kidney

I. Kidney transplantation

  1. Donor selection

    a. Major requirement is histocompatibility

  2. Pretransplantation donor—specific transfusions

    a. Desensitizes recipient to donor's tissue

    b. Identifies unfavorable response to donated organ by recipient

  3. Nursing management—preop

    a. Explain surgical procedure and follow-up care to client

    b. Show client where the donated kidney will be located (iliac fossa on opposite side of body from which the kidney was taken)

    c. Emphasize need for continued dialysis postop

    d. Use of immunosuppressive medications

    e. Need for infection prevention

    f. Pain management

    g. Pulmonary hygiene

    h. Maintaining integrity of vascular access

    i. Tubings and dressings, locations and purposes

  4. Nursing management—postop

    a. Monitor vital signs

    b. Monitor I and O—expect scant urine production for weeks postop

    c. Vascular access care

d. Observe for:

1) Hemorrhage

2) Shock

3) Rejection

a) Rejection—acute (days to months; decreased urine output, increased BUN and creatinine, fever, tenderness and swelling over graft site); chronic (months to years; gradual decrease in renal function, proteinuria, gradual increase in BUN and creatinine)

4) Infection

5) Pulmonary complications

6) Adverse effects of immunosuppressive and steroid therapies

e. Daily weights

f. Catheter care

g. Psychological support for donor and recipient

# Overview of Diuretics

**Table 9-5** Diuretic Medications

| MEDICATION | ADVERSE EFFECTS | NURSING CONSIDERATIONS |
|---|---|---|
| **Thiazide Diuretics** | | |
| Hydrochlorothiazide | Hypokalemia | Monitor electrolytes, especially potassium |
| Chlorothiazide | Hyperglycemia | I and O |
| | Blurred vision | Monitor BUN and creatinine |
| | Loss of $Na^+$ | Don't give at bedtime (hs) |
| | Dry mouth | Weigh client daily |
| | Hypotension | Encourage potassium-containing foods |
| **Potassium Sparing** | | |
| Spironolactone | Hyperkalemia | Used with other diuretics |
| | Hyponatremia | Give with meals |
| | Hepatic and renal damage | Avoid salt substitutes containing potassium |
| | Tinnitus | Monitor I and O |
| | Rash | |

*(Continued)*

**Table 9-5** Diuretic Medications (*Continued*)

| MEDICATION | ADVERSE EFFECTS | NURSING CONSIDERATIONS |
|---|---|---|
| **Loop Diuretics** | | |
| Furosemide<br>Ethacrynic acid | Hypotension<br>Hypokalemia<br>Hyperglycemia<br>GI upset<br>Weakness | Monitor BP, pulse rate, I and O<br>Monitor potassium<br>Give IV dose over 1–2 minutes → diuresis in 5–10 min<br>After PO dose, diuresis in about 30 min<br>Weigh client daily<br>Don't give at bedtime<br>Encourage potassium-containing foods |
| Bumetanide | Potassium depletion<br>Electrolyte imbalance<br>Hypovolemia<br>Ototoxicity | Supervise ambulation<br>Monitor blood pressure and pulse<br>Observe for signs of electrolyte imbalance |
| **Osmotic Diuretic** | | |
| Mannitol | Dry mouth<br>Thirst | I and O must be measured<br>Monitor vital signs<br>Monitor for electrolyte imbalance |
| **Thiazide-like Diuretics** | | |
| Chlorthalidone | Dizziness<br>Aplastic anemia<br>Orthostatic hypotension | Acts like a thiazide diuretic<br>Acts in 2–3 h, peak 2–6 h, lasts 2–3 days<br>Administer in A.M.<br>Monitor output, weight, BP, electrolytes<br>Increase $K^+$ in diet<br>Monitor glucose levels in diabetic clients<br>Change position slowly |
| **Action** | Thiazide—inhibits reabsorption of sodium and chloride in distal renal tubule | |
| | Loop—inhibits reabsorption of sodium and chloride in loop of Henle and distal renal tubules | |
| | Potassium sparing—blocks effect of aldosterone on renal tubules, causing loss of sodium and water and retention of potassium | |
| | Osmotic—pulls fluid from tissues due to hypertonic effect | |

(*Continued*)

**Table 9-5** Diuretic Medications (*Continued*)

| MEDICATION | ADVERSE EFFECTS | NURSING CONSIDERATIONS |
|---|---|---|
| **Indications** | Heart failure | |
| | Hypertension | |
| | Renal diseases | |
| | Diabetes insipidus | |
| | Reduction of osteoporosis in postmenopausal women | |
| **Adverse effects** | Dizziness, vertigo | |
| | Dry mouth | |
| | Orthostatic hypotension | |
| | Leukopenia | |
| | Polyuria, nocturia | |
| | Photosensitivity | |
| | Impotence | |
| | Hypokalemia (except for potassium sparing) | |
| | Hyponatremia | |
| | Various effects on calcium | |
| **Nursing considerations** | Take with food or milk | |
| | Take in A.M. | |
| | Monitor weight and electrolytes | |
| | Protect skin from the sun | |
| | Diet high in potassium for loop and thiazide diuretics | |
| | Limit potassium intake for potassium-sparing diuretics | |
| | Used as first-line medications for hypertension | |
| **Herbal interactions** | Licorice can promote potassium loss, causing hypokalemia | |
| | Aloe can decrease serum potassium level, causing hypokalemia | |
| | Ginkgo may increase blood pressure when taken with thiazide diuretics | |

**Table 9-6** Men's Health Medications

| MEDICATION | ADVERSE EFFECTS | NURSING CONSIDERATIONS |
|---|---|---|
| **Alpha-1 Adrenergic Blockers** | | |
| Terazosin | Dizziness<br>Headache<br>Weakness<br>Nasal congestion<br>Orthostatic hypotension | Used to decrease urinary urgency, hesitancy, nocturia in prostatic hyperplasia<br><br>Caution to change position slowly<br><br>Avoid alcohol, CNS depressants, hot showers due to orthostatic hypotension<br><br>Requires titration<br><br>Administer at bedtime due to risk of orthostatic hypotension<br><br>Effects may not be noted for 4 weeks |
| Tamsulosin | Dizziness<br>Headache | Used to decrease urinary urgency, hesitancy, nocturia in prostatic hyperplasia<br><br>Caution to change position slowly<br><br>Administer 30 min after same meal each day |
| **5-Alpha-Reductase Inhibitor** | | |
| Finasteride | Decreased libido<br>Impotence | Used to treat benign prostatic hyperplasia by slowing prostatic growth<br><br>May decrease serum PSA levels<br><br>6–12 months therapy required to determine if medication effective<br><br>May cause harm to male fetus; pregnant women should not be exposed to semen of partner taking finasteride and should not handle crushed medication<br><br>Monitor liver function tests |
| Dutasteride | Decreased libido<br>Impotence | Used to treat benign prostatic hyperplasia by slowing prostatic growth<br><br>May cause harm to male fetus; pregnant women should not be exposed to semen of partner taking dutasteride and should not handle crushed medication<br><br>Monitor liver function tests |

*(Continued)*

**Table 9-6** Diuretic Medications (*Continued*)

| MEDICATION | ADVERSE EFFECTS | NURSING CONSIDERATIONS |
|---|---|---|
| **Anti-Impotence** | | |
| Sildenafil<br>Vardenafil<br>Tadalafil | Headache<br><br>Flushing<br><br>Dyspepsia<br><br>Nasal congestion<br><br>Mild visual disturbance | Enhances blood flow to the corpus cavernosum to ensure erection to allow sexual intercourse<br><br>Should not take with nitrates in any form due to dramatic decrease in blood pressure<br><br>Usually taken 1 hour before sexual activity (sildenafil, vardenafil)<br><br>Tadalafil has longer duration of action (up to 36 hours)<br><br>Should not take more than 1 time per day<br><br>Notify health care provider if erection lasts longer than 4 hours |
| Saw palmetto | Urinary antiseptic used for short-term treatment of benign prostatic hypertrophy; may cause false-negative PSA test result | |

# End-of-Chapter Thinking Exercise

A middle-aged client is admitted to the emergency department (ED) after developing nausea and abdominal pain at home. The client also reports a headache and "fluttering in my chest." The client was recently diagnosed with renal insufficiency, chronic urinary tract infections (UTI), and benign prostatic hyperplasia (BPH). The client is currently taking trimethoprim/sulfamethoxazole 40/200 mg PO daily for prophylactic maintenance. Other medications include spironolactone 25 mg PO twice daily. The nurse reviews the electronic medical record to view the client's vital signs. Further assessment reveals that the client has an irregular heart rate and bilateral 2+ pedal edema. Vital signs below.

| VITAL SIGN | RESULTS |
|---|---|
| BP | 158/90 mm Hg |
| HR | 106 beats/minute, irregular |
| RR | 18 breaths/minute |
| T | 98.2°F (36.8°C) |
| Pain | 3/10 (abdomen) |
| SpO$_2$ | 93% on room air |

1. Which assessment finding **most** concerns the nurse? (Analyze Cues)

   1. Blood pressure
   2. Irregular heart rate
   3. Pulse oximetry reading
   4. Abdominal pain

2. The nurse notifies the health care provider of the situation and current assessment findings. Which electrolyte level is priority to monitor at this time? (Prioritize Hypothesis)

3. What does the nurse instruct the client about the client's diet? (Take Action)

# Thinking Exercise Explanations

1. Which assessment finding **most** concerns the nurse? (Analyze Cues)

   1. Blood pressure
   2. Irregular heart rate
   3. Pulse oximetry reading
   4. Abdominal pain

   The nurse would be most concerned about the client's heart rate and irregular rhythm. These findings indicate the client is experiencing a cardiac dysrhythmia. The blood pressure is elevated but is likely due to fluid retention and is not dangerously elevated at this time. The pulse oximetry reading is within normal limits, and the client is not exhibiting signs or symptoms of respiratory distress. The report of abdominal pain suggests hyperkalemia and will be addressed. The nurse is most concerned about findings related to the client's circulatory status and potential electrolyte imbalances associated with renal insufficiency and spironolactone.

2. The nurse notifies the physician of the situation and current assessment findings. Which electrolyte level is priority to monitor at this time? (Prioritize Hypothesis)

   - Potassium

   The client's symptoms of abdominal pain and irregular heart rate suggest the client may have developed hyperkalemia. A client with decreased kidney function is at risk for hyperkalemia. This client is also at risk for hyperkalemia due to taking a potassium-sparing diuretic (spironolactone).

3. What does the nurse instruct the client about the client's diet? (Take Action)

   - Limit sources of potassium (e.g., bananas, oranges, raisins, potatoes, spinach)
   - Limit the use of salt substitutes that contain potassium

   The client must limit sources of potassium in the diet. It is also important to point out that some salt substitutes contain potassium, so use of these replacements should also be limited.

# THE MUSCULOSKELETAL SYSTEM

# ALTERATIONS IN MUSCULOSKELETAL FUNCTION

## Mobility, Skin Integrity, Comfort, Client Education: Providing

### Low Back Pain

A. Predisposition

1. Herniated intervertebral disk; most commonly affecting L4–L5 or L5–S1 interspaces (*see* Figure 10-1)

2. Fracture of the spine

3. Spine dislocation

4. Osteoarthritis

5. Scoliosis

6. Tension

7. Poor posture and/or body mechanics

8. Lack of muscle tone

9. Degenerative disk disease

10. Obesity

11. Spinal stenosis—narrowing of spinal canal; osteoarthritis most common cause; compression of nerve roots and disk herniation

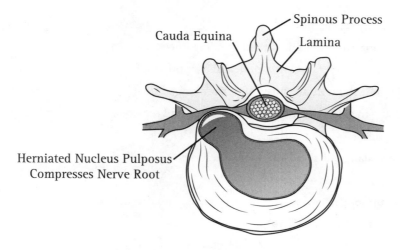

**Figure 10-1.** Herniated Intervertebral Disk

**B.** Diagnostic procedure

1. Myelography (not commonly done)

2. MRI, CT scan

3. Electromyogram (EMG)

4. Diskogram

**C.** Assessment

1. Pain—may be continuous

2. Depressed or absent Achilles tendon reflex; positive straight-leg raise test; numbness and paresthesias of leg

3. Guarded movement

4. Decreased ROM of spine

5. Diagnostic studies—x-ray, CT, myelogram, diskogram

**D.** Nursing management

1. To relieve pain and muscular spasm

   a. Administer appropriate medications (analgesics, NSAIDs, muscle relaxants, e.g., cyclobenzaprine)

   b. Apply moist heat/cool 20–30 minutes 4 times a day

   c. Bedrest; client in Fowler position with moderate hip and knee flexion

   d. Use firm mattress, bed board, or floor for back support

2. To regain normal elasticity of affected muscle

   a. Isometric exercises for abdominal muscles

   b. Daily exercise program

3. To return joint to normal function

   a. Assist with exercises for abdominal muscles

   b. ROM exercises

4. Good body mechanics

   a. Do not lean forward without bending knees

   b. Exercise under direction of health care provider

   c. Do not stand in one position for prolonged time

   d. Sleep in side-lying position with knees and hips bent

**E.** Client teaching

1. Exercise daily but avoid strenuous exercises

2. Correct posture at all times

3. Avoid prolonged sitting, standing, walking, and driving

4. Rest at intervals

5. Use hardboard for bed or firm mattress

6. Avoid prone position

7. Avoid straining or lifting heavy objects

**F.** Management specific to herniated lumbar disk

1. Conservative therapy—combination of medication, heat/ice therapy, ultrasound, transcutaneous electrical nerve stimulation (TENS)

2. Surgical therapy

   a. Percutaneous laser diskectomy; herniated portion of disk is lasered

   b. Diskectomy—partial removal of lamina

   c. Laminectomy—excision of a portion of the lamina to expose the affected disk for removal

   d. Laminectomy with fusion—involves several disk herniations; operation includes use of bone graft to strengthen the weakened vertebral column

   e. Postlaminectomy care

      1) Maintain body alignment

      2) Log roll every 2 h

      3) Calf exercises

      4) Assess for sensations and circulatory status, especially of lower extremities

      5) Monitor elimination

      6) Assist with ambulation

   f. Interbody cage fusion with bone graft

# Selected Musculoskeletal Trauma/Injuries and Disorders

**A.** Assessment

1. Contusions—injuries to soft tissue

   a. Ecchymosis

   b. Hematoma

2. Strains/sprains—pulled muscle/torn ligament

   a. Pain

   b. Swelling

3. Joint dislocations—displacement of joint bones; articulating surfaces lose all contact

   a. Pain

   b. Deformity

4. Fractures—break in continuity of bone (*see* Figure 10-2)

   a. Swelling

   b. Pallor, ecchymosis

   c. Loss of sensation to body parts

   d. Deformity

   e. Pain and/or acute tenderness

   f. Muscle spasms

   g. Loss of function

h.   Abnormal mobility

i.   Crepitus (grating sound on movement of ends of broken bone)

j.   Shortening of affected limb

k.   Decreased or absent pulses distal to injury

l.   Affected extremity colder than contralateral part

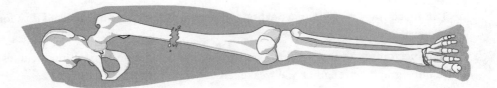

A.   Complete: break across entire cross-section of bone

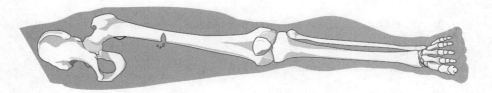

B.   Incomplete: break through portion of bone

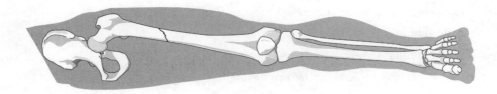

C.   Closed: no external communication

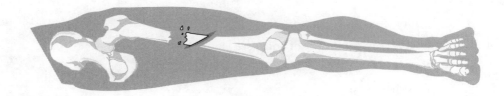

D.   Open: extends through skin

**Figure 10-2.** Types of Fractures

**B.** Types

1.  Avulsion—tearing away of a fragment of bone by a ligament or tendon pulling the fragment away

2.  Comminuted—a fracture in which the bone is crushed or broken into a number of pieces

3.  Greenstick—an incomplete fracture in which the bone is bent but fractured only on the outer arc of the bend

4.  Longitudinal—a fracture along the long axis of the bone

5.  Oblique—a slanted fracture of the shaft on the long axis of a bone

6.  Impacted—a bone break in which the adjacent fragmented ends of the fractured bone are wedged together

7.  Interarticular—a fracture within a movable joint

8.  Pathologic—a fracture resulting from a weakness in the bone tissue

9.  Spiral—a bone break in which the disruption of bone tissue is spiral, oblique, or transverse to the long axis of the bone

10. Stress—a fracture in the bones of the leg, ankle, or foot caused by repeated, prolonged, or abnormal weight-bearing stress (jogging, running, etc.)

11. Displaced—a traumatic bone break in which two ends of a fractured bone are separated (can cause an open or compound fracture)

**C.** Complications of fractures

1.  Types

    a.  Fat emboli—caused after fracture of long bones when fat globules move into bloodstream; may occlude major vessels; symptoms include shortness of breath, chest pain, anxiety, decreased oxygen saturation, chest petechiae

    b.  Hemorrhage

    c.  Delayed union—healing of fracture is slowed; caused by infection or distraction of fractured fragments; will see increase in bone pain

    d.  Nonunion—healing has not occurred 4–6 months after fracture; insufficient blood supply, repetitive stress on fracture site, infection, inadequate internal fixation; treated by bone grafting, internal fixation, electric bone stimulation

    e.  Sepsis

    f.  Compartment syndrome—high pressure within a muscle compartment of an extremity compromises circulation; pressure may be internal (bleeding) or external (casts); if left untreated, neuromuscular damage occurs within 4–6 hours; limb can become useless within 24–48 hours; will see unrelenting pain out of proportion to injury and unrelieved by pain medication, decreased pulse strength and pale cool extremity

    g.  Peripheral nerve damage

**D.** Nursing management

1. Contusions—treated with cold application for 24 h, followed by moist heat; apply elastic bandage

2. Strains/sprains—treated with rest and elevation of affected part; intermittent ice compresses for 24 h, followed by heat application; apply elastic pressure bandage; minimize use

3. Dislocations—considered an orthopedic emergency; treated with immobilization and reduction (e.g., the dislocated bone is brought back to its normal position, usually under anesthesia); bandages and splints are used to keep affected part immobile until healing occurs

4. Fractures

   a. Provide emergency care

     1) Immobilization before client is moved by use of splints; immobilize joint below and above fracture

     2) In an open fracture, cover the wound with sterile dressings or cleanest material available

     3) Emergency department—give narcotic adequate to relieve pain, except in presence of head injury

   b. Treatment

     1) Splinting/immobilization of the affected part to prevent soft tissue from being damaged by bony fragments

     2) Internal fixation—use of metal screws, plates, nails, and pins to stabilize reduced fractures

     3) Open reduction/surgical dissection and exposure of the fracture for reduction and alignment

5. Traction (*see* Figures 10-3 through 10-7)

   a. Purposes

     1) Immobilize fracture

     2) Alleviate pain and muscle spasm

     3) Prevent or correct deformities

     4) Promote healing

   b. Types of traction

     1) Skin (Buck extension, balanced suspension, Russell, pelvic traction)—noninvasive (does not penetrate the skin)

     2) Skeletal (halo fixation device, Crutchfield tongs)—invasive (penetrates the skin)

   c. Nursing management

     1) Maintain straight alignment of ropes and pulleys

     2) Assure that weights hang freely

     3) Frequently inspect skin for breakdown

4) Maintain position for countertraction

5) Encourage movement of unaffected areas

6) Investigate every report immediately and thoroughly

7) Maintain continuous pull

8) Clean pins with normal saline and sterile swabs 1–2 times/d

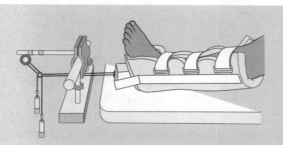

**Figure 10-3.** Buck Traction

Relieves muscular spasm of legs and back; if no fracture, may turn to either side; with fracture, turn to unaffected side. 8–20 lb used; 40 lb for scoliosis. Elevate foot of bed for countertraction. Use trapeze for moving. Place pillow beneath lower legs, not heel. Don't elevate knee gatch.

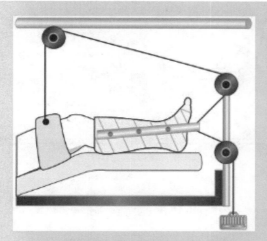

**Figure 10-4.** Russell Traction

"Pulls" contracted muscles; elevate foot of bed with shock blocks to provide countertraction; sling can be loosened for skin care; check popliteal pulse. Place pillows under lower leg. Make sure heel is off the bed. Must not turn from waist down. Lift client, not leg, to provide assistance.

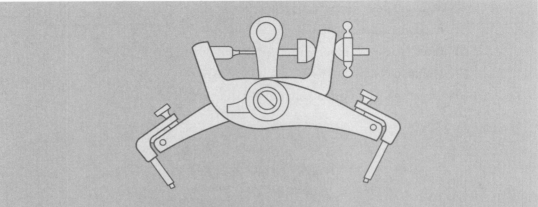

**Figure 10-5.** Cervical (Skull Tongs)

Realigns fracture of cervical vertebrae and relieves pressure on cervical nerve; never lift weights—traction must be continuous. No pillow under the head during feeding; hard to swallow, may need suctioning.

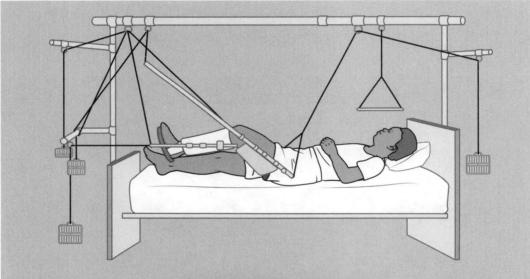

**Figure 10-6.** Balanced Suspension

Realigns fractures of the femur; uses pulley to create balanced suspension by countertraction to the top of the thigh splint. Thomas splint (positioned under anterior thigh) with Pearson attachment (supports leg from knee down) frequently used.

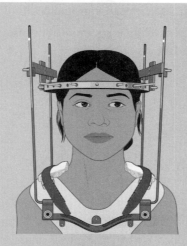

**Figure 10-7.** Halo Fixation Device (Vest)

Provides immobilization of cervical spine; pins inserted into skull are used to maintain traction; care of insertion site includes cleansing area around pins using sterile technique. If prescribed by health care provider, clean with sterile saline and sterile swabs 1–2 times/d.

6. Casting—provides rigid immobilization of affected body part for support and stability; may be plaster or fiberglass

   a. Immediate care

      1) Avoid covering cast until dry (48 h or longer); handle with palms, not fingertips (plaster cast)

      2) Avoid resting cast on hard surfaces or sharp edges

      3) Keep affected limb elevated above heart on soft surface until dry; no heat lamp

      4) Watch for danger signs (e.g., blueness or paleness, pain, numbness or tingling sensations on affected area); if present, elevate casted area; if it persists, contact health care provider

      5) Elevate arm cast above level of heart

   b. Intermediate care

      1) When cast is dry, client should be mobilized

      2) Encourage prescribed exercises (isometrics)

      3) Report to health care provider any break in cast or foul odor from cast

      4) Tell client not to scratch skin underneath cast; skin may break, and infection can set in

      5) If fiberglass cast gets wet, dry with hair dryer on cool setting

   c. After-cast care

      1) Wash skin gently

      2) Apply baby powder, cornstarch, or baby oil

      3) Have client gradually adjust to movement without support of cast

      4) Inform client that swelling is common after cast is removed; elevate limb and apply elastic bandage

# Fractured Hip

**A.** Assessment

  1. Leg shortened, adducted, externally rotated

  2. Pain

  3. Hematoma, ecchymosis

  4. Confirmed by x-rays

**B.** Gerontologic considerations—increased risk of vision and hearing deficits, orthostatic hypotension, medications; decreased fat and muscle mass; gait and balance problems

**C.** Diagnosis

  1. Commonly seen with older adult women with osteoporosis, postural hypotension, gait and balance problems, vision and hearing problems, medications, decreased fat and muscle mass

  2. Potential nursing diagnoses

    a. Impaired physical mobility

    b. Risk for peripheral neurovascular dysfunction

    c. Risk for impaired gas exchange

    d. Acute pain

**D.** Plan/implementation

  1. Total hip replacement—acetabulum, cartilage, and head of femur replaced with artificial joint (*see* Figure 10-8)

  2. Abduction of affected extremity (use splints, wedge pillow, or 2 or 3 pillows between legs)

  3. Turn client as ordered; keep heels off bed

  4. Ice to operative site

  5. Overbed trapeze to lift self onto fracture bedpan

  6. Prevention of thromboembolism—low-molecular-weight heparin (LMWH) and warfarin; do not sit for prolonged periods

  7. Initial ambulation with walker

  8. Crutch walking—three-point gait

  9. Chair with arms, wheelchair, semireclining toilet seat

  10. Medications—anticoagulants to prevent pulmonary embolism, antibiotics to prevent infection

  11. Don't sleep on operated side

  12. Don't flex hip more than 90°

  13. Use adaptive devices for dressing—extended handles, shoehorns

14. Report increased hip pain to health care provider immediately

15. Cleanse incision daily with mild soap and water; dry thoroughly

16. Inspect hip daily for redness, heat, drainage; if present, call health care provider immediately

17. Complications

    a. Dislocation of prosthesis

    b. Excessive wound drainage

    c. Thromboembolism

    d. Infection

18. Postoperative discharge teaching

    a. Maintain abduction

    b. Avoid stooping

    c. Do not sleep on operated side until directed to do so

    d. Flex hip only to 90°

    e. Never cross legs

    f. Avoid position of flexion during sexual activity

    g. Walking is excellent exercise; avoid overexertion

    h. In 3 mo, will be able to resume ADLs, except strenuous sports

19. Prevention

    a. Vitamin D and calcium supplementation

    b. Estrogen replacement therapy

    c. Bisphosphonates

    d. Aerobic and weight-bearing exercise

    e. Safety issues

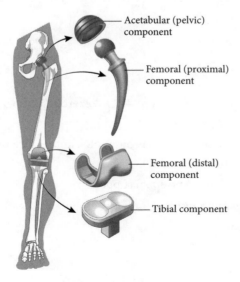

Acetabular (pelvic) component

Femoral (proximal) component

Femoral (distal) component

Tibial component

**Figure 10-8.** Total Hip and Knee Replacement

## Amputation

A.  Causes

   1.  Trauma

   2.  Peripheral vascular disease

   3.  Osteogenic sarcoma

   4.  Gerontologic considerations—decreased peripheral circulation, diabetic neuropathy, decreased immune response

B.  Types

   1.  Disarticulation—resection of an extremity through a joint

   2.  Above-the-knee amputation

   3.  Below-the-knee amputation

   4.  Guillotine or open surface

      a.  Amputation in which a straight, guillotine cut is made without skin flaps

      b.  Open amputation performed if infection is probable, developing, or recurrent (to allow drainage until the infection clears)

   5.  Closed or flap

      a.  Amputation in which one or two broad flaps of muscular and cutaneous tissue is/are retained to form a cover over the end of the bone

      b.  Performed when no infection is present

C.  Postoperative management (*see* Table 10-1)

   1.  Delayed prosthesis fitting—residual limb covered with figure-eight wrapping dressing and elastic bandage or residual limb socks; note if Penrose drain is inserted; reapply bandages every 4–6 hours

   2.  Immediate prosthesis fitting—residual limb covered with dressing and rigid plastic dressing; Penrose drains usually not inserted; rigid dressing helps prevent bleeding by compressing residual limb

D.  Nursing management

   1.  Prevent bleeding

   2.  Promote circulation

   3.  Prevent complications of immobility—ROM exercises, trapeze with overhead frame, prone position every 3–4 hours

   4.  Provide comfort and relieve pain—propranolol, antiseizure medications, and antispasmodics used for phantom limb pain

   5.  Provide psychological and emotional support

   6.  Client teaching regarding residual limb care

**Table 10-1** Postoperative Care of Amputation

| TYPE OF CARE | DELAYED PROSTHETIC FITTING | IMMEDIATE PROSTHETIC FITTING |
|---|---|---|
| Residual limb care | Observe dressings for signs of excessive bleeding; keep large tourniquet on hand to apply around residual limb in event of hemorrhage | Observe rigid dressing for signs of oozing; if blood stain appears, mark area and observe every 10 min for increase; report excessive oozing immediately to health care provider; provide cast care; guard against cast slipping off |
| Positioning | Elevate foot of the bed for the first few hours to hasten venous return and prevent edema; do not elevate on pillows—hip contracture may result | Lay residual limb flat on the bed; rigid cast acts to control swelling |
| Turning | Turn client to prone position for short time first postop day, then 30 min 2–3 times daily to prevent hip contracture; have client roll from side to side | Same; however, rigid cast acts to prevent both hip and joint contractures |
| Exercises | Have client start exercises to prevent contractures as soon as possible (1st or 2nd day postop), including active range of motion, especially of affected leg; strengthening exercises for upper extremities; hyperextension of residual limb | Exercises not as essential because rigid dressing prevents contractures; also early ambulation prevents all immobilization disabilities |
| Ambulation | Dangle and transfer client to wheelchair and back within 1st or 2nd day postop; crutch walking started as soon as client feels sufficiently strong | Dangle and ambulate client with walker for short period 1st day; increase length of ambulation each day; in physical therapy, client uses parallel bars, then crutches, then cane |
| Psychological support | Observe for signs of depression, despondency; remind depressed client that the prosthesis will be fitted when the wound heals | Observe for signs of depression; client is usually less depressed if awakens with prosthesis attached |
| Discharge | Teach residual limb care—inspect daily for abrasions, wash, expose to air, do not apply lotions, use only cotton or wool socks | Same |
| Comfort | Administer medication for pain; phantom limb pain possible; reality that limb is missing; client indicating that client wants the limb disposed of will help | Same |

## Diseases of the Musculoskeletal System

**A.** Rheumatoid arthritis (RA)

1. Description—systemic crippling condition characterized by inflammation of synovial membrane of the joints with periods of remission and exacerbation

2. History

   a. Autoimmunity

   b. Environmental factors

   c. Viral or streptococcal infection

   d. Genetic

3. Assessment

   a. Joint pain and swelling

   b. Limited joint movement

   c. Contractures; deformities

   d. Weakness, fatigue

   e. High fever and rheumatoid rash, particularly seen in juvenile RA (JRA)

   f. Nodules over bony prominences

   g. Ulnar deviation

   h. Periods of remissions and exacerbations

4. Diagnostic tests

   a. Blood studies

      1) Antistreptolysin O (ASO) titer

      2) Latex fixation—rheumatoid factor

      3) C-reactive protein

      4) Sedimentation rate

      5) ESR, antinuclear antibody (ANA)

   b. Aspiration of synovial fluid

   c. X-rays

5. Nursing management

   a. Relieve pain and discomfort

      1) Application of heat (e.g., warm tub baths; warm, moist compresses; paraffin dips)

      2) If inflammatory process is acute, application of cold packs or ice bags is sometimes effective

      3) Support joints with splints; cervical collar in late stages

      4) Administer analgesics and anti-inflammatory medications

      5) Administer disease-modifying antirheumatic medications (e.g., gold, hydroxychloroquine)

6) Administer immunosuppressive medications (e.g., methotrexate, azathioprine)

7) Administer antitumor necrosis medications (e.g., etanercept)

b. Promote rest and mobility

1) Proper positioning—avoid position flexion

2) Use firm mattress or bed board

3) ROM exercises as tolerated

4) Encourage independence and acceptance of limitations

c. Reduce inflammation—administer anti-inflammatory medications

d. Provide adequate dietary intake, appropriate diet for obesity

e. Provide operative care for clients undergoing musculoskeletal surgery (e.g., arthroplasty—total hip replacement)

f. Preoperative teaching

1) Teach partial weight-bearing use of crutches, isometric exercises, and transfer techniques

2) Familiarize client with overbed traction frame, trapeze, and abduction splint

g. Postoperative care

1) Position client flat in bed with affected extremity in abduction

2) Apply ice to operative area to reduce edema

3) Assess circulation of affected extremity

4) Administer medications to prevent postoperative complications

a) Pulmonary embolism—anticoagulants

b) Infection—antibiotics

5) Encourage active foot and ankle motion the day following surgery to prevent circulatory stasis

6) Help client ambulate gradually with walker, then crutches, using three-point gait

h. Postoperative discharge teaching

1) Maintain abduction

2) Avoid stooping

3) Do not sleep on operated side until directed to do so

4) Flex hip only to quarter circle

5) Never cross legs

6) Avoid position of flexion during sexual activity

7) Walking is excellent exercise; avoid overexertion

8) In 3 mo, will be able to resume ADLs, except strenuous sports

    **B.** Juvenile rheumatoid arthritis—(JRA)

       1. Pathophysiology—much the same as adult RA

       2. Characteristic clinical manifestations—same as RA, in addition:

          a. Intermittent fever and chills

          b. Rheumatoid rash (salmon pink, macular rash on chest, thighs, and upper arms)

          c. Iridocyclitis (inflammation of the iris and ciliary body)

          d. Growth restriction

       3. Diagnosis—latex fixation test for RA in adult is seldom positive for JRA

       4. Problems—same as RA plus impaired social and personality development

       5. Treatment and nursing management—same as RA; assist child in adjusting to chronic illness, and encourage regular ophthalmologic examination for iridocyclitis

    **C.** Ankylosing spondylitis (Marie-Strümpell disease)

       1. Description—chronic progressive disorder that primarily affects the spine

       2. Pathophysiology—synovitis, fibrosis, ankylosis of the vertebral joints

       3. Clinical manifestations

          a. Pain and stiffness

          b. Kyphosis

          c. Iritis

          d. Decreased respiratory function

       4. Diagnostic tests—x-rays (bony growths called syndesmophytes) that bridge the adjacent vertebrae are visible)

       5. Problems

          a. Alteration in comfort (pain)

          b. Decreased mobility

          c. Potential for respiratory difficulty

          d. Potential for poor body image and low self-esteem

       6. Treatment and nursing management

          a. Analgesics; promote comfort

          b. Anti-inflammatory medications, salicylates

          c. Administer disease-modifying antirheumatic medications (e.g., methotrexate)

          d. Administer antitumor necrosis medications (e.g., infliximab)

          e. Physical therapy, heat application

          f. Promote body alignment, especially of the spine

             1) Postural exercises

             2) Splinting; bracing

    g. Improve mobility

      1) ROM exercises

      2) Assist with ADLs

    h. Prevent respiratory complications

**D.** Degenerative joint disease (osteoarthritis)

  1. Description—nonsystemic, progressive degenerative condition that affects the joints; no remissions

  2. Pathophysiology—articular cartilage degenerates, new bone forms (spur), joint spaces close

  3. History

    a. Poor posture

    b. Trauma

    c. Stress on joints

    d. Obesity

    e. Smoking

  4. Assessment

    a. Muscular spasm, pain, limitation of motion, stiffness; impaired ADL performance

    b. Contractures, deformities

    c. Heberden nodes on fingers and Bouchard nodes of hand

    d. Obesity/debilitation

  5. Diagnostic test—x-rays and MRI of joints show narrowing of joint spaces, ESR, high-sensitivity C-reactive protein

  6. Risk factors

    a. Increased age—bone and joint changes

    b. Obesity and sedentary lifestyle

    c. Trauma to joints due to repetitive use

      1) Carpet installer

      2) Construction worker

      3) Farmer

      4) Sports injuries

  7. Nursing management

    a. Reduce pain and discomfort

      1) Balance rest with activity

      2) Administer analgesics and anti-inflammatory drugs (e.g., NSAIDs or acetaminophen), topical medication (e.g., lidocaine)

      3) Gerontologic considerations—increased risk of adverse effects with NSAIDs

      b.  Heat application or cold application

      c.  Maintain mobility

         1)  ROM

         2)  Encourage usual ADLs that involve using all joints

      d.  Provide adequate nutrition; obese clients should be put on appropriate diet

      e.  Complementary and alternative therapies—acupuncture, topical capsaicin, glucosamine, chondroitin

**E.**  Gout

    1.  Description—nonsystemic inflammation of the joints characterized by remissions and exacerbations

    2.  Pathophysiology—disturbed purine metabolism leads to elevated uric acid in the blood, causing tophi (deposits in the joints)

    3.  Predisposition—genetic defect of purine metabolism

      a.  Swollen, reddened, painful joints, often in the great toe

      b.  Limitation of motion

      c.  Deformity—tophi

    4.  Diagnostic tests

      a.  X-rays

      b.  Blood tests—WBC, sedimentation rate, uric acid level

      c.  Synovial aspiration

    5.  Nursing management

      a.  Relieve pain and discomfort

         1)  Rest affected joint

         2)  Administer analgesics

    6.  Reduce urate level in the blood

         1)  Eliminate purine food from diet, e.g., liver, sardines

         2)  Administer medication (colchicine, probenecid) (*see* Table 10-2)

**F.**  Bursitis

    1.  Description—inflammation of connective tissue sac between muscles, tendons, and bones, particularly affecting shoulder, elbow, and knee

    2.  History

      a.  Stress on joints

      b.  Toxins

      c.  Infections

    3.  Assessment

      a.  Pain

      b.  Decreased mobility, especially on abduction

**Table 10-2** Antigout Medications

| MEDICATION | ADVERSE EFFECTS | NURSING CONSIDERATIONS |
|---|---|---|
| Colchicine | GI upset<br>Agranulocytosis<br>Peripheral neuritis | Anti-inflammatory<br>Give with meals<br>Check CBC, I and O |
| Probenecid | Nausea, constipation<br>Skin rash | Reduces uric acid<br>Check BUN, renal function tests<br>Encourage fluids<br>Give with milk, food, antacids<br>Alkaline urine helps prevent renal uric acid stones |
| Sulfinpyrazone | Renal colic, peptic ulcer<br>Blood dyscrasias | Reduces uric acid in the blood<br>Check BUN, CBC, renal function tests<br>Encourage fluids<br>Give with food, milk, antacids |
| Allopurinol | GI upset<br>Headache, dizziness, drowsiness | Blocks formation of uric acid<br>Encourage fluids<br>Check I and O<br>Check CBC and renal function tests<br>Give with meals<br>Alkaline urine helps prevent renal uric acid stones |

4. Interventions
   a. Rest
   b. Immobilize affected joint by use of pillows, splints, slings
   c. Administer pain medication, muscle relaxants (diazepam), steroids, NSAIDs
   d. Apply heat/cold packs to decrease swelling
   e. Promote exercise (ROM)
   f. Assist in performance of ADLs by modifying activities relative to limitations
   g. Assist with cortisone injection, draining of bursas

**G.** Paget disease
   1. Description—disease of unknown cause characterized by enlargement of bones, bone deformities, and increasing vascularity of bones; typical client is male and older than 50 years
   2. Pathophysiology—bone resorption, disordered bone formation, vascularity of bone tissue

3. Assessment

   a. Pain and tenderness; long bone, spine, and rib pain

   b. Enlarged skull

   c. Kyphosis

   d. Bowed legs

   e. Waddling gait

   f. Decrease in height

   g. Pathologic fractures

4. Nursing management

   a. Administer analgesics

   b. Encourage rest

   c. Prevent pathological fractures by using safety precautions

   d. Administer specific medications to prevent bone destruction

**H.** Osteoporosis

1. Description—degenerative disease characterized by generalized loss of bone density and tensile strength

2. Pathophysiology—reduction in the amount of bone mass without change in mineral composition

3. History

   a. Age greater than 60

   b. Small framed and lean body build

   c. Caucasian or Asian race

   d. Decreased estrogen (menopause)

   e. Low calcium intake

   f. Vitamin D deficiency

   g. Malabsorptive disease of the GI tract

   h. Immobility

   i. Hyperthyroidism

   j. Hyperparathyroidism

   k. Prolonged use of steroids

   l. Older women—decreased bone mass, increased bone resorption after menopause, less calcium intake over lifetime

4. Assessment

   a. Lower back pain

   b. Kyphosis

   c. Decrease in height

5. Diagnostic tests—x-rays

6. Nursing management

   a. Provide optimal nutrition diet—high in calcium, protein, and vitamin D

   b. Teach about medications (*see* Table 10-3)

   c. Promote mobility and strength

      1) Encourage weight-bearing on the long bones

      2) ROM exercises

      3) Physiotherapy

   d. Prevent pathological fractures—safety precautions

   e. Promote comfort and relieve pain

      1) Bedrest

      2) Use of back brace or splint for support

      3) Use of bed boards or hard mattress

   f. Prevent bone resorption—administer calcitonin, a thyroid hormone that slows bone loss

**Table 10-3** Calcium and Vitamin D Medications

| | ADVERSE EFFECTS | NURSING CONSIDERATIONS |
|---|---|---|
| **Oral Calcium Medications** | | |
| Calcium carbonate<br>Calcium citrate | Chalky taste<br><br>Mild constipation<br><br>Alkalosis<br><br>Milk-alkali syndrome (with calcium carbonate) | Contraindicated in clients with a history of calcium renal calculi, hypercalcemia, or hypercalciuria<br><br>Assess BP and ECG; serum magnesium, potassium, and phosphorus; BUN; and serum creatinine as therapy begins<br><br>Monitor BP, ECG, electrolytes, and renal function<br><br>Monitor for signs and symptoms of hypercalcemia<br><br>Chewable tablets should be chewed well and taken with a full glass of water 30 minutes to 1 hour after meals |

(*Continued*)

**Table 10-3** Calcium and Vitamin D Medications (*Continued*)

| | ADVERSE EFFECTS | NURSING CONSIDERATIONS |
|---|---|---|
| **Other Medications** | | |
| Alendronate<br><br>Risedronate<br><br>Calcitonin salmon | Used in the prevention and treatment of osteoporosis and Paget disease | Prevents and treats osteoporosis<br><br>Longer-lasting treatment for Paget disease<br><br>Take in A.M. at least 30 min before other medication, food, water, or other liquids<br><br>Should sit up for 30 min after taking medication<br><br>Use sunscreen and wear protective clothing |

I. Osteomyelitis

  1. Description—infection of the bone, usually caused by *Staphylococcus aureus*, carried by the blood from a primary site of infection

  2. Pathophysiology—inflammation; abscess formation; necrosis of the bone

  3. History

    a. Chronic skin problems, e.g., pressure injury, gangrene

    b. Compound fractures

    c. Malnutrition

    d. Immunosuppression

  4. Assessment

    a. Pain

    b. Swelling, redness, warmth on affected area (localized infection)

    c. Fever (systemic infection)

  5. Diagnostic tests

    a. Leukocytosis

    b. Elevated sedimentation rate

    c. Culture and sensitivity

    d. X-ray of affected part

  6. Nursing management

    a. Promote comfort, relieve pain

      1) Bedrest

      2) Administer analgesics

3) Support affected extremity with pillows, splints to maintain proper body alignment

4) Provide cool environment and lightweight clothing

b. Reduce inflammatory process

1) Administer antibiotics and antipyretics

2) Avoid exercise and heat application to the affected area

3) Encourage fluid intake

4) Monitor I and O

c. Promote skin integrity

1) Asepsis

2) General skin care

3) Aseptic wound care

d. Provide emotional support

1) Allow for expression of fear and anxiety

2) Provide diversionary activities

e. Improve nutritional status

1) High-protein diet with sufficient carbohydrates, vitamins, and minerals

2) Small, frequent feedings

**J.** Osteomalacia

1. Description—decalcification of bones due to inadequate intake of vitamin D, absence of exposure to sunlight, intestinal malabsorption, chronic renal disease

2. Pathophysiology—calcium deficit leads to porosity and softening of the bones

3. Assessment

a. Bone pain and tenderness

b. Muscle weakness

c. Bowed legs

d. Kyphosis

4. Diagnostic tests—x-rays (porous bones)

5. Nursing interventions

a. Relief of pain

1) Administration of analgesics

2) Administration of herbal supplements (*see* Table 10-4)

3) Bedrest as needed

4) Maintain good body alignment

b. Promote mineralization of bone—administer vitamin D, calcium, and exposure to sunlight and/or ultraviolet irradiation

**Table 10-4** Herbal Supplements for Musculoskeletal System

| MEDICATION | ADVERSE EFFECTS | NURSING CONSIDERATIONS |
|---|---|---|
| Glucosamine | Nausea, heartburn, diarrhea | Antirheumatic<br><br>Contraindicated if shellfish allergy, client is pregnant or lactating<br><br>May worsen glycemic control<br><br>Must be taken on regular basis to be effective |
| Chondroitin | Headache<br><br>Restlessness<br><br>Nausea<br><br>Vomiting<br><br>Anorexia | Given alone or with glucosamine<br><br>Interactions with anticoagulants, NSAIDs, salicylates |

c. Promote safety

    1) Assist with performance of ADLs to prevent pathological fractures

    2) Regular medical follow-up

d. Instruct about high vitamin D foods (milk, eggs, vitamin D enriched cereals and bread products)

# End-of-Chapter Thinking Exercise

The emergency department (ED) nurse receives a report from emergency medical services (EMS). The client is an older adult female who slipped on a patch of ice this morning. The client lives alone; the fall was witnessed by a neighbor who called emergency medical services. While awaiting the client's arrival, the nurse reviews the client's electronic health record (EHR) from a recent admission with COVID-19. The client's past medical history (PMH) includes osteoporosis, paroxysmal vertigo, and diabetes mellitus. Home medications include calcium 600 mg PO BID, metformin 500 mg PO BID, aspirin 81 mg PO daily, and hydrochlorothiazide 12.5 mg PO daily. Prior to the admission with COVID-19, the client had no respiratory conditions but was discharged with an albuterol inhaler and a PO prednisone taper pack. The client arrives at the ED at 0930, and the nurse conducts the following assessment.

The client appears pale and is alert and oriented to person, place, and time but is slightly hard of hearing. The client states the fall occurred when going out to feed the cats. Skin cool, dry, and intact; lungs clear; and abdomen soft with hypoactive bowel sounds. Right lower leg externally rotated and shortened. Pedal pulses are palpable. The client reports pain 4/10 in right hip and leg—no visible right hip deformity. The client has an 18 gauge peripheral venous catheter infusing 0.9% NaCl at 75 mL/hr. BP 112/62, HR 78, RR 14, T 98.1°F (36.7°C).

1.   What risk factors does this client have for a fall causing a fracture? (Recognize Cues)

2.   Which assessment findings suggest the possibility of a right hip fracture? (Analyze Cues)

3.   Which interventions does the nurse implement? (Take Action)

# Thinking Exercise Explanations

1.  What risk factors does this client have for a fall causing a fracture? (Recognize Cues)

    - Age
    - Sex
    - Osteoporosis
    - Diuretic use
    - Paroxysmal vertigo
    - Sensory changes

    Older adults, especially females, are at a higher risk for a fall resulting in a fracture due to osteoporosis. Specifically in this client's case, the sensory change of hearing, the history of vertigo, and the use of a diuretic—which may cause orthostatic hypotension—are all potentially contributing factors.

2.  Which assessment findings suggest the possibility of a right hip fracture? (Analyze Cues)

    - Fall
    - Osteoporosis
    - Right lower leg externally rotated and shortened
    - Pain 4/10 in right hip and leg

    A known fall earlier in the day and a leg being externally rotated and shortened in an older adult client with osteoporosis suggest the possibility of a right hip fracture. Additional data, not present in this case, include the presence of a visible hematoma and/or ecchymosis over the hip/femur.

3.  Which interventions does the nurse implement? (Take Action)

    - Request an order for analgesics
    - Request an order for an x-ray of right hip and femur
    - Place an abduction wedge or pillow between the knees
    - Instruct the client on how to use the call light
    - Instruct the client not to attempt to get out of bed unassisted
    - Keep the client NPO until treatment plan is known

    The nurse should take actions to keep the client safe, which include instructing the client on how to use the call light, not to get out of bed without assistance, and placing an abduction wedge or pillow between the knees to prevent additional injury. In anticipation of surgery to repair the hip, the nurse should keep the client NPO until a diagnosis is made. Finally, the nurse should obtain an order for and administer IV pain medication.

[ CHAPTER 11 ]

# SENSORY AND NEUROLOGICAL FUNCTION

# SENSATION AND PERCEPTION FUNCTIONS

## Sensory Perception

## Anatomy And Physiology

A. Neuron (*see* Figure 11-1)

   1. Basic component of the nervous system

   2. Composed of cell body, axon, and dendrites

      a. Cell body is the center of metabolism

      b. Axons are long fibers that conduct impulses away from the cell body; there is usually one axon for each cell body

      c. Dendrites are short, unsheathed fibers that receive nerve impulses from other axons and transmit impulses to cell body

   3. Myelin sheath—covering that protects nerve fiber and facilitates the speed of impulse conduction

      a. Both axons and dendrites may or may not have myelin sheath

      b. Most axons leaving the central nervous system are heavily myelinated with Schwann cells

      c. Gaps in myelin sheath are termed nodes of Ranvier

      d. Gerontologic considerations—myelin sheath degeneration; decreased nerve conduction

   4. Primary function is transmission of nerve impulses

      a. Afferent (sensory) neurons: transmit impulses from peripheral receptors to the central nervous system

      b. Efferent (motor) neurons: transmit impulses from the central nervous system to muscles and organs

      c. Action potentials travel along axon; at end of nerve fiber, impulse is transmitted across junction between nerve cells (synapse) by chemical interaction

      d. Gerontologic considerations—less coordination of nerve impulse transmission; decreased ability to maintain blood pressure and body temperature; decreased sense of pain, touch, and temperature

   5. Neuroglia—glial cells

      a. Provide support, nourishment, and protection for neurons

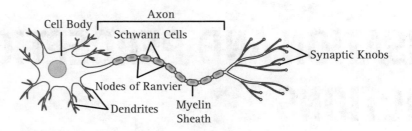

**Figure 11-1.** Anatomy and Physiology of the Neuron

**B.** Peripheral nervous system (PNS)—contains cranial nerves, spinal nerves, autonomic nervous system (unconscious reflexes), autonomic nervous system (ANS) sympathetic division (accelerates activity), and parasympathetic division (slows body processes)

**C.** Central nervous system (CNS)—contains brain and spinal cord (*see* Figure 11-2)

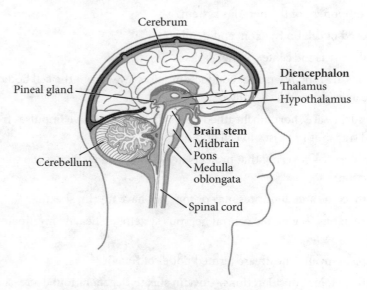

**Figure 11-2.** Central Nervous System (CNS)

1. Cerebrum—divided into left and right hemispheres by a longitudinal fissure; each cerebral hemisphere contains frontal, parietal, occipital, and temporal lobes; loss of neurons with aging; increased risk of Alzheimer's disease (*see* Figure 11-3)

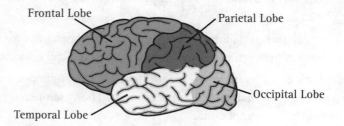

**Figure 11-3.** Divisions of the Brain

   a. Frontal lobes

      1) Precentral gyrus—motor function, contralateral movement: face, arm, leg, trunk

      2) Broca area—in the dominant hemisphere; responsible for the formation of words or speech

      3) Supplementary motor area—contralateral head and eye turning

      4) Prefrontal areas—personality, initiative

      5) Paracentral lobule—cortical inhibition of bladder and bowel

   b. Parietal lobes

      1) Important in concept of body image and awareness of external environment (ability to construct shapes)

      2) Postcentral gyrus—registers bodily sensations (temperature, touch, pressure, pain) from opposite side of body

   c. Occipital lobes—visual center; comprehension of written word

   d. Temporal lobes

      1) Dominant hearing of language; taste; smell

      2) Memory

      3) Wernicke speech area—recognition of language

2. Basal ganglia—regulate and integrate skeletal voluntary and autonomic motor activity originating in cerebral cortex

3. Diencephalon—connects the cerebrum and brain stem; contains several small structures, the most important of which are the thalamus and hypothalamus

   a. Thalamus—relay station for discrimination of sensation (pain, temperature, touch) received from the periphery; several nuclei in the thalamus, each with specific functions, such as integration of sensory stimuli necessary for abstract thinking and reasoning, vision, hearing; relay station for fibers going to the limbic system

   b. Hypothalamus—responsible for maintaining homeostasis through the secretion of hormones and central control of the autonomic nervous system

      1) Controls vital functions such as water balance, blood pressure, sleep, appetite, body temperature

      2) Affects some emotional responses (pleasure, fear)

      3) Control center for pituitary function

      4) Affects both divisions of the autonomic nervous system

   c. Limbic system influences affective (emotional) behaviors and basic drives such as sexual behavior, aggression

4. Brain stem—contains midbrain, pons, and medulla oblongata; extends from the cerebral hemispheres to the foramen magnum at the base of the skull

   a. Contains nuclei of the fifth, sixth, seventh, and eighth cranial nerves and ascending sensory and descending motor tracts

   b. Contains vital centers of respiratory, vasomotor, and cardiac functions

   c. Reticular formation—relays sensory information; controls vasomotor and respiratory activity

   d. Decreased number of neurons with aging

5. Ventricular system and cerebral spinal fluid (CSF)—supports and cushions the central nervous system

  a. Removes metabolic wastes

  b. Compensatory mechanisms for intracranial volume/pressure

  c. Produces 55 mL/d of CSF; 130–150 mL average amount in system; CSF production decreases with age

  d. Ventricles enlarge and widen with aging

6. Cranial meninges

  a. Dura mater—dense, fibrous, outermost layer serves as periosteum for cranial bones

  b. Arachnoid mater

    1) Delicate, avascular membrane lying under dura

    2) Surrounds brain loosely

    3) Subarachnoid spaces contain CSF, arteries, veins

    4) Contains arachnoid granulations that enable CSF to pass from subarachnoid space into the venous system

  c. Pia mater

    1) Most delicate and inner meningeal layer

    2) Barrier system

  d. Gerontologic considerations—increased subdural space due to cerebral atrophy

7. Cerebellum—control of muscle movement, balance, coordination; trunk mobility and equilibrium; decreased number of neurons with aging, increased problems with balance and coordination

8. Spinal cord—communications link between CNS and PNS; ascending pathways transmit sensory information, and descending pathways relay motor instructions

## Alterations in Neurological Function

A. Assessment—signs and symptoms

  1. Headache

  2. Dizziness

  3. Changes in level of consciousness

  4. Increased intracranial pressure

  5. Pupillary reactions—reaction to light, size

  6. Seizures—focal or generalized

  7. Changes in vital signs—increasing systolic BP, decreasing diastolic BP, bradycardia

  8. Hyperpyrexia

  9. Ocular movements—six cardinal fields of gaze

  10. Skeletal motor function; muscle strength

  11. Neurogenic bladder

12. Cranial nerve (CN) function (*see* Table 11-1)

13. Coma—Glasgow Coma Scale (*see* Table 11-2): score of 3–8 indicates severe head injury; score of 15 indicates client is alert and oriented

14. Verbal response

**Table 11-1** Cranial Nerve Assessment

| (#)/NERVE | FUNCTION | NORMAL FINDINGS | NURSING CONSIDERATIONS |
|---|---|---|---|
| (I) Olfactory | Sense of smell | Able to detect various odors in each nostril | Have client smell a nonirritating substance such as coffee or tobacco with eyes closed<br><br>Test each nostril separately |
| (II) Optic | Sense of vision | Clear (acute) vision near and distant | Snellen eye chart for far vision<br><br>Read newspaper for near vision<br><br>Ophthalmoscopic exam |
| (III) Oculomotor | Pupil constriction, raising of eyelids | Pupils equal in size and equally reactive to light | Observe for symmetry and eye-opening<br><br>Shine penlight into eye as client stares straight ahead<br><br>Assess with CN IV and CN VI; ask client to watch your finger as you move it toward their face<br><br>Instruct client to look up, down, inward and laterally |
| (IV) Trochlear | Downward and inward movement of eyes | Able to move eyes down and inward | (*See* Oculomotor, CN III); assess eye movement with CN III and CN VI |
| (V) Trigeminal | Motor—jaw movement<br><br>Sensory—sensation on the face and neck | Able to clench and relax jaw<br><br>Able to differentiate between various stimuli to the face and neck | Test with pin and wisp of cotton over each division on both sides of face<br><br>Ask client to open jaw, bite down, move jaw laterally against pressure<br><br>Stroke cornea with wisp of cotton |
| (VI) Abducens | Lateral movement of the eyes | Able to move eyes in all directions | (*See* Oculomotor, CN III); assess eye movement with CN III and CN IV |

(*Continued*)

**Table 11-1** Cranial Nerve Assessment (*Continued*)

| (#)/NERVE | FUNCTION | NORMAL FINDINGS | NURSING CONSIDERATIONS |
|---|---|---|---|
| (VII)<br>Facial | Motor—facial muscle movement<br><br>Sensory—taste on the anterior two-thirds of the tongue (sweet and salty) | Able to smile, whistle, wrinkle forehead<br><br>Able to differentiate tastes among various agents | Observe for facial symmetry after asking client to frown, smile, raise eyebrows, close eyelids against resistance, whistle, blow<br><br>Place sweet, sour, bitter, and salty substances on tongue |
| (VIII)<br>Acoustic | Sense of hearing and balance | Hearing intact<br><br>Balance maintained while walking | Test with watch ticking into ear, rubbing fingers together, Rinne test, Weber test<br><br>Test posture, standing with eyes closed<br><br>Otoscopic exam |
| (IX)<br>Glossopharyngeal | Motor—pharyngeal movement and swallowing Sensory—taste on posterior one-third of tongue (sour and bitter) | Gag reflex intact, able to swallow<br><br>Able to taste | Place sweet, sour, bitter, and salty substances on tongue<br><br>Note ability to swallow and handle secretions<br><br>Stimulate pharyngeal wall to elicit gag reflex |
| (X)<br>Vagus | Swallowing and speaking | Able to swallow and speak with a smooth voice | Inspect soft palate—instruct to say "ah"<br><br>Observe uvula for midline position<br><br>Rate quality of voice |
| (XI)<br>Spinal accessory | Motor—flexion and rotation of head; shrugging of shoulders | Able to flex and rotate head; able to shrug shoulders | Inspect and palpate sternocleidomastoid and trapezius muscles for size, contour, tone<br><br>Ask client to move head side to side against resistance and shrug shoulders against resistance |
| (XII)<br>Hypoglossal | Motor—tongue movements | Can move tongue side to side and stick it out symmetrically and in midline | Inspect tongue in mouth<br><br>Ask client to stick out tongue and move it quickly from side to side<br><br>Observe midline, symmetry, and rhythmic movement |

**Table 11-2** Glasgow Coma Scale

| Eyes Open | Spontaneously | 4 | | | | | | | | | | | | | | | | | | | | | | |
|---|---|---|---|---|---|---|---|---|---|---|---|---|---|---|---|---|---|---|---|---|---|---|---|---|
| | To speech | 3 | | | | | | | | | | | | | | | | | | | | | | |
| | To pain | 2 | | | | | | | | | | | | | | | | | | | | | | |
| | None | 1 | | | | | | | | | | | | | | | | | | | | | | |
| Best Verbal Response | Oriented | 5 | | | | | | | | | | | | | | | | | | | | | | |
| | Confused | 4 | | | | | | | | | | | | | | | | | | | | | | |
| | Inappropriate words | 3 | | | | | | | | | | | | | | | | | | | | | | |
| | Incomprehensible sounds | 2 | | | | | | | | | | | | | | | | | | | | | | |
| | None | 1 | | | | | | | | | | | | | | | | | | | | | | |
| Best Motor Response | Obeys commands | 6 | | | | | | | | | | | | | | | | | | | | | | |
| | Localizes pain | 5 | | | | | | | | | | | | | | | | | | | | | | |
| | Flexes to pain | 4 | | | | | | | | | | | | | | | | | | | | | | |
| | Flexor posture | 3 | | | | | | | | | | | | | | | | | | | | | | |
| | Extensor posture | 2 | | | | | | | | | | | | | | | | | | | | | | |
| | No response | 1 | | | | | | | | | | | | | | | | | | | | | | |

**B.** Specific conditions

   1. Loss of consciousness

      a. Assessment—unable to rouse client; use Glasgow Coma Scale to assess response to stimuli

      b. Management—caring for the unconscious client

         1) Protective measures

            a) Ensure adequate oxygenation and circulation

            b) Keep side rails in elevated position or mattress on floor

            c) Place in lateral recumbent position

            d) Maintain proper body alignment and range of motion (ROM)

            e) Prevent skin breakdown

            f) Maintain excretory function—catheter, stool softeners, laxatives, enemas

            g) Maintain fluid, electrolyte balance nutrition—IV, nasogastric feeding

            h) Explain all procedures—speak often to client

2. Increased intracranial pressure (ICP)

   a. Characteristics

      1) Causes

         a) Cerebral edema

         b) Hemorrhage

         c) Space-occupying lesions

      2) Complications

         a) Cerebral hypoxia

         b) Decreased cerebral perfusion

         c) Herniation—pupil dilation

      3) Early signs of developing increased intracranial pressure: first stimulates, then depresses vital signs

   b. Caring for the client with increased intracranial pressure

      1) Assess for altered level of consciousness (LOC)—often earliest sign of elevated ICP

         a) Confusion

         b) Restlessness

         c) Pupillary changes—blurred vision, diplopia, papilledema

      2) Maintain respiratory function and patent airway

      3) Observe seizure precautions

      4) Elevate head 15–30° to promote venous drainage from brain; monitor response to position change

      5) Avoid neck flexion and head rotation—support in cervical collar or neck rolls

      6) Reduce environmental stimuli

      7) Prevent the Valsalva maneuver; avoid coughing, sneezing, bending forward

      8) Administer stool softeners

      9) Teach client to exhale while turning or moving in bed

     10) Monitor vital signs hourly—be alert for widening pulse pressure

     11) Restrict fluids to 1,200–1,500 mL/d

     12) Administer medications (*see* Table 11-3)

         a) Osmotic diuretics (mannitol and furosemide) to reduce fluid volume

         b) Corticosteroid therapy (dexamethasone) to reduce cerebral edema

         c) Antiseizure medications—diazepam, phenytoin, phenobarbital

         d) Antipyretics

         e) Monitor during barbiturate coma

**Table 11-3** Anticonvulsant Medications

| MEDICATION | ADVERSE EFFECTS | NURSING CONSIDERATIONS |
|---|---|---|
| Clonazepam | Drowsiness<br>Dizziness<br>Confusion<br>Respiratory depression | Benzodiazepine<br>Do not discontinue suddenly<br>Avoid activities that require alertness |
| Diazepam | Drowsiness, ataxia<br>Hypotension<br>Tachycardia<br>Respiratory depression | IV push doses shouldn't exceed 2 mg/minute<br>Monitor vital signs–resuscitation equipment available if given IV<br>Alcohol increases CNS depression<br>After long-term use, withdrawal leads to symptoms such as vomiting, sweating, cramps, tremors, and possibly convulsions |
| Fosphenytoin | Drowsiness<br>Dizziness<br>Confusion<br>Leukopenia<br>Anemia | Used for tonic-clonic seizures, status epilepticus<br>Highly protein bound<br>Contact health care provider if rash develops |
| Levetiracetam | Dizziness<br>Suicidal ideation | Avoid alcohol<br>Avoid driving and activities that require alertness |
| Phenytoin sodium | Drowsiness, ataxia<br>Nystagmus<br>Blurred vision<br>Hirsutism<br>Lethargy<br>GI upset<br>Gingival hypertrophy | Give oral medication with at least 1/2 glass of water or with meals to minimize GI irritation<br>Inform client that red-brown or pink discoloration of sweat and urine may occur<br>IV administration may lead to cardiac arrest—have resuscitation equipment on hand<br>Never mix with any other medication or dextrose IV<br>Instruct in oral hygiene<br>Increase vitamin D intake, exposure to sunlight may be necessary with long-term use<br>Alcohol increases serum levels<br>Increased risk toxicity in older adults |

*(Continued)*

**Table 11-3** Anticonvulsant Medications (*Continued*)

| MEDICATION | ADVERSE EFFECTS | NURSING CONSIDERATIONS |
|---|---|---|
| Phenobarbital | Drowsiness, rash<br><br>GI upset<br><br>Initially constricts pupils<br><br>Respiratory depression<br><br>Ataxia | Monitor vital signs—resuscitation equipment should be available if given IV<br><br>Drowsiness diminishes after initial weeks of therapy<br><br>Don't take alcohol or perform hazardous activities<br><br>Nystagmus may indicate early toxicity<br><br>Sudden discontinuation may lead to withdrawal<br><br>Tolerance and dependence result from long-term use<br><br>Folic acid supplements are indicated for long-term use<br><br>Decreased cognitive function in older adults |
| Primidone | Drowsiness<br><br>Ataxia, diplopia<br><br>Nausea and vomiting | Don't discontinue use abruptly<br><br>Full therapeutic response may take 2 weeks<br><br>Shake liquid suspension well<br><br>Take with food if experiencing GI distress<br><br>Decreased cognitive function in older adults |
| Magnesium sulfate | Flushing<br><br>Sweating<br><br>Extreme thirst<br><br>Hypotension<br><br>Sedation, confusion | Monitor intake and output<br><br>Before each dose, deep-tendon reflexes should be tested<br><br>Vital signs should be monitored often during parenteral administration<br><br>Used for pregnancy-induced hypertension<br><br>Monitor magnesium levels |
| Valproic acid | Sedation<br><br>Tremor, ataxia<br><br>Nausea, vomiting<br><br>Prolonged bleeding time | Agent of choice in many seizure disorders of young children<br><br>Do not take with carbonated beverage<br><br>Take with food<br><br>Monitor platelets, bleeding time, and liver function tests |

(*Continued*)

**Table 11-3** Anticonvulsant Medications (*Continued*)

| MEDICATION | ADVERSE EFFECTS | NURSING CONSIDERATIONS |
|---|---|---|
| Carbamazepine | Myelosuppression<br><br>Dizziness, drowsiness<br><br>Ataxia<br><br>Diplopia, rash | Monitor intake and output<br><br>Supervise ambulation<br><br>Monitor CBC<br><br>Take with meals<br><br>Wear protective clothing due to photosensitivity<br><br>Multiple medication interactions |
| Gabapentin | Increased appetite<br><br>Ataxia<br><br>Irritability<br><br>Dizziness<br><br>Fatigue | Monitor weight and behavioral changes<br><br>Can also be used to treat postherpetic neuralgia other neuropathic pain, fibromyalgia, prophylaxis of migraine. |
| Lamotrigine | Diplopia<br><br>Headaches<br><br>Dizziness<br><br>Drowsiness<br><br>Ataxia<br><br>Nausea, vomiting<br><br>Life-threatening rash when given with valproic acid | Take divided doses with meals or just afterward to decrease adverse effects |
| Topiramate | Ataxia<br><br>Confusion<br><br>Dizziness<br><br>Fatigue<br><br>Vision problems | Adjunct therapy for intractable partial seizures<br><br>Increased risk for renal calculi<br><br>Stop medication immediately if eye problems—could lead to permanent damage |
| **Action** | Decreases flow of calcium and sodium across neuronal membranes | |
| **Indications** | Partial seizures: carbamazepine, phenobarbital, primidone, gabapentin, lamotrigine<br><br>Generalized tonic-clonic seizures: phenobarbital, primidone, carbamazepine<br><br>Absence seizures: ethosuximide<br><br>Status epilepticus: diazepam, lorazepam, phenytoin | |

*(Continued)*

**Table 11-3** Anticonvulsant Medications (*Continued*)

| MEDICATION | ADVERSE EFFECTS | NURSING CONSIDERATIONS |
|---|---|---|
| **Adverse effects** | Cardiovascular depression | |
| | Respiratory depression | |
| | Agranulocytosis | |
| | Aplastic anemia | |
| | Gingival hyperplasia (phenytoin) | |
| **Nursing considerations** | Tolerance develops with long-term use | |
| | Don't discontinue abruptly | |
| | Caution with use of medications that lower seizure threshold (monoamine oxidase [MAO] inhibitors) | |
| | Barbiturates and benzodiazepines also used as anticonvulsants | |
| | Increased risk reactions in older adults | |

3. Caring for the client demonstrating seizure activity (*see* Tables 11-4 and 11-5)
   a. Protect from injury
   b. Raise side rails or ease client to floor
   c. Keep bed in low position
   d. Pad side rails, place blanket or pillows alongside rails
   e. Loosen restrictive clothing
   f. Do not restrain, provide environment that will prevent injury
   g. Do not try to insert a bite block, padded tongue blade, or oral airway
   h. Protect yourself—client may flail arms
   i. Maintain adequate ventilation
      1) If possible, place client on one side with the head flexed forward to facilitate drainage of secretions
      2) Provide oxygen and suction equipment as needed; do not attempt to suction client during seizure
      3) If prescribed, administer oxygen by nasal cannula
   j. Monitor status
      1) Onset, duration, and pattern
      2) Level of consciousness (LOC)
      3) Vital signs
      4) Skin color
      5) Responses to interventions

6) Postseizure—check tongue, provide mouth care, raise head of bed to 30° angle, place in side-lying position

7) Administer medications: phenobarbital, diazepam, lorazepam, fosphenytoin

8) Check for adverse effects of phenytoin: gingival hyperplasia, dark urine

9) Provide description of seizures in record

k. Prevent sensory overload

1) Explain all tests and treatments to client

2) Promote rest and comfort

3) Be aware of cultural factors when providing nursing care

4) Provide privacy

5) Position noise-producing mechanical devices in a way that minimizes audibility

l. Complementary/alternative therapy

1) Ketogenic diet to prevent seizures

a) Diet high in fat and low in carbohydrates mimics effects of fasting and places the body in a constant state of ketosis

b) Suppresses many types of seizures, may be effective when other methods of seizure control have failed

**Table 11-4** Seizure Classifications

| FOCAL ONSET (AWARE/IMPAIRED AWARENESS) | GENERALIZED ONSET (IMPAIRED AWARENESS) | UNKNOWN ONSET (AWARE/IMPAIRED AWARENESS) |
|---|---|---|
| **Motor Onset** | **Motor Onset** | **Motor Onset** |
| Automatisms | Tonic-clonic | Tonic-clonic |
| Atonic | Myoclonic | Epileptic spasms |
| Clonic | Atonic | |
| Epileptic spasms | | |
| Hyperkinetic | | |
| Myoclonic | | |
| Tonic | | |
| **Nonmotor Onset (Absence)** | **Nonmotor Onset (Absence)** | **Nonmotor Onset (Absence)** |
| Autonomic behavior | Typical | Behavior arrest |
| Arrest | Atypical | |
| Cognitive | Myoclonic Eyelid–myoclonia | |
| Emotional | | |
| Sensory | | |

**Table 11-5** Seizure Definitions

| FOCAL ONSET | TYPES | CHARACTERISTICS |
|---|---|---|
| Motor seizure | Tonic-clonic | Begins with tonic phase<br>Immediate loss of consciousness<br>Clonic phase—rhythmic jerking of all extremities |
| | Myoclonic | Brief jerking of extremities |
| | Atonic | Sudden loss of muscle tone<br>Client falls |
| | Complex focal | Client blacks out for a few seconds<br>Automatism may occur |
| | Simple focal | Remains conscious, often reports aura |
| Nonmotor seizure | Absence, typical simple | Brief periods of consciousness like daydreaming, more common in children |
| | Absence, typical complex | Brief periods of loss of consciousness with some type of movement like blinking, chewing gestures |
| | Absence, atypical | Unaware, blank stare with movements like eye blinking, lip smacking; continue as adult; autonomic |

C. Prevent sensory deprivation

   1. Involve client in planning own care

   2. Encourage a variety of diversional activities

   3. Provide a continuous means of orientation, e.g., calendar, clock, television

D. Intracranial tumors

   1. Assessment—signs and symptoms vary, depending on location

     a. Motor deficits

     b. Language disturbances

     c. Hearing difficulties

     d. Visual disturbances

     e. Dizziness, coordination problems

     f. Paresthesias

     g. Seizures—frequently first presenting sign

     h. Personality disturbances

     i. Papilledema

     j. Headache

     k. Nausea and vomiting

l. Drowsiness

m. Changes in level of consciousness

2. Diagnostics (*see* Table 11-6)

**Table 11-6** Neurological Tests

| TEST | PURPOSE | PREPARATION/ TESTING | POSTTEST NURSING CARE |
|---|---|---|---|
| Cerebral angiography | Identifies aneurysms, vascular malformations, narrowed vessels | Informed consent<br><br>Explain procedure:<br><br>Lie flat; dye injection into femoral artery by needle/catheter; fluoroscopy and radiologic films taken after injection<br><br>Well hydrated<br><br>Preprocedure sedation<br><br>Skin prep, chosen site shaved<br><br>Mark peripheral pulses<br><br>May experience feeling of warmth and metallic taste when dye injected | Neurologic assessment every 15–30 min until vital signs are stable<br><br>Keep flat in bed 12–14 hours<br><br>Check puncture site every hour<br><br>Immobilize site for 6–8 hours<br><br>Assess distal pulses, color, and temperature<br><br>Observe symptoms of complications, allergic response to dye, puncture site hematoma<br><br>Force fluids, accurate intake and output |
| Lumbar puncture (LP) | Insertion of needle into subarachnoid space to obtain specimen, relieve pressure, inject dye or medications | Explain procedure<br><br>Informed consent<br><br>Procedure done at bedside or in treatment room<br><br>Positioned in lateral recumbent fetal position at edge of bed | Neurological assessment every<br><br>15–30 min until stable<br><br>Position flat for several hours<br><br>Encourage PO fluid to 3,000 mL<br><br>Oral analgesics for headache<br><br>Observe sterile dressing at insertion site for bleeding or drainage |

*(Continued)*

**Table 11-6** Neurological Tests (*Continued*)

| TEST | PURPOSE | PREPARATION/ TESTING | POSTTEST NURSING CARE |
|---|---|---|---|
| Electroencephalogram (EEG) | Records electrical activity of brain | Explain procedure<br><br>Procedure done by technician in a quiet room<br><br>Painless<br><br>Tranquilizer and stimulant medications withheld for 24-48 h pre-EEG<br><br>Stimulants such as caffeine, cola, and tea, cigarettes withheld for 24 h pre-EEG<br><br>May be asked to hyperventilate<br><br>3–4 min and watch bright, flashing light<br><br>Meals not withheld<br><br>May be kept awake night before test | Help client remove paste from hair<br><br>Administer prescribed medication withheld before EEG<br><br>Observe for seizure activity in seizure-prone clients |
| Magnetic resonance imaging (MRI) | Body parts visualized by magnetic energy | Screen client for pacemaker or metal parts in body; lie very still for 1 h | None |
| CT scan (computed tomography) | Detects hemorrhage, infarction, abscesses, tumors | Written consent<br><br>Explain procedure<br><br>Painless Immobile during exam<br><br>If contrast dye used, may experience flushed, warm face and metallic taste during injection | No specific intervention<br><br>Assess for allergic responses to contrast dye, e.g., rash, pruritus, urticaria<br><br>Encourage PO fluids |

(*Continued*)

**Table 11-6** Neurological Tests (*Continued*)

| TEST | PURPOSE | PREPARATION/ TESTING | POSTTEST NURSING CARE |
|---|---|---|---|
| Myelogram | Visualizes spinal column and subarachnoid space | Informed consent<br><br>Explain procedure<br><br>NPO for 4–6 h before test<br><br>Obtain allergy history<br><br>Phenothiazines, CNS depressants, and stimulants withheld for 48 h prior to test<br><br>Table will be moved to various positions during test | Neurologic assessment every 2–4 hours;<br><br>Bedrest with head of bed elevated 30–45° for 3 hr after procedure; assess for allergic responses to contrast dye, e.g., rash, pruritus, urticaria<br><br>Oral analgesics for headache<br><br>Encourage PO fluids<br><br>Assess for distended bladder<br><br>Inspect injection site |
| Positron emission tomography (PET) | Used to assess metabolic and physiologic function of brain; diagnose stroke,<br><br>brain tumor, epilepsy, Parkinson disease, head injury | Client inhales or is injected with radioactive substance, then is scanned<br><br>Tell client that dizziness, headache may be experienced<br><br>Teach relaxation exercises | No specific interventions |

3. Characteristics

   a. Types—classified according to location

     1) Supratentorial

     2) Infratentorial

   b. Causes—unknown

   c. Medical/surgical management—intracranial surgery (burr holes, craniotomy, cranioplasty), radiation

4. Nursing management—client undergoing neurosurgery

   a. Preoperative care

     1) Detailed neurological assessment for baseline data

     2) Head shave—prep of site

     3) Psychological support

     4) Prepare client for postoperative course

b. Postoperative care

1) Maintain patent airway

2) Elevate head of bed to a 30–45° angle—after supratentorial surgery

3) Position client flat on either side—after infratentorial surgery

4) Monitor vital and neurological signs

5) Observe for complications—respiratory difficulties, increased intracranial pressure, hyperthermia, meningitis, wound infection

6) Administer medications—corticosteroids, osmotic diuretics, mild analgesics, anticonvulsants, antibiotics, antipyretics, antiemetics, hormone replacement as needed; limited narcotics postop

**E.** Stroke

1. Assessment

a. F.A.S.T. warning signs to spot a stroke

- **F = Facial drooping**—Does one side of the face droop or is it numb? Ask the client to smile. Is the client's smile uneven?

- **A = Arm weakness**—Is one arm weak or numb? Ask the client to raise both arms. Does one arm drift downward?

- **S = Speech difficulty**—Is the client's speech slurred?

- **T = Time to call 911**

b. Confusion/disorientation

c. Changes in vital signs

d. Changes in neurological signs

e. Change in level of consciousness

f. Seizures

g. Aphasia—expressive, receptive, global

h. Hemiplegia (paralysis on one side of body), hemiparesis (weakness on one side of body)

i. Bladder and/or bowel incontinence

j. Headache, vomiting

k. Dysphagia—difficulty swallowing

l. Hemianopsia—loss of half of visual field

m. Decreased sensation/neglect syndrome

n. Emotional liability

2. Preventive measures—identify risk factors

a. Advanced age

b. Hypertension

c. Transient ischemic attacks (TIA)

d. Diabetes mellitus

  e. Smoking

  f. Obesity

  g. Elevated blood lipids

  h. Oral contraceptives

3. Characteristics

  a. Abrupt onset of neurological deficits resulting from interference with blood supply to the brain

  b. Causes

   1) Ischemic—blockage of cerebral flow from thrombosis, embolism

   2) Hemorrhagic—intracerebral, subarachnoid

4. Nursing management

  a. Immediate care

   1) Maintain patent airway

   2) Minimize activity

   3) Keep head in a midline, neutral position

   4) Maintain proper body alignment

   5) Keep side rails in upright position

   6) Administer thrombolytic therapy for ischemic stroke within 4 hours of start of symptoms if client meets criteria

  b. Intermediate care and rehabilitative needs

   1) Position for good body alignment and comfort

   2) Monitor elimination patterns

   3) Provide skin care

   4) Perform passive and/or active ROM exercises

   5) Orient to person, time, and place

   6) Move affected extremities slowly and gently; avoid pulling on affected arm

   7) Teach use of supportive devices—commode, trapeze, cane, etc.

   8) Address communication needs—e.g., supply pad and pencil, magic slate

  c. Gerontologic considerations—ability to perform ADLs, loss of independence, altered relationship with significant other

**F.** Organic brain syndrome

1. Assessment

  a. Acute organic brain syndrome

   1) Memory loss

   2) Confusion

   3) Delirium

   4) Hallucinations

   5) Delusions

    b. Chronic organic brain syndrome

      1) Memory deficit

      2) Deterioration of intellectual functioning

      3) Incoherent communication

      4) Irritability

      5) Mood swings

      6) Incontinence

      7) Unkempt appearance

2. Characteristics

    a. Acute organic brain syndrome—reversible condition

      1) Fluid and electrolyte imbalance

      2) Malnutrition

      3) Metabolic imbalance

      4) Trauma

      5) Infection

      6) Stress

    b. Chronic organic brain syndrome—irreversible condition

      1) Cerebral arteriosclerosis

      2) Tumor

      3) Korsakoff psychosis

      4) Alzheimer disease

    c. Nursing management

      1) Decrease disorientation by frequent reorientation

      2) Decrease confusion

      3) Reduce anxiety—provide calm environment

      4) Maximize independent functioning

      5) Refer to occupational therapy, as indicated

**G.** Intellectual delay (*see* Table 11-7)

1. Definition: subaverage intellectual function (IQ less than 70) with concurrent impairment in adaptive functioning; onset under the age of 18

2. Delay—general

    a. Assessment

      1) Sensory deficits

      2) Physical anomalies

      3) Delayed growth and development

**Table 11-7** Intellectual Delay

| CLASSIFICATION | IQ RANGE | PRESCHOOL GROWTH AND DEVELOPMENT | SCHOOL TRAINING AND EDUCATION | ADULT SOCIAL/ VOCATIONAL LEVEL |
|---|---|---|---|---|
| I. Mild | 55–70 | Slow to walk, feed self, and talk compared with other children | With special education, can learn reading and math skills for third- to sixth-grade level | Can achieve social/vocational self-maintenance<br><br>May need occasional psychosocial support |
| II. Moderate | 40–55 | Delays in motor development Can do some self-help activities | Responds to training Does not progress with reading or math skills<br><br>Poor communication skills | Sheltered, usually incapable of self-maintenance |
| III. Severe | 25–40 | Marked delay in development<br><br>May be able to help self minimally | Can profit from habit training<br><br>Has some understanding of speech | Dependent on others for care<br><br>Can conform to routine |
| IV. Profound | Under 25 | Significant delay, minimal-capacity functioning | May respond to skill training<br><br>Shows basic emotional responses | Incapable of self-maintenance, needs nursing care |

   b.  Characteristics

      1)  Lack of, or destruction of, brain cells

      2)  Causes—heredity, infection, fetal anoxia, cranial or chromosomal abnormalities, intracranial hemorrhage

   c.  Nursing management

      1)  Assist parents with adjustment

      2)  Provide sensory stimulation

      3)  Encourage socially acceptable behavior

      4)  Provide emotional support

      5)  Encourage school training, education, vocational development as appropriate

3. Down syndrome

    a. Assessment

        1) Mental capacity—IQ range from 20 to 70

        2) Marked hypotonia; short stature

        3) Altered physical development—epicanthal folds, low-set ears, protruding tongue, low nasal bridge

    b. Characteristics

        1) Trisomy 21—chromosomal abnormality involving an extra chromosome number 21

        2) Causes—unknown; associated with maternal age greater than 35

    c. Nursing management

        1) Provide stimulation—occupational therapy (OT), physical therapy (PT), special education

        2) Observe for signs of common physical problems: 30–40% have heart disease; 80% have hearing loss; respiratory infections are common

        3) Establish and maintain adequate nutrition, parental education and support

**H.** Learning delay

  1. Assessment

    a. Hyperkinesis (sometimes absent)

    b. Decreased attention span, i.e., attention deficit disorder (ADD) (*see* Table 11-8)

    c. Perceptual deficits

    d. Aggression/depression

  2. Characteristics—learning and behavioral disorders that occur because of CNS malfunctioning

    a. Neuropsychological testing—reveals individual differences

    b. Average to high IQ

  3. Nursing management

    a. Reduce frustration

    b. Special educational intervention; small class size

    c. Provide safety and security

    d. Administer medications, e.g., methylphenidate hydrochloride, dextroamphetamine sulfate

    e. Refer to appropriate resources—special education, parent support groups

**I.** Cranial nerve disorders

  1. Trigeminal neuralgia (tic douloureux) (see Table 11-9)

    a. Assessment

        1) Stabbing or burning facial pain—excruciating, unpredictable, and paroxysmal

        2) Twitching, grimacing of facial muscles

        3) Social isolation

 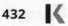

**Table 11-8** Attention Deficit Disorder Medications

| MEDICATION | ADVERSE EFFECTS | NURSING CONSIDERATIONS |
|---|---|---|
| Methylphenidate | Nervousness, palpitations<br><br>Insomnia<br><br>Tachycardia<br><br>Weight loss, growth suppression | May precipitate Tourette syndrome<br><br>Monitor CBC, platelet count<br><br>Has paradoxical calming effect in ADD<br><br>Monitor height/weight in children<br><br>Monitor BP<br><br>Avoid drinks with caffeine<br><br>Give at least 6 h before bedtime<br><br>Give pc |
| Dextroamphetamine sulfate | Insomnia<br><br>Tachycardia, palpitations | Controlled substance<br><br>May alter insulin needs<br><br>Give in A.M. to prevent insomnia<br><br>Don't use with MAO inhibitor (possible hypertensive crisis) |
| Dexmethylphenidate | Abdominal discomfort<br><br>Anorexia<br><br>Fever Nausea<br><br>Insomnia<br><br>Weight loss | Obtain baseline height and weight and monitor for growth restriction in children<br><br>Children are more likely to develop the adverse effects of abdominal pain, anorexia, insomnia, and weight loss<br><br>May lower the seizure threshold in those with a history of seizures<br><br>Do not administer in the afternoon or evening because it can cause insomnia<br><br>Monitor CBC, WBC count with differential, and platelet count |
| **Action** | Increase level of catecholamines in cerebral cortex and reticular activating system | |
| **Indications** | Attention deficit disorder (ADD)<br><br>Narcolepsy | |
| **Adverse effects** | Restlessness<br><br>Insomnia<br><br>Tremors<br><br>Tachycardia<br><br>Seizures | |
| **Nursing considerations** | Monitor growth rate in children | |

**Table 11-9** Cranial Nerve Disorders

| | TRIGEMINAL NEURALGIA (TIC DOULOUREUX) | BELL PALSY (FACIAL PARALYSIS) | ACOUSTIC NEUROMA |
|---|---|---|---|
| Assessment | Stabbing or burning facial pain—excruciating, unpredictable, paroxysmal<br><br>Twitching, grimacing of facial muscles | Inability to close eye<br><br>Decreased corneal reflex<br><br>Increased lacrimation<br><br>Speech difficulty<br><br>Loss of taste<br><br>Distortion of one side of face | Deafness—partial, initially<br><br>Dizziness<br><br>Vertigo<br><br>Tinnitus |
| Analysis | Type of neuralgia involving one or more branches of the fifth cranial nerve<br><br>Causes—infections of sinuses, teeth, mouth, or irritation of nerve from pressure | Peripheral involvement of the seventh cranial nerve<br><br>Predisposing factors—vascular ischemia, viral disease, edema, inflammatory reactions | Benign tumor of the eighth cranial nerve |
| Nursing considerations | Identify and avoid stimuli that exacerbate the attacks<br><br>Administer medications—carbamazepine and analgesics<br><br>Treatment—carbamazepine, alcohol injection to nerve, resection of the nerve, microvascular decompression<br><br>Avoid rubbing eye<br><br>Chew on opposite side of mouth | Protect head from cold or drafts<br><br>Administer analgesics<br><br>Assist with electrical stimulation<br><br>Teach isometric exercises for facial muscles (blow and suck from a straw)<br><br>Massage, warm packs<br><br>Provide emotional support for altered body image<br><br>Prevent corneal abrasions (artificial tears)<br><br>Treatment—electrical stimulation, analgesics, steroid therapy, antiviral medications<br><br>Recovery takes 3–5 wk | Treatment—surgical excision of tumor<br><br>Pre- and postoperative care for posterior fossa craniotomy<br><br>Comfort measures—assist with turning of head and neck |

   b. Characteristics

   1) Type of neuralgia involving one or more branches of the fifth cranial nerve (trigeminal)

   2) Causes—unknown; infections of sinuses, teeth, and mouth, irritation of nerve due to pressure are aggravating factors

   c. Nursing management

   1) Identify and avoid stimuli that exacerbate the attacks (light touch)

   2) Administer medications—carbamazepine and pain relievers when prescribed

   3) Administer appropriate diet

   4) Treatment—carbamazepine, alcohol injection to nerve, resection of the nerve, microvascular decompression

2. Bell palsy (facial paralysis)

   a. Assessment

   1) Inability of eye to close

   2) Increased lacrimation

   3) Speech difficulty

   4) Loss of taste

   5) Distortion of one side of face

   b. Characteristics

   1) Peripheral involvement of the seventh cranial nerve

   2) Causes—unknown; predisposing factors are vascular ischemia, viral disease, edema, inflammatory reactions

   c. Nursing management

   1) Comfort measures—protect head from cold or drafts, administer analgesics and appropriate diet

   2) Improve facial muscle tone—assist with electric stimulation, teach isometric exercises of face

   3) Provide emotional support for altered body image

   4) Prevent corneal abrasions

   5) Treatment—electrical stimulation, analgesics, steroid therapy

3. Acoustic neuroma

   a. Assessment

   1) Deafness—partial, initially

   2) Tinnitus

   3) Dizziness

      b. Characteristics

        1) Benign tumor of the vestibulocochlear nerve (cranial nerve VIII)

        2) Treatment—surgical excision of tumor

      c. Nursing management

        1) Pre- and postoperative care for posterior fossa craniotomy

        2) Comfort measures—assist with turning of head and neck

**J.** Head injury

  1. Assessment

    a. Battle sign (ecchymosis over mastoid bone may indicate a lower skull fracture); raccoon eyes (bruising around the eyes); rhinorrhea, otorrhea

    b. Concussion—transient mental confusion or loss of consciousness, headache, no residual neurological deficit, possible loss of memory surrounding event, long-term effects (lack of concentration, personality changes)

    c. Contusion—varies from slight depression of consciousness to coma, with decorticate posturing (flexion and internal rotation of forearms and hands) or decerebrate posturing (extension of arms and legs, pronation of arms, plantar flexion, opisthotonos), indicating deeper dysfunction, generalized cerebral edema

    d. Hemorrhage/hematoma

      1) Epidural—short period of unconsciousness followed by lucid interval with ipsilateral pupillary dilation, weakness of contralateral extremities, rapid neurologic deterioration

      2) Subdural—decreased level of consciousness, ipsilateral pupillary dilation, contralateral weakness, personality changes; increased risk with aging and chronic alcohol consumption

  2. Characteristics

    a. Theory—skull is a closed vault with a volume ratio of three components: brain tissue, blood, and CSF; sudden increase in any of these can cause brain dysfunction

    b. Ingestion of drugs and alcohol may delay manifestations of symptoms of damage

    c. Generalized brain swelling in response to injury

  3. Treatment

    a. Minor injury—repair CSF leak, scalp lacerations

    b. Penetrating wounds—surgical repair, antibiotics, and anticonvulsants

    c. Moderate to severe head injury—supportive care of the unconscious client, prophylactic anticonvulsants, prevent and control intracranial hypertension, prevent secondary brain damage from hypotension, prevent anemia, increased arterial carbon dioxide levels

4. Nursing management

   a. Management of increased intracranial pressure and cerebral edema

   b. Neurological assessment

   c. Administer glucocorticoids—dexamethasone, mannitol, furosemide

   d. Hypothermia—to decrease metabolic demands

   e. Barbiturate therapy—to decrease cerebral metabolic rate

   f. Minimal procedures, e.g., suctioning, turning, positioning (HOB elevated at 30° or more) in acute phase

   g. Prevention of complications of immobility

**K.** Spinal cord injury (*see* Table 11-10)

1. Assessment

   a. Loss of sensory function below injury

   b. Loss of motor function below injury

   c. Spinal shock symptoms

      1) Flaccid paralysis of skeletal muscles

      2) Complete loss of all sensation

      3) Suppression of somatic (pain, touch, temperature) and visceral reflexes

   d. Postural hypotension, bradycardia

   e. Circulatory problems—edema

   f. Alterations in normal thermoregulation

2. Extent of neurological deficit (*see* Table 11-10)

3. Characteristics

   a. Types of spinal cord injuries

      1) Concussion without direct trauma

      2) Penetrating wound or fracture dislocation

      3) Hemorrhage

      4) Compression of blood supply

   b. Categories of neurological deficit

      1) Complete—no voluntary motor activity or sensation below level of injury

      2) Incomplete—some voluntary motor activity or sensation below level of injury

      3) Paraplegia—thoracic vertebral injury or lower; lower extremities affected

      4) Tetraplegia (quadriplegia)—cervical vertebral injury; all four extremities involved

**Table 11-10** Spinal Cord Injury

| LEVEL OF INJURY | FUNCTIONAL ABILITY | SELF-CARE CAPABILITY |
|---|---|---|
| C3 and above | Inability to control muscles of breathing | Unable to care for self, life-sustaining ventilatory support essential |
| C4 | Movement of trapezius and sterno-cleidomastoid muscles, no upper extremity muscle function, minimal ventilatory capacity | Unable to care for self, may self-feed with powered devices (depending on respiratory function) |
| C5 | Neck movement, possible partial strength of shoulder and biceps | Can drive electric wheelchair, may be able to feed self with powered devices |
| C6 | Muscle function in C5 level; partial strength in pectoralis major | May self-propel a lightweight wheelchair, may feed self with devices, can write and care for self, can transfer from chair to bed |
| C7 | Muscle function in C6 level; no finger muscle power | Can dress lower extremities, minimal assistance needed, independence in wheelchair, can drive car with hand controls |
| C8 | Muscle function in C7 level; finger muscle power | Same as C7; in general, activities easier |
| T1–T4 | Good upper extremity muscle strength | Some independence from wheelchair, long leg braces for standing exercises |
| T5–L2 | Balance difficulties | Still requires wheelchair, limited ambulation with long leg braces and crutches |
| L3–L5 | Trunk-pelvis muscle function intact | May use crutches or canes for ambulation |
| L5–S3 | Waddling gait | Ambulation |

    c. Causes

      1) Trauma due to accidents—more common in young males

      2) Neoplasms

    d. Complication—autonomic dysreflexia, occurs with complete spinal cord injuries above T6; triggered by noxious stimuli below level of injury (full bladder, kinked catheter, full rectum, restrictive clothing)

e. Treatment

    1) Skeletal traction—Gardner-Wells, Crutchfield, Vinke tongs, halo traction

    2) Surgical stabilization—reduction and stabilization by fusion, wires, and plates

    3) Steroid therapy

    4) Hyperbaric oxygen therapy

    5) Antispasmodics (e.g., baclofen, diazepam)

4. Nursing management

  a. Ensure patent airway

  b. Maintenance of cardiovascular functioning

  c. Move client by log-rolling technique; use turning frames

  d. Provide good skin care

  e. Emotional support

  f. Ensure adequate nutrition

  g. Reduce aggravating factors that cause spasticity

  h. Bladder and bowel training

  i. Client and family education to cope with detailed care at home

5. Gerontologic concerns—fall prevention strategies; greater risk of complications after spinal cord injury (SCI)

**L.** Guillain-Barré syndrome

1. Assessment

  a. Diffuse inflammatory response occurring in peripheral nervous system, resulting in compression of nerve roots and peripheral nerves; demyelination occurs and slows or alters nerve conduction

  b. Possible etiologies

    1) Infective/viral

    2) Autoimmune response

    3) May follow immunizations

  c. Course

    1) Acute, rapid, ascending sensory and motor deficit that may stop at any level of CNS

    2) Protracted, develops slowly, regresses slowly

    3) Prolonged course with phases of deterioration and partial remission

2. Characteristics

  a. Abrupt onset of presenting signs

    1) Paresthesias/pain often occurring in stocking-and-glove distribution

    2) Motor losses symmetrical, usually beginning in lower extremities, then extend upward to include trunk, upper extremities, cranial nerves, and vasomotor function; deep-tendon reflexes disappear; respiratory muscle compromise

       3) Excessive or inadequate autonomic function

          a) Hypotension/tachycardia

          b) Vasomotor flushing

          c) Paralytic ileus

          d) Profuse sweating

       4) Plateau period—progress to peak severity between 2–4 weeks

       5) Recovery period—2 wk to 24 mo

3. Nursing management

    a. Intervention is symptomatic

    b. Steroids in acute phase

    c. Plasmapheresis, IV immunoglobulins, adrenocorticotropic hormone, corticosteroids

    d. Aggressive respiratory care

    e. Utilize principles of immobility

    f. Maintain adequate nutrition

    g. Physical therapy

    h. Pain-reducing measures

    i. Eye care

    j. Prevention of complications—UTI, aspiration, constipation, urinary retention

    k. Psychosocial

       1) Fear/anxiety

       2) Altered body image

**M.** Herpes zoster (shingles)

1. Assessment

    a. Herpesvirus; causative agent is identical to varicella (chickenpox)

    b. Results from reactivation of the varicella virus, which has remained dormant

    c. Most commonly affects (in descending order):

       1) Ophthalmic branch of the trigeminal nerve

       2) Thoracic branch

       3) Cervical branch

       4) Sacral branch

2. Characteristics

    a. Severe pain in specific dermatome for 1–2 d before skin changes

    b. Vesicular blisters on affected areas

    c. Muscle weakness in the affected area and distal to blisters

    d. Headache

3. Nursing management

   a. No specific treatment

      1) Analgesics

      2) Topical medication (e.g., permethrin, crotamiton)

      3) Antiviral medication (e.g., famciclovir, valacyclovir)

**N.** Ménière disease

1. Assessment

   a. Rare neurological syndrome manifested by recurrent attacks of vertigo with sensori-neural hearing loss

   b. Possible etiology—degeneration of the cochlear hair cells of the labyrinth

2. Characteristics

   a. Signs and symptoms

      1) Nausea and vomiting

      2) Incapacitating vertigo

      3) Tinnitus

      4) Feeling of pressure/fullness in the ear

      5) Fluctuating hearing loss (deafness after repeated episodes)

      6) Nystagmus

      7) Diagnostic tests—Weber and Rinne test, CT

   b. Course—attacks are recurrent several times a week with periods of remission lasting several years

3. Nursing management

   a. Antihistamines in acute phase (epinephrine, diphenhydramine)

   b. Antiemetics

   c. Bedrest during acute phase

   d. Provide protection when ambulatory

   e. Maintain adequate nutrition

**O.** Amyotrophic lateral sclerosis (Lou Gehrig disease)

1. Assessment

   a. Progressive, degenerative disease involving the lower motor neurons of the spinal cord and cerebral cortex; the voluntary motor system is particularly involved, with progressive degeneration of the corticospinal tract, leads to a mixture of spastic and atrophic changes in cranial and spinal musculature

   b. No specific pattern exists—involvement may vary in different parts of the same area

   c. Possible etiologies

      1) Genetic/familial

      2) Chronic (slow) viral infection

      3) Autoimmune disease

      4) Environmental factors

2. Characteristics

   a. Signs and symptoms

      1) Tongue fatigue/atrophy with fasciculations

      2) Nasal quality to speech/dysarthria

      3) Dysphagia/aspiration

      4) Muscular wasting/atrophy/spasticity

         a) Usually begins in upper extremities

         b) Distal portion affected first

         c) Fasciculations

      5) Emotional lability, cognitive dysfunction

      6) Respiratory insufficiency (usual cause of death)

      7) No alteration in autonomic, sensory, or mental function

3. Nursing management

   a. No known treatment proven effective

   b. Current approach remains supportive/symptomatic

   c. Apply principles of care of client with progressive, terminal disease

   d. Treat self-care deficits symptomatically

   e. Maintain adequate nutrition

   f. Physical therapy/speech therapy

   g. Adaptive home equipment

   h. Psychosocial support

   i. Administer riluzole—extends survival time; risk of liver toxicity

**P.** Encephalitis

1. Assessment

   a. Virus most common cause

   b. May be sequelae of:

      1) Viral disease, e.g., measles

      2) Prophylactic inoculations

      3) Obscure illness of viral origin

   c. Pathogens

      1) Arboviruses

         a) Eastern equine, Western equine, St. Louis, Powassan

         b) Reservoir in ticks, mosquitoes

      2) Enteroviruses—polio, ECHO, coxsackie

3) Other viruses (latent)

   a) Herpes simplex type 1

   b) Herpes zoster

   c) Mumps

   d) Cytomegalovirus, Epstein-Barr virus

   e) Rabies

4) Other

   a) Bacteria/spirochetes

   b) Fungal—*Cryptococcus*

   c) Protozoal, metazoal—malaria, toxoplasmosis

2. Characteristics

  a. Signs and symptoms

    1) Prodromal illness—headache, fever, myalgia, malaise, sore throat preceding onset of neurological signs

    2) Behavioral disturbances

    3) Alterations in consciousness from lethargy to coma

    4) Confusion/disorientation

    5) Bilateral motor/sensory deficits

    6) Seizures

    7) Meningeal signs

    8) Increased ICP

  b. CSF abnormalities

3. Management

  a. Medical management

    1) Symptomatic/supportive

    2) Antiserum—rabies

    3) Antiviral agents—adenine arabinoside (ARA-A), cytosine arabinoside (ARA-C), acyclovir

  b. Surgical management—decompression and necrotic tissue excision

  c. Nursing management

    1) Symptomatic care

    2) Prevent complications

**Q.** Meningitis

1. Assessment—access routes

  a. Blood—most common

    1) Septicemia/bacteremia

    2) Septic emboli—bacterial endocarditis, URI

    b. Direct pathogen invasion

       1) Traumatic—penetrating wounds, skull fracture, operative procedures

       2) Nontraumatic—secondary to otitis media, sinusitis, teeth infections

    c. Cerebrospinal fluid

       1) CSF leak—otorrhea, rhinorrhea

       2) Lumbar puncture

    d. Pathogens

       1) Bacteria—Gram-positive/negative organisms

       2) Virus—enteroviruses, mumps, measles

       3) Mycobacteria—*Mycobacterium tuberculosis*

       4) Fungal—*Cryptococcus neoformans*

       5) Spirochetes/parasites

    e. Host factors

       1) Immunoglobulin deficiency

       2) Long-term radiation therapy

       3) Immunosuppressive therapy

    f. Types

       1) Septic—organisms isolated by routine culture

       2) Aseptic—nonbacterial inflammatory disorder

2. Characteristics

    a. Signs and symptoms

       1) Headache/fever/photophobia

       2) Meningeal signs

          a) Nuchal rigidity

          b) Kernig sign—when hip flexed to 90°, complete extension of the knee is restricted and painful

          c) Brudzinski sign—attempts to flex the neck will produce flexion at knee and thigh

          d) Opisthotonic position—extensor rigidity, with legs hyperextended, forming an arc with the trunk

       3) Alterations in mental status—confusion to coma

       4) Seizures

       5) Infants

          a) Refusal of feedings

          b) Vomiting/diarrhea

          c) Bulging fontanelles

          d) Vacant stare

          e) High-pitched cry

3. Management

   a. Medical management

      1) Antibiotic therapy

      2) Antifungal therapy—amphotericin

      3) *Mycobacterium*—INH, streptomycin

      4) Viral—supportive therapy

   b. Surgical placement of ventricular catheter to drain CSF from ventricles

   c. Nursing management

      1) Decrease temperature

      2) Analgesia for headache

      3) Provide nonstimulating, dark environment

      4) Seizure precautions

      5) Monitor for shock and embolic complications

      6) Droplet precautions for *Haemophilus influenzae*, type b, and *Neisseria meningitidis*

**R.** Brain abscess

   1. Assessment

      a. Similar to meningitis assessment

      b. Asymptomatic until reaching considerable size if located in frontal or temporal lobe, mimics space-occupying lesion (e.g., a tumor)

   2. Characteristics

      a. Chills, fever

      b. Anorexia, malaise, lethargy

      c. Leukocytosis

      d. Meningeal signs

      e. Focal neurological signs—depending on area of lesion

         1) Seizures

         2) Motor/sensory deficits

         3) Visual disturbances

         4) Speech disturbances

         5) Personality changes

         6) Cranial nerve palsies

      f. Signs of increased intracranial pressure

      g. Increased white cell count, ESR

      h. CT, MRI

3. Management

   a. Nonsurgical—appropriate antibiotic therapy

   b. Surgical—extensive drainage and/or repeated aspiration

   c. Nursing care/goals—similar to meningitis/encephalitis

   d. Evaluation—minimal neurological deficit remains

**S.** Migraine headache

1. Assessment

   a. Prodromal—depression, irritability, feeling cold, food cravings, anorexia, change in activity level, increased urination

   b. Aura—light flashes and bright spots, numbness and tingling (lips, face, hands), mild confusion, drowsiness, dizziness, diplopia

   c. Headache—throbbing (often unilateral), photophobia, nausea, vomiting, 4–72 hours

   d. Recovery—pain gradually subsides, muscle aches in neck and scalp, sleep for extended period

2. Diagnosis

   a. Episodic events or acute attacks

   b. Seen more often in women before menses

   c. Familial disorders due to inherited vascular response to different chemicals

   d. Precipitating factors—stress, menstrual cycles, bright lights, depression, sleep deprivation, fatigue, foods containing tyramine, monosodium glutamate, nitrites, or milk products (aged cheese, processed foods); caffeine may trigger or may help alleviate attack

3. Plan/implementation

   a. Prevention and treatment

      1) Dietary modifications

      2) Medications

         a) Beta-blockers

         b) Triptan preparations—activate serotonin receptors

         c) Acetaminophen, NSAIDs

         d) Topiramate

         e) Ergotamines—dihydroergotamine (DHE); take at start of headache

4. Implementation

   a. Avoid triggers

   b. Comfort measures

   c. Quiet, dark environment

   d. Elevate head of bed 30°

5. Complementary/alternate therapy

    a. Riboflavin (vitamin $B_2$) supplement

        1) 400 mg daily may reduce the number and duration but not the severity of the headaches

        2) Take as an individual supplement

    b. Massage, meditation, relaxation techniques

**T.** Huntington disease

1. Assessment—rare, familial, progressive, degenerative disease passed from generation to generation (dominant inheritance)

2. Characteristics

    a. Depression and temper outbursts

    b. Choreiform movements

        1) Slight to severe restlessness

        2) Facial grimacing

        3) Arm movements

        4) Irregular leg movements

        5) Twisting, turning, struggling nature

        6) Tongue movements

        7) Person is in constant motion by end of disease progression

    c. Personality changes

        1) Irritability; demanding behavior

        2) Paranoia

        3) Memory loss

        4) Decreased intellectual function

        5) Dementia

        6) Psychosis seen at end stage

3. Management

    a. Therapeutic intervention

        1) Disease progresses until client is completely helpless and speechless

        2) Treatment is symptomatic

    b. Medication therapy—intended to reduce movement and subdue behavior changes

        1) Chlordiazepoxide

        2) Haloperidol

        3) Chlorpromazine

    c. Nursing management

        1) Supportive, symptomatic

        2) Genetic counseling for all family members

**U.** Parkinson disease

1. Description—chronic progressive disease; degeneration of dopamine-producing neurons in the substantia nigra of the midbrain, resulting in disturbed transmission of nerve impulses

2. Assessment

   a. Tremors (pill-rolling motion)

   b. Bradykinesia (loss of automatic movements)

   c. Restlessness

   d. Rigidity and propulsive gait

   e. Weakness

   f. Monotonous speech

   g. Increased salivation, dysphagia

   h. Depression, insomnia, dementia

   i. Masklike facial expression

   j. Constipation

   k. Urinary incontinence

3. Nursing management

   a. Promote rest, comfort, and sleep

   b. Keep client as functional and productive as possible

      1) Encourage finger exercises, e.g., typing, piano playing

      2) Range of motion (ROM) as appropriate

      3) Teach client ambulation modification, refer to physical therapy

         a) Goose-stepping walk

         b) Walk with wider base

         c) Concentrate on swinging arms while walking

         d) Turn around slowly, using small steps

         e) Look ahead, not down

   c. Promote family understanding of the disease

      1) Client's intellect is not impaired

      2) Sight and hearing are intact

      3) Disease is progressive but slow

   d. Refer for speech therapy, potential stereotactic surgery

   e. Administer medications for symptomatic relief (*see* Table 11-11)

   f. Other medications include ropinirole and pramipexole

   g. Antihistamines may also be used to manage tremors

4. Complementary/alternative therapy

   1) Coenzyme $Q_{10}$ supplements made naturally in the body; used by cells to produce energy and as an antioxidant

   2) 1,200 mg/d causes decreased deterioration in feedings, bathing, walking

 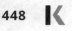

**Table 11-11** Parkinson Disease Medications

| MEDICATION | ADVERSE EFFECTS | NURSING CONSIDERATIONS |
|---|---|---|
| Apomorphine<br>Pramipexole<br>Ropinirole | Nausea<br><br>Dizziness<br><br>Constipation<br><br>Rhinitis<br><br>Sleepiness<br><br>Postural hypotension | A centrally acting dopamine agonist that reduces tremors and rigidity and improves movement, posture, and equilibrium<br><br>Overdose may require supportive measures to maintain BP<br><br>Monitor BP and heart rate and rhythm<br><br>Use cautiously in clients with a history of cardiac dysrhythmias, confusion, or hallucinations<br><br>Daily administration usually given in 3 divided doses |
| Benztropine mesylate<br>Trihexyphenidyl | Drowsiness, nausea, vomiting<br><br>Atropine-like effects—blurred vision, mydriasis<br><br>Antihistaminic effects—sedation, dizziness | Acts by lessening cholinergic effect of dopamine deficiency<br><br>Suppresses tremor of parkinsonism<br><br>Most adverse effects are reversed by changes in dosage<br><br>Additional drowsiness can occur with other CNS depressants |
| Levodopa | Nausea and vomiting, anorexia<br><br>Postural hypotension<br><br>Mental changes—confusion, agitation, mood alterations<br><br>Cardiac dysrhythmias<br><br>Twitching | Precursor of dopamine<br><br>Thought to restore dopamine levels in extrapyramidal centers<br><br>Administered in large, prolonged doses<br><br>Contraindicated in glaucoma, hemolytic anemia<br><br>Give with food<br><br>Monitor for postural hypotension<br><br>Avoid OTC meds that contain vitamin $B_6$ (pyridoxine); reverses effects |
| Bromocriptine mesylate | Dizziness, headache, hypotension<br><br>Tinnitus<br><br>Nausea, abdominal cramps<br><br>Pleural effusion<br><br>Orthostatic hypotension | Give with meals<br><br>May lead to early postpartum conception<br><br>Monitor cardiac, hepatic, renal, hematopoietic functions |

*(Continued)*

**Table 11-11** Parkinson Disease Medications (*Continued*)

| MEDICATION | ADVERSE EFFECTS | NURSING CONSIDERATIONS |
|---|---|---|
| Carbidopa–levodopa | Hemolytic anemia<br><br>Dystonic movements, ataxia<br><br>Orthostatic hypotension<br><br>Dysrhythmias<br><br>GI upset, dry mouth | Levodopa agent<br><br>Don't use with MAO inhibitors<br><br>Advise to change positions slowly<br><br>Take with food |
| Amantadine | CNS disturbances, hyperexcitability<br><br>Insomnia, vertigo, ataxia<br><br>Slurred speech, convulsions | |
| Selegiline<br><br>Rasagiline | Nausea, dyskinesia, agitation, rigidity | Inhibits MAO and increases dopamine levels |
| Entacapone<br><br>Tolcapone | Nausea, dyskinesia, agitation, rigidity | Used only with carbidopa-levodopa |

V.  Myasthenia gravis

   1.  Description—autoimmune process; deficiency of acetylcholine at myoneural junction

   2.  Assessment

      a.  Extreme skeletal muscle weakness, quickly produced by repeated movement but disappears following rest

      b.  Tiredness on slight exertion

      c.  Diplopia, ptosis

      d.  Impaired speech

      e.  Choking and aspiration of food

      f.  Respiratory distress

   3.  Diagnosis—Tensilon (edrophonium) test

   4.  Management

      a.  Medications

         1)  Anticholinergics

         2)  Corticosteroids, immunosuppressants

         3)  Surgical therapy—thymectomy

         4)  Plasmapheresis

b.  Nursing

1)  Promote comfort, rest, and sleep; balanced diet

2)  Relieve symptoms by administering medications (anticholinesterase, corticosteroids, immunosuppressants)

3)  Teach client

a)  Use of MedicAlert band

b)  Be aware of factors that may precipitate myasthenia crisis, e.g., infections, emotional stress, use of streptomycin or neomycin (which produce muscular weakness), surgery

c)  Be alert for myasthenia crisis—sudden inability to swallow, speak, or maintain a patent airway

**W.** Multiple sclerosis

1.  Description—chronic progressive disease characterized by demyelination and scarring throughout the brain and spinal cord

2.  History—onset between 15–50 y of age

a.  Viral

b.  Autoimmunity

c.  Genetic factors

3.  Assessment

a.  Ataxia

b.  Weakness

c.  Spasticity

d.  Vertigo, tinnitus

e.  Nystagmus, patchy blindness

f.  Chewing and swallowing difficulties

g.  Scanning speech

h.  Paresthesias

i.  Incontinence/retention of urine, constipation

j.  Emotional lability

k.  Sexual impairment

4.  Nursing management

a.  Promote comfort, rest, and sleep

b.  Promote maximum function, avoid stress

1)  Relaxation and coordination exercises

2)  Progressive resistance exercises, ROM

c.  Encourage fluid intake 2,000 mL/day

d. Administration of medications

1) Corticosteroids (e.g., methylprednisolone)

2) Immunosuppressive medications (e.g., cyclophosphamide)

3) Immune modulators (e.g., beta interferon)

4) Monoclonal antibody (e.g., natalizumab, glatiramer acetate)

e. Wide-based walk, use of cane or walker

f. Use of weighted bracelets and cuffs to stabilize upper extremities

g. Bladder and bowel training (care of indwelling urinary catheter if appropriate)

h. Self-help devices

i. Eye patch for diplopia

j. Occupational therapy

k. Nutritional therapy

l. Provide emotional support

m. Referrals—National Multiple Sclerosis Society

X. Alzheimer disease—chronic, progressive, degenerative disease characterized by a loss of memory, judgment, visuospatial perception, and personality

1. Etiology—changes in structure and chemistry of the brain; exact cause unknown

a. Structure—enlargement of the ventricles, widening of the cerebral sulci, narrowing of the gyri

b. Reduction in neurotransmitters

c. Vascular degeneration

2. Assessment

a. Stages—client may or may not progress through them in sequence

1) Early, Stage 1: forgets names, misplaces household items, short attention span, problems with judgment, decreased performance when stressed, decreased knowledge of current events, unable to travel alone to new destinations, inability to make decisions, increased confusion at night (sundowning), hoarding, wandering

2) Moderate, Stage 2: gross intellectual impairments; complete disorientation to time, place, and events; agitated; possible depression; loss of ability to care for self; speech and language deficits; visuospatial deficits

3) Severe, Stage 3: completely incapacitated, motor and verbal skills lost, general and focal neurological deficits, totally dependent in ADL

3. Nursing management

a. Structure the environment—prevent overstimulation, provide consistency, prepare client for changes in routine, reality and validation therapy, present change gradually

b. Promote independence in ADL—use occupational therapy as resource

c. Promote bowel and bladder continence—take client to bathroom frequently throughout the day, less frequently at night

d. Assist with facial recognition—encourage presence of family pictures and reminiscing

e. Medication therapy—use of donepezil and galantamine to improve cognitive function; also, antidepressants and other psychotropic medications may be appropriate to relieve hallucinations and delusions, promote sleep, N-methyl-D-aspartate (NMDA) receptor antagonists (e.g. memantine)

f. Severe—provide support; assist family to explore hospice support

4. Complementary/alternative therapy

a. Ingesting fish (a source of omega-3 fatty acids) one or more times per week may decrease the incidence of Alzheimer disease

b. Vitamin E 1,000 international units bid to delay loss of activities of daily living; progression to a rating score of 3 or death

c. *Ginkgo biloba* supplement

# ALTERATIONS IN VISION

## Sensory Perception, Client Education: Providing

## Anatomy of the Eye

(*see* Figure 11-4)

A. Three layers
   1. Sclera—fibrous outer coat
   2. Choroid—middle vascular coat
   3. Retina—inner nerve coat

B. Cornea
   1. Dome-like structure that forms most of the anterior portion of the eye
   2. Main refracting surface of the eye

C. Lens
   1. Lies behind pupil and iris
   2. Held in position by suspensory ligament attached to the ciliary body
   3. Elastic qualities allow accommodation to focus image on retina

D. Iris
   1. Colored portion of eye
   2. Attached around circumference by ciliary body
   3. Opening at center—pupil
   4. Controls the amount of light entering eye

E. Retina
   1. Innermost lining of the eye
   2. Contains rods and cones
      a. Rods function with colorless, twilight vision
      b. Cones function with perception of color and bright, daylight vision

c. Optic disk

1) Point of entrance of nerve and blood vessels

2) Blind spot

3) Most prominent structure visible on the fundus (retina lining at the back of eye)

a) Excessive pallor signals optic atrophy, a partial or complete destruction of the optic nerve

b) Excessive redness—may signal beginning papilledema inflammation

c) Papilledema (choked disks: severe form)

i) May be caused by inflammation

ii) May signal passive congestion from ICP

F. Gerontologic considerations

1. Cornea thickens and flattens; increased incidence of astigmatism

2. Lens thickens; decreased anterior chamber size; intraocular pressure increases; increased risk of glaucoma

3. Lens opacity increases; increased risk of cataracts

4. Retina degeneration—decreased visual acuity and color perception

5. Lacrimal apparatus—decreased tear production

6. Iris rigidity—smaller pupils; decreased response to light stimulation

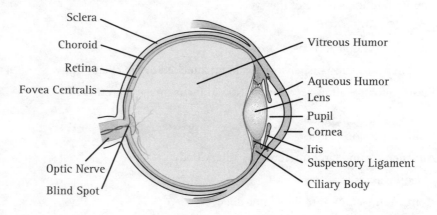

**Figure 11-4.** Anatomy of the Eye

# Visual Function

A. Assessment (*see* Table 11-12)

B. Signs and symptoms of eye problems

1. Redness, pain, and burning

2. Edema

3. Increased lacrimation and exudate

4. Headache

5. Nausea and vomiting

6. Squinting

7. Visual disturbances

8. Disorders of accommodation (*see* Table 11-13)

**Table 11-12** Visual Function Tests

| TEST | PROCEDURE | CLIENT PREPARATION |
|------|-----------|-------------------|
| Tonometry—measures intraocular pressure | Cornea is anesthetized<br><br>Tonometer registers degree of indentation on cornea when pressure is applied<br><br>Pressure increased in glaucoma | Client will be recumbent or sitting<br><br>Remove contact lenses<br><br>Advise not to squint, cough, or hold breath during the procedure |
| Visual fields—measurement of range of vision (perimetry) | Client is seated a measured distance from chart of concentric circles<br><br>Client is asked to fix eyes on a point on a chart at center of circle<br><br>Client instructed to indicate when client first sees pointer; this point is recorded as a point in field of vision<br><br>This procedure is repeated around 360° of a circle<br><br>Normal visual fields for each eye are approximately a 50° angle superiorly, 90° laterally, 70° inferiorly, and 60° medially | None |
| Snellen test—test of visual acuity | Client stands 20 ft from chart of letters<br><br>One eye is covered at a time<br><br>Client reads chart to smallest letter visible<br><br>Test results indicate comparison of distance at which this client reads to what normal eye sees at 20 ft | None |

**Table 11-13** Disorders of Accommodation

| TYPES | NURSING CONSIDERATIONS |
| --- | --- |
| Myopia (nearsightedness)—light rays refract at a point in front of the retina | Corrective lenses |
| Hyperopia (farsightedness)—light rays refract behind the retina | Corrective lenses |
| Presbyopia with aging | Commonly occurs after age 35 Corrective lenses |
| Astigmatism—uneven curvature of cornea causing blurring of vision | Corrective lenses |

C. Treatments

  1. Eye irrigation—method

     a. Tilt head back and toward the side of affected area

     b. Allow irrigating fluid to flow from the inner to the outer canthus

     c. Use a small bulb syringe or eyedropper to dispense fluid

     d. Place small basin close to head to collect excess fluid and drainage

  2. Eyedrop instillation (*see* Table 11-14)

     1) Wash hands before instillation

     2) Do not allow dropper to touch eye

     3) Do not allow drops from eye to flow across nose into opposite eye

     a. Tilt head back and look up; pull lid down

     b. Place drops into center of lower conjunctival sac

        1) Instruct client not to squeeze eye

        2) Teach client to blink between drops

     c. To prevent systemic absorption, press the inner canthus near the bridge of the nose for 1–2 minutes

     d. Equipment must be sterile

**Table 11-14** Instillation of Eyedrops

| A. | Equipment must be sterile.<br><br>Teach handwashing before instillation.<br>Do not allow dropper to touch eye.<br>Do not allow drops from one eye to flow across nose or into opposite eye. |
|---|---|
| B. | Tile head back.<br><br>Allow overflow to go out temporal side of eye. |
| C. | Place drops into lower conjunctival sac.<br><br>Instruct client not to squeeze eye.<br>Teach client to blink between drops. |
| D. | To prevent systemic absorption, press the inner angle of eye after instillation. |

**D.** Nursing management of eye emergencies

1. Prevent eye injuries
   a. Provide safe toys
   b. Use of eye protectors when working with chemicals, tools
   c. Use of eye protectors during sports
   d. Protect eyes from ultraviolet light
   e. Instructions for first aid
2. Emergency treatment
   a. Burns (*see* Table 11-15)
   b. Trauma (*see* Table 11-16)

**Table 11-15** Burns of the Eye

| TYPES | NURSING CONSIDERATIONS |
|---|---|
| Chemical:<br><br>Acids, cleansers, insecticides | Eye irrigation with copious amounts of water for 15–20 min |
| Radiation:<br><br>Sun, lightning, eclipses | Prevention—use of eye shields |
| Thermal:<br><br>Hot metals, liquids, other occupational hazards | Use of goggles to protect the cornea; patching; analgesics |

**Table 11-16** Eye Trauma

| TYPES | NURSING CONSIDERATIONS |
|---|---|
| Nonpenetrating—abrasions | Eye patch for 24 h |
| Nonpenetrating—contusions | Cold compresses, analgesics |
| Penetrating—pointed or sharp objects | Cover with patch; refer to surgeon |

# Loss of Visual Function

A.  Assessment

    1.  Adjustment to vision loss depends upon:

        a.  Age of onset

        b.  Degree of suddenness

    2.  Principles of working with blind persons

        a.  Facilitate normal lifestyle patterns

            1)  Adapted household equipment

            2)  Books and newspapers with large print for partially sighted

            3)  Provide information concerning aids for the blind

            4)  Braille

            5)  Canes

            6)  Guide dogs

            7)  Facilitate developmental patterns

            8)  Encourage social development

            9)  Provide for education and employment

    3.  Nursing management of the blind client

        a.  Enhance communication

            1)  Address client by name

            2)  Always introduce self

            3)  State reason for being there

            4)  Inform client when leaving the room

        b.  Provide sense of safety and security

            1)  Explain all procedures in detail

            2)  Keep furniture arrangement consistent

            3)  Provide handrail

            4)  Doors should never be half open

            5)  Have client follow attendant when walking by lightly touching attendant's elbow (half step ahead)

            6)  Instruct client in use of lightweight walking stick when walking alone

c. Foster sense of independence

　　1) Provide assistance only when needed

　　2) Identify food and location on plate or tray

　　3) Encourage recreational and leisure time activities

## Care for the Client Undergoing Eye Surgery

**A.** Preoperative care

　1. Assessment of visual acuity

　2. Preparation of periorbital area

　3. Orientation to surroundings

　4. Preoperative teaching—prepare for postoperative course

　5. Teach postop necessity to avoid straining with stool, stooping

**B.** Postoperative care

　1. Observe for complications—hemorrhage, sharp pain, infection

　2. Avoid sneezing, coughing, straining with stool, bending down

　3. Protect from injury; restrict activity

　4. Keep signal bell within reach

　5. Administer medications as ordered; medication for nausea, vomiting, restlessness

　6. Shield worn for protective purposes

　7. Discharge teaching—avoid stooping or straining at stool; use proper body mechanics

## Selected Disorders of the Eye

**A.** Detached retina

　1. History

　　a. Flashes of light

　　b. Blurred or "sooty" vision, "floaters"

　　c. Sensation of particles moving in line of vision

　　d. Delineated areas of vision blank

　　e. A feeling of a curtain coming up or down

　　f. Loss of vision

　　g. Confusion, apprehension

　2. Characteristics

　　a. Separation of the retina from the choroid

　　b. Cause

　　　1) Trauma

　　　2) Aging process

　　　3) Diabetes

　　　4) Tumors

      c.  Medical management

         1)  Sedatives and tranquilizers

         2)  Surgery—retina to adhere to choroid

   3.  Nursing management

      a.  Bedrest, do not bend forward, avoid excessive movements

      b.  Affected eye or both eyes may be patched to decrease movement of eye(s)

      c.  Specific positioning—area of detachment should be in the dependent position

      d.  Take precautions to avoid bumping head, moving eyes rapidly, or rapidly jerking the head

      e.  Hair washing delayed for 1 wk

      f.  Avoid strenuous activity for 3 mo

**B.**  Cataracts

   1.  History

      a.  Objects appear distorted and blurred

      b.  Annoying glare

      c.  Pupil changes from black to gray to milky white

   2.  Assessment

      a.  Partial or total opacity of the normally transparent crystalline lens

      b.  Cause

         1)  Congenital

         2)  Trauma

         3)  Aging process

         4)  Associated with diabetes mellitus, intraocular surgery

         5)  Medications—steroid therapy

      c.  Surgical management—laser surgery

         1)  Extracapsular extraction—cut through the anterior capsule to express the opaque lens material

         2)  Intracapsular extraction (method of choice)—removal of entire lens and capsule

         3)  Lens implantation

   3.  Nursing management

      a.  Observe for postoperative complications

         1)  Hemorrhage

         2)  Increased intraocular pressure

         3)  Slipped suture(s)

         4)  If lens implant, pupil should remain constricted; if aphakic, pupil remains dilated

      b.  Avoid straining and no heavy lifting

      c.  Bend from the knees only to pick up things

    d. Instruct about instillation of eyedrops, use of night shields

    e. Protect eye from bright lights

    f. Adjustments needed in perception if aphakic

    g. Diversional activities

**C.** Glaucoma

  1. Assessment

    a. Cloudy, blurry, or loss of vision

    b. Artificial lights appear to have rainbows or halos around them

    c. Loss of vision

    d. Decreased peripheral vision

    e. Pain, headache

    f. Nausea, vomiting

    g. Tonometer readings exceed normal intraocular pressure (10–21 mm Hg)

  2. Characteristics

    a. Abnormal increase in intraocular pressure leading to visual disability and blindness—obstruction of outflow of aqueous humor

    b. Types

      1) Angle closure (closed-angle); sudden onset, emergency

      2) Open-angle (primary); most common; blockage of aqueous humor flow

    c. Causes

      1) Closed-angle glaucoma—associated with ocular diseases, trauma

      2) Open-angle glaucoma—associated with aging, heredity, retinal vein occlusion

    d. Treatment of closed-angle glaucoma (*see* Table 11-17)

      1) Medications—miotics, carbonic anhydrase inhibitors, oral glycerin and mannitol

      2) Surgery

    e. Treatment of open-angle glaucoma

      1) Medications—miotics, carbonic anhydrase inhibitors, anticholinesterase beta-blocking agents, adrenergic agonists, prostaglandin agonists

      2) Surgery—laser trabeculoplasty, standard glaucoma surgery

    f. Common nursing diagnosis—sensory/perceptual/visual alteration

  3. Nursing management

    a. Compliance with medical therapy

    b. Avoid tight clothing (e.g., collars)

    c. Reduce external stimuli

    d. Avoid heavy lifting, straining at stool

    e. Avoid use of mydriatics

**Table 11-17** Eye Medications

| MEDICATION | ADVERSE EFFECTS | NURSING CONSIDERATIONS |
|---|---|---|
| Methylcellulose | Eye irritation if excess is allowed to dry on eyelids | Lubricant<br><br>Use eyewash to rinse eyelids of "sandy" sensation felt after administration |
| Polyvinyl alcohol | Blurred vision<br><br>Burning | Artificial tears<br><br>Applied to contact lenses before insertion |
| Tetrahydrozoline | Cardiac irregularities<br><br>Pupillary dilation, increased intraocular pressure<br><br>Transient stinging | Used for ocular congestion, irritation, allergic conditions<br><br>Rebound congestion may occur with frequent or prolonged use<br><br>Apply light pressure on lacrimal sac for 1 min following instillation |
| Timolol maleate | Eye irritation<br><br>Hypotension | Beta-blocking agent<br><br>Reduces intraocular pressure in management of glaucoma<br><br>Apply light pressure on lacrimal sac for 1 min following instillation<br><br>Monitor BP and pulse |
| **Action** | Causes vasoconstriction by local adrenergic action | |
| **Indications** | Ocular irritation | |
| **Adverse effects** | Headache<br><br>Dizziness<br><br>Transient stinging in eye<br><br>Pupillary dilation<br><br>Photophobia | |
| **Nursing considerations** | Apply light pressure on lacrimal sac for 1 min after instilling drops<br><br>Rebound congestion may occur with prolonged use | |

f.  Educate public to five danger signs of glaucoma:

1)  Brow arching

2)  Halos around lights

3)  Blurry vision

4)  Diminished peripheral vision

5)  Headache or eye pain

# ALTERATIONS IN HEARING

## Sensory Perception, Client Education: Providing

## Anatomy and Physiology of Ear

(*see* Figure 11-5)

A. External ear

1. Pinna or auricle
2. External acoustic meatus
3. External auditory canal

B. Middle ear

1. Located in temporal bone
2. Contains ossicles
   a. Malleus
   b. Incus
   c. Stapes
3. Eustachian tube—connects middle ear to the throat and assists in equalizing pressure in middle ear
4. Physiology of sound
   a. Sound waves enter external auditory canal to tympanic membrane
   b. Tympanic membrane vibrates, triggering ossicles (malleus, incus, stapes)
   c. Vibration transmitted to oval window to acoustic nerve and brain

C. Inner ear

1. Contains vestibule, semicircular canals, and cochlea (labyrinth)
2. Movement of the sensory hairs signals changes in position; aids in maintaining stable posture

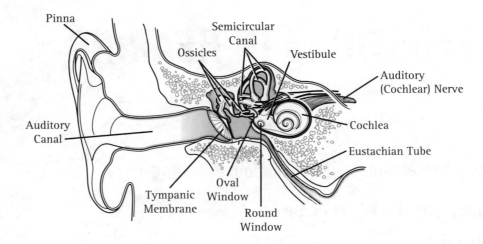

**Figure 11-5.** Anatomy and Physiology of the Ear

    **D.**  Gerontologic considerations

        1.  Ear canal narrows

        2.  Cerumen glands atrophy; dried cerumen

        3.  Tympanic membrane flexibility decreases; decreased sound transmission in middle ear

        4.  Decreased ability to hear high-frequency sounds

## Alterations in Function

    **A.**  Assessment

        1.  Signs and symptoms

            a.  Pain, fever

            b.  Headache

            c.  Discharge

            d.  Altered growth and development

            e.  Personality changes, e.g., irritability, depression, suspiciousness, withdrawal

        2.  Diagnostics

            a.  Audiogram—quantitative, i.e., degree of loss

            b.  Tuning fork—qualitative, i.e., type of loss

    **B.**  Types of hearing loss

        1.  Conductive loss—disorder in auditory canal, eardrum, or ossicles

            a.  Causes

                1)  Infection

                2)  Inflammation

                3)  Foreign body

                4)  Trauma

            b.  Complications—meningitis resulting from initial infection

c. Management

1) Heat

2) Antibiotics

3) Ear drops, ointments, irrigation

4) Surgery

5) Hearing aid

2. Perceptive (sensorineural loss)—due to disorder of the organ of Corti or the auditory nerve

   a. Causes

      1) Congenital—maternal exposure to communicable disease

      2) Infection, medication toxicity

      3) Trauma

      4) Labyrinth dysfunction—Ménière disease

   b. Complications

      1) Vertigo

      2) Tinnitus

      3) Vomiting

   c. Management

      1) Medication

      2) Surgery

      3) Combined loss—conductive and sensorineural

      4) Psychogenic loss—functional

**C.** Nursing management of ear infections

1. Ear irrigation—method

   a. Tilt head toward side of affected ear; gently direct stream of fluid against sides of canal

   b. After procedure, instruct client to lie on affected side to facilitate drainage

   c. Contraindicated if there is evidence of swelling or tenderness

2. Ear drop instillation—method

   a. Position the affected ear uppermost

   b. Pull outer ear upward and backward for preschoolers through adults (3 years of age and older)

   c. Pull outer ear downward and backward for infants and toddlers (under 3 years of age)

   d. Place drops so they run down the wall of ear canal

   e. Have client lie on unaffected ear to encourage absorption

    **D.**  Nursing management for clients undergoing ear surgery

        1.  Preoperative care

           a.  Assessment of preoperative symptoms

           b.  Prep depends on nature of incision

           c.  Encourage client to wash hair prior to surgery

           d.  Teaching—expect postoperative hearing loss and discuss need for special position of operative ear as ordered

        2.  Postoperative care

           a.  Reinforce dressing only; avoid nose blowing, sneezing, and coughing

           b.  Observe for possible complications

               1)  Facial nerve damage—may be transient

               2)  Infection

               3)  Vertigo, tinnitus

               4)  Do not apply pressure if bleeding is noted on internal ear surgery—notify health care provider immediately

               5)  Administer medications

               6)  Provide for client safety

           c.  Discharge teaching—avoid getting water into ear, flying, drafts, crowds, exercise caution around people with respiratory infections

## Selected Disorders

    **A.**  Acute otitis media

        1.  Assessment

           a.  Fever, chills

           b.  Headache

           c.  Ringing in ears

           d.  Deafness

           e.  Sharp pain

           f.  Head rolling, crying, ear tugging (child)

           g.  Nausea, vomiting

           h.  Red, bulging tympanic membrane

        2.  Characteristics

           a.  Infection of middle ear

           b.  Cause—pathogenic organisms, i.e., bacteria and viruses

    c.  Complications

        1)  Chronic otitis media—children more susceptible due to short eustachian tube

        2)  Residual deafness

        3)  Perforation of tympanic membrane

        4)  Cholesteatoma growth

        5)  Mastoiditis or meningitis

    d.  Medical and surgical management

        1)  Antibiotics—organism specific

        2)  Antihistamines for allergies

        3)  Nasal decongestants

        4)  Ventilatory tubes—inserted into eustachian tube for continuous ventilation

        5)  Myringotomy—tympanic membrane incision to relieve pressure and release purulent fluid

    e.  Nursing management

        1)  Administer medication as ordered

        2)  Report persistent symptoms to health care provider

        3)  Following a myringotomy—no water can be allowed to enter the ear

        4)  Bedrest if temperature is elevated

        5)  Position on side of involved ear to promote drainage

**B.**  Mastoiditis

  1.  Assessment

    a.  Fever, chills

    b.  Headache, dizziness

    c.  Deafness

    d.  Auricle discharge

    e.  Pain, tenderness

    f.  Stiff neck

    g.  Facial paralysis

    h.  Vomiting

    i.  Can cause meningitis

  2.  Characteristics

    a.  Inflammation of mastoid

    b.  Cause—middle ear infection

  3.  Medical/surgical treatment

    a.  Antibiotic therapy

    b.  Mastoidectomy—removal of mastoid cells

4. Nursing management

   a. Observe for postoperative complications

      1) Facial nerve injury—facial paralysis

      2) Infection

      3) Vertigo

   b. Administer medications as ordered

**C.** Ménière disease

  1. Assessment

   a. Decreased hearing on involved side

   b. Tinnitus

   c. Headache, nystagmus, rapid eye movements

   d. Vertigo

   e. Anxiety

   f. Nausea, vomiting

  2. Characteristics

   a. Dilation of the membrane of the labyrinth

   b. Complication—hearing loss

   c. Medical and nursing management

      1) Salt-free and neutral ash diet (Furstenberg diet)—restrict water and salt intake

      2) Symptomatic treatment, i.e., antiemetics, antihistamines, vasodilators, antivertigo medications, diuretics

      3) Decompression of endolymphatic sac with Teflon shunt (method of choice)

      4) Total labyrinthectomy—last resort with the possible complication of Bell palsy

      5) Cochlear implant

      6) Client education

         a) Need to slow down body movements—jerking or sudden movements may precipitate attack

         b) Need for self-protection and to lie down when an attack takes place

         c) If driving, pull over and stop car

         d) Occupational counseling—if occupation involves operating machinery

# End-of-Chapter Thinking Exercise

(0700) The nurse receives a handoff report on a young adult client in the intensive care unit (ICU). The client was admitted last night following a motor vehicle collision with a tree. The car rolled and the client, who was the driver, was not wearing a seatbelt. The client sustained a closed head injury and fractured left radius and ulna that will require surgical repair as soon as there is an opening on the surgery schedule. The client was unconscious at the scene but upon arrival to the emergency department (ED) responded to painful stimuli with a Glasgow Coma Scale (GCS) of 12 and bilaterally sluggish pupillary response. Toxicology screening revealed an elevated blood alcohol level. When admitted to the ICU, the client was alert and oriented to person, place, and time but did not recall the accident. Seizure precautions were initiated. The client reported a headache of 6/10 and left arm pain 10/10. Morphine sulfate 2 mg IVP given at 0610. IV 0.9% NaCl at 100 mL/hr to a 20 gauge IV in the right forearm.

(0720) The nurse assesses the client and finds the client unresponsive with vital signs below.

| VITAL SIGNS | 0400 | 0720 |
|---|---|---|
| BP | 162/84 | 178/54 |
| HR | 72 | 56 |
| RR | 20 | 13, irregular |
| T | 98.8°F (37.1°C) | 99.4°F (37.4°C) |
| SpO$_2$ | 98% on room air | 94% on room air |

1. Which assessment findings at 0720 indicate a possible increase in intracranial pressure (ICP)? (Analyze Cues)

2. Which actions does the nurse take? (Take Action)

3. IV mannitol is administered at 0735. An ICP catheter is placed at 0800 with an initial reading of 27 mm Hg. Surgical repair of the client's arm fractures is put on hold. Throughout the nurse's 12-hour shift, the client's condition stabilizes. What criteria does the nurse use to determine that the client is improving? (Evaluate Outcomes)

# Thinking Exercise Explanations

1. Which assessment findings indicate a possible increase in intracranial pressure (ICP)? (Analyze Cues)

   • Change in level of consciousness (LOC)

   • Widening pulse pressure (increasing systolic, decreasing diastolic)

   • Bradycardia

   • Irregular respirations

   An early sign of increased ICP is a change in LOC. If ICP is not managed, vital signs will deteriorate and affect perfusion to the brain and other vital organs. Widening pulse pressure, bradycardia, and irregular respirations (i.e., Cushing triad) indicate increased ICP.

2. Which actions does the nurse take? (Take Action)

   • Notify the health care provider

   • Ensure the head of bed (HOB) is 15–30°

   • Obtain supplies for ICP catheter insertion

   • Ensure seizure precautions are in place

   • Reduce environmental stimuli

   • Continue monitoring vital signs and LOC

   The nurse should immediately contact the health care provider as this is an emergent situation. Ensuring the HOB is elevated (up to 30°), implementing seizure precautions, reducing environmental stimuli, and anticipating ICP catheter placement are all intended to ensure the client's safety. Ongoing monitoring of vital signs and LOC will provide the nurse with timely data to evaluate the client's condition and take additional action if necessary.

3. IV mannitol is administered at 0735. An ICP catheter is placed at 0800 with an initial reading of 27 mm Hg. Surgical repair of the client's arm fractures is put on hold. Throughout the nurse's 12-hour shift, the client's condition stabilizes. What criteria does the nurse use to determine that the client is improving? (Evaluate Outcomes)

   • Stabilizing vital signs, for example, BP 150/72, HR 72, respirations 16 and regular

   • Improving LOC, for example, rouses to verbal stimuli and obeys commands

   • Improving ICP readings, closer to the normal range of 5–15 mm Hg

   • Improving pupillary response, for example, bilateral pupils now briskly reactive to light

   The nurse needs to continue closely monitoring the client using the above parameters.

# ONCOLOGY

# CANCER

## Cellular Regulation, Comfort

## Cancer

A group of many diseases of multiple causes that can arise in any cell that is able to evade regulatory controls over cell proliferation and differentiation

A. Assessment

   1. American Cancer Society warning signs

      a. <u>C</u>hange in bowel, bladder habits

      b. <u>A</u> sore that does not heal

      c. <u>U</u>nusual bleeding or discharge from any body orifice

      d. <u>T</u>hickening or a lump in the breast or elsewhere

      e. <u>I</u>ndigestion or difficulty in swallowing

      f. <u>O</u>bvious change in a wart or mole

      g. <u>N</u>agging cough or hoarseness

B. Etiology

   1. Defect in cellular proliferation

      a. Proliferation is indiscriminate and continuous

      b. Continuous growth of tumor mass: pyramid effect

   2. Defect in cellular differentiation

      a. Oncogenes interfere with normal cell expression, causing cells to be malignant

      b. Cells regain fetal appearance and function

      c. Some cells produce hormones; others produce proteins

   3. Development of cancer (multifactorial)

      a. Physical

         1) Radiation—excessive exposure to sunlight, ultraviolet radiation, and ionizing radiation

         2) Chronic irritation

         3) Foreign bodies

b.  Malignancies correlated with physical factors

1)  Leukemias

2)  Lymphoma

3)  Thyroid cancer

4)  Bone cancer

5)  Lung cancer (asbestos related)

c.  Chemical

1)  Food additives, e.g., nitrates

2)  Dietary factors

3)  Pharmaceutical, e.g., stilbestrol

4)  Smoking

5)  Alcohol

d.  Malignancies correlated with chemical factors

1)  Vaginal cancer

2)  Acute myelogenous leukemia

3)  Non-Hodgkin lymphoma

4)  Multiple myeloma

5)  Lung cancer

e.  Genetic

1)  Strong predisposition

2)  Inherited chromosomal abnormalities

f.  Cancers with a genetic component

1)  Lung cancer

2)  Breast cancer

3)  Leukemia

4)  Uterine cancer

5)  Colon cancer

6)  Neuroblastoma

g.  Viral—incorporated into cell genesis

1)  DNA and RNA viruses induce malignancies

2)  Epstein-Barr virus, Burkitt lymphoma

h.  Stress—inhibits immune surveillance system

4.  Classifications

a.  Carcinoma/adenocarcinoma—epithelial tissue

b.  Sarcoma—connective tissue

c.  Lymphoma—lymphoid tissue

d.  Leukemia—blood-forming tissue (WBCs and platelets)

e. Multiple myeloma—plasma

f. Neuroblastoma—nerve cells

g. Meningeal sarcoma—meninges

C. Nursing management

1. Chemotherapy (*see* Tables 12-1 through 12-8)

2. Radiotherapy—gamma, beta, and alpha rays

a. External radiation (e.g., cobalt); external beam (teletherapy)

1) Leave radiology markings intact on skin

2) Avoid creams or lotions, deodorants, perfumes (only vitamin A and D ointment permitted)

3) Use lukewarm water to cleanse area

4) Assess skin for redness, cracking

5) Administer antiemetics for nausea, analgesics for pain

6) Observe skin, mucous membranes, and hair follicles for adverse effects

7) No hot water bottle, tape; don't expose area to cold or sunlight

8) Wear cotton clothing

**Table 12-1** Antineoplastic Medications: Alkylating Agents

| | |
|---|---|
| **Example** | Cyclophosphamide |
| **Actions** | Interferes with rapidly reproducing cell DNA |
| **Indications** | Leukemia |
| | Multiple myeloma |
| **Adverse effects** | Bone marrow suppression |
| | Nausea, vomiting |
| | Stomatitis |
| | Alopecia |
| | Gonadal suppression |
| | Renal toxicity (cisplatin) |
| | Ototoxicity (Cisplatin) |
| **Nursing considerations** | Used with other chemotherapeutic agents |
| | Check hematopoietic function weekly |
| | Encourage fluids (10-12 glasses/day) |

**Table 12-2** Antineoplastic Medications: Antimetabolites

| | |
|---|---|
| **Examples** | Fluorouracil |
| | Mercaptopurine |
| | Methotrexate |
| **Actions** | Closely resembles normal metabolites, "counterfeits" fool cells; cell division halted |
| **Indications** | Acute lymphatic leukemia |
| | Rheumatoid arthritis |
| | Psoriasis |
| | Cancer of colon, breast, stomach, pancreas |
| | Sickle cell anemia |
| **Adverse effects** | Nausea, vomiting |
| | Diarrhea |
| | Oral ulceration |
| | Hepatic dysfunction |
| | Bone marrow suppression |
| | Renal dysfunction |
| | Alopecia |
| **Nursing considerations** | Monitor hematopoietic function |
| | Good mouth care |
| | Small frequent feedings |
| | Counsel about body image changes (alopecia); provide wig |
| | Good skin care |
| | Photosensitivity precautions |
| | Infection control precautions |

**Table 12-3** Antineoplastic Medications: Antitumor Antibiotics

| Examples | Dactinomycin |
| --- | --- |
| | Doxorubicin |
| **Actions** | Interferes with DNA and RNA synthesis |
| **Indications** | Hodgkin disease |
| | Non-Hodgkin lymphoma |
| | Leukemia |
| | Many cancers |
| **Adverse effects** | Bone marrow depression |
| | Nausea, vomiting |
| | Alopecia |
| | Stomatitis |
| | Heart damage |
| | Septic shock |
| **Nursing considerations** | Monitor closely for septicemic reactions |
| | Monitor for manifestations of extravasation at injection site (severe pain or burning that lasts minutes to hours, redness after injection is completed, ulceration after 48 hours) Instruct client that urine and tears may be red in color |
| | Monitor for signs of heart failure |

**Table 12-4** Antineoplastic Medications: Hormonal Agents

| Examples | Antiestrogen: |
| --- | --- |
| |     Tamoxifen |
| | Aromatase inhibitors: |
| |     Anastrozole |
| |     Letrozole |
| |     Exemestane |
| | Gonadotropin-releasing hormone agonist: |
| |     Leuprolide |
| | Gonadotropin-releasing hormone antagonist: |
| |     Degarelix |

*(Continued)*

**Table 12-4** Antineoplastic Medications: Hormonal Agents (*Continued*)

| Actions | Tamoxifen—antiestrogen (competes with estrogen to bind at estrogen receptor sites on malignant cells) |
|---|---|
| | Leuprolide—progestin (causes tumor cell regression by unknown mechanism) |
| | Testolactone—androgen (used for palliation in advanced breast cancer) |
| **Indications** | Breast cancer |
| **Adverse effects** | Hypercalcemia |
| | Jaundice |
| | Increased appetite |
| | Masculinization or feminization |
| | Sodium and fluid retention |
| | Nausea, vomiting |
| | Hot flashes |
| | Vaginal dryness |
| **Nursing considerations** | Baseline and periodic gyn exams |
| | Not given IV |
| | Discuss pregnancy prevention |

**Table 12-5** Antineoplastic Medications: Vinca Alkaloids

| Examples | Vinblastine sulfate |
|---|---|
| | Vincristine sulfate |
| **Actions** | Interferes with cell division |
| **Indications** | Hodgkin disease |
| | Lymphoma |
| | Cancers |
| **Adverse effects** | Bone marrow suppression (mild with vincristine) |
| | Neuropathies (vincristine) |
| | Stomatitis |
| **Nursing considerations** | Same as antitumor antibiotics |

**Table 12-6** Antineoplastic Medications: DNA Topoisomerase

| Examples | Irinotecan |
| --- | --- |
| | Topotecan |
| Actions | Binds to enzyme that breaks the DNA strands |
| Indications | Ovary, lung, colon, and rectal cancers |
| Adverse effects | Bone marrow suppression |
| | Diarrhea |
| | Nausea, vomiting |
| | Hepatotoxicity |

**Table 12-7** Antineoplastic Medications: Overview

| MEDICATION | ADVERSE EFFECTS | NURSING CONSIDERATIONS |
| --- | --- | --- |
| **Alkylating Agents** | | |
| Busulfan | Bone marrow depression | Check CBC (applies to all medications in this table) |
| | | Most chemotherapy causes stomatitis and requires extra fluids to flush system |
| Chlorambucil | Nausea, vomiting, bone marrow depression, sterility | Monitor for infection |
| | | Avoid IM injections when platelet count is low to minimize bleeding |
| Cyclophosphamide | Alopecia, bone marrow depression, hemorrhagic cystitis, dermatitis, hyperkalemia, hypoglycemia, amenorrhea | Report hematuria, force fluids |
| | | Monitor for infection |
| | | Give antiemetics |
| **Platinum Compound** | | |
| Cisplatin | Anaphylactic-type reaction, seizures, hearing loss, renal toxicity, leukopenia, thrombocytopenia | Monitor dosing |
| | | Assess frequently for ototoxicity assess for renal toxicity |
| **Antimetabolites** | | |
| Fluorouracil | Nausea, stomatitis, GI ulceration, diarrhea, bone marrow depression, liver dysfunction, alopecia | Monitor for infection |
| | | Avoid extravasation |

*(Continued)*

**Table 12-7** Antineoplastic Medications: Overview (*Continued*)

| MEDICATION | ADVERSE EFFECTS | NURSING CONSIDERATIONS |
|---|---|---|
| Methotrexate | Oral and GI ulceration, liver damage, bone marrow depression, stomatitis, alopecia, bloody diarrhea, fatigue | Good mouth care, avoid alcohol<br><br>Monitor hepatic and renal function tests |
| Mercaptopurine | Liver damage, bone marrow depression, infection, alopecia, abdominal bleeding | Check liver function tests |
| Cytarabine | Hematologic abnormalities, nausea, vomiting, rash, weight loss | Force fluids<br><br>Good oral hygiene |
| Hydroxyurea | Bone marrow depression, GI symptoms, rash | Teach client to report toxic GI symptoms promptly |
| **Antibiotic Antineoplastics** | | |
| Doxorubicin | Red urine, nausea, vomiting, stomatitis, alopecia, cardiotoxicity, blisters, bone marrow depression | Check EKG, avoid IV infiltration<br><br>Monitor vital signs closely<br><br>Good mouth care |
| Bleomycin | Nausea, vomiting, alopecia, edema of hands, pulmonary fibrosis, fever, bone marrow depression | Observe for pulmonary complications<br><br>Treat fever with acetaminophen<br><br>Check breath sounds frequently |
| Dactinomycin | Nausea, bone marrow depression | Give antiemetic before administration |
| **Vinca Alkaloids** | | |
| Vinblastine | Nausea, vomiting, stomatitis, alopecia, loss of reflexes, bone marrow depression | Avoid IV infiltration and extravasation<br><br>Give antiemetic before administration<br><br>Acute bronchospasm can occur if given IV<br><br>Allopurinol given to increase excretion and decrease buildup of urates (uric acid) |
| Vincristine | Peripheral neuritis, loss of reflexes, bone marrow depression, alopecia, GI symptoms | Avoid IV infiltration and extravasation<br><br>Check reflexes, motor and sensory function<br><br>Allopurinol given to increase excretion and decrease buildup of urates (uric acid) |

(*Continued*)

**Table 12-7** Antineoplastic Medications: Overview (*Continued*)

| MEDICATION | ADVERSE EFFECTS | NURSING CONSIDERATIONS |
|---|---|---|
| **Hormonal Agents** | | |
| Tamoxifen | Transient fall in WBC or platelets, hypercalcemia, bone pain | Check CBC<br><br>Monitor serum calcium<br><br>Nonsteroidal antiestrogen |

**Table 12-8** Antineoplastic Medications: Nursing Implications for Adverse Effects

| | |
|---|---|
| Bone marrow suppression | Monitor bleeding—bleeding gums, bruising, petechiae, guaiac stools, urine, and emesis<br><br>Avoid IM injections and rectal temperatures<br><br>Apply pressure to venipuncture sites |
| Nausea, vomiting | Monitor intake and output ratios, appetite, and nutritional intake<br><br>Prophylactic antiemetics as ordered<br><br>Smaller, more frequent meals |
| Altered immunologic response | Prevent infection by handwashing<br><br>Timely reporting of alterations in vital signs or symptoms indicating possible infection |
| Impaired oral mucous membrane; stomatitis | Oral hygiene measures |
| Fatigue | Encourage rest and discuss measures to conserve energy<br><br>Use relaxation techniques, mental imagery |

b. Internal radiation (e.g., cesium, radium, gold); brachytherapy

   1) Sealed source—mechanically positioned source of radioactive material placed in body cavity or tumor

      a) Lead container and long-handled forceps in room in event of dislodged source

      b) Save all dressings, bed linens until source is removed; then discard dressings and linens as usual

      c) Urine, feces, and linens not radioactive

      d) Do not stand close to or in line with radioactive source

      e) Client on bedrest while implant in place

      f) Position of source verified by radiography

      2) Unsealed source of radiation—unsealed liquid given orally or instilled in body cavity (e.g., iodine [$^{131}$I])

         a) All body fluids contaminated

         b) Greatest danger from body fluids during first 24–96 h

      3) Nursing management for client with internal radiation

         a) Assign client to private room

         b) Place "Caution: Radioactive Material" sign on door

         c) Wear dosimeter film badge at all times when interacting with client (offers no protection but measures amount of exposure; each nurse has individual badge)

         d) Do not assign pregnant nurse to client

         e) Rotate staff caring for client

         f) Organize tasks so limited time is spent in client's room

         g) Limit visitors

         h) Encourage client to do own care

         i) Provide shield in room

         j) Use antiemetics for nausea

         k) Consider body image (e.g., alopecia)

         l) Provide comfort measures, analgesic for pain

         m) Provide good nutrition

3. Skin care

   a. Avoid use of soaps, powders, lotions

   b. Wear cotton, loose-fitting clothing

4. Mouth care

   a. Stomatitis—develops 5–14 d after chemotherapy begins

   b. Symptoms—erythema, ulcers, bleeding

   c. Oral rinses with saline or soft-bristled toothbrush

   d. Avoid hot (temperature) or spicy foods

   e. Topical antifungals and anesthetics

5. Hair care

   a. Alopecia commonly seen, alters body image; alopecia temporary

   b. Assist with wig or hairpiece

   c. Scarves, hats

6. Nutritional changes

   a. Anorexia, nausea, and vomiting commonly seen with chemotherapy

   b. Malabsorption and cachexia (wasting) common

   c. Make meals appealing to senses

   d. Conform diet to client preferences and nutritional needs

  e. Small, frequent meals with additional supplements between meals (high-calorie, high-protein diet)

  f. Encourage fluids but limit at mealtimes

  g. Perform oral hygiene and provide relief of pain before mealtime

  h. TPN as needed

 7. Neutropenic precautions—prevent infection among clients with immunosuppression

  a. Assess skin integrity every 8 h; auscultate breath sounds, presence of cough, sore throat; check temperature every 4 h; report if greater than 101°F (38°C); monitor CBC and differential daily

  b. Private when possible

  c. Thorough hand hygiene before entering client's room

  d. Allow no staff with cold or sore throat to care for client

  e. No fresh flowers or standing water

  f. Clean room daily

  g. Low microbial diet; no fresh salads, unpeeled fresh fruits or vegetables

  h. Deep breathe every 4 h

  i. Meticulous body hygiene

  j. Inspect IV site, meticulous IV site care

 8. Pain relief—three-step ladder approach

  a. For mild pain—nonnarcotic meds (acetaminophen) along with antiemetics, antidepressants, glucocorticoids

  b. For moderate pain—weak narcotics (codeine) and nonnarcotics

  c. For severe pain—strong narcotics (morphine)

  d. Give pain meds on regularly scheduled basis (preventative approach), additional analgesics given for breakthrough pain

 9. Activity level

  a. Alternate rest and activity

  b. Maintain normal lifestyle

10. Psychosocial issues

  a. Encourage participation in self-care and decision making

  b. Provide referral to support groups, organizations

  c. Hospice care

11. Complementary/alternative therapy

  a. Vitamin E administered with cisplatin decreases the incidence and severity of treatment-associated neurotoxicity

[ SECTION 2 ]

# LEUKEMIA

## Cellular Regulation, Coagulation

## Leukemia

Fatal neoplastic disease that involves the blood-forming tissues of the bone marrow, spleen, and lymph nodes

A. Outstanding characteristic—abnormal, uncontrolled, and destructive proliferation of one type of white cell and its precursors

B. Classification of the leukemias

1. Acute leukemia—rapid onset and progresses to a fatal termination within days to months; more common among children and young adults

2. Chronic leukemia—gradual onset with a slower, more protracted course; more common between ages 25–60

C. Assessment

1. Severe infection (e.g., ulcerations of the mouth and throat, pneumonia, septicemia)— high leukocyte count (15,000–500,000/microL or higher), immature or abnormal, and consequently are unable to fight and destroy microorganisms

2. Anemia accompanied by fatigue, lethargy, hypoxia, and hemorrhage (e.g., gum bleeding, ecchymoses, petechiae, retinal hemorrhages) due to thrombocytopenia—occurs because rapidly proliferating leukocytes "crowd out" the developing erythrocytes and thrombocytes, bone and joint pain

3. Enlarged organs cause pressure on adjacent structures (e.g., splenomegaly, hepatomegaly, lymphadenopathy, bone marrow hypercellularity)—distention of tissues occurs from accumulation of high numbers of white cells

4. Increased metabolic rate accompanied by weakness, pallor, and weight loss

   a. Increased production of leukocytes requires large amounts of amino acids and vitamins

   b. Increased destruction of cells leads to increased release of metabolic wastes, which must be disposed of by the body

5. Uric acid stones, which cause renal pain, obstruction, and infection—uric acid is released as a result of the destruction of large numbers of leukocytes by antileukemic medications

6. Renal insufficiency with uremia as a late development—abnormal leukocytes infiltrate into the kidneys

7. Central nervous system symptoms (e.g., headache, disorientation, convulsions)—abnormal white cells infiltrate into the brain and nervous system

8. Diagnosis

   a. Elevated leukocyte count with a "shift to the left" (presence of large numbers of immature neutrophils)

   b. A differential leukocyte count in which one type of white cell is overwhelmingly predominant

   c. A bone marrow specimen that contains massive numbers of leukocytes

   d. A blood smear that reveals many "blast" cells

   e. The presence of anemia, bleeding, tenderness, sternal tenderness, and organ enlargement

**D.** Factors associated with development of leukemia

   1. Viruses

   2. Ionizing radiation

   3. Genetic predisposition

   4. Absorption of certain chemicals (e.g., benzene, pyridine, and aniline dyes)

**E.** Nursing management

   1. Monitor for signs of bleeding, e.g., petechiae, bruising, bleeding gums; follow bleeding precautions

   2. Monitor for signs of infection, e.g., changes in vital signs, chills

   3. Provide mouth care

   4. Provide high-calorie, high-vitamin diet

   5. Provide frequent feedings of soft, easy-to-eat foods

   6. Provide antiemetics, as ordered, for nausea and vomiting

   7. Neutropenic precautions if necessary

   8. Strict handwashing

   9. Prevent skin breakdown

   10. Administer and monitor blood transfusions (whole blood, platelets)

   11. Administer medications, as ordered, and observe for adverse effects

       a. Chemotherapy

          1) Nausea, vomiting, diarrhea

          2) Stomatitis, alopecia, skin reactions

          3) Bone marrow depression

       b. Radiation or radioisotope therapy—bone marrow transplants

# SKIN CANCER

## Cellular Regulation, Skin Integrity

## Skin Cancer

A. Assessment

   1. Basal cell carcinoma—small, waxy nodule on sun-exposed areas of body (e.g., face); may ulcerate and crust

   2. Squamous cell carcinoma—rough, thick, scaly tumor seen on arms or face

   3. Malignant melanoma—variegated color (brown, black mixed with gray or white) circular lesion with irregular edges seen on trunk or legs

B. Types

   1. Basal cell carcinoma—most common type of skin cancer; rarely metastasizes but commonly recurs

   2. Squamous cell carcinoma—may metastasize to blood or lymph

   3. Malignant melanoma—most lethal of skin cancers; frequently seen in ages 20–45; highest risk persons with fair complexions, blue eyes, red or blond hair, and freckles; metastasizes to bone, liver, spleen, CNS, lungs, lymph

   4. Diagnosed by skin lesion biopsy

C. Nursing management

   1. Postop care following surgical excision

   2. Teach prevention

      a. Avoid exposure to sun 10 A.M. to 3 P.M.

      b. Use sunscreen with solar protection factor (SPF) to block harmful rays (especially important for children)

      c. Reapply sunscreen after swimming or prolonged time in sun

      d. Use lip balm with sunscreen protection

      e. Wear hat when outdoors

      f. Do not use tanning lamps or booths

      g. Teach client to examine skin surfaces monthly

3. Teach how to identify danger signs of melanoma—change in size, color, shape of mole or surrounding skin

4. Chemotherapy for metastases

5. Complementary/alternative therapy

   a. Fish oil, vitamin E from food, normal levels of selenium, green tea, and soy may decrease risk of melanoma

   b. Nonsteroidal anti-inflammatory drugs (NSAIDs) may reduce risk of melanoma

# INTRACRANIAL TUMORS

## Intracranial Regulation, Cellular Regulation

## Intracranial Tumors

A. Assessment—signs and symptoms vary depending on location

1. Motor deficits

2. Language disturbances

3. Hearing difficulties (temporal lobe), visual disturbances (occipital lobe)

4. Dizziness, paresthesia (cerebellum), coordination problems

5. Seizures (motor cortex)—frequently first presenting sign

6. Personality disturbances (frontal lobe)

7. Papilledema

8. Nausea and vomiting

9. Drowsiness, changes in level of consciousness

B. Types

1. Types—classified according to location

a. Supratentorial—incision usually behind hairline; surgery within the cerebral hemisphere

b. Infratentorial—incision made at nape of neck around occipital lobe; surgery within brain stem and cerebellum

2. Causes—unknown

3. Medical/surgical management—intracranial surgery (burr holes, craniotomy, cranioplasty), radiation

C. Nursing management

1. Preoperative care

a. Detailed neurological assessment for baseline data

b. Head shave—prep site

c. Psychological support

d. Prepare client for postoperative course

2. Postoperative care

   a. Maintain patent airway

   b. Elevate head of bed 30–45° after supratentorial surgery

   c. Position client flat and lateral on either side after infratentorial surgery

   d. Monitor vital and neurological signs

   e. Observe for complications—respiratory difficulties, increased intracranial pressure, hyperthermia, meningitis, wound infection

   f. Administer medications—corticosteroids, osmotic diuretics, mild analgesics, anticonvulsants, antibiotics, antipyretics, antiemetics, hormone replacement as needed; limited narcotics postoperatively (masks changes in LOC)

# PANCREATIC TUMORS

## Metabolism, Cellular Regulation

## PANCREATIC TUMORS

A. Assessment

   1. Weight loss

   2. Vague upper or midabdominal discomfort

   3. Abnormal glucose tolerance test (hyperglycemia)

   4. Jaundice, clay-colored stools, dark urine

B. Types

   1. Tumors may arise from any portion of the pancreas (head or tail); each has unique clinical manifestations

C. Diagnostic tests—CT, CT-guided needle biopsy, MRI

D. Nursing/medical management

   1. Medical

      a. High-calorie, bland, low-fat diet; small, frequent feedings

      b. Avoid alcohol

      c. Anticholinergics

      d. Chemotherapy, radiation therapy, stent placement

   2. Surgery (Whipple procedure)—removal of head of pancreas, distal portion of common bile duct, the duodenum, and part of the stomach

   3. Postop care

      a. Monitor for peritonitis and intestinal obstruction

      b. Monitor for hypotension

      c. Monitor for steatorrhea

      d. Administer pancreatic enzymes

      e. Monitor for diabetes mellitus

# CARCINOMA OF THE LARYNX

## Gas Exchange, Cellular Regulation

## Carcinoma of the Larynx

A. Assessment
1. Pain radiating to the ears
2. Hoarseness, dysphagia, foul breath
3. Dyspnea
4. Enlarged cervical nodes
5. Hemoptysis

B. Diagnostic tests
1. Laryngoscopy, bronchoscopy
2. Biopsy
3. CT, MRI
4. X-rays

C. Causes
1. Industrial chemicals
2. Cigarette smoking and alcohol use
3. Straining of the vocal cords
4. Chronic laryngitis
5. Family predisposition

D. Nursing management
1. Caring for the client with a laryngectomy or laser surgery
   a. Preoperative care
      1) Explain compensatory methods of communication
      2) Referral to speech therapy
   b. Postoperative care
      1) Laryngectomy care—stoma care, suction
      2) Place in semi-Fowler position
      3) Turn, cough, and deep breathe
      4) Nasogastric gastrostomy or jejunostomy enteral nutrition

       5) Provide humidified oxygen

       6) Suction oral secretions

       7) Monitor condition of skin flap

  c. Observe for postoperative complications after laryngectomy

       1) Respiratory difficulties

       2) Fistula formation

       3) Rupture of carotid artery

       4) Stenosis of trachea

  d. Monitor weight, food intake, and fluid I and O

  e. Communication for total laryngectomy clients

       1) Esophageal speech

       2) Artificial larynx—commonly used mechanical device for speech

       3) Radiation therapy—small, localized cancers; sore throat, increased hoarseness, dysphagia

       4) Chemotherapy—alone or with radiation therapy and surgery

# End-of-Chapter Thinking Exercise

(1245) The charge nurse receives notice that a client who is currently in the radiation oncology department will be admitted following insertion of internal radiation (brachytherapy) into a tumor in the client's right breast.

(1300) The client is admitted to a private room on the oncology floor, and an assessment is completed. The client is a 46-year-old mother of two teenage sons and a 4-month-old baby girl. Upon arrival to the room, the client is alert and oriented to person, place, and time. The client tearfully states, "I know this was the right thing to do, but it's going to be so hard not seeing my kids for 5 days." Emotional support is provided. Lungs clear, abdomen soft, bedpan used, voided 400 mL clear yellow urine. Right breast dressing 2″ × 2″ dry and intact; client denies pain stating, "They numbed it really well." An 18 gauge IV with 0.45% NaCl infusing at 75 mL/hr is located in left forearm without redness or edema. Asking for lunch; advised client the diet order is to start with clear liquids and advance as tolerated. Review of orders indicates the client will be in the hospital for 5 days, the implant will be removed, and then the client will be discharged. Vital signs are below.

| VITAL SIGN | 1300 | 1830 |
| --- | --- | --- |
| BP | 162/94 mm Hg | 134/72 mm Hg |
| HR | 104 beats/minute | 82 beats/minute |
| RR | 24 breaths/minute | 14 breaths/minute |
| T | 98.2°F (36.8°C) | 99.1°F (37.3°C) |
| Pain | 0/10 | 2/10 |
| SpO$_2$ | 98% on room air | 97% on room air |

1. The nurse is precepting a new graduate nurse and asks the new graduate nurse to review the policy on brachytherapy and prepare the client teaching instructions. What does the new graduate nurse plan to teach the client? (Generate Solutions)

2. The new graduate nurse provides education to the client, who states, "I don't want someone to get cancer from taking care of me." Which action does the new graduate nurse take? (Take Action)

3. The new graduate nurse arranges a video chat with the client and family. Client was given lorazepam 0.5 mg PO at 1700. At 1830, the nurse obtains the client's vital signs and notes that the client is resting comfortably. Which findings indicate the plan of care has been effective? (Evaluate Outcomes)

# Thinking Exercise Explanations

1. The nurse is precepting a new graduate nurse and asks the new graduate nurse to review the policy on brachytherapy and prepare the client teaching instructions. What does the new graduate nurse plan to teach the client? (Generate Solutions)

   - Remain on bedrest to maintain the proper position of the internal radiation implant
   - Adults can visit for short periods of time, but children and/or pregnant persons should not spend time with the client
   - Bed linens will be placed in a linen cart and kept in the room until the radiation implant is removed
   - The lead screen is to remain between the client and the door
   - A "Caution: Radioactive Material" sign will be placed on the door

   It is important for the client to understand the teaching points so that safety is maintained and the staff and visitors have limited exposure to the radioactive material.

2. The new graduate nurse provides education to the client who states, "I don't want someone to get cancer from taking care of me." Which action does the new graduate nurse take? (Take Action)

   - Provide reassurance to the client that the staff will wear lead aprons and dosimeters to minimize and measure their exposure to radiation
   - Actively listen to the client
   - Assess the client's need for an antianxiety medication
   - Offer to help the client video chat with her spouse and children using an electronic tablet maintained on the unit
   - Relay the client's comments as well as the actions taken to the nurse

   Listening to the client's concerns and evaluating client understanding is key for the nurse to plan appropriate care. Determining that the client misunderstood the original teaching points allows the nurse to clarify and take actions to help alleviate the client's anxiety.

3. The new graduate nurse arranges a video chat with the client and family. Client was given lorazepam 0.5 mg PO at 1700. At 1830, the nurse obtains the client's vital signs and notes that the client is resting comfortably. Which findings indicate the plan of care has been effective? (Evaluate Outcomes)

   - The client accepted the antianxiety medication and was resting
   - The client's BP, HR, RR have therapeutically decreased
   - The client's temperature should be closely monitored, as the client is at risk for infection
   - The client remained in bed and used a call light for assistance with the bedpan
   - The client was able to "see" her family while keeping them safe

   Based on the 1830 vital signs, the client is experiencing mild pain. The nurse should consider the future need for a mild analgesic. Evaluating the outcomes and making adjustments to the plan of care will help the nurse to provide the most effective and supportive care to the client undergoing brachytherapy.

# [ CHAPTER 13 ]

# MATERNITY AND GYNECOLOGICAL NURSING

# THE REPRODUCTIVE SYSTEM

## Reproduction, Sexuality, Client Education: Providing Human Reproduction

A. Female

1. Anatomy

   a. External structures

      1) Mons veneris—fat pad covered with pubic hair, over symphysis pubis

      2) Labia majora—crescent-shaped fatty tissue containing folds of skin; extends down from mons veneris to perineum

      3) Labia minora—narrow folds of hairless skin between labia majora and vagina

      4) Clitoris—short, sensitive, erectile tissue; anterior junction of the vulva

      5) Perineum—area between vaginal opening and anus composed of muscles and fascia that support pelvic structures

      6) Hymen—membranous tissue over vaginal opening

      7) Urethral opening—beneath clitoris

   b. Internal organs and structures

      1) Ovaries—small oval organs located on each side of the uterus in the upper part of the pelvis; function in the development and expulsion of ova

      2) Fallopian tubes (oviduct)—two tubes, each closely adjoining an ovary

         a) Each has two openings—one into the abdominal cavity and one into the uterine cavity

         b) Function to conduct the released ovum from the ovary to the uterus

      3) Uterus—hollow, pear-shaped, thick-walled muscular structure, located between the bladder and the rectum in the pelvic cavity

         a) Composed of three sections: fundus, body, and cervix

         b) Consists of:

            i) The myometrium—involuntary muscle fibers that provide for expansion and support during pregnancy and for expulsion of fetus and control of hemorrhage during labor and delivery

ii) The endometrium—highly vascular lining that provides for implantation of fertilized ovum, shed during menstruation

c) During labor, expels the products of conception

4) Vagina—distensible mucous membrane–lined passage (birth canal) located between the bladder and rectum

5) Pelvis—the bony ring through which the fetus passes during labor and delivery; consists of four united bones (two hip or innominate bones, the sacrum, and the coccyx) between the trunk and the thighs

a) Pelvic types

i) Gynecoid—classic female pelvis inlet, well-rounded (oval); ideal for delivery

ii) Android—resembling a male pelvis, narrow and heart shaped; usually requires cesarean section or difficult forceps delivery

iii) Platypelloid—flat, broad pelvis; usually not adequate for vaginal delivery

iv) Anthropoid—similar to pelvis of anthropoid ape; long, deep, and narrow; usually adequate for vaginal delivery

b) Measurements—may be obtained by internal and external pelvic examination (using a pelvimeter), x-ray pelvimetry (used rarely in pregnancy and only late in third trimester or in labor), and ultrasound

6) Breasts—pair of accessory glands of female reproduction responsible for lactation

a) Externally covered by skin with darker-colored nipple and areola containing Montgomery's glands that lubricate the nipples

b) Internally contain the alveoli that produce the colostrum (premilk) and breast milk late in pregnancy and after delivery as well as lactiferous or mammary ducts to eject the milk

2. Physiology

a. Menstrual cycle—four phases (dates assume a 28-d cycle)

1) Menstrual phase (days 1–5)—degeneration and discharge of most of endometrium if conception does not occur

2) Proliferative phase (days 6–14)—graafian follicle is approaching maximum development in ovary (follicular fluid contains estrogen, which is responsible for the thickening of the endometrium)

3) Secretory/luteal phase (days 14–28)—corpus luteum secretes progesterone, which changes the character of the uterine lining to prepare for implantation of fertilized ovum

4) Ischemic phase—occurs if fertilization does not occur; corpus luteum degenerates; decrease in estrogen and progesterone levels; menstrual flow begins

  b. Hormonal control of menstrual cycle—pituitary gland

  1) Anterior lobe: follicle-stimulating hormone (FSH) rises slightly in the proliferative phase until just before ovulation, when both FSH and luteinizing hormone (LH) rise rapidly, triggering the rupture of the follicle

  2) Posterior lobe: secretes oxytocin and causes uterine contractions

  c. Menstrual irregularities

  1) Amenorrhea—absence of menstrual flow when normally expected; may result from congenital abnormalities, physical or emotional disorders, hormonal disturbances, and most often, pregnancy

  2) Oligomenorrhea—scanty flow

  3) Menorrhagia—excessive flow

  4) Dysmenorrhea—painful menstruation

  d. Menopause—cessation of menses and fertility, average age 50 years old

  1) Assessment—may be symptoms associated with hormonal changes, e.g., lighter or heavier flow before cessation, hot flashes and night sweats, emotional disturbances, atrophy of genitals, and decreased bladder support

  2) Management—estrogen replacement therapy (ERT), contraindicated if client/family has history of uterine or breast cancer, hypertension, or thromboembolic disease; Kegel exercises for strengthening pelvic muscle support, supplemental calcium (1 g hs) to slow osteoporosis, regular exercise, and good nutrition

  3) Complementary/alternative therapy

  a) Black cohosh

  i) Relieves hot flashes

  ii) May increase hypotensive effect of antihypertensives

  iii) Do not take for more than 6 months

3. Nursing management during female reproductive cycle

  a. Assessment

  1) Client's understanding of anatomy and the importance of periodic pelvic examinations and Pap smears

  2) Assist with pelvic examination, cultures, and Pap smear—advise no douching for at least 12 h prior to test, have client empty bladder just before exam, place client in lithotomy position

  b. Interventions

  1) Appropriate information and referrals

  2) Less emphasis on monthly breast self-exam (BSE) but more important to develop breast self-awareness; this involves becoming familiar with how breasts look and feel; many women do this through performing breast self-exams

  3) Instruct client in breast self-examination

  a) Perform examination one week after the onset of each menstrual period; if nonmenstruating, a routine monthly time, e.g., the first day of the month

       b)   Inspect breasts in the mirror first with arms at sides, second with arms above head, and third with hands on hips, always looking for asymmetry, changes in skin color or texture, dimpling, or retractions

       c)   While lying on the back and using a circular motion of the fingertips in a circular pattern around breast and into the axilla, palpate all of the tissue to detect unusual growths

       d)   Examine nipples for discharge

    4)   Contraception—assess understanding, desired form, risk factors (*see* Table 13-1)

**B.**   Normal male anatomy

    1.   External organs and structures

      a.   Scrotum—external pouch containing the testes, epididymis, and vas deferens at a slightly lower temperature than normal body temperature

      b.   Penis—organ of copulation composed of erectile tissue; allows for passage of urine and semen

    2.   Internal organs of reproduction

      a.   Testes—site of testosterone and sperm production; sperm produced continuously from puberty

      b.   Canal system

        1)   Seminiferous tubules—site of sperm production

        2)   Vas deferens—sperm storage and transport

        3)   Interstitial cells—secrete testosterone

        4)   Urethra—passage for ejaculate as well as urine

      c.   Prostate gland—accessory gland of male reproduction that enhances the transmission of sperm

**Table 13-1** Methods of Contraception

| METHOD | NURSING CONSIDERATIONS |
|---|---|
| Oral contraceptives—"the pill" | 1. Action—inhibits the release of FSH, resulting in anovulatory menstrual cycles; close to 100% effective. |
| | 2. Adverse effects—nausea and vomiting (usually occurring the first 3 months), increased susceptibility to vaginal infections. |
| | 3. Contraindications—hypertension, thromboembolic disease, and history of circulatory disease, varicosities, or diabetes mellitus. |
| | 4. Teaching—swallow whole at the same time each day. One missed pill should be taken as soon as remembered that day or two taken the next day; more than one missed pill requires use of another method of birth control for the rest of the cycle. Consume adequate amounts of vitamin B. Report severe/persistent chest pain, cough, and/or shortness of breath. Report severe abdominal pain, dizziness, weakness, and/or numbness. Report eye or speech problems, and report severe leg pain. |

*(Continued)*

**Table 13-1** Methods of Contraception (*Continued*)

| METHOD | NURSING CONSIDERATIONS |
|---|---|
| Hormone injections—medroxy-progesterone estradiol | Injectable progestin that prevents ovulation for 12 weeks. Convenient because it is unrelated to coitus (requires no action at the time of intercourse) and is 99.7% effective. Injections must be given every 12 weeks. The site should not be massaged after the injection because this accelerates the absorption and decreases the effectiveness time. Menstrual irregularity, spotting, and breakthrough bleeding are common. |
| | Return to fertility is 6 to 12 months |
| | A monthly injectable contraceptive. Similar to oral contraceptives in chemical formulation but has the advantage of monthly rather than daily dosing. Provides effective, immediate contraception within 5 days of the last normal menstrual period (LNMP) |
| | Menstrual periods less painful and with less blood loss. Return to fertility is 2–4 months |
| Intrauterine device (IUD) | 1. Action—presumed either to cause degeneration of the fertilized egg or render the uterine wall impervious to implantation; nearly 100% effective. |
| | 2. Inserted by health care provider during the client's menstrual period when the cervix is dilated. |
| | 3. Adverse effects—cramping or excessive menstrual flow (for 2–3 months); can cause infection. |
| | 4. Teaching—check for presence of the IUD string routinely, especially after each menstrual period. Report unusual cramping, late period, abnormal spotting/bleeding, abdominal pain or pain with intercourse, exposure to STDs, infection, and missing/shorter/longer IUD string. |
| Condom—rubber sheath applied over the penis | 1. Action—prevents the ejaculate and sperm from entering the vagina; helps prevent sexually transmitted disease; effective if properly used; OTC. |
| | 2. Teaching—apply to erect penis with room at the tip every time before vaginal penetration. Use a water-based lubricant, e.g., K-Y jelly, never petroleum-based lubricant. Hold the rim when withdrawing the penis from the vagina. If the condom breaks, partner should use contraceptive foam or cream immediately. |
| Female (vaginal) condom | Allows the woman some protection from disease without relying on the male condom. The device is a polyurethane pouch inserted into the vagina, with flexible rings at both ends. The closed end with its ring functions as a diaphragm. The open end with its ring partially covers the perineum. The female condom should not be used at the same time that the male partner is using a condom. Failure rates are high with the female condom, at about 21%. Increased risk of infections. |

(*Continued*)

**Table 13-1** Methods of Contraception (*Continued*)

| METHOD | NURSING CONSIDERATIONS |
| --- | --- |
| Diaphragm—flexible rubber ring with a latex-covered dome inserted into the vagina, tucked behind the pubic bone, and released to cover the cervix | 1. Action—prevents the sperm from entering the cervix; highly effective if used correctly.<br>2. Must be fitted by health care provider, and the method of inserting must be practiced by the client before use.<br>3. Risk—urinary tract infection (UTI) and toxic shock syndrome (TSS).<br>4. Teaching—diaphragm should not be inserted more than 6 hours prior to coitus; best used in conjunction with a spermicidal gel applied to rim and inside the dome before inserting. Additional spermicide is necessary if coitus is repeated. Remove at least once in 24 hours to decrease risk of toxic shock syndrome; report symptoms of UTI and TSS. |
| Vaginal spermicides (vaginal cream, foam, jellies) | 1. Action—interferes with the viability of sperm and prevents their entry into the cervix; OTC.<br>2. Teaching—must be inserted before each act of intercourse; report symptoms of allergic reaction to the chemical. |
| Natural family planning (rhythm method, basal body temperature, cervical mucus method) | 1. Action—periodic abstinence from intercourse during fertile period; based on the regularity of ovulation; has variable effectiveness.<br>2. Teaching—fertile period may be determined by a drop in basal body temperature before and a slight rise after ovulation and/or by a change in cervical mucus from thick, cloudy, and sticky during nonfertile period to more abundant, clear, thin, stretchy, and slippery as ovulation occurs. |
| Coitus interruptus | Action—man withdraws his penis before ejaculation to avoid depositing sperm into vagina; has variable effectiveness. |
| Sterilization | 1. Vasectomy (male)—terminates the passage of sperm through the vas deferens.<br>2. Usually done in health care provider's office under local anesthesia; permanent and 100% effective.<br>3. Teaching—postprocedure discomfort and swelling may be relieved by mild analgesic, ice packs, and scrotal support. Sterility not complete until the proximal vas deferens is free of sperm (about 3 months); another method of birth control must be used until two sperm-free semen analyses. Success of reversal by vasovasostomy varies from 30-85%.<br>4. Tubal ligation (female)—fallopian tubes are tied and/or cauterized through an abdominal incision, laparoscopy, or minilaparotomy.<br>5. Teaching—usual postop care and instructions; intercourse may be resumed after bleeding ceases.<br>6. Success of reversal by reconstruction of the fallopian tubes is 40-75%. |

3. Nursing management of male reproduction

   a. Assessment—client's knowledge of reproduction

   b. Teach testicular self-examination

      1) Support testes in palm of one hand, and roll each testis between the thumb and forefinger

      2) Best palpated in the shower when cremaster muscles are relaxed and testes are pendulous

      3) Report any changes in color and shape, lumps, or swelling

# Assessment and Diagnostic Tools—Female

**A.** Culdoscopy—lighted tube inserted through vagina to directly examine ovaries, fallopian tubes, uterus, and small intestines; used to rule out ectopic pregnancy, evaluate ovarian disorders and pelvic masses (see Table 13-2)

   1. Local anesthetic and/or light sedation

   2. Knee-chest position during procedure

   3. Air entering the abdominal cavity during the procedure can cause irritation of the phrenic nerve of the diaphragm; client may report severe shoulder pain when she sits up; postprocedure the client should be positioned on her abdomen with a pillow underneath to expel the air

   4. Postprocedure—assess vital signs; observe for vaginal bleeding; offer analgesic and/or back rub to relieve temporary discomfort; instruct client to avoid douching and intercourse for 2 wk

**B.** Colposcopy—colposcope (magnifies tissue) inserted into the vagina through the speculum to observe tissues for color, shape, vasculature, and lesions

**C.** Laparoscopy—lighted laparoscope inserted through an incision beneath the umbilicus to view structures in the pelvic cavity; done under general anesthesia

   1. A straight or indwelling urinary catheter is inserted to maintain bladder decompression

   2. Carbon dioxide may be introduced to distend the abdomen and enhance visualization

   3. At the end of the procedure, the $CO_2$ is released and the incision is covered with a dressing

   4. After the procedure, routine postoperative care is provided; client may be out of bed and have a regular diet as tolerated

**D.** Smears—done to identify infectious processes, the presence of abnormal cells, and hormonal changes

**E.** Cultures—taken from exudate of the vagina, cervix, or breast to diagnose syphilis, gonorrhea, genital herpes, chlamydia (requires laboratory-prepared media), or mastitis

**F.** Biopsies—samples of tissue are taken to confirm or locate a malignant lesion

   1. Cervical—to detect cancer of the cervix

      a. Punch biopsy may be done as office procedure without anesthesia; cone biopsy requires anesthesia in an operating room

      b. Postprocedural tampon for vaginal packing is left in place for 8–24 h

**Table 13-2** Female Reproductive System: Diagnostic Tests and Procedures

| STANDARD TESTS | CLIENT PREPARATION | NURSING CONSIDERATIONS |
|---|---|---|
| Culdoscopy—visualization of ovaries, fallopian tubes, uterus via lighted tube inserted into vagina and through cul-de-sac | Local anesthetic and/or light sedation | Knee-chest position during procedure<br><br>Position on abdomen after procedure<br><br>Observe for vaginal bleeding<br><br>Avoid douching and intercourse for 2 wk |
| Colposcopy—visualization of cervix and vaginal tissues for color, shape by using a lighted scope | Similar to pelvic exam<br><br>Performed between menstrual periods<br><br>Takes 20 min | Lithotomy position<br><br>Cervix is washed with dilute acetic acid |
| Laparoscopy—visualization of pelvic cavity through an incision beneath the umbilicus to view structures | Carbon dioxide introduced to enhance visualization<br><br>General anesthesia<br><br>Indwelling urinary catheter inserted for bladder decompression | Out of bed after procedure<br><br>Regular diet |
| Cultures and smears—samples of tissues are taken to identify infectious processes or abnormal cells | No anesthetic needed | *Chlamydia* smear needs media preparation by laboratory |
| Papanicolaou (Pap) test microscopic—examination of cervical cells | No vaginal intercourse or douching 24 hours before test | Lithotomy position<br><br>Client in mid-menstrual cycle<br><br>Manage discomfort |
| Biopsy—sample tissue taken to identify unusual cells | No anesthesia<br><br>May have cramping sensation<br><br>Expect restrictions on intercourse, douching, and swimming for 3 d | Provide written instructions<br><br>Refrain from douching and intercourse |

2. Endometrial—usually an office procedure with or without anesthesia; afterward the client is allowed to rest until cramping stops and advised to refrain from douching and intercourse until discharge stops

3. Dilation and curettage (D and C)—cervix dilated and the uterus scraped for biopsy tissue or aspirated for bleeding tissue

4. Breast biopsy—obtained by incision or aspiration under general or local anesthesia

**G.** Radiographic examinations—to detect abnormal tissue, presence and position of structures, patency of ducts

    1. Mammography—used to detect tumors of the breast before clinical symptoms appear; no cream, powder, or deodorant is to be used before the test

    2. Thermography—detects changes in circulation in breast tissue: increased heat in areas of increased blood supply indicates a tumor process

## Problems of the Female Reproductive Tract

(*see* Table 13-3)

**A.** Infectious processes

    1. Vaginal

        a. Simple vaginitis—characterized by a yellow discharge, itching, burning, and edema; treated with dilute vinegar douche, antibiotics, sitz baths

        b. Nonspecific vaginitis (*Gardnerella*)—presumed to be bacterial

            1) Gray-white discharge with foul/fishy odor; itching; "clue" cells on saline wet slide

            2) May be treated locally with sulfa vaginal cream; more commonly with oral metronidazole, tetracycline (both of which are contraindicated in pregnancy), or ampicillin

        c. *Candida albicans*—overgrowth of vaginal yeast

            1) Odorless, cheesy white discharge; itching, inflamed vagina and perineum

            2) Treated with topical clotrimazole, nystatin, or oral (fluconazole)

        d. *Trichomonas vaginalis*—protozoan infection

            1) Profuse green/yellow/white, malodorous, frothy discharge; irritated genitalia, itching; "strawberry" cervix

            2) Client and partner(s) are treated with metronidazole and advised to use a condom during intercourse; concurrent alcohol ingestion with metronidazole causes severe GI symptoms (disulfiram-type reaction)

        e. Atrophic vaginitis—occurs after menopause

            1) Pale, thin, dry mucosa; itching; dyspareunia

            2) Treated with topical estrogen cream, water-soluble vaginal lubricants, and sometimes antibiotic vaginal suppositories and ointments

    2. Toxic shock syndrome (TSS)

        a. Characterized by sudden onset of high fever, vomiting, diarrhea, drop in systolic blood pressure, diffuse sunburn-like macular red rash, later desquamation of palms and soles; usually *Staphylococcus aureus*

        b. Potential involvement of kidneys, CNS, gastrointestinal system, hematological system, and/or cardiovascular system; therefore, early diagnosis and treatment are important

        c. Managed with antibiotics, fluid and electrolyte replacement, education about tampon use

**Table 13-3** Problems of the Reproductive Tract

| DISORDER | ASSESSMENT | NURSING CONSIDERATIONS |
|---|---|---|
| Infertility | Inability to conceive after a year of unprotected intercourse<br><br>Tests include check of tubal patency, sperm<br><br>Affects approximately 10–15% of all couples analysis | Support and assist clients through tests<br><br>Allow expression of feelings and refer to support groups as needed<br><br>Alternatives include artificial insemination, in vitro fertilization, adoption |
| Simple vaginitis | Yellow discharge, itching, burning | Douche, antibiotics, sitz baths |
| Atrophic vaginitis | Occurs after menopause<br><br>Pale, thin, dry mucosa, itching, dyspareunia | Treated with topical estrogen cream, water-soluble vaginal lubricants, antibiotic vaginal suppositories and ointments |
| *Candida albicans* | Odorless, cheesy white discharge<br><br>Itching, inflamed vagina and perineum | Topical clotrimazole, fluconazole, nystatin |
| Toxic shock syndrome (TSS) | Sudden-onset fever, vomiting, diarrhea, drop in systolic blood pressure, and erythematous rash on palms and soles | Early diagnosis critical to avoid involvement with other organ systems<br><br>Managed with antibiotics, fluid and electrolyte replacement<br><br>Educate about use of tampons |
| Pelvic inflammatory disease (PID) | Local infection spreads to the fallopian tubes, ovaries, and other organs<br><br>Malaise, fever, abdominal pain, leukocytosis, and vaginal discharge | Managed with antibiotics, fluid and electrolyte replacement, warm douches to increase circulation, rest<br><br>Can cause adhesions that produce sterility |
| Mastitis | Reddened, inflamed breast<br><br>Exudate from nipple<br><br>Fever, fatigue, leukocytosis, pain | Systemic antibiotics, warm packs to promote drainage, rest, breast support |
| Fibrocystic changes | Multiple cyst development<br><br>Free-moving, tender, enlarged during menstrual period and about 1 wk before | Review importance and technique of breast self-exam<br><br>Provide frequent monitoring for changes<br><br>Prepare for possibility of aspiration, biopsy, or surgery<br><br>Diet changes and vitamin supplements<br><br>Benign but associated with increased risk of breast cancer |

*(Continued)*

**Table 13-3** Problems of the Reproductive Tract (*Continued*)

| DISORDER | ASSESSMENT | NURSING CONSIDERATIONS |
|---|---|---|
| Cancer of the cervix | Early—asymptomatic<br><br>Later—abnormal bleeding, especially postcoital | Preparation for tests, biopsy<br><br>Internal radiation therapy<br><br>Pap smear |
| Breast cancer | Small, fixed, painless lump<br><br>Rash, or in more advanced cases, change in color, puckering or dimpling of skin, pain and/or tenderness, nipple retraction or discharge<br><br>Axillary adenopathy | Mammography screening<br><br>Prepare for surgery and/or radiation, chemotherapy |
| Uterine fibroids (myomas) | Low-back pain, fertility problems<br><br>Menorrhagia | Benign tumors of myometrium<br><br>Size and symptoms determine action<br><br>Prepare for possible hysterectomy (removal of uterus) or myomectomy (partial resection of uterus) |
| Uterine displacement/ prolapse | Weak pelvic support, sometimes after menopause<br><br>Pain, menstrual interruption, fertility problems<br><br>Urinary incontinence | Kegel exercises—isometric exercises of the muscle that controls urine flow (pubococcygeus, or PC muscle) can improve pelvic musculature support<br><br>Pessary—device inserted into vagina that gives support to uterus in cases of retroversion or prolapse; must be inserted and rechecked by health professional<br><br>Surgical intervention—colporrhaphy (suturing fascia and musculature to support prolapsed structures) |
| Endometriosis | Found in colon, ovaries, supporting ligaments<br><br>Causes inflammation and pain<br><br>Causes dysmenorrhea and infertility, backache<br><br>Most common in young nulliparous women | Advise client that oral contraceptives suppress endometrial buildup or that surgical removal of tissue is possible<br><br>Inform client that symptoms abate after childbirth and lactation |

*(Continued)*

**Table 13-3** Problems of the Reproductive Tract (*Continued*)

| DISORDER | ASSESSMENT | NURSING CONSIDERATIONS |
|---|---|---|
| Uterine cancer | Watery discharge, irregular menstrual bleeding, menorrhagia<br><br>Diagnosed by endometrial biopsy or curettage | Internal radiation implants—must restrict movements; bedrest with air mattress<br><br>Enema, douche, low-residue diet, ample fluids<br><br>Indwelling catheter and fracture pan for elimination<br><br>Visitors and professionals wear protective garments and limit exposure time<br><br>Dislodged implant must be handled with special tongs and placed in lead-lined container for removal; call hospital radiation therapy specialist first<br><br>Hysterectomy:<br><br>    Subtotal—removal of fundus only<br><br>    Total—removal of the uterus (vagina remains intact)<br><br>    Total abdominal hysterectomy with bilateral salpingo-oophorectomy (TAH-BSO)—removal of uterus, fallopian tubes, and ovaries<br><br>    Radical—removal of lymph nodes as well as TAH-BSO<br><br>    Assess for hemorrhage, infection, thrombophlebitis; if ovaries removed, estrogen replacement therapy (ERT) may be needed |
| Ovarian cyst | Pelvic discomfort<br><br>Palpable during routine exam | May do biopsy or removal to prevent necrosis<br><br>Monitor by sonography |
| Ovarian cancer | Family history of ovarian cancer; client history of breast, bowel, endometrial cancer; nulliparity; infertility; heavy menses; palpation of abdominal mass (late sign); diagnosis by ultrasound, CT, x-ray, IVP | Surgical removal, chemotherapy, staging of tumor after removal<br><br>Foster verbalization of feelings, ensure continuity of care, encourage support systems |
| Orchitis (male) | Complication of mumps, virus, STD; may cause sterility, pain, and swelling | Prophylactic gamma globulin if exposed to mumps virus<br><br>Administration of medications specific for organism<br><br>Ice packs to reduce swelling, scrotal support, bedrest |
| Prostatitis (male) | May be complication of lower UTIs<br><br>Acute—fever, chills, dysuria, purulent penile discharge; elevated WBC and bacteria in urine<br><br>Chronic—backache; urinary frequency; enlarged, firm, slightly tender prostate | Antibiotics, sitz baths<br><br>Increased fluid intake<br><br>Activities to drain the prostate |

(*Continued*)

**Table 13-3** Problems of the Reproductive Tract (*Continued*)

| DISORDER | ASSESSMENT | NURSING CONSIDERATIONS |
|---|---|---|
| Benign prostatic hyperplasia (BPH) (male) | Enlargement of the glandular and cellular tissue of the prostate, resulting in compression on the urethra and urinary retention; most often in men over 50 y old<br><br>Dysuria, frequency, urgency, decreased urinary stream, hesitancy, and nocturia; later symptoms may be cystitis, hydronephrosis, or urinary calculi<br><br>KUB, x-ray, IVP, and cystoscopy demonstrate prostate enlargement and urinary tract changes | Preoperative:<br><br>Promote urinary drainage<br><br>Assure nutrition<br><br>Correct fluid and electrolyte balance<br><br>Antibiotics<br><br>Acid-ash diet to treat infection<br><br>Postoperative:<br><br>Assure patency of three-way indwelling urinary catheter; may have continuous irrigation with normal saline to remove clots<br><br>If traction on catheter (pulled taut and taped to abdomen or leg to prevent bleeding), keep client's leg straight<br><br>Monitor drainage (should be reddish pink that progresses to clear)<br><br>Discourage attempts to void around catheter; control/treat bladder spasms<br><br>Teach bladder retraining by contracting and relaxing sphincter; instruct to avoid heavy lifting, straining at bowel movement, prolonged travel; inform about potential for impotence, and discuss alternative ways of expressing sexuality |
| Prostate cancer (male) | Urinary urgency, frequency, retention<br><br>Back pain or pain radiating down leg | Hormonal and chemotherapy; surgical removal |
| Phimosis | Stenosis of the distal foreskin of the penis, resulting in an inability to retract the foreskin in the uncircumcised male<br><br>Associated symptoms include urinary retention and balanitis (inflammation of the glans penis) | Physiologic phimosis is present in infants and young children because the foreskin normally is not retractable until ages 3–5 years; in adults, phimosis is frequently associated with adhesions due to recurrent inflammation and infection |
| Inguinal hernia | Protrusion of a bowel loop through the inguinal ring; usually soft and painless; usually decreases or disappears (reduces) with gentle pressure | With the client in the supine position, gentle pressure on the visible hernia causes the bowel loop to return to the abdominal cavity; direct assessment of an inguinal hernia requires the examiner to insert a finger into the inguinal canal and ask the client to strain or cough, causing the bowel loop to be palpable; hernias that fail to reduce require immediate medical attention |

(*Continued*)

**Table 13-3** Problems of the Reproductive Tract (*Continued*)

| DISORDER | ASSESSMENT | NURSING CONSIDERATIONS |
|---|---|---|
| Varicocele | Abnormal dilation and tortuosity of the veins along the spermatic cord<br><br>Client may report a pulling sensation, dull ache, or scrotal pain; the veins above the testis may be palpated as a thickened area in the scrotum | Cause is often multifactorial but is thought to be caused by differences in venous drainage between the right and left sides; most commonly affects boys and young men, and most often on the left side; is a cause of male infertility because of increased testicular pressure |
| Testicular cancer | Painless testicular mass discovered by the client on self-examination or by the sexual partner; if pain is an initial symptom, usually indicates that the mass has caused bleeding within the testicle or has caused testicular torsion | Most common malignancy in men 20–34 years of age; those at greatest risk have a history of undescended testicle(s) at birth (cryptorchidism); teaching and practice of testicular self-examination (TSE) is critically important in early detection |

3. Pelvic inflammatory disease (PID)—local infection, usually gonorrhea and/or chlamydia, spreads to the fallopian tubes, ovaries, and other organs

   a. Characterized by lower-abdominal pain and tenderness, malaise, fever, leukocytosis, and purulent vaginal discharge

   b. Potential to cause adhesions that produce sterility and contribute to ectopic pregnancy

   c. Risk factors include 20 years old or younger, multiple sexual partners, IUD, vaginal douching, smoking, history of STDs, history of PID

   d. Management includes noting amount, color, and odor of drainage; systemic antibiotics; warm douches to increase circulation and promote drainage; rest and comfort measures; STD prevention

B. Problems related to the breast

   1. Fibrocystic disease

      a. Characterized by multiple soft, tender, freely moving cysts that become enlarged during menstruation and subside during pregnancy, lactation, or after menopause

      b. Management includes aspiration to relieve discomfort and instructing the client to report to the health care provider any changes in shape or size

   2. Hypoplasia or hyperplasia of the breast—may affect a woman's self-concept; cosmetic surgery may be done to increase or reduce breast size

      a. Augmentation mammoplasty—inserts are placed under breast tissue

      b. Reduction mammoplasty—excessive tissue removed and the nipple is relocated

   3. Mastitis—infection of the breast (occurring most often during lactation) caused by inadequate cleanliness of the breast, infection in the infant, blood-borne infections, or plugged lactiferous ducts

a. Characterized by reddened, inflamed, and tender breasts; exudate from the nipple; fever, fatigue, leukocytosis; and pain from stagnation of milk

b. Management includes administering systemic antibiotics, warm packs to promote drainage, and instructing the client to wear a brassiere to support the breasts

4. Cancer of the breast—rapidly growing tumor

a. Assessment—small, immobile, painless lump; rash; or in more advanced cases, change in color, puckering or dimpling of skin, pain and/or tenderness, nipple retraction or discharge; axillary adenopathy; detection by mammography

b. Risk factors include family history of mother, sister, or daughter developing pre-menopausal breast cancer; age greater than 50; menses beginning age less than 12; no children; first pregnancy occurs age greater than 30; menopause age greater than 55

c. May be managed by surgery, radiation therapy, and/or chemotherapy

d. Types of mastectomies

1) Partial (lumpectomy)—removal of involved tissue while preserving contour and muscle function; usually followed by radiation

2) Subcutaneous (adenomastectomy)—removal of breast tissue but skin and nipple remain intact; used with premalignant lesions

3) Simple—removal of the entire breast; a skin flap may be left for cosmetic reconstruction

4) Radical—removal of the breast as well as the major and minor pectoral muscles, all lymph nodes, fat, and fascia; a skin graft may be used to cover the area

5) Modified radical—removal of all of above except the major and minor pectoral muscles

6) Extended radical—the chest wall is resected as well as all of above

7) Super-radical—the sternum is split and lymph nodes are dissected from the mediastinum

e. Nursing care in addition to routine postop care

1) Inspect dressing and incision for bleeding

2) To prevent lymphedema (pooling of lymph circulation in involved arm), elevate it on a pillow, turn client to back and unaffected side; avoid constricting clothing and using the arm for blood pressure measurement, IVs, injections, blood draws

3) To prevent muscle contractures, encourage an exercise program with gradual progression from those that do not stress the incision to adduction and external rotation

4) Promote acceptance of new body image by providing emotional support

C. Problems of the uterus

1. Fibroids (myomas)—benign tumors on the myometrium

a. Assessment—backache, constipation, menorrhagia, and pain

b. May predispose to uterine cancer

    c. Management includes hysterectomy (surgical removal of the uterus) or myomectomy (partial resection of the uterus)

2. Uterine displacements—caused by weakening of pelvic muscles; may be retrograde (retroversion and/or retroflexion) or forward displacement (anteversion and/or anteflexion)

    a. Assessment—discomfort, dysmenorrhea

    b. May contribute to infertility

    c. Management includes muscle-strengthening exercises, insertion of a pessary, or surgery to shorten the muscles

3. Uterine prolapse—collapse of the uterus into the vagina due to weakened pelvic musculature

    a. Assessment—urinary incontinence, retention, constipation, backache, and vaginal discharge

    b. Management by insertion of a pessary or by surgical removal of the uterus

4. Cancer of the cervix—malignant tumor cells invade the cervix

    a. Assessment—often asymptomatic; with invasion, the primary sign is painless vaginal bleeding; later a watery, foul-smelling discharge progressively becomes darker; irregular menstrual bleeding and menorrhagia; confirmed positive Pap smear and positive cervical biopsy

    b. Risk factors include family history of mother, sister, or daughter developing premenopausal breast cancer; age greater than 50 years; menses begin before age 12; no children or first pregnancy occurs after age 30; menopause after age 55; human papilloma virus (HPV) infection, multiple sex partners

    c. Loop electrosurgical excision procedure (LEEP); laser therapy, cryotherapy, conization

    d. Managed by intravaginal radiation implants to deter tumor growth and metastatic invasion or by hysterectomy

    e. Types of hysterectomy

        1) Subtotal—removal of the fundus only

        2) Total—removal of the uterus (vagina remains intact)

        3) Hysterosalpingo-oophorectomy—removal of the uterus, fallopian tubes, and ovaries

        4) Radical—removal of the lymph nodes in addition to the uterus, fallopian tubes, and ovaries

    f. Nursing care—appropriate for internal radiation therapy or routine preoperative and postoperative care of client with malignancy

5. Uterine (endometrial) cancer—slowly growing malignancy most often occurring postmenopausally

    a. Assessment—usually asymptomatic during early development; primary symptom is postmenopausal vaginal bleeding, followed by low pelvic and lower-back pain, palpable uterine mass; diagnosis by endometrial biopsy

    b. Risk factors include age greater than 55, postmenopausal bleeding, obesity, diabetes mellitus, hypertension, unopposed estrogen-replacement therapy

    c. Management includes internal and sometimes external radiation therapy; surgery (*see* Cancer of the Cervix); chemotherapy in advanced cases, hormonal therapy

**D.** Problems related to the ovaries

  1. Ovarian cysts—benign tumors (rare after menopause); may or may not be painful; surgical removal may be recommended during fertile years for cysts larger than 8 cm

  2. Ovarian cancer—leading cause of death from female reproductive malignancies because of rapid growth and spread and lack of early symptoms; related to excessive exposure to estrogen

    a. Assessment—family history of ovarian cancer, client history of breast cancer, *BRCA1* and *BRCA2* genetic mutations, bowel cancer, endometrial cancer, nulliparity, infertility, heavy menses, palpation of abdominal mass (late sign); diagnosis by ultrasound, CT, x-ray, IVP

    b. Management—Elective salpingo-oophorectomy, hysterectomy, chemotherapy, staging of tumor after removal

    c. Nursing care—foster verbalization of feelings, continuity of care, encourage support systems

**E.** Other alterations of female reproductive structures

  1. Endometriosis—proliferation of aberrant endometrial tissue in the uterus, ovaries, fallopian tubes, and within the abdominal cavity and vagina

    a. Assessment—backache, menstrual irregularities, and increasing dysmenorrhea

    b. May potentially cause adhesions, which can result in sterility

    c. Management includes hormonal contraceptives (ovulation is the stimulus for the proliferation of tissue), NSAIDs, gonadotropin-releasing hormone (GnRH) agonists (e.g., leuprolide)

  2. Cancer of the vulva—rarely occurring tumor

  3. Cystocele—protrusion of the bladder through the vaginal wall

    a. Assessment—interference with voiding and stress incontinence

    b. Management includes Kegel exercises; surgery (anterior colporrhaphy) to surgically shorten the muscles that support the bladder

  4. Rectocele—protrusion of the rectum through the vaginal wall characterized by rectal pressure, heaviness, and hemorrhoids; Kegel exercises; pelvic support with pessaries; surgical repair

## Assessment and Diagnostic Tools—Male

**A.** Cystoscopy—insertion of a lighted cystoscope through the urethra to the bladder; used to visualize the prostate and bladder; to remove tumors, stones, prostate tissue; to implant radium

  1. Pretest nursing care—routine preop care; may be general anesthesia requiring client NPO or local anesthesia

    2. Posttest nursing care—monitor I and O and vital signs (VS); check for more than pink-tinged hematuria and large clots; provide warm sitz baths and mild analgesics for discomfort; report signs and symptoms of infection

**B.** Prostatic smear—detects microorganisms or tumor cells in the prostate; health care provider massages the prostate through the rectum, and the client voids into a sterile specimen container

**C.** Testicular biopsy—to detect abnormal cells and presence of sperm, obtained by incision or aspiration

**D.** Prostatic acid phosphatase—blood test used to detect prostatic cancer

**E.** Prostate-specific antigen (PSA)—another blood test used to detect prostatic cancer

## Problems of the Male Reproductive Tract

**A.** Infection

    1. Testicular (orchitis)—complication of mumps, virus, STD; may cause sterility

        a. Assessment—pain and swelling

        b. Management—administration of prophylactic gamma globulin if exposed to mump virus; administration of medications specific for organism; ice packs to reduce swelling; bedrest; scrotal support

    2. Prostatitis—may be complication of lower UTIs

        a. Assessment

            1) Acute fever, chills, dysuria, purulent penile discharge; elevated WBC and bacteria in urine

            2) Chronic—backache, urinary frequency; enlarged, firm, slightly tender prostate

        b. Management—antibiotics, sitz baths, increased fluid intake, activities to drain the prostate

2. Problems of the prostate

    1. Benign prostatic hyperplasia (BPH)—enlargement of the glandular and cellular tissue of the prostate, resulting in compression on the urethra and urinary retention; most often in men over 50 y old

        a. Assessment—dysuria, frequency, urgency, decreased urinary stream, hesitancy, and nocturia; later symptoms may be cystitis, hydronephrosis, or urinary calculi; KUB x-ray, IVP, and cystoscopy demonstrate prostate enlargement and urinary tract changes

        b. Management—prostatic massage to reduce prostatic congestion and surgical intervention (suprapubic prostatectomy, retropubic prostatectomy, perineal approach, transurethral resection [TURP], radical prostatectomy)

        c. Medications—5-alpha reductase inhibitor (e.g., finasteride); alpha-blocking agents (e.g., tamsulosin)

        d. Complementary and alternative therapies—saw palmetto extract, lycopene

        e. Nursing care

1) Preoperative—promote urinary drainage, assure nutrition, and correct fluid and electrolyte balance; antibiotics and acid-ash diet to treat infection

2) Postoperative

   a) Assure patency of three-way indwelling urinary catheter, may be continuous irrigation to remove clots; if traction on catheter (pulled taut and taped to abdomen or leg to prevent bleeding), keep leg straight, monitor drainage (should be reddish pink initially, progresses to clear)

   b) Discourage attempts to void around catheter; control/treat bladder spasms

   c) Teach bladder retraining by contracting and relaxing sphincter; instruct to avoid heavy lifting, straining at bowel movement, prolonged travel; inform about potential for impotence complications, and discuss alternative ways of expressing sexuality

2. Cancer—proliferation of cells originating in the posterior lobe of the prostate

   a. Assessment—urinary urgency, frequency, and retention; back pain or pain radiating down the leg; stony hard prostate with irregularities or indurations by palpation; confirmation by biopsy

   b. Diagnosis—prostatic-specific antigen serum biomarker, ultrasound biopsy

   c. Management—hormonal and chemotherapy (palliative measures to relieve pain and retard metastasis) and/or surgical intervention (removal of the prostate gland and, if there is metastasis, the seminal vesicles and part of the urethra)

   d. Nursing care as appropriate to the management plan

## Problems of Infertility

Inability to conceive after at least one year of regular unprotected sexual intercourse; may be related to female, male, or most often, to multiple factors or conditions in both

A. Factors in the male

   1. Conditions

      a. Anatomical abnormalities of the penis, urethra, prostate, or seminal vesicle difficulties

      b. Testicular infection (orchitis); varicosities, abnormalities, e.g., cryptorchidism (undescended testicles); retrograde ejaculation; hypospadias (placement of urethral meatus on underside of penis) and/or chordee (painful downward curvature of penis with erection), torsion (twisting of spermatic cord causing ischemia and, eventually, necrosis of testis; surgical emergency)

      c. Illnesses, surgeries, and/or medications

      d. Social factors, e.g., stress, smoking, alcohol, and/or drugs, nutritional inadequacies

      e. Spermatozoal abnormalities

2. Specific tests

    a. Semen analysis/sperm adequacy—evaluates the quantity, number, motility, and morphology of sperm

    b. Postcoital test evaluates for sperm placement, receptivity of cervical mucus, and ability of sperm to migrate

**B.** Factors in the female

    1. Anatomical defects of the vagina, cervix, uterus, tubes, ovaries

    2. Endocrine abnormalities, e.g., pituitary dysfunction, deficient estrogen or progesterone

    3. Endometriosis/endometritis

    4. Social factors, e.g., coital problems

    5. Chronic disease states

    6. Immunologic reactions to sperm

**C.** Specific tests

    1. Basal body temperature and cervical mucus for estimate of ovulation and hormonal assessment of ovulatory function

    2. Hysterosalpingogram—x-ray with radiopaque substance to evaluate tubal patency; may be therapeutic by removing tubal obstruction

    3. Pelvic ultrasound

    4. Laparoscopy

**D.** Nursing management

    1. Assessment

        a. Obtain detailed health, sexual, reproductive, psychosocial, and family history

        b. Assist with complete physical examination

        c. Provide information, rationale, and instructions for the tests; reinforce necessity to comply with scheduled tests

    2. Encourage couple to relate feelings; support groups may be helpful

    3. Discuss appropriate alternatives

        a. Artificial insemination by partner and/or donor

        b. In vitro fertilization

        c. Adoption

        d. Accepting childlessness

## Sexually Transmitted Infections (STI)

**A.** Definition—contagious disease spread by contact during sexual intercourse

**B.** Overall picture

    1. Prevention involves education and contact investigation

    2. Measures to control spread include prophylactic vaccine development

**C.** Signs of sexually transmitted infections (*see* Table 13-4)

**Table 13-4** Sexually Transmitted Infections

| TYPE | SYMPTOMS | DIAGNOSTIC TESTS | TRANSMISSION AND INCUBATION | NURSING CONSIDERATIONS |
|------|----------|------------------|------------------------------|------------------------|
| Syphilis | Stage 1: painless chancre disappears within 4 weeks | Venereal Disease Research laboratory (VDRL), rapid plasma reagin (RPR), fluorescent treponemal antibody absorption test<br><br>(FTA-ABS), Microhemagglutination assay for Treponema pallidum (MHA-TP)<br><br>(to confirm syphilis when VDRL and RPR are positive)<br><br>Darkfield microscopy | Mucous membrane or skin; congenital; kissing, sexual contact<br><br>10–90 days | Prevention—condoms<br><br>Treat with penicillin G IM |
| | Stage 2: copper-colored rash on palms and soles; low-grade fever | | | For penicillin allergy—erythromycin for 10–15 days<br><br>Ceftriaxone and tetracyclines (nonpregnant females) |
| | Stage 3: cardiac and CNS dysfunction | | | Retest for cure<br><br>Abstinence from sexual activity until treatment complete<br><br>Reportable disease |
| Gonorrhea | Thick discharge from vagina or urethra<br><br>Frequently asymptomatic in females<br><br>If female has symptoms, usually has purulent discharge, dysuria, and dyspareunia (painful intercourse)<br><br>Symptoms in male include painful urination and a yellow-green discharge | Culture of discharge from cervix or urethra<br><br>Positive results for other STD diagnostic tests | Mucous membrane or skin; congenital; vaginal, orogenital, anogenital sexual activity<br><br>2–7 days | IM ceftriaxone 1 time and PO doxycycline bid for 1 week; azithromycin<br><br>IM aqueous penicillin with PO probenecid (to delay penicillin urinary excretion); PO azithromycin or doxycycline is used to treat chlamydia, which coexists in 45% of cases<br><br>Spectinomycin if allergy to ceftriaxone<br><br>Monitor for complications, pelvic inflammatory disease |

*(Continued)*

**Table 13-4** Sexually Transmitted Infections (*Continued*)

| TYPE | SYMPTOMS | DIAGNOSTIC TESTS | TRANSMISSION AND INCUBATION | NURSING CONSIDERATIONS |
|---|---|---|---|---|
| Genital herpes (HSV-2) | Painful vesicular genital lesions<br><br>Difficulty voiding<br><br>Recurrence in times of stress, infection, menses | Direct examination of cells<br><br>HSV antibodies | Mucous membrane or skin; congenital<br><br>Virus can survive on objects such as towels<br><br>3–14 days | Acyclovir (not cure)<br><br>Emotional support<br><br>Sitz baths<br><br>Local medication<br><br>Notification of contacts<br><br>Monitor Pap smears on regular basis—increased incidence of cancer of cervix<br><br>Precautions about vaginal delivery |
| Chlamydia | Men—dysuria, frequent urination, watery discharge<br><br>Women—may be asymptomatic, thick discharge with acrid odor, pelvic pain, yellow-colored discharge; painful menses | Direct examination of cells<br><br>Enzyme-linked ELISA | Mucous membrane; sexual contact<br><br>1–3 weeks | Notification of contacts<br><br>May cause sterility<br><br>Treat with azithromycin, doxycycline, erythromycin |
| Condylomata acuminata (genital warts) | Initially single, small papillary lesion spreads into large, cauliflower-like cluster on perineum and/or vagina or penis; may be itching/burning | Direct exam<br><br>Biopsy<br><br>HPV | Majority due to human papilloma virus (HPV)<br><br>Mucous membrane; sexual contact; congenital<br><br>1–3 months | Curettage, cryotherapy with liquid nitrogen or podophyllin resin<br><br>Keratolytic agents<br><br>Avoid intimate sexual contact until lesions are healed<br><br>Strong association with incidence of genital dysplasia and cervical carcinoma<br><br>Atypical, pigmented, or persistent warts should be biopsied<br><br>Notify contacts |

# CHILDBEARING—ANTEPARTUM CARE

## Reproduction

### Fertilization—Union of Ovum and Spermatozoon

A. Cells of the human body develop from chromosomes

1. Normal human cell tissue contains 46 chromosomes—22 pairs of homologous autosomes (any chromosome other than a sex chromosome) and one pair of sex chromosomes; one chromosome of each pair of chromosomes is received from the mother and the other one from the father

2. Sex determination occurs at the moment of conception as a result of the sex chromosome contributed by the male; an X-carrying sperm fertilizing the ovum produces a female (XX), a Y-carrying sperm produces a male (XY)

3. Aberrations in the number of chromosomes result in abnormal offspring or spontaneous abortion

B. Process of fertilization (conception)—only one sperm penetrates ovum

1. Usually occurs in the outer third of the fallopian tube

2. Implantation usually occurs in the upper part of the uterus about 7–10 d after fertilization when the developing zygote burrows into the endometrium, which has undergone changes to provide for its nourishment and is now called the decidua

3. There are 3 groups of cells in the developing embryo

   a. Outer layer (ectoderm)—develops into the following structures: hair, nails, sebaceous glands, sweat glands, epithelium of nasal and oral passages

   b. Middle layer (mesoderm)—develops into the following structures: muscles, bones, sexual structures, heart, kidneys, teeth dentin

   c. Inner layer (endoderm)—develops into the following: epithelium of digestive tract, respiratory tract, bladder

## Structures of Pregnancy

A. Fetal membranes—2 layers

1. Amnion—the smooth, slippery membrane enclosing the fluid-filled space that develops around the embryo (the "bag of waters") wherein the fetus floats and moves

   a. Fluid functions to maintain fetal temperature and cushion the fetus from injury

      b. At full term, contains about 500–1,000 mL of clear, slightly yellowish liquid with a characteristic but not foul odor; later in the pregnancy, fetus contributes to the fluid through urine excretion and absorbs from it by swallowing; hydramnios or polyhydramnios (greater than 2,000 mL) or oligohydramnios (less than 500 mL) indicate an abnormal process

  2. Chorion—the outer membrane that gives rise to the placenta, which is formed by the union of chorionic villi and decidua basalis

**B.** The umbilical cord—connects the placenta and the fetus; is about 20 inches in length and about 0.75 inch in diameter; contains two arteries and one large vein

**C.** Placenta—organ of pregnancy that permits an exchange across two closed vascular systems by diffusion, active transport, pinocytosis, and leakage (which allows for a slight mixing of blood)

  1. Functions

      a. Transfers nutrients from maternal bloodstream by a number of mechanisms

      b. Transfer of oxygen from mother to fetus by diffusion

      c. Removes waste products of fetal metabolism into mother's bloodstream, from which these will be excreted

      d. Produces hormones of pregnancy

        1) Early in pregnancy, human chorionic gonadotropin supports the corpus luteum in the continued production of progesterone and estrogen necessary for the maintenance of the secretory phase of the endometrium

        2) After the second month of pregnancy, the placenta takes over the production of estrogen and progesterone from the ovaries

        3) High levels of estrogen and progesterone during gestation also function to suppress the secretion of prolactin from the anterior pituitary gland, thereby delaying the onset of lactation until after delivery of the placenta, when the estrogen and progesterone levels drop significantly

      e. Passes antibodies to fetus from mother

      f. Provides a barrier to some but not all harmful substances; microorganisms, especially viruses, and medications may cross

  2. Perfusion (blood flow) is influenced by:

      a. Maternal BP

      b. Condition of maternal blood vessels

      c. Uterine contractions have inhibiting effect

      d. Maternal position, i.e., in supine position the gravid uterus compresses the inferior vena cava and descending aorta, causing reduced venous return and cardiac output, which may cause hypotension and decreased blood flow to the brain (dizziness, pallor, clamminess), the kidneys, and placenta (decreased fetal heart rate); corrected by left side-lying

# Fetal Development

**A.** Stages (*see* Table 13-5)

  1. Ovum (10–14 d)—implantation

    a. hCG is secreted by cells of chorionic villi to ensure continued estrogen and progesterone secretion; progesterone is absolutely necessary for implantation and maintenance of decidua

    b. Possible abnormal events

      1) Spontaneous abortion/ectopic pregnancy

      2) Maternal infection (e.g., rubella), resulting in multiple anomalies

      3) Genetic defects before 3 wk may result in spontaneous abortion

  2. Embryo (13 d through 8 wk)—organ development

    a. Cell growth and tissue differentiation, resulting in formation of all body systems

    b. Possible abnormal events

      1) Time of highest mortality

      2) Malformations related to genetic defects, poor maternal health, teratogens (nongenetic factors that can cause fetal malformations)

  3. Fetus (9 wk to term)—refinement of organ systems

    a. Growth in body size and organ maturity

    b. Possible abnormal events

      1) Preterm delivery (before 38 wk)—prognosis dependent on CNS maturity to maintain body temperature and respirations, lung development, and availability of clinical technology

      2) Intrauterine growth restriction (IUGR) or small for gestational age (SGA)

      3) Poor organ system development

**Table 13-5** Fetal Development

| AGE | SIZE | DEVELOPMENTAL FACTORS |
| --- | --- | --- |
| 4 wk | 0.25 in | Recognizable traces of all organs; heart formed and beating; backbone bent with head touching tip of tail |
| 8 wk | 1 in | Head very large in proportion to rest of body; some discernible facial features<br>Tail less prominent<br>Some movement |
| 12 wk | 3 in<br>1–1.6 oz | All organ systems are formed<br>Well-differentiated genitals; rudimentary kidneys that secrete urine<br>Able to suck and swallow |
| 16 wk | 6 in<br>4 oz | External genitalia obvious; able to distinguish sex; meconium in bowel |
| 20 wk | 10 in<br>10 oz | Fetal heartbeat can be heard; fetal movement should be felt by mother<br>Fine hairs over body (lanugo) |
| 24 wk | 12 in<br>1.5 lb | Skin red, wrinkled, little fat<br>Body well proportioned and covered with vernix caseosa |
| 28 wk | 14–15 in<br>2.5 lb | Skin is wrinkled<br>If born at this time, may survive with respiratory support and intensive care |
| 32 wk | 16.5 in | Most infants would survive if born; may need support for respiratory system |
| 36 wk | 16–19 in<br>5.5–6 lb | Lanugo disappearing<br>Deposits of subcutaneous fat<br>Chances of survival good; may require some special care |
| 40 wk | 20 in<br>6.5–7.5 lb | Full term; full development<br>Most lanugo has disappeared; vernix caseosa only in skin creases and folds |

# Maternal Adaptations in Pregnancy

A. Anatomical

　1. Uterus—changes in size, structure, and position to become a thin-walled, muscular, abdominal organ capable of containing the fetus, placenta, and amniotic fluid

　　a. In the early months of pregnancy, growth is partly due to formation of new muscle fibers and enlargement of pre-existing muscle fibers

　　b. After the first trimester, the increase in size is partly mechanical due to the pressure of the developing fetus

　　c. The full-term pregnant uterus and its contents weigh about 12 lb

2. Cervix—undergoes increased blood supply, edema, and hyperplasia of the cervical glands contributing to:

    a. Softening (Goodell's sign) about 6 wk

    b. A blue-violet color (Chadwick's sign) about 6–8 wk

    c. Increased friability (bleeds easily after Pap smear and intercourse)

    d. Distention of cervical mucosa glands with mucus, creating a tenacious "mucous plug" that seals the endocervical canal and inhibits the ascent of bacteria and other substances into the uterus

3. Vagina and external genital organs—enlarge, soften, thicken, and develop blue-violet hue as a result of increased vasculature

    a. Vaginal secretions become alkaline, causing an increased risk of vaginitis

    b. Connective tissue loosens in preparation for labor and delivery

4. Breasts—enlarge early in pregnancy, causing progressive feelings of heaviness, fullness, and tenderness; the nipple and areola become larger, darker in color; blood vessels enlarge and become prominent beneath the skin

5. Body mass—changes with weight gain; total desirable weight gain in pregnancy (for average woman) is about 23–28 lb; 3–4 lb (1.36–1.81 kg) during the first trimester, followed by an average of slightly less than one pound per week for the rest of the pregnancy

6. Skin

    a. Pink or reddish streaks (striae gravidarum) may occur on breasts, abdomen, buttocks, and/or thighs as a result of fat deposits, which cause stretching of the skin

    b. Increased pigmentation can occur on the face as blotchy brown areas on the forehead and cheeks (chloasma or "mask of pregnancy") and on the abdomen as dark line from the symphysis pubis to the umbilicus (linea nigra)

    c. Minute vascular spiders may occur

    d. The umbilicus is pushed outward, and by about the seventh month, its depression disappears and becomes a darkened area on the abdominal wall

    e. Sweat and sebaceous glands are more active

7. Musculoskeletal

    a. Change in the center of gravity, decreased muscle tone, and increased weight-bearing cause an accelerated lumbosacral curve, which may lead to lower-back pain and difficulty with locomotion

    b. Progesterone-produced relaxation and increased mobility of the pelvic joints may cause discomfort and difficulty in walking

    c. The vertical abdominal muscles may separate (diastasis recti)

**B.** Physiological

   1. Hormonal

      a. Placental

         1) Estrogen—enlargement of uterus, breasts, genitals; growth of glandular tissue, ducts, alveoli, and nipples of breasts; fat deposition; increased elasticity of connective tissue; altered thyroid function; altered nutrient metabolism; sodium and water retention by kidneys; hypercoagulability of blood; vascular changes

         2) Progesterone—development of decidua; decreased contractility of the uterus; decreased gastric motility (sphincters relaxed); increased sensitivity to $CO_2$ in respiratory center; decreased tone of smooth muscle; development of secretory portions of lobular-alveolar system in breasts; sodium excretion

         3) Human chorionic somatomammotropin and human placental lactogen; anabolic effect; insulin antagonist

      b. Pituitary gland

         1) Anterior lobe secretes prolactin hormone after delivery of the placenta

         2) Posterior lobe secretes oxytocin during labor and lactation

   2. Blood—total blood volume in body increases during pregnancy by about 30%; normal blood pressure is maintained by peripheral vasodilation

      a. RBC production increases; WBC count increases; clotting factors increase while fibrinolytic activity decreases

      b. Hemoglobin and hematocrit levels decrease slightly in response to hemodilution (increased plasma content); hemoglobin less than 10 g/dL or hematocrit less than 35% may indicate anemia

      c. The increased blood volume creates the need for the heart to pump more blood through the aorta (about 50% more blood per minute), resulting in increased heart rate; occasional palpitations (possibly due to sympathetic nervous imbalance in the early months of pregnancy or to intra-abdominal pressure of the enlarged uterus toward the end of the pregnancy)

   3. Respiration—in the later months of pregnancy, the enlarged uterus causes the diaphragm to be displaced upward, putting pressure on the lungs and causing shortness of breath

   4. Digestion

      a. Nausea and vomiting may occur in the first trimester; vomiting that is excessive or persists beyond this time (hyperemesis gravidarum) may require medical management; appetite usually improves as pregnancy advances

      b. Progesterone-induced relaxation of smooth muscle tone, reduction in total acidity of gastric juices, and pressure from the growing uterus may cause heartburn, flatulence, and constipation

      c. Aversions or cravings for certain foods or unusual substances (e.g., pica) may occur

      d. Carbohydrate metabolism is profoundly affected to meet growth and development needs of fetus and the metabolic needs of mother to support tissue expansion

1) The first half of pregnancy

   a) Maternal glucose is moved across the placenta by active transport, causing maternal glucose levels to fall slightly; maternal pancreas responds by decreasing production of insulin

   b) Maternal insulin does not cross the placenta

   c) By 8 wk, the fetus's own insulin production is consistent with the amount of glucose received from the mother

2) The second half of pregnancy—the placental hormones impede the mother's ability to utilize insulin; the resulting demand for added insulin can be met by a normally functioning pancreas

5. Urinary system

   a. Urinary output is increased and has a low specific gravity; possible tendency to excrete glucose; reabsorption of sodium and decreased water output (latter half of pregnancy) is a compensatory mechanism to maintain increased blood volume

   b. Ureters become dilated (especially the right ureter) due to the pressure of the enlarged uterus; the dilated ureters are unable to propel urine as efficiently, resulting in stasis of urine and possible urinary tract infection

   c. Bladder—urinary frequency may occur early in pregnancy and later again when "lightening" occurs, result of increased pressure on the bladder from the enlarged uterus

**C.** Psychological

1. First trimester—maternal ambivalence, even in planned pregnancy, is usual; there may be some anticipation and concern related to fears and fantasies about the pregnancy

2. Second trimester—usually increased maternal feelings of physical and emotional well-being; mother is often described as self-absorbed and introverted

3. Third trimester—possible new fears related to labor and delivery and fantasies about the appearance of the baby; feelings of awkwardness, clumsiness, and decreased femininity related to changes in body image

4. Paternal reactions—may parallel those of mother; some may experience physical symptoms of pregnancy (couvade syndrome)

5. Adaptation of siblings—age and experience related

# Prenatal Assessment

**A.** Verifying pregnancy

1. Signs and symptoms

   a. Presumptive—suspicion not proof; predominantly subjective; amenorrhea, nausea/vomiting ("morning sickness"), breast sensitivity, fatigue/lassitude, quickening (maternal perception of fetal movement occurring between 16–20 wk of gestation)

   b. Probable—increased suspicion but still no proof; no subjective data; uterine enlargement, souffle, and contractions; positive urine pregnancy tests

   c. Positive—definite signs of pregnancy; no subjective data; fetal heartbeat (about 8 wk by fetal Doppler and by 20 wk auscultation), palpation of fetal movement, outline of fetal skeleton by sonogram or x-ray (done only if absolutely necessary late in pregnancy)

2. Pregnancy test—human chorionic gonadotropin (hCG)

   a. Immunologic tests can detect hCG in woman's urine by 2 wk after missed period; cannot measure the amount of hCG; false readings may occur with inappropriate timing, handling error, or some medications

**B.** Estimated date of birth (EDB) or estimated date of delivery (term pregnancy is 38–42 wk)

1. Naegle's rule: add 7 days to the first day of the last menstrual period (LMP), subtract 3 months, and add 1 year, except if LMP is in the first 3 months of the year (EDB = LMP + 7 days − 3 months + 1 year); assumes a 28-d cycle and no recent use of oral contraceptive

2. Measurement of fundal height from the top of symphysis pubis to the top of the fundus with a flexible, nonstretchable tape measure to be used as a gross estimate of dates

   a. Level of symphysis between 12–14 wk

   b. At the umbilicus about 20 wk (measures 20 cm)

   c. Rises about 1 cm/wk until 36 wk, after which it varies

**C.** History

1. Initial visit

   a. Obstetrical

      1) Gravida—the total number of pregnancies regardless of duration (includes present pregnancy)

      2) Para—number of past pregnancies that have gone beyond the period of viability (capability of the fetus to survive outside of the uterus; currently considered any time after 20-wk gestation), regardless of the number of fetuses or whether the infant was born alive or dead

      3) Abortion—pregnancy that terminates before the period of viability

   b. Health factors that may influence course of pregnancy

      1) Past/concurrent illnesses, surgeries, medications (possible teratogens)

      2) Reproductive factors, e.g., menstrual pattern or problems, contraception, infections

      3) Personal, social, cultural, marital, sexual, environmental, educational, occupational, drugs (including alcohol), cigarette smoking, caffeine (coffee, tea, colas), exercise factors

      4) Nutritional—prepregnancy weight (may indicate long-term malnutrition and depleted nutrient stores), recent weight gain or loss (may denote at-risk situation), adequacy of diet, vitamin supplements

2. Interim history

    a. Frequency, intensity, and management of discomforts of pregnancy

    b. Abnormal signs and symptoms or risk factors

    c. Changes in emotional, financial, marital status

    d. Nutritional status

        1) Weight gain should be within expected parameters; based on prepregnancy weight

        2) Increased nutrient requirements

            a) Calories—300 kcal/d; may need adjustment for prepregnant under/overweight

            b) There should be no attempt at weight reduction during pregnancy

            c) Carbohydrates—needed to prevent unsuitable use of fats/proteins for added energy needs; important to avoid "empty" calorie sources

            d) Proteins to 60 g/d; additional increase for adolescent/multiple pregnancies; efficient use requires complete protein (contains all essential amino acids; animal sources) or protein source complemented with other protein sources, e.g., legumes, grains, nuts

            e) Iron—to a total of 30 mg/d of elemental iron; usually requires supplement

            f) Calcium to 1,200 mg/d; best obtained from dairy products; if milk is disliked or poorly tolerated, calcium supplement may be necessary

            g) Sodium—should not be restricted without serious indication; excess should be discouraged

        3) 24-h recall/diet diary may be used to evaluate high-risk woman

**D.** Physical assessment

    1. Initial visit—complete physical exam

        a. Breast exam—nipple formation using "pinch test" in which the areola is pinched gently and pushed in with the examiner's thumb and forefinger; an everted or normal nipple will protrude, an inverted nipple will look flat or turned inward, indicating potential difficulty with breast feeding

        b. Pelvic exam—Pap smear; culture for gonorrhea and herpes if appropriate; smear for chlamydia; bimanual (palpation of reproductive organs between abdominal and vaginal hands) to establish uterine size, consistency, and contour; pelvic measurements

    2. Routine visits—every 4 wk until 32 wk, then every 2 wk until 36 wk, then weekly until delivery to monitor vital signs, weight, fetal heart tones, fundal height and outline

**E.** Laboratory screening

    1. Initially and at routine visits, urine dipstick for glucose, protein (pregnancy-induced hypertension and UTI)

    2. Gonorrhea/chlamydia (GC) culture at 1st prenatal visit for all, may be retested at 36 weeks if the woman tested positive previously, has a new sex partner, or has multiple sex partners

3. Maternal serum alpha-fetoprotein (AFP) at 16–18 wk to identify risk of neural tube defect in fetus

4. Glucose screening between 24–28 wk to detect gestational diabetes

5. Rh antibody titers checked in 1st trimester, at 28 weeks gestation, and more frequently as directed per health care provider

F. Discomforts associated with pregnancy (*see* Table 13-6)

**Table 13-6** Discomforts of Pregnancy

| ASSESSMENT | NURSING CONSIDERATIONS |
|---|---|
| Nausea and vomiting (morning sickness) | May occur any time of day<br>Eat dry crackers on arising<br>Eat small, frequent meals |
| Constipation, hemorrhoids | Bulk foods, fiber<br>Generous fluid intake<br>Encourage regularity, routine |
| Leg cramps | Increase calcium intake<br>Flex feet, local heat |
| Breast soreness | Well-fitting bra<br>Bra may be worn at night |
| Backache | Emphasize posture<br>Careful lifting<br>Good shoes |
| Heartburn | Small, frequent meals<br>Antacids—avoid those containing phosphorus<br>Decrease amount of fatty and fried foods |
| Dizziness | Slow, deliberate movements<br>Support stockings<br>Monitor intake |
| Vertigo, light-headedness | Vena cava or supine hypotensive syndrome<br>Turn on left side |
| Urinary frequency | Kegel exercises<br>Decrease fluids before bed<br>Report signs of infection |

1. First trimester
   a. Nausea and vomiting ("morning sickness") related to altered hormone levels and metabolic changes; advise small snacks of dry crackers before arising, small feedings of bland food, milk; avoid strong odors and greasy foods
   b. Urinary frequency and urgency without dysuria; fluid intake should not be restricted
   c. Increased vaginal discharge; manage with good hygiene (but no douching) and loose-fitting cotton underwear; report signs or symptoms of vaginitis
   d. Breast soreness due to hormonal changes; suggest wearing a well-fitting, supportive brassiere
   e. Headache due to tension from emotional and physical stresses at any time during pregnancy; provide reassurance, suggest relaxation techniques; inform client to report persistent and/or severe episodes

2. Second and third trimesters
   a. Heartburn may be related to tension and vomiting in early pregnancy, progesterone-induced decreased motility and relaxation of the cardiac sphincter, displacement of the stomach by the growing uterus; encourage small, frequent meals and discourage overeating, ingesting fried/fatty foods, lying down soon after eating, use of sodium bicarbonate (would interfere with sodium balance)
   b. Constipation related to progesterone-induced hypoperistalsis, compression/displacement of the bowel by the enlarging uterus, poor food choices, lack of fluids, and/or iron supplementation; advise bulk foods, fruits and vegetables, exercise, and generous fluid intake; avoid laxatives
   c. Hemorrhoids due to pelvic congestion related to pressure from enlarged uterus; suggest regulation of bowel habits, gentle reinsertion into rectum with use of lubricant, relief measures, e.g., ice packs, topical ointments, sitz baths, lying down with legs elevated
   d. Uterine contractions (Braxton-Hicks) due to tension on the round ligaments as a result of displacement of the uterus; instruct client to rest, change position or activity
   e. Backache due to increased spinal curvature; educate the client on the importance of good posture; pelvic tilt exercises
   f. Faintness related to vasomotor lability or postural hypotension; instruct the client to use slow, deliberate movements when rising, avoid prolonged standing and warm, stuffy environments; elastic hose may be needed
   g. Leg cramps related to pressure on the nerves supplying the lower extremities, aggravated by poor peripheral circulation or fatigue; instruct the client to increase calcium and decrease phosphorus intake; encourage dorsiflexion of feet

h. Ankle edema related to decreased venous return from lower extremities, instruct the client to avoid wearing anything that constricts blood flow, elevate legs when sitting or resting, and dorsiflex feet when sitting or standing for any length of time; medical management if edema persists in A.M., is pitting, involves the face, or associated with elevated BP, proteinuria, persistent headaches

i. Varicosities of extremities or vulva related to uterine compression of venous return, increased vein wall distensibility from progesterone-initiated relaxation, or inherited tendency; suggest elevating legs frequently, avoid sitting with legs crossed, standing/sitting for long periods of time, or wearing constrictive clothing; support/elastic stockings may be helpful

## Fetal Assessment

A. Fetal heart rate (FHR)—a significant predictor of fetal well-being; should be monitored at all routine prenatal and any acute care visits; may be referred to as fetal heart tones (FHT)

B. Fetal movements (FM)—a regular pattern of 10 movements in one hour is a good indicator of fetal well-being; less than 10 movements in a 3-h period should be reported

# LABOR AND DELIVERY

## Fluid/Electrolyte Balance, Comfort, Perfusion, Emotional Process

## Labor and Delivery

A. Critical factors affecting the process of labor

1. Passage (maternal)—size and type of pelvis, ability of the cervix to efface and dilate, and distensibility of vagina and introitus

2. Passenger (fetal)

   a. Size—primarily related to fetal skull

   b. Fetopelvic relationships

      1) Lie—relationship of spine of fetus to spine of mother; longitudinal (parallel), transverse (right angles), oblique (slight angle off a true transverse lie)

      2) Presentation—part of fetus that presents to (enters) maternal pelvic inlet

         a) Cephalic/vertex—head presentation (greater than 95% of labors)

         b) Breech presentation (3–4%)

            i)   Frank (most common)—flexion of hips and extension of knees

            ii)  Complete—flexion of hips and knees

            iii) Footling/incomplete—extension of hips and knees

         c) Shoulder (transverse lie)—rare

      3) Attitude—relationship of fetal parts to each other; usually flexion of head and extremities on chest and abdomen to accommodate to shape of uterine cavity

      4) Position—relationship of fetal reference point to mother's pelvis (*see* Figure 13-1)

         a) Fetal reference point

            i)   Vertex presentation—dependent upon degree of flexion of fetal head on chest; full flexion—occiput (O); full extension—chin (M); moderate extension—brow (B)

            ii)  Breech presentation—sacrum (S)

            iii) Shoulder presentation—scapula (SC)

         b) Maternal pelvis is designated per her right/left and anterior/posterior

         c) Expressed as standard three-letter abbreviation; e.g., LOA = left occiput anterior, indicating vertex presentation with fetal occiput on mother's left side toward the front of her pelvis; to find best location for FHR assessment, determine the location of the fetal back; weeks of gestation may alter the location as well (*see* Figure 13-1)

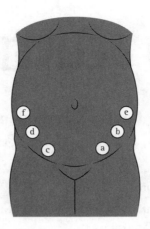

**Figure 13-1.** Determining Position

    a)    LOA—left occiput anterior, most common; FHR best heard below umbilicus on mother's left side

    b)    LOP—left occiput posterior

    c)    ROA—right occiput anterior

    d)    ROP—right occiput posterior

    e)    LSA—left sacrum anterior

    f)    RSA—right sacrum anterior

5)    Station—level of presenting part of fetus in relation to imaginary line between ischial spines (0 station) in midpelvis of mother (*see* Figure 13-2)

    a)    −5 to −1 indicates a presenting part above 0 station (floating); +1 to +5 indicates a presenting part below 0 station

    b)    Engagement—when the presenting part is at 0 station

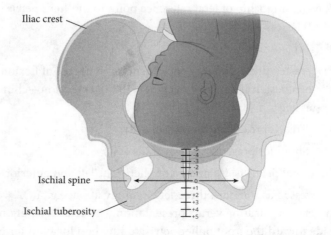

**Figure 13-2.** Station of Presenting Part

3. Powers—force expelling the fetus and placenta

   a. Primary—involuntary uterine contractions

      1) Three phases

         a) Increment—steep crescent slope from beginning of a contraction until its peak

         b) Acme/peak—strongest intensity

         c) Decrement—diminishing intensity

      2) Characteristics of contractions

         a) Frequency—time frame in minutes from the beginning of one contraction to the beginning of the next one; frequency of less than every 2 min should be reported

         b) Duration—time frame in seconds from the beginning of a contraction to its completion; greater than 90 seconds should be reported because of potential risk of uterine rupture or fetal distress

         c) Intensity—the strength of a contraction at acme; may be assessed by subjective description from the woman, palpation (mild contraction would feel like the tip of the nose, moderate like the chin, strong like the forehead), or electronic intrauterine pressure catheter (IUPC)

   b. Secondary—voluntary bearing-down efforts

4. Psychological state of the woman—fear and anxiety may lead to increased perception of pain and impede progress of labor; preparation and support for childbirth may enhance coping efforts

   a. Preparation for childbirth education about the birthing process and methods to decrease discomfort and tension

      1) Relaxation of voluntary muscles

      2) Distraction, focal point, imagery

      3) Breathing techniques with each contraction

         a) Always begin and end with "cleansing" or "relaxing" breath (inhale deeply through nose and exhale passively through relaxed, pursed lips)

         b) Hyperventilation—may cause maternal respiratory alkalosis and compromise fetal oxygenation; characterized by light-headedness, dizziness, tingling of fingers and/or circumoral numbness; managed by having woman breathe into her cupped hands or a paper bag

   b. Support person/"coach" should be involved in the formal preparation

5. Position (maternal)

   a. Side-lying enhances blood flow to the utero-feto-placental unit and maternal kidneys

   b. Upright (standing, walking, squatting) enlists gravity to aid in fetal descent through the birth canal

   c. Frequent changes relieve fatigue and improve circulation

B. Cardinal mechanisms/movements of labor in vertex presentation—usually flow smoothly and often overlap; failure to accomplish one or more usually requires obstetrical intervention

1. Descent—progress through the maternal pelvis; continuous throughout labor
2. Flexion—as a result of resistance from maternal pelvis and musculature, the head flexes so that a smaller diameter enters pelvis
3. Internal rotation—head rotates from occiput transverse or oblique position (usual position as it enters the pelvis) to anterior/posterior at pelvic outlet; head is under symphysis pubis and neck is twisted
4. Extension—the head is moved backward as it proceeds under the symphysis pubis and baby is born by extension over the perineum
5. Restitution and external rotation—movement of head to align itself with face and shoulders (restitution) and then rotation bringing shoulders into anteroposterior diameter appears as one movement
6. Expulsion—first the anterior shoulder under the symphysis pubis, then the posterior shoulder over the perineum, followed rapidly by the rest of the body; time of birth is recorded at this point

C. Signs and symptoms of labor

1. Impending—may begin several weeks prior to labor
   a. Lightening—settling of uterus and fetal-presenting part into pelvis; sensation of decreased abdominal distention
   b. Increased Braxton-Hicks contractions (mild, intermittent, irregular, abdominal contractions); decrease/disappear with activity
   c. May be heightened anxiety, anticipation, and fatigue
   d. Weight loss of about 2–3 lb 3–4 d before onset of labor; related to changes in estrogen and progesterone levels
   e. Increased vaginal mucus discharge
   f. Fetal movements may appear less active
   g. May be episodes of false labor (*see* Table 13-7)

**Table 13-7** True Versus False Labor

| TRUE | FALSE |
|---|---|
| Cervix progressively effaced and dilated | Cervical changes do not occur |
| Contractions—regular with increasing frequency (shortened intervals), duration, and intensity | Contractions—irregular with usually no change in frequency, duration, or intensity |
| Discomfort radiates from back around the abdomen | Discomfort is usually abdominal |
| Contractions do not decrease with rest | Contractions may lessen with activity or rest |

2. Onset

   a. Expulsion of mucous plug; pink/brown-tinged discharge (bloody show)

   b. Regular contractions increasing in frequency, duration, and intensity

   c. Spontaneous rupture of membranes (SROM) may occur before or during labor

      1) Check FHR by auscultation for 1 min and with next contraction

      2) May be a gush or trickle; report strong/foul odor (infection), meconium stained (in vertex presentation, may indicate fetal anoxia) or wine colored (indicative of premature separation of placenta)

      3) Questionable leakage of amniotic fluids should be tested for alkalinity to differentiate from urine

         a) Nitrazine tape turns blue/gray/green (alkaline); urine (acidic) does not change the yellow color

         b) A mixture of cervical mucus and amniotic fluid dried on a slide looks like crystallized ferns by microscopic examination

   d. Cervical changes

      1) Effacement—thinning and shortening of the cervix during late pregnancy and/or labor; measured in percentages (100% is fully effaced)

      2) Dilation—opening and enlargement of the cervical canal; measured in centimeters 0–10 cm (10 cm is fully dilated)

**D.** Stages of labor

1. First stage (dilating stage)—from onset of regular contractions to full dilation; averages 13–18 h for nulliparas and 8–9 h for multiparas

   a. Latent phase (0–3 cm)—the cervix begins effacing and dilating, and contractions become increasingly stronger and more frequent; nulliparas 7–10 h and multiparas 5–6 h

   b. Active phase (4–7 cm)—more rapid dilation of cervix and descent of presenting part; approximately 3–4 h for both

   c. Transition (8–10 cm)—contractions may be every 2–3 min and last 60–90 s; should not be more than 3 h for nulliparas or 1 h for multiparas

      1) May be accompanied by irritability and restlessness, hyperventilation, and dark heavy show as well as leg cramps, nausea/vomiting, hiccups, belching

      2) Possible rectal pressure creating a desire to push; should discourage before full dilation because it may cause maternal exhaustion and both cervical and fetal trauma

2. Second stage (complete cervical dilation to delivery of fetus)—from complete dilation of cervix to delivery of the baby; averages 2 h for nulliparas and 20 min for multiparas

   a. Contractions are now severe, lasting 60–90 s at 2–3 min intervals

b. Bearing down/pushing increases intra-abdominal pressure from voluntary contraction of maternal abdominal muscles and pushes the presenting part against the pelvic floor, causing a stretching, burning sensation and bulging of the perineum; "crowning" occurs when the presenting part appears at the vaginal orifice, distending the vulva

c. Timing of transfer to delivery room

1) Nulliparas—during second stage when the presenting part begins to distend the perineum

2) Multiparas—at the end of first stage when the cervix is dilated 8–9 cm

d. Delivery

1) Normal spontaneous vaginal delivery

a) The mother is encouraged not to push as the head is delivered; the neonate cries (or is encouraged to do so to expand the lungs); if the cord is encircling the neck (nuchal cord), it is gently slipped over the head

b) Episiotomy (a surgical incision of the perineum) may be done at the end of the second stage of labor to facilitate delivery and to avoid laceration of the perineum

2) Assisted deliveries

a) Forceps—two double-curved, spoonlike articulated blades used to extract the fetal head; indicated if mother cannot push fetus out or if compromised maternal/fecal status in late second stage; contraindicated in cephalopelvic disproportion (CPD)

b) Vacuum extractor—delivery with use of a suction device that is applied to the fetal scalp for traction; used in prolonged second stage; contraindicated in CPD and face/breech presentation

e. A difficult stage for the fetus because of possible trauma or asphyxia as it passes through the birth canal

3. Third stage (birth and delivery of placenta)—from delivery of the baby to delivery of the placenta; if more than 30 min, placenta is considered retained

a. Separation of placenta from the uterine wall evidenced by a change in the fundus from discoid to globular shape as it becomes firm and rises in the abdomen, a sudden gush/trickle of blood, and lengthening of the umbilical cord

b. Expulsion of the placenta through the vagina by uterine contractions and pushing by mother or by gentle traction on the umbilical cord

c. Contraction of the uterus following delivery controls uterine hemorrhage and produces placental separation; if necessary, oxytocin or methylergonovine maleate may be administered to help contract the uterus

4. Fourth stage—immediate recovery period from delivery of placenta to stabilization of maternal systemic responses and contraction of the uterus; from 1–4 h

   a. Mother begins to readjust to nonpregnant state

   b. Areas of concern include discomfort due to contraction of uterus (afterpain) and/or episiotomy, fatigue or exhaustion, hunger, thirst, excessive bleeding, bladder distention, parent-newborn interaction

E. Pharmacological control of discomfort (*see* Table 13-8)

1. Principles of use—minimize pain without increasing risk to mother or fetus; type of pain relief is influenced by length of gestation, maternal choice, mother's emotional status, response to pain, previous history with analgesics or anesthesia, and general character of labor process

   a. Timing of administration

      1) Before 5 cm (latent phase)—may retard or stop labor

      2) From 5–7 cm (early active phase)—may aid relaxation

      3) After 8 cm (transition phase)—may result in respiratory depression requiring resuscitative measures in sedated neonate

   b. Because most medications cross the placental barrier, FHR is taken frequently before and after administration of medication

2. Systemic analgesia—functions through alleviation of sensation of pain or enhancement of threshold for pain

   a. Narcotics

      1) Morphine—Rapidly crosses the placenta, causing decrease in FHR variability

      2) Fentanyl—less nausea, vomiting, and respiratory depression than meperidine

      3) Mixed narcotic agonist-antagonist compounds (butorphanol [IM/IV], nalbuphine [IV/IM/SC])—analgesia while decreasing adverse effects but can still produce respiratory depression, nausea and vomiting, light-headedness

      4) Narcotic antagonist (opioid antagonist)—counteracts respiratory depressant effects; may be administered to mother IM/IV 5–15 min prior to delivery or to neonate IV via umbilical vein immediately after birth

      Note: Narcotic antagonist given to a woman who is addicted to narcotics may cause immediate withdrawal symptoms

   b. Antiemetics—used to decrease nausea, vomiting, and anxiety

      1) Hydroxyzine—can increase effectiveness of opioid; decreases anxiety and nausea/vomiting (N/V); cannot be given IV

      2) Promethazine—reduces N/V; can cause sedation; may contribute to maternal hypotension

**Table 13-8** Common Analgesics and Anesthetics of Labor and Delivery

| MEDICATION | ADVERSE EFFECTS | NURSING CONSIDERATIONS |
|---|---|---|
| Morphine | Hypotension<br><br>Bradycardia<br><br>Respiratory depression | Sedates<br><br>Anxiety relief<br><br>Pain control<br><br>Do not administer within 2 h of expected delivery<br><br>Have naloxone available for newborn |
| Nalbuphine | Respiratory depression | Causes less N/V for the mother |
| Lidocaine | Confusion<br><br>Tremors<br><br>Restlessness<br><br>Hypotension<br><br>Dysrhythmias<br><br>Tinnitus<br><br>Blurred vision | Regional nerve block<br><br>Relieves uterine or perineal pain<br><br>If subarachnoid space used, keep client flat for 6–8 h |
| Opioid Antagonists | | |
| Naloxone hydrochloride | Tachycardia<br><br>Hypertension<br><br>Tremors | IV into umbilical vein for neonates<br><br>Endotracheal (ET) if neonate is intubated (0.01 mg/kg)<br><br>Reverses narcotic depression |

3. Local anesthetics—used to provide nerve blockage in specific areas

   a. Subarachnoid block/"saddle block" (nerves from S1–S4)—anesthetizes perineum, lower pelvis, and upper thighs; diminishes pushing efforts; high incidence of maternal hypotension and potential for fetal hypoxia

   b. Pudendal nerve block—local anesthetic is injected into pudendal nerves; provides pain relief in lower vagina, vulva, and perineum

   c. Neuraxial analgesia/anesthesia—produces a loss of sensation or, with opioid use, pain control; does not interfere with the process of labor; provided by epidural, intrathecal, and/or spinal injection

1) Epidural block—affects the entire pelvis by blocking impulses at level of T12 through S5; may be administered continuously through tubing left in place; incidence of maternal hypotension may be minimized if 500–1,000 mL of IV fluid is infused at a rapid rate prior to administration and mother is maintained in side-lying position

   a) There must be vigilant monitoring of maternal BP and FHR every 1–2 min × 15 min and every 10–15 min thereafter

   b) Treatment of maternal hypotension includes:

      i) Mild/moderate—place mother in left lateral position, increase the rate of IV fluid; administer oxygen by mask

      ii) Severe/prolonged—place mother in Trendelenburg position for 2–3 min

2) Combined spinal-epidural—provides rapid onset of pain relief; maternal motor function unimpaired

3) Patient-controlled epidural analgesia (PCEA)—placement of an indwelling epidural catheter is completed and the mother can control the amount of analgesia provided

d. General anesthesia—used for emergency cesarean births; all agents cross the placental barrier, so fetal depression is of concern

**F.** Fetal monitoring during labor and delivery

1. Fetal heart rate

   a. Methods

      1) Periodic auscultation of the fetal heart by fetoscope (stethoscope adapted to amplify sound) or fetal Doppler (ultrasound stethoscope) during contractions and for 30 s beyond; best heard over fetal back

      2) Electronic fetal monitoring (EFM)—continuous monitoring providing audio and visual recordings as well as tracing strips

         a) External—indirect, noninvasive method using a lubricated (water-soluble gel) ultrasound transducer attached to the abdomen

         b) Internal—small electrode attached to the fetal scalp; indicated for high-risk maternity client, problematic labor, or with oxytocin use; requires ROM, cervical dilation of at least 2 cm, and presenting part can be reached

   b. Alterations in fetal heart rate

      1) Rate

         a) Normal—120–160 beats per minute (bpm) during a 10-minute period, excluding fetal heart rate measured during a contraction

         b) Tachycardia (greater than 160 bpm)—associated with prematurity, maternal fever, fetal activity, or fetal hypoxia/infection, medications; if continued for greater than 10 minutes or accompanied by late deceleration, indicates fetal distress

    c)   Bradycardia (less than 110 bpm)—associated with fetal hypoxia, maternal medications/hypotension, prolonged cord compression, congenital heart lesions; persistent bradycardia or persistent drop of 20 beats per min below baseline may indicate cord compression or separation of the placenta

2)  Variability—beat-to-beat fluctuations; measured by internal EFM only

    a)   Absent (fluctuation range undetectable)—may be associated with fetal sleep state, fetal prematurity, reaction to medications, congenital anomalies, hypoxia, acidosis

    b)   Minimal (fluctuation range less than 5 bpm)—loss of the baseline (beat-to-beat variation) or "smoothing out" of the baseline is often a prelude to neonatal death

    c)   Moderate (fluctuation range of 6–25 bpm)—normal; indicates fetus is well-developed and oxygenated

    d)   Marked (fluctuation range greater than 25 bpm)—causes may be cord prolapse or compression, maternal hypotension, uterine hyperstimulation, abruptio placentae

3)  Periodic changes

    a)   Accelerations—elevation of fetal heart rate more than 15 bpm above the baseline lasting more than 15 seconds and less than 2 minutes; reassuring and commonly seen with fetal movement

    b)   Decelerations—transient fall in fetal heart rate; classified as early, late, or variable

        i)   Early—characterized by gradual decrease in fetal heart rate; nadir (lowest point) coincides with the peak of the contraction; most often uniform mirror image of contraction on tracing; associated with head compression, commonly in second stage with pushing

        ii)   Late—transitory decrease in fetal heart rate; smooth and symmetrical decrease; characterized by nadir occurring after the peak of the contraction; return to baseline does not occur until contraction is over; indicative of fetal hypoxia because of deficient placental perfusion

        iii)   Variable deceleration—transient U/V/M–shaped reduction occurring at any time before, during, or after contraction; indicative of cord compression, which may be relieved by change in mother's position; ominous if repetitive, prolonged, severe, or has slow return to baseline

    c)   Nursing interventions

        i)   For early decelerations—evaluate fetal station and maternal dilation and effacement; usually no intervention is required

        ii)   For late decelerations (at the first sign of abnormal tracing)—position mother lying on left side (if no change, move to other side, Trendelenburg, or knee/chest position); administer oxygen by mask, start IV or increase flow rate, stop oxytocin if appropriate; if the pattern persists, fetal scalp blood sampling for acidosis (pH greater than 7.25 is normal, 7.20–7.24 is considered preacidotic—repeat in 10–15 min; 7.2 or less indicates serious acidosis; prepare for cesarean section)

    iii)   For variable decelerations—reposition the mother to relieve pressure on the cord

**G.** Intrapartum nursing management

1. Stage 1

   a. Maternal

      1)  Monitor vital signs, fluid and electrolyte balance, frequency, duration, and intensity of uterine contractions and degree of discomfort (hourly, at minimum); urine protein and glucose with every voiding; laboratory results; preparedness; ROM

      2)  Provide comfort measures—e.g., positioning, back massage/effleurage (light abdominal stroking in rhythm with breathing during a contraction to ease mild/moderate discomfort), warm/cold compresses, ice chips

      3)  Support coping measures—reassure, explain procedures, reinforce/teach breathing techniques, relaxation, focal point

      4)  Assist support person

   b. Fetal—monitor status

2. Stage 2

   a. Maternal

      1)  Monitor physical status; assess progress of labor, perineal and rectal bulging, increased vaginal show

      2)  Assist in techniques to foster expulsion—encourage bearing down with focus on vaginal orifice (discourage breath holding for more than 5 s), position squatting, side-lying, Fowler as appropriate

      3)  Provide comfort measures; support coping measures; assist support person

   b. Fetus/neonate

      1)  Monitor fetal heart rate and regularity

      2)  Provide immediate neonatal care

         a)  Mucus is removed by bulb syringe immediately after the head is delivered (mouth before nose to avoid aspiration)

         b)  After delivery of the full body, the cord is clamped twice and cut between the clamps

         c)  Record time of birth

         d)  Inspect cord for two arteries and one vein

         e)  Dry and wrap neonate to prevent heat loss

3. Stage 3

a. Maternal—observe for signs and symptoms of placental separation; assess amount of blood loss; monitor blood pressure, pulse, and fundus frequently

b. Neonate

1) Apgar scores at 1 and 5 min to evaluate condition at birth (*see* Table 13-9)

a) Based on five signs: heartbeat, respiratory effort, muscle tone, reflex irritability, color

b) Each sign rated 0–2 (2 is top score); all the scores are added for total score

c) 7–10 (good condition) should do well in normal neonatal nursery; 4–6 (fair condition) may require close observation; 0–3 (extremely poor condition) resuscitation and intensive care are required

**Table 13-9** Apgar Score

|  | 0 | 1 | 2 |
|---|---|---|---|
| Heart rate | Absent | Slow (less than 100 bpm) | Normal (greater than 100 bpm) |
| Respiratory effort | Absent | Slow, irregular, weak cry | Good cry |
| Muscle tone | Flaccid | Some flexion of extremities | Well flexed |
| Reflexes | No response | Grimace | Vigorous cry |
| Color | Blue, pale | Body pink, extremities blue | Completely pink |
| **TOTAL** _____ | | | |

2) Maintain temperature—minimize exposure to environmental heat loss (evaporation, radiation, conduction, convection); skin to skin with mother or at 97.5–99°F (36.4–37.2°C) skin temperature

3) Weigh and measure neonate

4) Place identification band on neonate; footprint neonate and fingerprint mother

5) Record time of first void and stool (meconium) after delivery; monitor physical status

6) Initiate parent-child interaction

7) Instill prophylactic eye ointment—legally required to prevent conjunctival gonococcal infection that could lead to blindness in the neonate; 0.5% erythromycin

8) Administer intramuscular phytonadione (vitamin K)—for first 3–4 d of life, the neonate is unable to synthesize vitamin K, which is necessary for blood clotting and coagulation

4. Stage 4 (*see* Table 13-10)

    a. Monitor maternal blood pressure and pulse; uterine contractility tone and location; amount and color of lochia, presence of clots; condition of episiotomy every 15 min × 4

    b. Monitor bladder function

    c. Provide comfort

    d. Evaluate parental interaction

**Table 13-10** Fourth Stage of Labor

| FIRST 1–2 H | | NURSING CONSIDERATIONS |
|---|---|---|
| Vital signs (BP, pulse) | q 15 min | Follow protocol until stable |
| Fundus | q 15 min | Position—at the level of the umbilicus for the first 12 h, then descends by one fingerbreadth each succeeding day, pelvic organ usually by day 10 |
| Lochia (color, volume) | q 15 min | Lochia (endometrial sloughing)—day 1-3 rubra (bloody with fleshy odor; may be clots); day 4-9 serosa (pink/brown with fleshy odor); day 10+ alba (yellow/white); at no time should there be a foul odor (indicates infection) |
| Urinary | Measure first void | May have urethral edema, urine retention |
| Bonding | Encourage interaction | Emphasize touch, eye contact |

# POSTPARTUM

## Fluid/Electrolyte Balance

## From Stage 4 Until 6 Weeks After Delivery

A.  Involution—(uterus reduced to prepregnant size)

   1.  Fundus—midline, firm, height

      a.  Position—at the level of the umbilicus for the first 12 h, then descends by one finger-breadth each succeeding day, pelvic organ usually by day 10

      b.  If deviations, check bladder and have client void; if deviations continue, massage fundus

   2.  Lochia (endometrial sloughing)—day 1–3 rubra (bloody with fleshy odor; may be clots); day 4–9 serosa (pink/brown with fleshy odor); day 10+ alba (yellow/white); at no time should there be a foul odor (indicates infection)

      a.  Blood loss greater than 500 mL after a vaginal birth or 1,000 mL after a cesarean birth.

      b.  Moderate amount of blood flow is greater than 4 inches but less than 6 inches of flow on the peri-pad within 1 hour (approximately 25–50 mL)

      c.  Large amount of blood flow is greater than 6 inches to saturated peri-pad within 1 hour (approximately 50–80 mL)

      d.  Accurate measurement of blood loss is accomplished by weighing peri-pad

B.  Perineum—possible discomfort, swelling, and/or ecchymosis

   1.  Managed with analgesics and/or topical anesthetics, ice packs for first 12–24 h and then 20-min sitz baths 3–4 times/d, tightening buttocks before sitting

   2.  Monitor episiotomy/laceration (see postoperative care)—teach techniques to prevent infection, e.g., change pads on regular basis, peri care (cleaning from front to back using peri-bottle or surgigator after each voiding and bowel movement), sitz baths

C.  Breasts—progress from soft to filling with potential for engorgement (vascular congestion related to increased blood and lymph supply; breasts are larger, firmer, and painful)

   1.  Nonnursing woman—suppress lactation

      a.  Mechanical methods—tight-fitting brassiere, ice packs, minimize breast stimulation

   2.  Nursing woman—successful lactation is dependent on infant sucking and maternal production and delivery of milk (letdown/milk ejection reflex); monitor and teach preventive measures for potential problems (*see* Table 13-11)

**Table 13-11** Lactation Principles

| BREAST CARE—ANTEPARTUM AND POSTPARTUM | INITIATING BREAST FEEDING |
|---|---|
| Soap on nipples should be avoided during bathing to prevent dryness | Relaxed position of mother is essential—support dependent arm with pillow |
| Redness or swelling can indicate infection and should always be investigated | Alternate which breast is offered first at each feeding |
| | Five minutes on each breast is sufficient at first—teach proper way to break suction |
| | Most of the areola should be in infant's mouth to ensure proper sucking |

    a.  Nipple irritation/cracking

       1)  Nipple care—clean with warm water, no soap, and dry thoroughly; absorbent breast pads if leaking occurs; apply breast milk to nipples and areola after each feeding and air dry; apply warm compresses after each feeding and air dry

       2)  Position nipple so that infant's mouth covers a large portion of the areola, and release infant's mouth from nipple by inserting finger to break suction

       3)  Rotate breast feeding positions

    b.  Engorgement—nurse frequently (every 0.5–3 h) and long enough to empty breasts completely (evidenced by sucking without swallowing); warm shower or compresses to stimulate letdown; alternate starting breast at each feeding; mild analgesic 20 min before feeding and ice packs between feedings for pronounced discomfort

    c.  Plugged ducts—area of tenderness and lumpiness often associated with engorgement; may be relieved by heat and massage prior to feeding

    d.  Expression of breast milk—to collect milk for supplemental feedings, to relieve breast fullness or to build milk supply; may be manually expressed or pumped by a device and refrigerated up to 4 days or frozen in plastic bottles (to maintain stability of all elements) in refrigerator freezer for 6 months ideally but up to 12 months is acceptable; thawed breast milk should never be refrozen

    e.  Medications—most medications/drugs cross into breast milk; check with health care provider before taking any medication

**D.**  Elimination

    1.  Urinary—increased output (postpartum diuresis), urethral trauma, decreased bladder sensation, and inability to void in the recumbent position may cause bladder distention, incomplete emptying, and/or urinary stasis, increasing the risk of uterine relaxation and hemorrhage and/or UTI; monitor I and O and encourage voiding every 24 h (early ambulation and pouring warm water over perineum); catheterization may be necessary if no voiding after 8 h

2. GI—bowel sluggishness, decreased abdominal muscle tone, perineal discomfort may lead to constipation; managed by early ambulation, increased dietary fiber and hydration, stool softeners

**E.** Afterpains—cramps due to uterine contractions; last 2–3 d; more common in multipara and with nursing; may be relieved by lying on abdomen with small pillow, heat, ambulation, mild analgesic (if breast feeding, 1 h before nursing)

**F.** Rubella vaccine—for susceptible woman; Rho(D) immune globulin intramuscular (IGIM) as appropriate

**G.** Psychosocial adjustment

1. Attachment/bonding—influenced by maternal psychosocial-cultural factors, infant health status, temperament, behaviors, and circumstances of the prenatal, intrapartum, postpartum, and neonatal course; evidenced initially by touching and cuddling, naming, "en face" positioning for direct eye contact, later by reciprocity and rhythmicity in maternal-infant interaction

2. Phases of adjustment

   a. "Taking in"/dependency (day 1–2 after delivery)—preoccupied with self and own needs (food and sleep); talkative and passive; follows directions and is hesitant about making decisions; retells perceptions of birth experience

   b. "Taking hold"/dependency-independency (by day 3)—performing self-care; expresses concern for self and baby; open to instructions

   c. "Letting go"/independence (evident by weeks 5–6)—assuming new role and responsibilities; may be grief for relinquished roles; adjustment to accommodate for infant in family

3. "Postpartum blues" (day 3–7)—normal occurrence of "roller-coaster" emotions, weeping, "let-down feeling"; usually relieved with emotional support and rest/sleep; report if prolonged or later onset

4. Sexual activities—abstain from intercourse until episiotomy is healed and lochia has ceased (usually 3–4 wk); may be affected by fatigue, fear of discomfort, leakage of breast milk, concern about another pregnancy; assess and discuss couple's desire for and understanding about contraceptive methods; breast feeding does not give adequate protection, and oral contraceptives should not be used during breast feeding

[ SECTION 5 ]

# THE NEONATE

## Gas Exchange, Fluid/Electrolyte Balance

### Assessment—physical examination

**A.** Measurements at term

1. Weight—6–9 lb (2,750–4,082 g); normal 5–10% weight loss in first few days should be regained in 1–2 wk

2. Length—19–21 in (48–53 cm)

3. Head circumference—13–14 in (33–35 cm); one-fourth body length

4. Chest—12–13 in (30.5-33 cm); 1 in (2.54 cm) less than head circumference

**B.** Vital signs

1. Temperature

   a. Rectal not recommended as routine because of potential for rectal mucosa irritation and increased risk of perforation

   b. Axillary—97.7–98.6°F (36.5–37°C); thermometer should remain in place at least 3 min unless an electronic thermometer is used

2. Apical rate—100 bpm (sleep); 120–140 bpm (awake); up to 180 bpm (crying); assessed by auscultation for 1 full minute when infant not crying

3. Respirations—30–60/min; primarily diaphragmatic and abdominal synchronous with chest movements; may be short periods (less than 15 s) of apnea; since neonate is an obligatory nose breather, it is important to keep nose and mouth clear

4. Blood pressure—averages 65/41 mm Hg (arm and calf) in full-term resting neonate; thigh blood pressure may be 4–8 mm Hg higher than arm or calf blood pressure

**C.** Posture

1. Maintains fetal position for several days

2. Resistance to extension of extremities

**D.** Skin—sensitive to drying

1. Erythematous (beefy red) color for a few hours after birth; then pink or as expected for racial background; acrocyanosis (bluish discoloration of hands and feet) is normal for 24 h

2. Vernix caseosa—protective gray-white fatty substance of cheesy consistency covering the fetal/newborn skin; do not attempt vigorous removal

3. Lanugo—light distribution of downy, fine hair may be over the shoulders, forehead, and cheeks; extensive amount is indicative of prematurity

4. Milia—distended sebaceous glands appearing as tiny, white, pinpoint papules on forehead, nose, cheeks, and chin of neonate that disappear spontaneously in a few days or weeks

5. Pigmentation

   a. Slate gray nevus (congenital dermal melanocytosis)—bluish gray or dark nonelevated pigmentation area over the lower back and buttocks present at birth in some infants, (African American, Hispanic, Asian)

   b. Birthmarks

      1) Telangiectatic nevi ("stork bites")—cluster of small, flat, red, localized areas of capillary dilatation usually on eyelids, nose, nape of neck; can be blanched by the pressure of the finger; usually fade during infancy

      2) Nevus vasculosus (strawberry mark)—raised, demarcated, dark red, rough-surfaced capillary hemangioma in dermal and subdural layers; grows rapidly for several months and then begins to fade; usually disappears by 7 y old

      3) Nevus flammeus (port wine stain)—reddish, usually flat discoloration commonly on the face or neck; does not grow and does not fade

E. Head—may appear asymmetrical because of overriding of cranial bones during labor and delivery (molding); head lag less than 45°

   1. Fontanels—"soft spots" at junction of cranial bones

      a. Anterior fontanel—diamond shaped, easily felt, usually open and flat (may be moderate bulging with crying/stooling); sustained bulging occurs with increased intracranial pressure, depression with dehydration; may be slight pulsation; closes by 18 mo of age

      b. Posterior—triangular, not easily palpated; closes between 8–12 wk of life

   2. Cephalohematoma—collection of blood under the periosteum of a cranial bone appearing 1–2 d; does not cross suture line; disappears in weeks to months

   3. Caput succedaneum—localized soft swelling of the scalp often associated with a long and difficult birth; present at birth; overrides the suture line; fluid is reabsorbed within hours to days after delivery

   4. Face—symmetrical distribution and movement of all features; asymmetry may signify paralysis of facial cranial nerve (Bell palsy)

   5. Eyes—may be edematous; yellow-white drainage associated with silver nitrate drops (chemical conjunctivitis), which should disappear in 1–2 d without treatment; areas of subconjunctival hemorrhage

   6. Mouth—sucks well when stimulated; hard and soft palate intact when examined with clean-gloved finger

   7. Ears—tops (pinnae) should be parallel with the inner and outer canthi of eyes; low-set ears are associated with chromosomal abnormalities, intellectual delay, and/or internal organ abnormalities; hearing is evaluated by an arousal response to loud or moderately loud noise unaccompanied by vibration

F. Chest—breast engorgement lasting up to 2 wk may occur in both males and females

**G.** Abdomen

1. Cylindrical and slightly protuberant

2. Umbilical cord—initially white and gelatinous, shriveled and black by 2–3 d, falls off within 1–2 wk; foul-smelling discharge is indicative of infection and requires immediate treatment to prevent septicemia

3. First stool is dark green or black and is tarry (meconium), passed within 12–24 h; followed by thin brown-green transitional stools for first 2–3 d; then 1–2 formed pale yellow stools/day with formula feeding or loose golden yellow stools with every feeding for breast feeding

**H.** Genitourinary—urine is present in bladder at birth, but neonate may not void for 12–24 h (may be brick-red spots on diaper from passage of uric acid crystals); thereafter usually voids pale yellow urine 6–10 times/d

1. Female—labia relatively large and approximated; may be normal thick white discharge; a white cheeselike substance (smegma and/or blood tinge [pseudomenstruation])

2. Male—testes can be palpated in scrotum

**I.** Trunk and extremities

1. Arms and legs symmetric in shape and function

2. Hips abduct to greater than 60°; symmetric inguinal and buttock creases indicating no hip dislocation

3. Foot in straight line

**J.** Reflexes

1. Rooting and sucking—turns toward any object touching/stroking cheek/mouth, opens mouth, and sucks rhythmically when finger/nipple is inserted into mouth (usually disappears by 4–7 mo)

2. Pupillary—constriction on exposure to light

3. Palmar grasp—pressure on palm elicits grasp (fades by 3–4 mo)

4. Plantar grasp—pressure on sole behind toes elicits flexion (lessens by 8 mo)

5. Tonic neck—fencing position; lying on back with head turned on one side, arm and leg on that side of body will be in extension while extremities on opposite side will be flexed (disappears by 3–4 mo)

6. Moro—elicited by sudden disturbance in the infant's immediate environment, body will stiffen, arms in tense extension followed by embrace gesture with thumb and index finger in a "c" formation (disappears after 3–4 mo)

7. Positive—supporting; infant will stiffen legs and appear to stand when held upright

8. Stepping reflex—when held upright with one foot touching a flat surface, will step alternatingly (generally fades by 4 weeks)

9. Babinski's sign—stroking the sole of the foot from heel upward across ball of foot will cause all toes to fan (reverts to usual adult response by 24 mo)

## Routine Care

A. Monitor vital signs at least once per shift

B. Begin and monitor feeding schedule

    1. Before initiating first formula feeding, check for readiness (active bowel sounds, absence of abdominal distention, and lusty cry) and for absence of gagging, choking, regurgitating associated with tracheoesophageal fistula or esophageal atresia by giving a small amount of sterile water (glucose is irritating to lungs)

    2. Because colostrum is readily absorbed by the gastrointestinal system, breast feeding may be started immediately after birth

C. Umbilical cord care—clean cord daily, following health care provider prescription; no tub baths until cord falls off; fold diapers below to maintain dry area; report redness, drainage, foul odor

D. Care of penis

    1. Uncircumcised—do not force retraction of foreskin (complete separation of foreskin and glans penis takes 3–5 y); parents should be told to *gently* test for retraction occasionally during the bath and, when it has occurred, *gently* clean glans with soap and water

    2. Circumcised (surgical removal of prepuce/foreskin)

        a. Ensure signed permission before procedure; provide pain control during and after procedure

        b. Postprocedure monitor for bleeding and voiding, apply A and D ointment (lanolin/petrolatum) or petroleum jelly (except when Plastibell is used)

        c. Teach parents to clean area with warm water squeezed over penis and dry gently; a whitish yellow exudate is normal and should not be removed; if Plastibell is used, report to health care provider if it has not fallen off in about 8 d

E. Administer prophylactic medications

    1. Eye prophylaxis—0.5% erythromycin or 1% tetracycline immediately after birth

    2. IM phytonadione (vitamin K)—neonate unable to synthesize vitamin K immediately after birth

[ SECTION 6 ]

# CHILDBEARING—MATERNAL COMPLICATIONS

## Coagulation, Perfusion, Infection

### Monitoring Fetal Status

A. Ultrasonography—(visualizes the fetus, placenta, amniotic fluid) can diagnose a pregnancy in the first 6 wk and monitor fetal growth and intrauterine environment throughout the course of pregnancy; adjunct to amniocentesis; no known harmful effects to mother and fetus; woman must drink fluid and not void prior to test

B. Amniocentesis—amniotic fluid is aspirated by a needle inserted through the abdominal and uterine walls; indicated early in pregnancy (14–17 wk) to detect inborn errors of metabolism, chromosomal abnormalities, open neural tube defect (NTD); determine sex of fetus and sex-linked disorders after 28 wk; determine lung maturity after 30 wk

   1. Indicated for pregnant women 35 y and older; couples who already have had a child with a genetic disorder; one or both parents affected with a genetic disorder; mothers who are carriers for X-linked disorders

   2. Prior to the procedure, the client's bladder should be emptied; ultrasonography (x-ray only if necessary) is used to avoid trauma from the needle

   3. Postprocedure, monitor for signs and symptoms of hemorrhage, labor, premature separation of placenta, fetal distress, amniotic fluid embolism, infection, inadvertent injury to maternal intestines/bladder or fetus; Rho(D) immune globulin intramuscular (IGIM) is indicated for Rh-negative mothers

C. Chorionic villus sampling (CVS)—transcervical aspiration of chorionic villi that allows for first-trimester (8–12 wk) diagnosing of genetic disorders (Down syndrome, sickle cell anemia, phenylketonuria [PKU], Duchenne muscular dystrophy), comparable to amniocentesis (except for NTD); preprocedure: there should be full bladder; ultrasound is used as in amniocentesis; postprocedure: precautions as for amniocentesis

D. Estriol levels—serial 24-h maternal urine samples or serum specimens to determine fetoplacental status; falling levels usually indicate deterioration

E. Nonstress test (NST)—evaluates FHR by electronic fetal monitor (EFM) in response to fetal movement (FM); as early as 27 wk; woman should eat 2 h before and may be given snacks during to enhance FM; monitor for maternal hypotension

   1. Indicated 1–2 times/wk for high-risk pregnancy

2. Interpretation

    a. Reactive—FHR accelerations of 15 or more bpm lasting 15 or more seconds with at least 2 FM in a 20-min period; monitor NST 1–2 times/wk

    b. Nonreactive—any one of the above criteria is not met; continue EFM and additional testing; immediate delivery may be necessary; report decelerations

    c. Unsatisfactory—inadequate FM despite snacks/gentle pushing baby/vibroacoustic stimulation or unable to interpret data; repeat NST within 24 h

**F.** Biophysical profile—assessment of fetal breathing movements, body movements, muscle tone, amniotic fluid volume by ultrasound, and FHR reactivity by NST; with a score of 0–2 for each, 8–10 is considered normal

**G.** Contraction/stress test (CCT/OCT)—evaluates FHR in response to contractions initiated by endogenous (nipple stimulation) or exogenous oxytocin (IV); after 28 wk; woman in semi-Fowler or side-lying position

    1. Indications—intrauterine growth restriction (IUGR), diabetes, postdates (greater than 42 wk), nonreactive NST, abnormal biophysical profile

    2. Contraindications—third-trimester bleeding, previous cesarean delivery (C/S) with classic incision, potential for preterm labor

    3. Interpretation

        a. Negative—no late decelerations with at least three contractions lasting 40–60 s in a 10-min period; repeat as necessary or in 1 wk

        b. Positive—late decelerations with at least 50% of contractions; potential fetal risk and cesarean may be necessary

        c. Suspicious—late decelerations in less than half of contractions; other testing and/or repeat stress test in 24 h

        d. Unsatisfactory—inadequate contraction pattern or tracing; continue test or repeat after mother rests

**H.** Percutaneous umbilical blood sampling (PUBS)—second- and third-trimester method to aspirate cord blood (location identified by ultrasound) to test for genetic conditions, chromosomal abnormalities, fetal infections, hemolytic or hematological disorders

## Prenatal

**A.** Factors associated with increased risk—lack of prenatal care, age less than 18 or older than 35, conception within two months of previous delivery, fifth or subsequent delivery, prepregnant weight 20% more or less than normal and/or minimal or no weight gain, fetal anomaly

**B.** Adolescence—may be interference with normal physical growth and maturation, lack of family acceptance or support, isolation from peers, delayed/no prenatal care, and increased medical and obstetrical risks; requires support for feelings, assistance with decision making, regular monitoring of health status, instruction in nutrition

**C.** Substance use/abuse

1. Drugs (including alcohol)—may be increased risk of maternal nutritional deficits, sexually transmitted infections (STIs), AIDS, delayed/no prenatal care, withdrawal symptoms, and fetal intrauterine growth restriction (IUGR), anomalies, spontaneous abortions, death, signs and symptoms of withdrawal or addiction in neonate; educate, reinforce, counsel, and/or refer as necessary; emphasize that a safe level of alcohol has not been identified

2. Cigarettes—increased incidence of intrauterine growth restriction (IUGR), preterm births, low Apgar scores, spontaneous abortions, sudden infant death syndrome (SIDS); as with drugs

**D.** Infections

1. Urinary tract infections (UTIs)—characterized by urinary frequency and urgency, dysuria, and sometimes hematuria and manifested in upper tract by fever, malaise, anorexia, nausea, abdominal/back pain; confirmed by greater than 100,000/mL bacterial colony count by mid-stream urine; sometimes asymptomatic; treated with sulfa-based medications and ampicillin

2. TORCH test series—group of maternal systemic infections that can be transmitted across the placenta or by ascending infection (after ROM) to the fetus; infection early in pregnancy may produce significant and devastating fetal deformities, whereas later infection may result in overwhelming active systemic disease and/or CNS involvement, causing severe neurological impairment or death of newborn

   a. **T**oxoplasmosis (protozoa; transplacental to fetus)—discourage eating undercooked meat and handling cat litter box

   b. **O**ther

      1) Syphilis

      2) Varicella/shingles (transplacental to fetus or droplet to newborn)—caution susceptible woman about contact with the disease and zoster immune globulin for exposure

      3) Group B beta-hemolytic *Streptococcus* (direct or indirect to fetus during labor and delivery)—treated with penicillin

      4) Hepatitis B (transplacental and contact with secretions during delivery)—screen and immunize maternal carriers; treat newborn with HBIg

      5) AIDS (as with hepatitis)—titers in newborn may be passive transfer of maternal antibodies or active antibody formation

   c. **R**ubella (transplacental)—prenatal testing required by law; caution susceptible woman about contact; vaccine is not given during pregnancy

   d. **C**ytomegalovirus (CMV)—transmitted in body fluids; detected by antibody/serological testing

   e. **H**erpes type 2 (transplacental, ascending infection within 4–6 h after ROM or contact during delivery if active lesions)—cesarean delivery if active lesions

**E.** Bleeding

1. Early (before 20 wk)

a. Spontaneous abortion characterized by painless (may be cramping) dark or bright red vaginal bleeding (*see* Table 13-12)

**Table 13-12** Clinical Classifications of Spontaneous Abortion

| TYPE | ASSESSMENT | NURSING CONSIDERATIONS |
|---|---|---|
| Threatened | Vaginal bleeding and cramping<br><br>Soft uterus, cervix closed | Ultrasound for intrauterine sac, quantitative hCG<br><br>Decrease activity for 24–48 h, avoid stress, no sexual intercourse for 2 wk after bleeding stops<br><br>Monitor amount and character of bleeding; report clots, tissue, foul odor |
| Inevitable, if cervical dilation cannot be prevented | Persistent symptoms, hemorrhage, moderate to severe cramping<br><br>Cervical dilatation and effacement | Monitor for hemorrhage (save and count pads) and infection; if persistent or increased symptoms, D and C<br><br>Emotional support for grief and loss |
| Incomplete | Persistent symptoms, expulsion of part of products of conception | Administer IV/blood, oxytocin<br><br>D and C or suction evacuation |
| Complete | As above, except no retained tissue | Possible methylergonovine; no other treatment if no evidence of hemorrhage or infection |
| Missed—fetus dies in utero but is not expelled | May be none/some abating of above symptoms<br><br>Cervix is closed<br><br>If retained greater than 6 wk, increased risk of infection, disseminated intravascular coagulation (DIC), and emotional distress | D and C evacuation within 4-6 wk<br><br>After 12 wk, dilate cervix with several applications of prostaglandin gel or suppositories of laminaria (dried sterilized seaweed that expands with cervical secretions) |
| Habitual—3 or more | May be incompetent cervix, infertility | Cerclage (encircling cervix with suture) |

b. Ectopic pregnancy—implantation outside uterus (commonly in fallopian tube), potentially life-threatening to mother

1) Characterized by unilateral lower-quadrant pain after 4–6 wk of normal signs and symptoms of pregnancy; bleeding may be gradual oozing to frank bleeding; may be palpable unilateral mass in adnexa; low hCG levels; rigid and tender abdomen; signs and symptoms of hemorrhage

2) Necessary to be alert for signs and symptoms—investigate risk factors especially PID, multiple sexual partners, recurrent episodes of gonorrhea, infertility

3) Management—monitor Hb and Hct, ultrasound for adnexal mass, may be culdocentesis (indicated by nonclotting blood), laparoscopy and/or laparotomy; adequate blood replacement (type and X match, IV with large-bore needle); prepare for surgery; postoperatively, monitor for infection and paralytic ileus, support for emotional distress, Rho(D) immune globulin intramuscular (IGIM) for Rh-negative woman

2. Late in pregnancy

a. Placenta previa—may be low-lying in lower segment, marginal at border of internal cervical os, or partial or complete obstruction of the os

1) Characterized by painless vaginal bleeding, which is usually slight at first and increases in subsequent unpredictable episodes; usually soft and nontender abdomen

2) Management

a) Hospitalization initially—bedrest side-lying position for at least 72 h; ultrasound to locate placenta; no vaginal/rectal exam unless delivery would not be a problem (if becomes necessary, must be done in OR under sterile conditions); amniocentesis for lung maturity; monitor for changes in bleeding and fetal status; daily Hb and Hct; 2 units of cross-matched blood available

b) Home if bleeding ceases and pregnancy to be maintained—limit activity; no douching, enemas, coitus; monitor FM; NST at least every 1–2 wk

c) Delivery by cesarean if evidence of fetal maturity, excessive bleeding, active labor, other complications

b. Abruptio placentae—premature separation of normally implanted placenta; may be marginal (near edge) with dark red vaginal bleeding or central (at center) with concealed bleeding; life-threatening to fetus and mother

1) Characterized by abdominal pain; uterine rigidity and tenderness; rapid signs and symptoms of maternal shock and/or fetal distress

2) Manage signs and symptoms; prepare for immediate delivery, usually cesarean section

3) Postoperatively monitor for complications

a) Infection

b) Renal failure

c) Disseminated intravascular coagulation (DIC)—massive hemorrhage initiates coagulation process causing massive numbers of clots in peripheral vessels (may result in tissue damage from multiple thrombi), which in turn stimulate fibrinolytic activity, resulting in decreased platelet and fibrinogen levels and signs and symptoms of local generalized bleeding (increased vaginal blood flow, oozing IV site, ecchymosis, hematuria, etc.); monitor PT, PTT, and Hct; protect from injury; no IM injections; early anticoagulant therapy is controversial

3. Hydatidiform mole—degenerative anomaly of chorionic villi characterized by elevated hCG levels, uterine size greater than expected for dates, no FHR, minimal dark red/brown vaginal bleeding with passage of grapelike clusters and no fetus by ultrasound, possibly increased nausea and vomiting and associated pregnancy-induced hypertension; treated with curettage to completely remove all molar tissue, which can become malignant; pregnancy is discouraged for 1 y, and hCG levels are monitored during that time (if continue to be elevated, may require hysterectomy and chemotherapy)

F. Diabetes mellitus—interaction of diabetes and pregnancy may cause serious problems for mother and fetus/newborn

1. Classification

a. Type 1

b. Type 2

c. Gestational diabetes (GDM)

d. Impaired glucose tolerance (IGT)

2. Effect of diabetes on pregnancy—long-standing diabetes and/or poor control before conception can increase risk of maternal infections, pregnancy-induced hypertension (PIH), hydramnios (greater than 2,000 mL amniotic fluid) and consequent preterm labor, macrosomia (large for gestational age but may have immature organ systems), and in more severe cases, congenital anomalies, IUGR, prematurity, and respiratory distress syndrome (RDS) in neonate; untreated ketoacidosis can cause coma and death of mother and fetus

3. Gestational diabetes—usually normal response to glucose load before and after pregnancy; abnormal response is usually noted after 20 wk, when insulin need accelerates and brings about symptoms; some gravidas will need exogenous insulin but majority are controlled by diet; oral hypoglycemics must not be used because they may be teratogenic and increase the risk of neonatal hypoglycemia

4. Assessment

a. Risk factors for GDM—obesity, family history of diabetes; client history of gestational diabetes, hypertension/PIH, recurrent UTIs, monilial vaginitis, polyhydramnios; previously large infant (9 lb/4,000 g or more), previously unexplained death/anomaly or stillbirths; glycosuria, proteinuria on two or more occasions

b. Diabetes screening—at 24–28 wk for all gravidas

1) Screen blood glucose level 1 h after 50 g concentrated glucose solution

2) Three-hour glucose tolerance test; normal findings—fasting blood sugar (FBS): less than 92 mg/dL (5.1mmol/L); 1 h: less than 180 mg/dL (9 mmol/L); 2 h: less than 153 mg/dL (8.5 mmol/L); 3 h: less than 140 mg/dL (7.8 mmol/L)

3) If two or more abnormal findings, significant for diabetes

c. Glycosylated hemoglobin (HbA1c)—measures control over the past 3 mo; elevations (greater than 6–8%) in first trimester are associated with increased risk of congenital anomaly and spontaneous abortion; in the last trimester with macrosomia

5. Management—requires close medical and obstetrical supervision throughout the pregnancy, strict insulin regulation to maintain blood glucose levels between 60–110 g/dL (3.3–6.1 mmol/L) to prevent hyperglycemia or hypoglycemia, routine home glucose monitoring, regulated physical activity, and diet individualized to diabetic and pregnancy needs

**G.** Hypertension

1. Pre-existing hypertension (HTN)—diagnosed and treated before the 20th week of pregnancy; requires strict medical and obstetrical management (see Table 13-13)

2. Gestational hypertension—characterized by hypertension (systolic pressure greater than 140 mm Hg and/or diastolic pressure greater than 90 mm Hg) without proteinuria after 20 weeks gestation and resolving by 12 weeks postpartum; treated with frequent evaluation of BP and protein in urine (see Table 13-13)

3. Pre-eclampsia and eclampsia (see Tables 13-13 and 13-14)

a. Assessment—increased risk in African Americans, greater than 35-y-old or less than 17-y-old primigravida, multiple fetuses or history of diabetes and renal disease, family history of PIH; prenatal screening at each visit for symptomatology

**Table 13-13** Hypertensive States of Pregnancy Medications

| MEDICATION | ADVERSE EFFECTS | NURSING CONSIDERATIONS |
|---|---|---|
| Magnesium sulfate | Flushing, sweating<br><br>Symptoms of toxicity: sudden drop in BP, respirations less than 12/min, urinary output less than 25–30 mL/hr, decreased/absent DTRs, toxic serum levels | CNS depressant, anticonvulsant<br><br>Monitor BP, pulse (P), respirations (R), FHR at least every 15 min; magnesium sulfate levels and DTR prior to administration; mental status frequently; have resuscitation equipment and calcium gluconate/chloride (antidote) in room |
| Hydralazine | Tachycardia, palpitations<br><br>Headache<br><br>Nausea and vomiting<br><br>Orthostatic hypotension | Vasodilator<br><br>Maintain diastolic BP<br><br>90–100 mm Hg for adequate uteroplacental flow; monitor FHT and neonatal status |
| Diazepam | Risk of neonatal depression if given within 24 h of delivery | Sedative, anticonvulsant<br><br>Monitor FHT and neonatal status |
| Methyldopa | May mask symptoms of pre-eclampsia; risk of maternal orthostatic hypotension and decreased pulse and BP in neonate for 2–3 d<br><br>Hemolytic anemia | Used for chronic HTN<br><br>Monitor maternal, fetal, and neonatal vital signs<br><br>Monitor maternal mental status |
| Propranolol | Decreased heart rate, depression, hypoglycemia | Take apical rate before giving<br><br>Monitor BP, EKG |

**Table 13-14** Characteristics of Pre-Eclampsia and Eclampsia

| CONDITION | BP | PROTEINURIA | SEIZURES | HYPERREFLEXIA | OTHER |
|---|---|---|---|---|---|
| Mild pre-eclampsia | Greater than 140/90 mm Hg after 20 weeks gestation | 300 mg/L per 24 h<br><br>Greater than 1+ random sample | No | No | Mild facial edema<br><br>Weight gain (greater than 4.5 lb/wk) |
| Severe pre-eclampsia | Greater than 160/110 mm Hg | Greater than 500 mg/L per 24 h<br><br>Greater than 3+ random sample | No | Yes | Headache<br><br>Oliguria<br><br>Blurred vision<br><br>RUQ pain<br><br>Thrombocytopenia<br><br>Hemolysis, elevated liver enzymes, low platelet count) (HELLP) |
| Eclampsia | Greater than 160/110 mm Hg | Marked proteinuria | Yes | No | Same as severe pre-eclampsia<br><br>Severe headache<br><br>Renal failure<br><br>Cerebral hemorrhage |

**Table 13-15** Pre-Eclampsia and Eclampsia Treatment

| CONDITION | TREATMENT |
|---|---|
| Mild pre-eclampsia | Bedrest in left lateral position |
| | Monitor BP daily |
| | 8 oz water 6–8 times/day |
| | Frequent follow-up |
| Severe pre-eclampsia | Depends on fetal age and severity |
| | Only cure is delivery of fetus (induction of labor) |
| | Control BP (hydralazine), prevent seizures (magnesium sulfate) |
| | Prevent long-term morbidity and maternal mortality |
| | Emotional support if delivery prior to age of viability |
| Eclampsia (medical emergency) | Support through seizures and potential coma |
| | Ensure patent airway, $O_2$ support |
| | DIC management |
| | Delivery of fetus |
| | Emotional support if delivery prior to age of viability |
| | In cases of severe hypertension, seizures may still occur 24–48 h postpartum; monitor magnesium sulfate or hydralazine if continued postpartum |

# Cardiac Disease

A. Assessment

　　1. Chest pain

　　2. Dyspnea on exertion; dyspnea at rest; edema

　　3. Monitor vital signs and do EKG as heart lesion (especially those of the mitral valve) may become aggravated by pregnancy

B. Treatment of heart disease in pregnancy is determined by the functional capacity of the heart, and type of delivery will be influenced by the mother's status and the condition of fetus

C. Nursing management

　　1. Encourage rest and adequate nutrition during pregnancy

　　2. Encourage moderation in physical activity

　　3. Explain importance of avoidance and early treatment of upper-respiratory infections

　　4. Be alert for signs of heart failure: increase of dyspnea; tachycardia; weight gain

　　5. Monitor activity level

# Precipitous Delivery Outside Hospital Setting

A.  Assessment

   1.  Determine that transport to hospital/birthing center is not possible

   2.  Evaluate mother's cognitive status and explain actions

B.  Nursing management

   1.  Remain with client; do not attempt to prevent birth

   2.  Prepare sterile or clean environment

   3.  Support infant's head; apply slight perineal pressure to control speed of delivery

   4.  Slip nuchal cord, if present, over head

   5.  Gently rotate infant externally as head emerges

   6.  Deliver shoulders, trunk, holding head downward to facilitate drainage

   7.  Dry baby and place on mother's abdomen

   8.  Hold placenta as delivered (keep level with newborn heart or tie the umbilical cord)

   9.  Wrap infant in blanket and put to breast

   10. Check for bleeding and fundal tone

   11. Comfort mother and family; arrange transport to hospital

# CHILDBEARING–NEONATAL COMPLICATIONS

## Fluid/Electrolyte Balance, Gas Exchange, Infection

### High-Risk Childbearing–Neonatal

A. Antepartum risk factor

  1. Maternal history

    a. Smoking, alcoholism

    b. Infection

    c. Psychosocial problems

  2. Risk factors—fetal

    a. Birth asphyxia

    b. Preterm birth (characteristics)

      1) Little subcutaneous fat

      2) Hair—fine and feathery (lanugo)

      3) Poor resistance to infection

      4) Sole of foot smooth and fine

      5) Limbs—relaxed and extended

      6) Weak, underdeveloped muscles

      7) Weak sucking and swallowing

      8) Absorption problems

      9) Ear cartilage poorly developed—ears fold easily

      10) Female—clitoris is prominent; labia majora poorly developed

      11) Male—scrotum underdeveloped; minimal rugae

      12) Immature respiratory system

      13) Potential impairment of renal functioning

      14) Grasp reflex—grasp is weak

    c. Post-term birth—more than 42 wk gestation

    d. Small for gestational age (SGA)—birth weight below 10th percentile expected for gestational age

      1) Characteristics

        a) Reduced subcutaneous fat; loose and dry skin; sparse scalp hair

        b) Diminished muscle mass

          c)   Sunken abdomen (should be well-rounded)

          d)   Thin, yellowish, dry, dull umbilical cord

          e)   Wide skull sutures (inadequate bone growth)

          f)   Chronic intrauterine hypoxia

      2)  Large for gestational age (LGA)—birth weight 4,000 g or more

          a)   Congenital anomalies

          b)   Apgar score less than 7

          c)   Early or severe jaundice

             i)   Develops in first 24 h

             ii)   Bilirubin levels above 15 mg/100 mL in a full-term newborn

**B.**  Assessment of problems

   1.  Actual and potential problems of high-risk infants

      a.  Difficulty initiating and maintaining respirations (preterm, postterm, SGA)

      b.  Malnutrition (preterm, postterm, SGA)

      c.  Poor thermoregulation (preterm, postterm, SGA)

      d.  CNS trauma (preterm, postterm, SGA, and LGA)

      e.  Diminished resistance to infection (preterm, SGA)

      f.  Musculoskeletal immaturity (preterm, SGA)

      g.  Difficulty maintaining renal function (preterm)

      h.  Hematologic problems (preterm)

      i.  Fetopelvic disproportion—leading to possible birth trauma and asphyxia (LGA)

      j.  Hypoglycemia (LGA, SGA)

**C.**  Selected neonatal disorders

   1.  Respiratory distress syndrome—deficiency of surfactant in the immature lung

      a.  Assessment

        1)  Labored breathing—retractions, tachypnea, expiratory grunting, nasal flaring

        2)  Cyanosis

        3)  Development of flaccidness, unresponsiveness, apneic episodes

        4)  Breathing satisfactory immediately after birth; distress develops 6–8 h or 2–3 d after birth

        5)  Carries highest risk of long-term neurological complications

        6)  $PO_2$ less than 50 mm Hg; $pCO_2$ greater than 60 mm Hg

      b.  Nursing management

        1)  Maintain neutral thermal environment to conserve utilization of oxygen

        2)  Provide respiratory support

          a)   Oxygen therapy

          b)   Maintain patent airway with frequent suctioning

          c)   Place in side-lying position with roll under neck for hyperextension to facilitate open airway

d) Positive end-expiratory pressure (PEEP) or CPAP—keep prongs in place; high-frequency ventilation

3) Provide adequate hydration and caloric intake with gavage feeding and/or parenteral nutrition (if respiratory rate is increased); minimizes risk of aspiration

2. Perinatal asphyxia—periods of hypoxia during the birthing process

a. Assessment of problem

1) Meconium staining

2) Abnormal respirations with cyanosis and decreased respiratory rate

3) Possible intracranial hemorrhage manifested by bradycardia, reduced responsiveness, convulsions

4) Predisposing conditions

a) SGA infant

b) Maternal history of heavy cigarette smoking; pre-eclampsia–eclampsia; multiple gestations

b. Basic causes of asphyxia

1) Asphyxia caused by obstructed airway

2) Nonresponse of respiratory center in the brain

3) Atelectasis—areas of collapsed alveoli

4) Respiratory distress syndrome

5) Pneumothorax or interstitial emphysema—air admitted and trapped between air sacs, preventing full lung expansion

3. Miscellaneous conditions affecting the respiratory system

a. Agenesis—absence of one part of lung

b. Diaphragmatic hernia—abdominal organs/intestines push into the thoracic cavity

c. Congenital malformations of the heart and great vessels

d. Cysts in the thoracic cavity

e. Choanal atresia—obstruction of the posterior nares; infant mouth breathes; may become cyanotic at feedings; surgery may be indicated

f. Congenital laryngeal stridor—crowing inspiration caused by a flabby epiglottis; severe deformity may necessitate tracheotomy and/or laryngoplasty

4. Cold stress

a. Assessment of cold stress

1) Temperature instability to suboptimal levels

2) Oxygen consumption and energy are diverted from maintaining normal brain cell and cardiac functions and growth to thermogenesis

3) Development of respiratory and metabolic acidosis

b. Nursing management

1) Alter environment to increase infant's temperature

2) Monitor temperature

    3) Observe for signs of cold stress

       a) Mottling of skin or cyanosis

       b) Abnormal blood gases (acidosis), hypoxia

5. Hypoglycemia—blood glucose less than 30–35 mg/dL (1.7–1.9 mmol/L) in term infants (normal 40–80 mg/dL [2.2-4.4 mmol/L])

  a. Infants at risk

    1) Low-birth-weight or dysmature infants

    2) Infant of diabetic mother

    3) Infant of pre-eclamptic–eclamptic mother

    4) Cold-stressed infants

  b. Assessment—jitteriness, irregular respiratory effort, cyanosis, weak and high-pitched cry, lethargy, eye-rolling, seizures

  c. Nursing intervention

    1) Perform frequent blood glucose test

    2) Initiate early feeding either orally or with appropriate parenteral fluid

    3) Administer glucose carefully to avoid rebound hypoglycemia

6. Neonatal hypovolemic shock

  a. Assessment

    1) Characteristic symptoms similar to asphyxia except that heart rate and respiratory rate are increased

    2) May be caused by placenta previa, placenta abruptio, or bleeding from umbilical cord

    3) Anemia may be caused by hypovolemia

  b. Nursing management

    1) Monitor vital signs, especially blood pressure

    2) Immediate transfusion

7. Neonatal sepsis

  a. Assessment

    1) Temperature instability

    2) Poor sucking, vomiting, diarrhea

    3) Lethargy, convulsive activity

    4) Lack of weight gain, dehydration

    5) Predisposing factors

       a) Maternal signs and symptoms of infection

       b) Premature rupture of membranes

       c) Prolonged labor or delivery by cesarean section or forceps

  b. Nursing management

    1) Early identification of symptoms

2) Administration of prophylactic antibiotics as ordered

3) Maintain clean environment for neonate

8. Hyperbilirubinemia

a. Physiologic jaundice (icterus)—yellow coloration of skin and eyes

1) Normal after first 24 h of life

2) Caused by infant's inability to clear away waste of RBC destruction previously done via placental circulation, resolving cephalohematoma

9. Pathologic jaundice (hemolytic anemia)

a. May appear during first 24 h of life

b. Lasts longer than 7 d in full-term or 10 d in preterm infants

c. Higher than acceptable bilirubin levels

d. Associated conditions include immature liver, increased rate of hemolysis due to Rh incompatibility, cephalohematoma, cold stress, asphyxia, hypoglycemia, low serum albumin levels

e. Treated by phototherapy or exchange transfusions

10. Breast milk jaundice

a. Presence of an enzyme in milk of some women inhibits the enzyme (glucuronyl transferase) needed for bilirubin conjugation

b. Occurs in small proportion of infants

c. Early onset

1) Onset 2–4 days

2) Caused by decreased milk intake because milk supply not established

3) Encourage mother to breast feed 10–12 times/day; do not give water supplements

d. Late onset

1) Onset 5–7 days

2) Caused by less frequent stooling; possible factors in breast milk preventing bilirubin conjugation

3) Increase frequency of breast feeding; no water supplements; monitor bilirubin levels; phototherapy if needed

11. Rh incompatibility

a. Rh (−) mother produces antibodies against Rh (+) fetal blood cells, causing excessive hemolysis

b. Mother sensitized during first pregnancy by Rh (+) fetal cells

c. Mother may receive Rho(D) immune globulin intramuscular (IGIM) postdelivery or postabortion to prevent disease in newborn

1) Rho(D) immune globulin intramuscular (IGIM)—Rh immunoglobulin; not useful in women already sensitized and who have Rh antibodies

2) Given IM, not into fatty tissues or IV

d.  Nursing management

1)  Early determination of onset

2)  Phototherapy with fluorescent lighting—alters the nature of bilirubin to aid excretion (bilirubin excreted in stool); infant's eyes and genitals must be covered

3)  Exchange transfusion if indicated—removes serum bilirubin and maternal hemolytic antibodies

4)  Parental education and reassurance

12. Hemolytic disease of newborn (erythroblastosis fetalis)

a.  Assessment

1)  Jaundice within 24 h of birth

2)  Serum bilirubin level elevates rapidly

3)  Hematocrit decreased, anemia due to hemolysis of large number of erythrocytes

4)  Coombs test—detects antibodies attached to circulating erythrocytes, performed on cord blood sample

b.  Causes

1)  Destruction of RBCs from antigen-antibody reaction

2)  Baby's Rh antigens enter mother; mother produces antibodies; antibodies re-enter baby and cause hemolysis and jaundice

3)  Rare during first pregnancy

c.  Nursing management

1)  Assist in early identification

2)  Phototherapy with fluorescent lighting—alters nature of bilirubin to aid excretion; infant's eyes and genitals must be covered

3)  Exchange transfusion if indicated—removes bilirubin and maternal hemolytic antibodies

13. Necrotizing enterocolitis

a.  Assessment

1)  Feeding intolerance, bile-colored vomiting, abdominal distension

2)  Blood in stool

3)  Temperature instability

4)  Hypothermia

5)  Lethargy

6)  Onset 4–10 d after feeding started

7)  Diagnostics

a)  Hematest—positive stools

b)  Abdominal radiograph shows air in bowel wall

b.  Nursing management

1)  Stop oral feedings; NPO; insert nasogastric tube; observe for 24–48 h

2)  Administer antibiotics and intravenous fluids as ordered

       3)  Handle infant carefully; avoid tight diapering

       4)  Provide caloric needs via TPN or small oral feedings

       5)  Careful handwashing

14.  Infant of addicted mother/Neonatal Abstinence Syndrome (NAS)

    a.  Assessment

       1)  High-pitched cry, hyperreflexivity, decreased sleep

       2)  Diaphoresis, tachypnea, excessive mucus

       3)  Vomiting, uncoordinated sucking, nonnutritive sucking

       4)  Drug withdrawal from narcotics, barbiturates, or cocaine; may manifest as early as 12–24 h after birth, up to 7–10 d after delivery

    b.  Nursing management

       1)  Assess muscle tone, irritability, vital signs

       2)  Administer phenobarbital as ordered

       3)  Report symptoms of respiratory distress

       4)  Reduce environmental stimulation

       5)  Provide adequate nutrition/fluids; provide pacifier for nonnutritive sucking

       6)  Monitor mother/child interactions

15.  Disorders of the eye

    a.  Retinopathy of prematurity—a cause of blindness in premature infants

       1)  Assessment—ensure that all infants born less than 36 wk or less than 4.4 lb (2,000 g) at birth have eye exam by qualified provider

       2)  Characteristics

          a)  High concentrations of oxygen cause the premature infant's retinal vessels to constrict, causing blindness

          b)  Sometimes occurs when oxygen concentrations are greater than 40% and when used for longer than 48–72 h in infants

          c)  Planning and implementation

             i)  Use minimum amount of oxygen

            ii)  Monitor $PO_2$ continuously

           iii)  Maintain $PO_2$ level within normal limits

           iv)  Administer vitamin E as ordered; thought to affect tissue response to oxygen

    b.  Conjunctivitis of the newborn

       1)  Assessment—redness and swelling of the eyelids with exudate from the eyes

       2)  Characteristics

          a)  Caused by gonococcus organism

          b)  Milder form develops from the silver nitrate instilled in the eyes at birth

    3)  Nursing management

        a)  Observe for inflammation and exudate from eyes 24–48 h after birth

        b)  Observe for purulent discharge

        c)  Administer silver nitrate prophylactically as ordered

        d)  Administer antibiotic therapy as ordered

  c.  Strabismus

    1)  Assessment—eyes do not function as a unit because of an imbalance of the extraocular muscles

        a)  Visible deviation of eye

        b)  Diplopia

        c)  Child tilts head or squints to focus

    2)  Nursing management

        a)  Therapy

            i)  Developing visual acuity in both eyes

           ii)  Developing coordinate function

        b)  Nonsurgical intervention begins no later than age 6

            i)  Occlusion of unaffected eye to strengthen weaker eye

           ii)  Corrective lenses combined with other therapy to improve acuity

          iii)  Orthoptic exercises designed to strengthen eye muscles

        c)  Surgery on rectus muscles of eye

16.  Congenital malformations of the urinary tract (*see* Table 13-16)

**Table 13-16** Congenital Malformations of the Urinary Tract

| ASSESSMENT | ANALYSIS | NURSING CONSIDERATIONS |
| --- | --- | --- |
| Epispadias | Urethral opening on dorsal surface of the penis | No circumcision—foreskin used in surgical repair |
| Hypospadias | Male urethral opening on the ventral surface of penis, or female urethral opening in vagina | No circumcision—foreskin used in surgical repair |
| Horseshoe kidney | Kidneys are fused at lower poles | Hydronephrosis can develop<br><br>Surgical correction |
| Urethral duplication | Two separate ureters from one kidney | Recurrent UTIs<br><br>Surgical correction |
| Hydroureter | Ureter dilatation | Urinary diversion is indicated |
| Bladder exstrophy | Posterior and lateral surfaces of the bladder are exposed; often seen with epispadias | Immediate reconstructive surgery to close bladder and abdominal wall |

**D.** Basic concepts of management (general for high-risk newborn)

1. Resuscitate immediately

2. Provide warmth—use incubator for thermoregulation

3. Support respiratory function

   a. Provide air or oxygen as indicated; use caution with oxygen concentrations above 40% due to risk of retinopathy of prematurity (ROP)

   b. Provide humidity

   c. Suction

   d. Position

4. Maintain fluid and electrolyte balance—administer parenteral fluids as indicated

5. Meet nutritional needs

6. Monitor infant's condition

   a. Vital signs—temperature, apical pulse, respiratory rate

   b. Intake and output

   c. Skin—color, turgor

   d. CNS symptoms

      1) Fontanels—bulging, flat

      2) Convulsions

      3) Reflexes

7. Observe for signs of infection

8. Prevent skin breakdown

9. Promote healthy parent-child relationship

**E.** Absence of complications of oxygen therapy

1. Retinopathy of prematurity

   a. Occurs primarily in premature infants

   b. High concentrations of oxygen cause damage to the retinal blood supply

   c. The best prophylaxis is to reduce the oxygen concentration to the minimum in amount and time of exposure

2. Chronic lung disease

   a. Pathologic process that develops in the lungs of infants with hyaline membrane disease who have required assisted ventilation

   b. The disease is characterized by changes and/or damage to the lungs

   c. No specific treatment aside from oxygen therapy and other supportive measures; most infants recover by 6 mo to 1 y of age

   **F.** Absence of complications associated with nutrition

    1. Neonatal necrotizing enterocolitis (NEC)

     a. Serious condition, usually of preterm infant, speculated to be related to vascular compromise of the gastrointestinal tract (possibly related to hypoxia or sepsis); result of above is damage to the GI tract

     b. Nonspecific clinical signs include lethargy, vomiting, distended (often shiny) abdomen, blood in stools or gastric contents, and absence of bowel sounds

     c. Treatment includes discontinuation of all oral feedings, institution of abdominal decompression via nasogastric suction, and administration of systemic antibiotics

     d. Complications include bowel perforation requiring surgical resection and creation of ileostomy or colostomy

   **G.** Weight gain

   **H.** Active parent-child interaction

# End-of-Chapter Thinking Exercise

(0530) The postpartum nurse receives a report on a 32-year-old female (gravida 4, para 3) who received an epidural anesthetic and then vaginally delivered a male infant at 29 weeks gestation at 0415. The infant is stable in the NICU at the same hospital. The client was started on magnesium sulfate with a 2 gm bolus IV. The client is now receiving magnesium sulfate 750 mg/hour via continuous infusion to prevent seizure activity. The client also has an IV of 0.9% NaCl at 100 mL/hour infusing through a 20 gauge IV in the right hand.

(0600) Client received from labor and delivery via stretcher. Alert and oriented to person, place, and time. Most recent set of vital signs below. Fundus firm at umbilical line, moderate amount of lochia, perineum intact. Lungs are clear, indwelling urinary catheter in place and draining amber-colored urine. IV 0.9% NaCl at 100 mL/hour and magnesium sulfate at 750 mg/hour infusing. IV line to right hand without redness, edema, or coolness. Spouse in NICU and client tearfully asking, "Is my baby OK? Why can't I see him?" Informed spouse that nurse will call the NICU for an update.

| VITAL SIGN | 0445 | 0600 |
|---|---|---|
| BP | 184/112 mm Hg | 178/92 mm Hg |
| HR | 108 beats/minute | 100 beats/minute |
| RR | 16 breaths/minute | 12 breaths/minute |
| T | 98.2°F (36.8°C) | 99.1°F (37.3°C) |
| Pain | 0/10 | 0/10 |
| SpO$_2$ | 98% on room air | 97% on room air |

1. Which assessment findings concern the postpartum nurse? (Recognize Cues)

2. Which interventions are appropriate for the nurse to include in the plan of care? (Generate Solutions)

3. At 1005, the nurse obtains the client's vital signs.

| VITAL SIGNS 1005 |
|---|
| BP 90/58 mm Hg |
| P 68 beats/minute |
| R 8 breaths/minute |
| T 99.4°F (37.4°C) |
| SpO$_2$ 93% on room air |

The client's arms are trembling, and while the client's eyes are open, there is no response to verbal stimuli. The nurse will immediately contact the physician and anticipate holding the magnesium sulfate, administering calcium gluconate, and continuously monitoring the client's response.

If magnesium sulfate was effective, which findings would the nurse have expected for this client? (Evaluate Outcomes)

# Thinking Exercise Explanations

1. Which assessment findings concern the nurse? (Recognize Cues)

   - BP
   - HR
   - Tearful and anxious client (receiving magnesium sulfate infusion)

   Magnesium sulfate in the immediate postoperative period is used to treat eclampsia and prevent seizure activity as vital signs are monitored and stabilized.

2. Which interventions are appropriate for the nurse to include in the plan of care? (Generate Solutions)

   - Continue frequent assessment of vital signs and level of consciousness (refer to agency policy/protocol when administering magnesium sulfate)
   - Maintain seizure precautions
   - Dim the lights and decrease sensory stimuli
   - Obtain an order for serum magnesium levels to monitor for toxicity (regarding frequency, refer to agency policy/protocol)
   - Assess deep tendon reflexes (DTR) per agency policy/protocol when administering magnesium sulfate
   - Ensure resuscitation equipment is readily available
   - Ensure access to calcium gluconate/chloride
   - Monitor for adverse effects of magnesium sulfate:
     - Flushing
     - Diaphoresis
     - Sudden drop in BP
     - RR <12 breaths/minute
     - Urinary output <25–30 mL/hour
     - Decreased or absent DTRs

   Magnesium sulfate is a potentially dangerous medication and requires monitoring for seizures, serum toxicity, decrease in DTRs, changes in vital signs, and/or low urinary output. The nurse should also ensure that the client and any visitors are aware of the need to decrease sensory stimuli (loud noises, bright lights, numerous visitors, etc.) to decrease the chance of seizures.

3. At 1005, the nurse obtains the client's vital signs.

| VITAL SIGNS 1005 |
| --- |
| BP 90/58 mm Hg |
| P 68 beats/minute |
| R 8 breaths/minute |
| T 99.4°F (37.4°C) |
| SpO$_2$ 93% on room air |

The client's arms are trembling, and while the client's eyes are open, there is no response to verbal stimuli. The nurse will immediately contact the physician and anticipate holding the magnesium sulfate, administering calcium gluconate, and continuously monitoring the client's response.

If magnesium sulfate was effective, which findings would the nurse have expected for this client? (Evaluate Outcomes)

- Absence of seizure activity
- Absence of headache, visual disturbances, epigastric pain
- No deteriorations in level of consciousness
- 2+ DTRs (normal)
- Urinary output greater than 30 mL/hr
- Normal maternal blood pressure, respiratory rate (hypotension, bradypnea are concerning)

# [ CHAPTER 14 ]

# PEDIATRIC NURSING

| SECTIONS | CONCEPTS COVERED |
|---|---|
| 1. Growth and Development | Table 14-1. Overview of Erickson Developmental Tasks Throughout the Life Span |
| | Table 14-2. Infant Growth and Development |
| | Table 14-3. Toddler Growth and Development |
| | Table 14-4. Preschool Growth and Development |
| | Table 14-5. School-Age Growth and Development |
| | Table 14-6. Adolescent Growth and Development |
| | Table 14-7. Young Adulthood Growth and Development |
| | Table 14-8. Middle Adulthood Growth and Development |
| | Table 14-9. Late Adulthood Growth and Development |
| 2. Pediatric Assessment/Wellness | Table 14-10. Age-Appropriate Preparation for Health Care Procedures |
| | Table 14-11. Nursing Considerations for the Child Receiving Immunizations |
| | Table 14-12. Common Communicable Diseases of Childhood |
| | Table 14-13. Teaching Prevention of Accidental Poisoning in Children |
| 3. Alterations in Pediatric Health | Figure 14-1. Logan Bow |
| | Figure 14-2. Esophageal Atresia and Tracheoesophageal Fistula |
| | Figure 14-3. Ventriculoperitoneal Shunt |
| | Table 14-14. Congenital Heart Anomalies |
| | Figure 14-4. Types of Spina Bifida |
| | Figure 14-5. Developmental Dysplasia of the Hip (DDH) |
| | Figure 14-6. Pavlik Harness |
| | Figure 14-7. Hip Spica Cast |
| | Figure 14-8. Casting for Talipes Equinovarus |
| | Figure 14-9. Scoliosis |

[ SECTION 1 ]

# GROWTH AND DEVELOPMENT

## Growth and Development

## Phases of Growth and Development

(Ages may vary by theorist and source)

A. Process—sequence is orderly and predictable; rate tends to be variable within (more quickly/slowly) and between (earlier/later) individuals

  1. Growth—increase in size (height and weight); tends to be cyclical, more rapid in utero, during infancy, and adolescence

  2. Development—maturation of physiological and psychosocial systems to more complex states

    a. Developmental tasks—skills and competencies associated with each developmental stage that have an effect on subsequent stages of development

    b. Developmental milestone—standard of reference by which to compare the child's development at specific ages

    c. Developmental delay(s)—variable of development that lags behind the range of a given age

B. Theoretical approaches to development

  1. Erikson (psychosocial approach) (*see* Table 14-1)

    a. Social development

    b. Role of play in development

**Table 14-1** Overview of Erikson Developmental Tasks Throughout the Life Span

| AGE | STAGE | ERIKSON TASK | POSITIVE OUTCOME | NEGATIVE OUTCOME |
|---|---|---|---|---|
| Birth–1 year | Infancy | Trust vs. mistrust | Trusts self and others | Demonstrates an inability to trust; withdrawal, isolation |
| 1–3 y | Toddler | Autonomy vs. shame and doubt | Exercises self-control and influences the environment directly | Demonstrates defiance and negativism |
| 3–6 y | Preschool | Initiative vs. guilt | Begins to evaluate own behavior; learns limits on influence in the environment | Demonstrates fearful, pessimistic behaviors; lacks self-confidence |
| 6–12 y | School-age | Industry vs. inferiority | Develops a sense of confidence; uses creative energies to influence the environment | Demonstrates feelings of inadequacy, mediocrity, and self-doubt |
| 12–20 y | Adolescence | Identity vs. role confusion | Develops a coherent sense of self; plans for a future of work/education | Demonstrates an inability to develop personal and vocational identity |
| 20–45 y | Young adulthood | Intimacy vs. isolation | Develops connections to work and intimate relationships | Demonstrates an avoidance of intimacy and vocational/career commitments |
| 45–65 y | Middle adulthood | Generativity vs. stagnation | Involved with established family; expands personal creativity and productivity | Demonstrates lack of interests, commitments; preoccupation with self-centered concerns |
| 65 plus | Late adulthood | Integrity vs. despair | Identification of life as meaningful | Demonstrates fear of death; life lacks meaning |

2. Piaget (cognitive approach)—four stages

    a. Sensorimotor—birth to 2 y old

        1) Simple incremental learning—begins with reflex activity progressing to repetitive behavior, then to imitative behavior

        2) Increased level of curiosity

        3) Sense of self as differentiated and separate from environment

        4) Increasing awareness of object permanence (things exist even if not visible)

    b. Preoperational—2 to 7 y old

        1) Thinking and learning are concrete and tangible, based on what is seen, heard, felt, experienced; cannot make generalizations/deductions

        2) Toward the end of this stage, reasoning is more intuitive; beginning understanding of size, mass, time

    c. Concrete operations—7 to 11 y old

        1) Increasingly logical and coherent in thinking; solves problems in concrete manner

        2) Able to sort, classify, collect, order, and organize facts about the environment

        3) Can manage a number of aspects of a situation at one time but not yet able to deal with abstractions

        4) Can consider other points of view

    d. Formal operations—12 to 15 y old

        1) Able to deal with abstractions and abstract symbols

        2) Flexible and adaptable

        3) Can problem-solve, develop hypotheses, test them, and arrive at conclusions

        4) Questions and examines moral, ethical, religious, and social issues as beginning definition of self as an adult

3. Freud (psychological approach)—experiences at different stages influence personality traits

    a. Oral (birth to 1 y)—pessimism/optimism, trust/suspiciousness

    b. Anal (1 to 3 y)—retentiveness/overgenerosity, rigidity/laxity, constrictedness/expansiveness, stubbornness/acquiescence, orderliness/messiness

    c. Phallic (3 to 6 y)—brashness/bashfulness, gaiety/sadness, stylishness/plainness, gregariousness/isolation

    d. Latency (6 to 12 y)—elaboration of previously acquired traits

    e. Genital (12+ y)—preparation for forming relationships and marriage

**C.** Chronological phases

1. Prenatal—conception until birth; rapid growth and development

2. Neonatal—birth until 4 wk of age; adjustment to extrauterine life

3. Infancy—4 wk to 12 or 18 mo (upright locomotion); rapid and incremental growth and motor, cognitive, and social development (*see* Table 14-2)

**Table 14-2** Infant Growth and Development

| 1 MO | 7 MO |
|---|---|
| Head sags | Sits for short periods using hands for support |
| Turns head side to side when prone | Transfers toys from hand to hand |
| Lifts head momentarily from bed | Fear of strangers begins to appear |
| | Lability of mood (abrupt mood shifts) |
| | Responds to name |
| **2 MO** | **8 MO** |
| Closing of posterior fontanel | Anxiety with strangers |
| Diminished tonic neck and Moro reflexes | Regular patterns of elimination |
| Able to turn from side to back | Sits unsupported |
| Eyes begin to follow a moving object | Beginning pincer grasp |
| Social smile first appears | Makes consonant sounds |
| | Responds to word "no" |
| **3 MO** | **9 MO** |
| Can hold rattle | Elevates self to sitting position |
| Head held erect, steady | Creeps on hands and knees |
| Follows objects to 180° | Develops preference for dominant hand |
| Smiles in mother's presence | Rudimentary imitative expression |
| Laughs audibly | Responds to parental anger |
| **4 MO** | **10 MO** |
| Rolls back to side | Crawls well |
| Brings objects to mouth | Pulls self to standing position with support |
| Evidence of pleasure in social contact | Brings hands together |
| Drooling | Vocalizes one or two words |
| Moro reflex absent after 3–4 mo | |
| **5 MO** | **11 MO** |
| Birth weight usually doubled | Erect standing posture with support |
| Takes objects presented to them | Walks holding on to furniture |
| Teething may begin | Drops objects and expects it to be picked up |
| Smiles at mirror image | Plays peekaboo |
| | Shakes head for "no" |

*(Continued)*

**Table 14.2** Infant Growth and Development (*Continued*)

| 6 MO | 12 MO |
|---|---|
| Average weight gain of 3–5 oz per week during second 6 mo | Birth weight usually tripled |
| Can hold bottle | Needs help while walking |
| Can turn from back to stomach | Sits from standing position without assistance |
| Early ability to distinguish and recognize parents and strangers | Eats with fingers |
| Can chew and bite | Usually says 3–5 words in addition to "mama" and "dada" |
| | May need "security blanket" or favorite toy |
| **AGE-APPROPRIATE TOYS** ||
| Birth to 2 months | Mobiles |
| 2–4 mo | Rattles, cradle gym |
| 4–6 mo | Brightly colored toys (small enough to grasp, large enough for safety) |
| 6–9 mo | Large toys with bright colors, movable parts, and noisemakers |
| 9–12 mo | Books with large pictures, large push-pull toys, teddy bears |

4. Toddler—12 or 18 mo to 3 y; slowed growth; marked physical and personality development characterized by profound activity, curiosity, and negativism (*see* Table 14-3)

 a. Physical—birth weight quadrupled by 2.5 years; height grows about 8 in (20.3 cm); pulse 110, respirations 26, BP 85/37–91/49; 20 teeth by 2.5 years; has sphincter control needed for toilet training; appetite lessens because of decreased growth needs

 b. Motor—walks well forward and backward, stoops and recovers, climbs, runs, jumps in place, throws overhand, voluntarily releases hand, uses spoon, drinks from cup, scribbles

 c. Psychosocial—indicates wants by behaviors other than crying, may have temper tantrums; increases vocabulary from 10–20 words to about 900 at 3 y; imitates, helps with household chores; points to body parts, recognizes animals; almost dressing/undressing with help at 18–24 mo (cannot zipper, button, tie shoes); attachment to "security blanket"/stuffed animal

 d. Play—parallel play; appropriate toys include push-pull toys, riding toys, workbench, toy hammers, drums, pots and pans, blocks, puzzles with very few large pieces, finger paints, crayons, dolls/stuffed animals

 e. Stresses—separation from parents (bedtime may be seen as desertion); alteration in environment/routine/rituals (expect regression/temper tantrums); toilet training; loud noises/animals

f. Safety—accidents (i.e., motor vehicle, burns, poisoning, falls, choking/suffocation [round, cylindrical, and pliable objects, such as balloons, are most dangerous]) are leading cause of death because of continued clumsiness associated with increased mobility as well as striving for independence and heightened curiosity accompanied by the ability to open things but without cognitive ability to understand potential dangers; requires vigilant childproofing and supervision while promoting independence; child restraint in motor vehicles is absolute necessity

g. Three phases of separation anxiety

1) Protest—cries/screams for parents; inconsolable by others

2) Despair—crying ends; less active; uninterested in food/play; clutches "security" object if available

3) Denial—appears adjusted; evidences interest in environment; ignores parent when they return; resigned, not contented

**Table 14-3** Toddler Growth and Development

| 15 MO | 24 MO |
|---|---|
| Walks alone | Early efforts at jumping |
| Crawls up stairs | Builds 6- to 7-block tower |
| Builds 2-block tower | Turns book pages one at a time |
| Throws objects | 300-word vocabulary |
| Grasps spoon | Obeys easy commands |
| Names commonplace objects | Parallel play |
| **18 MO** | **30 MO** |
| Anterior fontanel usually closed | Walks on tiptoe |
| Walks backward | Jumps with both feet |
| Climbs stairs | Builds 8-block tower |
| Scribbles | Stands on one foot |
| Builds 3-block tower | Has sphincter control for toilet training |
| Oral vocabulary—10 or more words | |
| Great at mimicry | |
| **AGE-APPROPRIATE TOYS** | |
| Push-pull toys | |
| Low rocking horses | |
| Dolls | |
| Stuffed animals | |

5. Preschool—3 to 6 y; steady growth and development distinguished by acquisition of language, social skills, and imagination as well as enhanced self-control and mastery (*see* Table 14-4)

   a. Physical—weight increases 4–6 lb/y (1.8–2.7 kg/y); birth length doubled by 4 y; pulse 90–100, respirations 24–25, BP 85–100/60–70; permanent molars appear behind deciduous teeth, maximum potential for amblyopia/"lazy eye" (reduced visual acuity in one eye); handedness is established

   b. Motor—rides tricycle; walks up (3 y) then down (4 y) stairs alternating feet; hops on one foot, tandem walks; draws circle, then cross, then triangle; dresses with assistance, then with supervision, then alone

   c. Psychosocial—knows first name, then age, then last name; uses plurals and three-word sentences, progressing to complex sentences, follows directions, counts; knows simple songs, names of colors, coins, meaning of many words; asks inquisitive questions; evidence of gender-specific behavior by 5 y; becomes more eager to please; may develop imaginary playmates

**Table 14-4** Preschool Growth and Development

| 3 YEARS | 5 YEARS |
|---|---|
| Copies a circle | Runs well |
| Builds bridge with 3 cubes | Jumps rope |
| Less negativistic than toddler, decreased tantrums | Dresses without help |
| Rides tricycle | 2,100-word vocabulary |
| Jumps off bottom step | Tolerates increasing periods of separation from parents |
| Undresses without help | Beginnings of cooperative play |
| 900-word vocabulary, uses sentences | Gender-specific behavior |
| Increased attention span | Skips on alternate feet |
| **4 YEARS** | Ties shoes |
| Climbs and jumps well | |
| Laces shoes | |
| Brushes teeth | |
| 1,500-word vocabulary | |
| Skips and hops on one foot | |
| Throws overhead | |
| May have imaginary friend | |
| **AGE-APPROPRIATE TOYS AND ACTIVITIES** | |
| Child imitative of adult patterns and roles | |
| Offer playground materials, housekeeping toys, coloring books, tricycles with helmet | |

d. Play—associative/interactive/cooperative play; appropriate toys include tricycles and playground equipment; construction sets, illustrated books, puzzles, modeling clay, paints/crayons, simple games; imitative and dramatic play (dress-up, doll house, puppets); supervised TV

e. Stresses—illogical fears (inanimate objects, the dark, ghosts); separation from parents, may be evidenced as anorexia, insomnia, continued quiet crying, and/or aggression; bodily injury, mutilation (fear that puncture will not close and insides will leak out), and pain; intrusive procedures are threatening

f. Safety—similar to toddler; can understand and learn about potential dangers; in motor vehicles, shoulder harness and lap belt appropriate when child is 40 lb, 40 in, or 4 y old

6. School-age—6 to 11 or 12 y; constant progress in physical, mental, and social development; skill, competency, and self-concept (*see* Table 14-5)

**Table 14-5** School-Age Growth and Development

| 6 YEARS | 9 YEARS |
|---|---|
| Self-centered | Skillful manual work possible |
| Extreme sensitivity to criticism | Conflicts between adult authorities and peer group |
| Begins losing temporary teeth | Better behaved |
| Appearance of first permanent teeth | Conflict between needs for independence and dependence |
| Ties knots | Likes school |
| Develops concepts of numbers | |
| Takes bath without supervision | |
| **7 YEARS** | |
| Temporal perception improving | **10–12 YEARS** |
| Increased self-reliance for basic activities | Remainder of teeth (except wisdom) erupt |
| Team games/sports/organizations | Uses telephone |
| Develops concept of time | Responds to advertising |
| Boys prefer playing with boys and girls with girls | Increasingly responsible |
| **8 YEARS** | More selective when choosing friends |
| Friends sought out actively | Develops beginning of interest in opposite sex |
| Eye development generally complete | Loves conversation |
| Movements more graceful | Raises pets |
| Helps with household chores | |
| **Age-Appropriate Toys, Games, and Activities** | |
| Construction toys, use of tools, household serving tools, table game sports | |
| Participation in repair, building, and mechanical activities, household chores | |

a. Physical—continued slow growth; begins losing temporary teeth early in this phase and has all permanent teeth, except final molars, by the end; bone growth exceeds that of muscles and ligaments, resulting in susceptibility to injuries/fractures

b. Motor—skips, skates, tumbles, tandem walks backward, prints progressing to script, ties knots and then bows

c. Psychosocial—has significant peer relationships, assumes complete responsibility for personal care; school occupies most of time and has social as well as cognitive impact; developing morality, dominated by moral realism with strict sense of right/wrong until 9 y, then development of moral autonomy recognizing different points of view; able to acknowledge own strengths and weaknesses; developing modesty

d. Play—cooperative group play with leader and organized rules/rituals; usual activities include team games/sports/organizations; board games, books, swimming, hiking, bicycling, skating

e. Stresses—possible school phobia; fear of death, disease/injury, punishment

f. Safety—decreasing incidence of accidents except for injuries associated with sports/activities, requires appropriate supervision and education about proper use and maintenance of equipment and hazards of risk taking

7. Adolescence—approximately 11 or 12 to 18 or 20 y (depending on sex and individual rate); rapid and dynamic biological, physical, and personality maturation characterized by emotional and family turmoil, leading to redefinition of self-concept and establishment of independence (*see* Table 14-6)

**Table 14-6** Adolescent Growth and Development

| PHYSICAL DEVELOPMENT—PUBERTY |
| --- |
| Attainment of sexual maturity |
| Rapid alterations in height and weight |
| Girls develop more rapidly than boys |
| Onset may be related to hypothalamic activity, which influences pituitary gland to secrete hormones affecting testes and ovaries |
| Testes and ovaries produce hormones (androgens and estrogens) that determine development of secondary sexual characteristics |
| Pimples or acne related to increased sebaceous gland activity |
| Increased sweat production |
| Weight gain proportionally greater than height gain during early stages |
| Initial problems in coordination—appearance of clumsiness related to rapid, unsynchronized growth of many systems |
| Rapid growth may cause easy fatigue |
| Preoccupation with physical appearance |

*(Continued)*

**Table 14.6** Infant Growth and Development (*Continued*)

| MALE CHANGES |
|---|
| Increase in genital size |
| Breast swelling |
| Appearance of pubic, facial, axillary, and chest hair |
| Deepening voice |
| Production of functional sperm |
| Nocturnal emissions |

| FEMALE CHANGES |
|---|
| Increase in pelvic diameter |
| Breast development |
| Altered nature of vaginal secretions |
| Appearance of axillary and pubic hair |
| Menarche—first menstrual period |

| PHYSICAL DEVELOPMENT—ADOLESCENT |
|---|
| More complete development of secondary sexual characteristics |
| Improved motor coordination |
| Wisdom teeth appear (ages 17–21) |

| PSYCHOSEXUAL DEVELOPMENT |
|---|
| Masturbation as expression of sexual tension |
| Sexual fantasies |
| Experimental sexual intercourse |

| PSYCHOSOCIAL DEVELOPMENT |
|---|
| Preoccupied with rapid body changes, what is "normal" |
| Conformity to peer pressure |
| Moody |
| Increased daydreaming |
| Increased independence |
| Moving toward a mature sexual identity |

a. Physical—vital signs approach adult levels; wisdom teeth appear about 17–21 y; puberty is related to hormonal changes and is universal in pattern but not rate (females tend to develop earlier than males)

1) Growth spurt occurs early

   a) Girls—height increases approximately 3 in/y, slows dramatically at menarche, and ceases around age 16; fat is deposited in thighs, hips, and breasts; pelvis broadens

   b) Boys—height increases 4 in/y starting about age 13 and slows in late teens; weight doubles between 12 and 18 y old, related to increased muscle mass; broader chest

2) Sweat production and increased body odor result from increased apocrine gland activity; acne may occur related to increased sebaceous gland activity

3) Sexual characteristics and functioning develop

   a) Females

      i) Increase in pelvic diameter

      ii) Breast development—bud stage with protuberant areola; complete about time of menarche

      iii) Nature of vaginal secretions changes

      iv) Axillary and pubic hair appear

      v) Menarche—first menstrual period occurs around 12.5 y; for first 1–2 y anovulatory, frequently irregular menses

   b) Males

      i) Increase in genital size beginning about 13 y is first sign of sexual maturation; continues until reproductive maturity (age 17–18)

      ii) Possible temporary breast swelling of short duration

      iii) Pubic, facial, axillary, and chest hair appear

      iv) Voice deepens

      v) Production of functional sperm

      vi) Nocturnal emissions—normal physiologic reflex to ejaculate buildup of semen occurring during sleep; masturbation increases as a way to release semen

      vii) Motor—often clumsiness associated with growth spurt, motor ability is at adult levels

b. Psychosocial

1) Early—preoccupied with changing body; ambivalent relationship with parents/authority figures; seeking peer affiliations; may begin "dating"; wide and intense mood swings; limited capability for abstract thinking; seeking to identify values

2)   Middle—very self-centered; rich fantasy life; idealistic; major conflicts with parents/authority figures; strong identification with peer group; multiple "love"/sexual relationships (homosexuality is recognized by this time); tends to be more introspective and withdrawn; enhanced ability for abstract reasoning; concerned with philosophical, political, and social issues

3)   Late—established body image; irreversible sexual identity and gender role definition; independent from and less conflict with parents/authority figures; establishing stable individual friendships with both sexes and committed intimacy relationship; more stability in emotions; able to think abstractly; develops life philosophy (values, beliefs); makes occupational decisions

c.   Activities—primarily peer group oriented

d.   Stresses—threat of loss of control, fear of altered body image; separation primarily from peer group

e.   Safety—accidents, especially related to motor vehicles, sports, firearms, homicide, and suicide are leading causes of death; may be significantly related to drug and/or alcohol use; education is paramount

8.   Early and middle adulthood—18 or 20 to 65 y; developmental state and function characterized by self-sufficiency in pursuit of occupation/vocation and defined interpersonal relationships (*see* Tables 14-7 and 14-8)

a.   Physical/cognitive—stabilized growth state (weight is variable) and functioning, refines formal operational abilities, undergoes menopause, begins physical/physiological degeneration

b.   Psychosocial—develops self-sufficiency, pursues vocation/occupation, has intense interpersonal relationships (most frequently marriage and children)

9.   Late adulthood—65 years until death (*see* Table 14-9)

a.   Physical/cognitive—has general slowing of physical and cognitive functioning

b.   Psychosocial—needs to establish highest degree of independence (self-sufficiency) physically possible by adapting environment to ability; reflects on life accomplishments, events, and experiences; continues interpersonal relationships despite changes and loss

**D.**   Factors affecting growth and development

1.   Genetic defects

a.   Increased risk in certain groups of people, e.g., African Americans for sickle cell disease, Northern European descendants of Ashkenazic Jews for Tay-Sachs disease, Mediterranean ancestry for thalassemia; couples with a history of a child with a defect; family history of a structural abnormality or systemic disease that may be hereditary; prospective parents who are closely blood related; women over 40

**Table 14-7** Young Adulthood Growth and Development

| 20 TO 35 YEARS | 35 TO 40 YEARS | 40 TO 45 YEARS |
|---|---|---|
| Decreased hero worship | Period of discovery, rediscovery of interests and goals | (There is some overlap in years) |
| Increased reality | Increased sense of urgency | Self-questioning |
| Independent from parents | Life more serious | Fear of middle age and aging |
| Possible marriage, partnership | Major goals to accomplish | Reappraises the past |
| Realization that everything is not black or white, some "gray" areas | Plateaus at work and marriage, partnership | Discards unrealistic goals |
| Looks toward future, hopes for success | Sense of satisfaction | Potential changes of work, marriage, partnership |
| Peak intelligence, memory | | "Sandwich" generation—concerned with children and aging parents |
| Maximum problem-solving ability | | Increased awareness of mortality |
| | | Potential loss of significant others |

**Table 14-8** Middle Adulthood Growth and Development

| 45 TO 55 YEARS | 55 TO 60 YEARS | 60 TO 65 YEARS |
|---|---|---|
| Graying hair, wrinkling skin | (There is some overlap in years) | Increasingly forgetful |
| Evaluates past | Increasing physical decline | Accepts limitations |
| Pains and muscle aches | Sets new goals | Modification of lifestyle |
| Reassessment | Defines value of life, self | Decreased power |
| Realization—future shorter time span than past | Assesses legacies— professional, personal | Retirement |
| Menopause | Serenity and fulfillment | Less restricted time, able to choose different activities |
| Decreased sensory acuity | Balance between old and young | |
| Powerful, policy makers, leaders | Accepts changes of aging | |
| Relates to older and younger generations | | |

**Table 14-9** Late Adulthood Growth and Development

| 65 TO 80 YEARS | GREATER THAN 80 YEARS |
|---|---|
| Physical decline | Signs of aging very evident |
| Loss of significant others | Few significant relationships |
| Appraisal of life | Withdrawal, risk of isolation |
| Appearance of chronic diseases | Self-concern |
| Reconciliation of goals and achievements | Acceptance of death, faces mortality |
| Changing social roles | Increased losses |
| | Decreased abilities |

b. Chromosomal alteration—may be numeric or structural

1) Down syndrome (trisomy 21)—increased in women over 35 y; characterized by a small, round head with flattened occiput; low-set ears; large fat pads at the nape of a short neck; protruding tongue; small mouth and high palate; epicanthal folds with slanted eyes; hypotonic muscles with hypermobility of joints; short, broad hands with inward-curved little finger; transverse simian palmar crease; mental deficiencies

2) Turner syndrome (female with only one X)—characterized by stunted growth, fibrous streaks in ovaries, usually infertile, no intellectual impairment; occasionally perceptual problems

3) Klinefelter syndrome (male with extra X)—normal intelligence to mild intellectual delay; usually infertile

c. Autosomal defects—defects occurring in any chromosome pair other than the sex chromosomes

1) Autosomal dominant—union of normal parent with affected parent; the affected parent has a 50% chance of passing on the abnormal gene in each pregnancy; *BRCA1* and *BRCA2* breast cancer, type 2 diabetes, Marfan syndrome, polycystic kidney disease

2) Autosomal recessive—requires transmission of abnormal gene from both parents for expression of condition; cystic fibrosis, sickle cell disease

3) Sex-linked transmission traits—trait carried on a sex chromosome (usually the X chromosome); may be dominant or recessive, but recessive is more prevalent; e.g., hemophilia, color blindness

      d. Inborn errors of metabolism—disorders of protein, fat, or carbohydrate metabolism reflecting absent or defective enzymes that generally follow a recessive pattern of inheritance

          1) Phenylketonuria (PKU)—disorder due to autosomal recessive gene, creating a deficiency in the liver enzyme phenylalanine hydroxylase, which metabolizes the amino acid phenylalanine; results in metabolic accumulation in blood; toxic to brain cells

          2) Tay-Sachs disease—autosomal recessive trait resulting from a deficiency of hexosaminidase A, resulting in apathy, regression in motor and social development, and decreased vision

          3) Cystic fibrosis (mucoviscidosis or fibrocystic disease of the pancreas)—an autosomal recessive trait characterized by generalized involvement of exocrine glands, resulting in altered viscosity of mucus-secreting glands throughout the body

  2. Racial and ethnic influences

  3. Environment—may influence development more than genetic factors

      a. Family's socioeconomic factors

      b. Adequate nutrition

      c. Climate

  4. Intrapersonal factors

      a. State of health

      b. Emotional state

**E.** Assessment of growth and development

  1. Growth

      a. Repeated measurements must be done and recorded accurately on a regular basis to establish pattern and identify deviations; at least five times in first year and then yearly at every well-child visit and sick-child visit as appropriate

      b. Assessing length/height—infant or toddler positioned supine on exam table with legs extended is measured from crown of head to heels using flexible, nonstretchable tape while another person maintains child's position; for the older child, standing measurement is easier and more accurate

      c. Standardized growth chart

          1) Individual's length/height, weight, and head and chest circumference (until 3 y) are assessed in relation to general population, to previous pattern, and to each other

          2) Necessary to re-evaluate and report measurements greater than 97th percentile and less than 3rd percentile or deviations from established pattern

2. Development—evaluates current developmental function, identifies need for follow-up, helps parents to understand the child's behavior and prepare for new experiences, and provides basis for anticipatory guidance

   a. Evaluation should include all the subsystems of development, biophysical (gross and fine motor), cognitive, language, social, affective

   b. Developmental tools

      1) Denver II—evaluates children from birth to 6 y in four skill areas: personal-social, fine motor, language, gross motor

         a) Age adjusted for prematurity by subtracting the number of months preterm

         b) Questionable value in testing children of minority/ethnic groups

      2) Revised Prescreening Developmental Questionnaire (R-PDQ)—paper and pencil questionnaire from the Denver II for parents to answer to prescreen children

3. Muscular coordination and control—proceeds in head-to-toe (cephalocaudal), trunk-to-periphery (proximodistal), gross to fine developmental pattern

4. Intellectual—related to genetic potentialities and environment; intelligence tests used to determine IQ; mental age divided by chronological age multiplied by 100

# PEDIATRIC ASSESSMENT/WELLNESS

## Health Promotion, Client Education: Providing

## Pediatric Assessment

A. Subjective—health history

1. Serves not only to gather information but also to build trust/rapport, establish focus of examination/labwork, enhance knowledge base of caregivers, and to offer support

2. Format

    a. Indirect interview—open-ended questioning

        1) Advantages—may provide opportunity for greater exploration of underlying issues/concerns, for more complex description(s), and for therapeutic responses

        2) Disadvantages—may be time-consuming, require sorting through unnecessary/irrelevant information and allow parent to avoid area of concern

    b. Direct questioning—promotes specific responses to specific questions, used especially when time factor is important but tends to inhibit exploration

    c. Questionnaire may be done before visit but must be reviewed with client/caregiver

3. Approach

    a. Child and parent together—provides opportunity to observe parent-child interaction, time for child to get used to practitioner, and opportunity for older child to contribute to interview but may inhibit completeness/accuracy of history

    b. Child and parent separately—provides for more complete discussion of sensitive issues, especially with adolescent; confidentiality should be ensured except in potential situations of harm to self (suicide) or another person by the informant

    c. Avoid "talking down" to child/adolescent, making statements/promises that cannot be accomplished, e.g., "I won't hurt you"; sudden/exaggerated movements and/or staring at young child

B. Physical examination

1. Setting—ensure privacy, comfort, and adequate time

2. Approach

    a. Quiet voice with slow and easy approach appropriate to age of child

    b. Introduce self—use full name and title, clarify role/function, and explain rationale of process for eliciting information

c. Use complete names except with child/adolescent or when adult is well-known and/or gives permission for first name use

3. Examination—utilize same basic skills and techniques; however, the order may vary according to age of child to ensure the safety and comfort of child and to provide for ease of examination and accuracy of finding(s) (*see* Table 14-10)

a. Wash hands before exam for cleanliness and to warm hands

b. Basic tools and skills

   1) Observation/inspection—appearance, behavior, activity, interaction with parent; careful visual examination of an area

   2) Palpation

     a) Fine tactile details—fingertip pads

     b) Temperature—back/dorsum of hand

     c) Vibration—palm/palmar surface of fingers

**Table 14-10** Age-Appropriate Preparation for Health Care Procedures

| AGE | SPECIAL NEEDS | TYPICAL FEARS |
|---|---|---|
| Newborn | Include parents / Mommy restraint | Loud noises / Sudden movements |
| 6–12 mo | Model desired behavior | Strangers, heights |
| Toddler | Simple explanations / Use distractions / Allow choices | Separation from parents / Animals, strangers / Change in environments |
| Preschool | Encourage understanding by playing with puppets, dolls / Demonstrate equipment / Talk at child's eye level | Separation from parents / Ghosts / Scary people |
| School-age | Allow questions / Explain why / Allow to handle equipment | Dark, injury / Being alone / Death |
| Adolescent | Explain long-term benefit / Accept regression / Provide privacy | Social incompetence / War, accidents / Death |

3) Percussion—assess density

    a) Direct—sinus cavity

    b) Indirect/bimanual—resonance (lungs), tympany (gas filled, e.g., stomach), dull (organ tissue), flat (bone)

4) Auscultation

    a) Diaphragm—firmly against surface for high-frequency sounds

    b) Bell—lightly against surface for low-frequency sounds

c. Age-related factors—position, undressing, and sequence of exam

1) Infant and toddler

    a) Take full advantage of opportunities as they arise; when child is quiet, examine lungs, heart, and abdomen

    b) Observe child's activities while they are in waiting and exam rooms

    c) Key to success is distraction—test for developmental milestones in the form of a game before performing general exam

    d) May examine neonate and infant on table until approximately 6 mo, thereafter, on parent's lap; do invasive procedures (ears and throat) last

    e) Uncooperative child must be adequately restrained during invasive procedures to prevent injury

2) Young child

    a) Remove clothing as examination progresses

    b) Allow child to choose between possible alternatives but do not request child's permission to do something if child really has no choice

    c) Do the more invasive/uncomfortable procedures last, protecting child as mentioned

    d) May be helpful to play games

3) Preschool age/early school-age child

    a) Encourage child to remove their own clothing (children usually like to keep on underwear and socks); note dexterity

    b) Allow child to choose position for exam

    c) May be helpful to involve child, encourage handling appropriate equipment, allow listening to own heart

4) School-age child

    a) Respect modesty—offer gown to any child beyond early childhood

    b) Explain each step and allow child to participate actively

    c) Can proceed in usual head-to-toe sequence; if child is sick, assess healthy areas first

        5) Adolescent

           a) Paramount to provide for privacy and modesty; best to examine genitalia last

           b) Reassure about normalcy of findings as appropriate

           c) Provide health teaching as exam progresses

**C.** Vital signs

    1. Temperature

        a. Rectally provides precise diagnosis of fever but is contraindicated if less than 1 month of age (due to risk of rectal perforation), diarrhea, recent rectal surgery, ano-rectal lesions, receiving chemotherapy

        b. Rectally if recent/current vomiting, child unable to keep mouth closed

        c. Axillary if rectal irritation/diarrhea in young child; however, axillary readings may be insensitive and inconsistent

        d. Intra-auricular probe allows rapid, noninvasive reading when appropriate

    2. Heart rate—apical/radial counted for 1 full minute; assess rate and rhythm; PMI in infant is just lateral to nipple; with growth, gradually more medial

    3. Respirations—rate and rhythm; note signs and symptoms of respiratory distress, grunting, flaring, retracting

    4. Blood pressure—usually after 3 y old

        a. Methods

           1) Auscultation

           2) Palpation

           3) Doppler

        b. Size of cuff important—should be one-half to two-thirds of area of extremity; too narrow—abnormally high reading; too wide—abnormally low reading

**D.** Routine lab work

    1. Hb/Hct—at 6–9 mo, between 12–18 mo, and during adolescence

    2. Urinalysis—after toilet trained and when necessary for signs and symptoms

    3. Lead screening—at 12 months (6 months if high-risk)

    4. Sickle cell screening—after 6 mo in high-risk populations (sickledex)

    5. Tuberculosis (tine, Mantoux)—after 12 mo old

## Immunizations (See Table 14-11)

**A.** Recommended Child and Adolescent Immunization Schedule for ages 18 years or younger, United States, 2022

https://www.cdc.gov/vaccines/schedules/hcp/imz/child-adolescent.html

**B.** Catch-Up Immunization Schedule for Children and Adolescents who start late or who are more than 1 month behind, United States, 2022

https://www.cdc.gov/vaccines/schedules/hcp/imz/catchup.html

**Table 14-11** Nursing Considerations for the Child Receiving Immunizations

| NAME | ROUTE | NURSING CONSIDERATIONS |
|---|---|---|
| DTaP (diphtheria, tetanus, pertussis) | IM anterior or lateral thigh (No IMs in gluteal muscle until after child is walking) | Potential adverse effects include fever within 24–48 h, swelling, redness, soreness at injection site<br><br>More serious adverse effects—continuous screaming, convulsions, high fever, loss of consciousness<br><br>Do not administer if there is past history of serious reaction |
| MMR (measles, mumps, rubella) | SC anterior or lateral thigh | Potential adverse effects include rash, fever, and arthritis; may occur 10 d to 2 wk after vaccination<br><br>May give DTaP, MMR, and IPV at same time if family has history of not keeping appointments for vaccinations<br><br>Contraindicated with allergies to neomycin<br><br>Is live attenuated vaccine |
| IPV (polio) | IM | Reactions very rare |
| HB (hepatitis B) | IM vastus lateralis or deltoid | Should not be given into dorsogluteal site<br><br>Mild local tenderness at injection site |
| Tuberculosis test | Intradermal | May be given 4–6 y and 11–16 y if in high-prevalence areas<br><br>Evaluated in 48–72 h<br><br>PPD (purified protein derivative) 0.1 mL<br><br>Tine test (multiple puncture) less accurate |
| TD (tetanus/diphtheria booster) | IM anterior or lateral thigh | Repeat every 10 y<br><br>Contraindicated in moderate or severe illness |
| Live attenuated rubella | SC anterior or lateral thigh | Give once only to women who are antibody-negative for rubella and if pregnancy can be prevented for 3 mo postvaccination |
| Live attenuated mumps | SC | Give once<br><br>Prevention of orchitis (and therefore sterility) in susceptible males |

For Recommended Immunization Schedule for persons aged 0 through 18 years, go to: http://www.cdc.gov/vaccines/schedules/hcp/imz/child-adolescent.html

For Catch-up Immunization Schedule for persons age 4 months through 18 years who start late or who are more than 1 month behind, go to: http://www.cdc.gov/vaccines/schedules/hcp/imz/catchup.html

For Recommended Adult Immunization Schedule, by vaccine and age group, go to: http://www. cdc.gov/vaccines/schedules/hcp/imz/adult.html

C. Overall contraindications to immunizations

1. Severe febrile illness

2. Live viruses should not be given to anyone with altered immune system, e.g., undergoing chemotherapy, radiation, or with immunologic deficiency

3. Previous allergic response to a vaccine

4. Recently acquired passive immunity, e.g., blood transfusion, immunoglobulin

## Common Childhood Problems

A. Common communicable disease (*see* Table 14-12)

**Table 14-12** Common Communicable Diseases of Childhood

| NAME/ INCUBATION | TRANSMISSION/CLINICAL PICTURE | NURSING CONSIDERATIONS |
|---|---|---|
| Chickenpox (varicella) 13–17 days | Prodromal: slight fever, malaise, anorexia<br><br>Rash is pruritic, begins as macule, then papule, and then vesicle with successive crops of all three stages present at any one time; lymphadenopathy; elevated temperature<br><br>Transmission: spread by direct contact, airborne, contaminated object | Isolation until all vesicles are crusted; communicable from 1–2 days before rash<br><br>Avoid use of aspirin due to association with Reye syndrome; use acetaminophen and/or ibuprofen<br><br>Topical application of calamine lotion or baking soda baths<br><br>Airborne and contact precautions in hospital |
| Diphtheria 2–5 days | Prodromal: resembles common cold<br><br>Low-grade fever, hoarseness, malaise, pharyngeal lymphadenitis; characteristic white/gray pharyngeal membrane<br><br>Transmission: direct contact with a carrier, infected client contaminated articles | Contact and droplet precautions until two successive negative nose and throat cultures are obtained<br><br>Complete bedrest; watch for signs of respiratory distress and obstruction; provide for humidification, suctioning, and tracheostomy as needed; severe cases can lead to sepsis and death<br><br>Administer antitoxin therapy |
| Pertussis (whooping cough) 5–21 days, usually 10 | Prodromal: upper respiratory infection for 1–2 weeks<br><br>Severe cough with high-pitched "whooping" sound, especially at night, lasts 4–6 weeks; vomiting<br><br>Transmission: direct contact, droplet, contaminated articles | Hospitalization for infants; bedrest and hydration<br><br>Complications: pneumonia, weight loss, dehydration, hemorrhage, hernia, airway obstruction<br><br>Maintain high humidity and restful environment; suction; oxygen<br><br>Administer erythromycin and pertussis immune globulin |

(Continued)

**Table 14.12** Common Communicable Diseases of Childhood (*Continued*)

| | | |
|---|---|---|
| Rubella (German measles)<br><br>14–21 days | Prodromal: none in children, low fever and sore throat in adolescent<br><br>Maculopapular rash appears first on face and then on rest of the body<br><br>Symptoms subside first day after rash<br><br>Transmission: droplet spread and contaminated articles | Contact precautions<br><br>Isolate child from potentially pregnant women<br><br>Comfort measures; antipyretics and analgesics<br><br>Rare complications include arthritis and encephalitis<br><br>Droplet precautions<br><br>Risk of fetal deformity |
| Rubeola<br><br>10–20 days | Prodromal: fever and malaise followed by cough and Koplik's spots on buccal mucosa<br><br>Erythematous maculopapular rash with face first affected; turns brown after 3 days when symptoms subside<br><br>Transmission: direct contact with droplets | Isolate until 5th day; maintain bedrest during first 3–4 days<br><br>Institute airborne and seizure precautions<br><br>Antipyretics, dim lights; humidifier for room<br><br>Keep skin clean and maintain hydration |
| Scarlet fever<br><br>2–4 days | Prodromal: high fever with vomiting, chills, malaise, followed by enlarged tonsils covered with exudate, strawberry tongue<br><br>Rash: red tiny lesions that become generalized and then desquamate; rash appears within 24 hours<br><br>Transmission: droplet spread or contaminated articles<br><br>Group A beta-hemolytic streptococci | Droplet precautions for 24 hours after start of antibiotics<br><br>Ensure compliance with oral antibiotic therapy<br><br>Bedrest during febrile phase<br><br>Analgesics for sore throat<br><br>Encourage fluids, soft diet<br><br>Administer penicillin or erythromycin |
| Mononucleosis<br><br>4–6 weeks | Malaise, fever, enlarged lymph nodes, sore throat, flulike aches, low-grade temperature<br><br>Highest incidence 15–30 years old<br><br>Transmission: direct contact with oral secretions, unknown | Advise family members to avoid contact with saliva (cups, silverware) for about 3 months<br><br>Treatment is rest and good nutrition; strenuous exercise is to be avoided to prevent spleen rupture<br><br>Complications include encephalitis and spleen rupture |
| Tonsillitis (streptococcal) | Fever, white exudate on tonsils<br><br>Positive culture for group A *Streptococcus* (group A strep) | Antibiotics<br><br>Teach parents serious potential complications: rheumatic fever, glomerulonephritis |
| Mumps<br><br>14–21 days | Malaise, headache, fever, parotid gland swelling<br><br>Transmission: direct contact with saliva, droplet | Isolation before and after appearance of swelling<br><br>Soft, bland diet<br><br>Complications: deafness, meningitis, encephalitis, sterility |

    **B.** Poison control/prevention

      1. Assessment

        a. Airway, breathing, circulation (ABC)—treat the client first, then the poison

        b. Identify poison—amount ingested, time of ingestion; save vomitus

        c. Diagnostics

          1) Urine and serum analysis

          2) Long-bone x-rays if suspect lead deposits

          3) CAT scan, EEG

      2. Nursing management

        a. Prevention—most toxic ingestions are acute (*see* Table 14-13)

          1) Childproofing—store all potentially poisonous substances in locked, out-of-reach area

          2) Increased awareness of precipitating factors

            a) Growth and development characteristics—under/overestimating the capabilities of the child

            b) Changes in household routine

            c) Conditions that increase emotional tension of family members

**Table 14-13** Teaching Prevention of Accidental Poisoning in Children

| ACTION | RATIONALE |
|---|---|
| Proper storage—locked cabinets | Once child can crawl, can investigate cabinets and ingest contents of bottles |
| Never take medicine in front of children | Children are interested in anything their parents take and will mimic taking medicine |
| Never leave medication in purse, on table, or on kitchen counter | Children will investigate area and ingest bottle contents |
| Never refer to medicine as candy | Increases interest in taking medicine when unsupervised |
| Leave medicines, cleaning supplies in original containers | Pill boxes, soda bottles increase attractiveness and inhibit identification of substance should poisoning occur |
| Provide activities and play materials for children | Encourages child's interest without endangering them |
| Teach need for supervision of small children | Small children cannot foresee potential harm and need protection |

b. Instructions for caretaker in case of suspected poison ingestion

1) Recognize signs and symptoms of accidental poisoning—change in child's appearance/behavior; presence of unusual substances in child's mouth, hands, play area; burns, blisters, and/or suspicious odor around child's mouth; open/empty containers in child's possession

2) Initiate steps to stop exposure

3) Call Poison Control Center—be prepared to provide information

   a) Substance—name, time, amount, route

   b) Child—condition, age, weight

4) Save any substance, vomitus, stool, urine

5) Induce vomiting if indicated by Poison Control Center

c. Emergency care in a health care facility

1) Basic life support

   a) Respiratory—intubate if comatose, seizing, or no gag reflex; frequent blood gases

   b) Circulation—IV fluids; maintain fluid and electrolyte balance; cardiac monitor: essential for comatose child and with tricyclic antidepressant or phenothiazine ingestion

2) Gastric lavage and aspiration—client is intubated and positioned head down and on left side; large oro/nasogastric tube inserted, and repeated irrigations of normal saline instilled until clear; not more than 10 mL/kg; must be done within 60 minutes

3) Activated charcoal—absorbs compounds, forming a nonabsorbable complex; 5–10 g for each gram of toxin

   a) Give within 1 h of ingestion and after emetic

   b) Mix with water to make a syrup; given PO or via gastric tube

d. Hasten elimination

1) Cathartic—to speed substance through lower GI tract; not recommended

2) Diuretics—for substances eliminated by kidneys

3) Chelation—heavy metals (e.g., mercury, lead, and arsenic) are not readily eliminated from body; progressive buildup leads to toxicity; a chelating agent binds with the heavy metal, forming a complex that can be eliminated by kidneys, peritoneal hemodialysis (e.g., deferoxamine, dimercaprol, calcium EDTA)

e. Prevent recurrence—crisis intervention with nonjudgmental approach; acknowledge difficulty in maintaining constant supervision; explore contributory factors; discuss and educate about growth and development influences as well as passive (child restraint closures) and active safety measures

    **C.** Common substances that cause poisoning

      1. Aspirin (salicylate)—products containing aspirin

        a. Assessment

          1) Tinnitus, nausea, sweating, dizziness, headache

          2) Change in mental status

          3) Increased temperature, hyperventilation (respiratory alkalosis)

          4) Later, metabolic acidosis and respiratory acidosis, bleeding, and hypovolemia

        b. Effects

          1) Toxicity begins at doses of 150–200 mg/kg; 4 gm may be fatal to child

            a) Altered acid-base balance (respiratory alkalosis) due to increased respiratory rate

            b) Increased metabolism causes greater $O_2$ consumption, $CO_2$, and heat production

            c) Metabolic acidosis results in hyperkalemia, dehydration, and kidney failure

            d) May result in decreased prothrombin formation and decreased platelet aggregation, causing bleeding

        c. Nursing management

          1) Induce vomiting; initiate gastric lavage with activated charcoal

          2) Monitor vital signs and laboratory values

          3) Maintain IV hydration and electrolyte replacement; monitor I and O, skin turgor, fontanels, urinary specific gravity, serum potassium (hypokalemia may occur with correct of condition)

          4) Reduce temperature—tepid water baths or hypothermia blankets; prone to seizures

          5) Vitamin K, if needed, for bleeding disorder; guaiac of vomitus/stools

          6) IV sodium bicarbonate enhances excretion

      2. Acetaminophen overdose

        a. Assessment

          1) First 2 h, nausea and vomiting, sweating, pallor, hypothermia, slow-weak pulse

          2) Followed by latent period (1–1.5 d) when symptoms abate

          3) If no treatment, hepatic involvement occurs (may last up to 1 wk) with RUQ pain, jaundice, confusion, stupor, coagulation abnormalities

          4) Diagnostic tests—serum acetaminophen levels at least 4 h after ingestion; liver function tests (AST, ALT) and kidney function tests (creatinine, BUN)—change in renal and liver function is a late sign

        b. Effects

          1) Toxicity begins at 150 mg/kg

          2) Major risk is hepatic necrosis

c. Nursing management

1) Induce vomiting

2) *N*-acetylcysteine—specific antidote; most effective in 8–10 hours; must be given within 24 hrs; given PO every 4 hours × 72 hrs or IV × 3 doses

3) Maintain hydration; monitor output

4) Monitor liver and kidney function

3. Lead toxicity (plumbism)

a. Assessment

1) Physical symptoms

a) Irritability

b) Sleepiness, decreased activity

c) Nausea, vomiting, abdominal pain

d) Constipation

e) Decreased activity

f) Increased intracranial pressure (e.g., seizures and motor dysfunction)

2) Environmental sources

a) Flaking, lead-based paint (primary source)

b) Crumbling plaster

c) Odor of lead-based gasoline

d) Pottery with lead glaze

e) Lead solder in pipes

3) Diagnostic tests

a) Blood lead level—there is no safe level of lead in the blood; public health action is recommended with blood levels above 5 mcg/dL (0.24 mcmol/L)

b) Erythrocyte protoporphyrin (EP) level

c) CBC—anemia

d) X-rays (long bone/GI)—may show radiopaque material, "lead lines"

e) Calcium disodium mobilization/provocative test—to evaluate degree of stored lead; lead levels are measured in urine collected over a specific time after injection of calcium disodium

b. Analysis

1) Child—practice of pica (habitual and compulsive ingestion of nonfood substances); children absorb more lead than adults; paint chips taste sweet

2) Pathology—lead is slowly excreted by kidneys and GI tract; stored in inert form in long bones; chronic ingestion affects many body systems

a) Hematological—blocks formation of hemoglobin, leading to microcytic anemia (initial sign) and increased erythrocyte protoporphyrin (EP)

b) Renal—toxic to kidney tubules, allowing an abnormal excretion of protein, glucose, amino acids, phosphates

        c)  CNS—increases membrane permeability, resulting in fluid shifts into brain tissue, cell ischemia, and destruction causing neurological and intellectual deficiencies with low-dose exposure; with high-dose exposure, intellectual delay, convulsions, and death (lead encephalopathy)

  c.  Nursing management

    1)  Chelating agent—promotes lead excretion in urine and stool; dimercaprol (BAL in oil), calcium disodium EDTA; succimer; deferoxamine

      a)  Maintain hydration

      b)  Identify sources of lead and institute de-leading procedures; involve local housing authorities as needed

      c)  Instruct parents about supervision for pica and ways to encourage other activities for the child

# ALTERATIONS IN PEDIATRIC HEALTH

## Mobility, Intracranial Regulation, Elimination

### Interventions for the Hospitalized Child

A. Prevent or minimize the effects of separation on the child

1. Encourage parental involvement in child's care, especially through rooming-in facilities

2. Assign the same nurse to care for the child

3. Provide objects that re-create familiar surroundings (e.g., toys from home)

B. Observe for alterations in parenting

1. Behavior patterns of parents and child

2. Identify healthy relationships and unhealthy relationships, e.g., failure to thrive; indications of child abuse

C. Educate parents on proper health care for children

1. Pediatrician visits; immunization schedules; childhood diseases

2. Review diet and exercise patterns

### Selected Disorders—Infants

A. Cleft lip and palate

1. Definition—congenital malformation

   a. Cleft lip—small or large fissure in facial process of upper lip or up to nasal septum, including anterior maxilla

   b. Cleft palate—midline, bilateral, or unilateral fissures in hard and soft palate

2. Basic concepts

   a. Lip is usually repaired during first weeks of life

   b. Palate is usually repaired before child develops altered speech patterns (between 12–18 months)

3. Clinical manifestations

   a. Parents will have strong reaction to birth of infant with defect—provide support and information

   b. Assess infant's ability to suck

4. Nursing management

a. Preoperative

1) Maintain adequate nutrition

2) Feed with soft nipple, special lamb's nipple, Breck feeder, or cup

b. Postoperative

1) Maintain airway

a) Observe for respiratory distress

b) Provide suction equipment and endotracheal tube at bedside

2) Guard suture line

a) Keep suture line clean and dry

b) Use lip-protective devices, i.e., Logan bow device (*see* Figure 14-1) or tape as ordered

c) Maintain side-lying position on unaffected side

d) Minimize crying with comfort measures—rocking, cuddling

e) Use restraints as needed

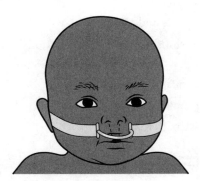

**Figure 14-1.** Logan Bow

3) Provide nutrition

a) Use feeding techniques to minimize trauma—usually very slow to feed

b) Burp baby frequently during feedings

4) Facilitate parents' positive response to child

5) Provide referrals to speech therapy and orthodontists as needed

**B.** Colic (in infants)

1. Definition—abdominal cramps

2. Assessment

a. Abrupt onset of crying with loud screams commonly lasting 3 hours and occurring at least 3 times/week, clenched fists, and legs drawn up to abdomen

b. Flatus or belching during the vigorous crying spells

c. Symptoms worse in early evening and night

3. Analysis

   a. Most frequent in infants of low birth weight

   b. Usually disappears by 3 mo of age

   c. Excessive air swallowing

      1) Too rapid feeding

      2) Too vigorous sucking on small nipple holes or an empty bottle

   d. Excessive carbohydrate intake—causes increased fermentation and production of gas

   e. Indigestion from overfeeding

   f. Insufficient emotional satisfaction

4. Nursing management

   a. Enemas, suppositories, and rectal tubes to relieve distention

   b. Frequent burping of baby during and after feedings

   c. Modification of amount and type of formula

   d. Local application of heat to abdomen

   e. Additional cuddling and closeness

   f. Medications—e.g., antispasmodics for relief

C. Pyloric stenosis

   1. Definition—obstruction of the passageway from the stomach to the duodenum due to enlargement of the sphincter muscle, sometimes twice its normal size

   2. Basic concepts

      a. Inflammation and edema can reduce the size of the opening until there is complete obstruction

      b. Infants usually asymptomatic until the second to fourth week after birth; then, regurgitation develops into projectile vomiting; most frequently seen in Caucasian, male, full-term infants

   3. Clinical manifestations

      a. Upper gastrointestinal x-rays reveal delayed gastric emptying and elongated pyloric channel

      b. Signs of pyloric stenosis include projectile vomiting, weight loss, constipation, dehydration, olive-sized tumor, visible peristaltic waves from left upper quadrant (LUQ) to right upper quadrant (RUQ)

   4. Nursing management

      a. Preoperative

         1) Prevent regurgitation and vomiting

            a) Give small, frequent feedings

            b) Position upright after feedings

            c) Keep quiet environment after feeding

2) Monitor for complications—alkalosis, hypokalemia, dehydration, and shock

3) Support parents

a) Allow verbalization of parents' anxieties

b) Instruct parents on expected progress and behavior

b. Postoperative

1) Check incision site; keep incision site clean and dry

2) Provide parenteral fluids at ordered rate

3) Monitor warmth

4) Small, frequent feedings of glucose water or electrolyte solution 4–6 hours post-operatively; advance diet gradually

5) If clear fluids retained, start formula 24 hours post op

**D.** Esophageal atresia and tracheoesophageal fistula

1. Definition—malformations of the esophagus, often with associated anomalies of the heart or genitourinary systems (*see* Figure 14-2)

2. History

a. During the fifth week of embryological development, the embryonic foregut must lengthen and separate into trachea and esophagus; defects in this development result in blind pouches and/or fistulas

b. In almost 90% of tracheoesophageal defects, the esophagus ends in a blind pouch and the trachea has a short segment attaching it to the stomach (*see* panel A in Figure 14-2); the second most common defect is seen in panel B, and the defects seen in panels C and D are very rare

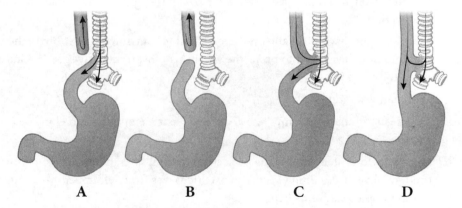

A          B          C          D

**Figure 14-2.** Esophageal Atresia and Tracheoesophageal Fistula

3. Assessment

a. Excessive saliva

b. Stomach distention

c. Choking

d. Coughing

e. Cyanosis

4. Nursing management

   a. Preoperative

      1) Position to prevent saliva aspiration

      2) Facilitate gastrostomy drainage

   b. Postoperative

      1) Care for incision site—observe for inflammation

      2) Prevent pulmonary complications—suction and position

      3) Provide TPN until gastrectomy or oral feedings tolerated

**E.** Strabismus

  1. Assessment—eyes do not function as a unit because of an imbalance of the extraocular muscles

   a. Visible deviation of eye

   b. Diplopia

   c. Child tilts head or squints to focus

  2. Management

   a. Therapy

      1) Developing visual acuity in both eyes

      2) Developing coordinate function

   b. Nonsurgical intervention begins no later than age 6

      1) Occlusion of unaffected eye to strengthen weaker eye

      2) Corrective lenses combined with other therapy to improve acuity

      3) Orthoptic exercises designed to strengthen eye muscles

**F.** Hydrocephalus

  1. Assessment

   a. Congenital or acquired condition characterized by an increase in the accumulation of CSF within the ventricular system and subsequent increase in ventricular pressure

  2. Etiology

   a. Neoplasm

   b. Aqueductal stenosis—stenosis/obstructions in ventricular system

   c. Spina bifida

   d. Congenital cysts/vascular malformations

   e. Meningitis

   f. Head trauma

   g. Intraventricular hemorrhage in premature infants

   h. Idiopathic

3. Types

   a. Communicating—due to increased production of CSF or impaired absorption of CSF

   b. Noncommunicating—due to obstruction/blockage of CSF circulation between ventricles and subarachnoid

4. Characteristics

   a. Signs and symptoms

      1) Fronto-occipital circumference increasing at abnormally fast rate

      2) Splint sutures and widened fontanels

      3) Prominent forehead

      4) Dilated scalp veins

      5) Distended/tense fontanels

      6) Sunset eyes, nystagmus

      7) Irritability, vomiting

      8) Unusual somnolence

      9) Convulsions

      10) High-pitched cry

5. Nursing/medical management

   a. Operative management

      1) Ventriculoperitoneal shunt—ventricles to peritoneal cavity (*see* Figure 14-3)

      2) Ventricular atrial shunt—ventricles to right atrium

      3) Ventricular drainage—external

      4) Discharge planning/community referral

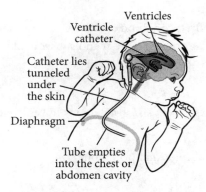

**Figure 14-3.** Ventriculoperitoneal Shunt

   b. Nursing care

      1) Observation of shunt functioning/malfunction

      2) Shunt modified as child grows

      3) Observe for increased intracranial pressure and signs of shunt infection (irritability, high-pitched cry, lethargy)

4) Postoperative positioning—on unoperated side in flat position; do not hold infant with head elevated

5) Continual testing for developmental abnormalities/intellectual delay

6) Continual testing for developmental abnormalities and cognitive deficiencies

7) Discharge planning/community referral

8) Teach parents about increased risk for allergies if myelomeningocele present

**G.** Congenital heart anomalies (*see* Table 14-14)

1. Assessment/symptoms

2. History—predisposing factors

a. Rubella during pregnancy

b. Maternal alcoholism

c. Maternal age over 40 y

d. Maternal diabetes

e. Sibling with heart disease

f. Parent with congenital heart disease

g. Other congenital anomalies

**Table 14-14** Congenital Heart Anomalies

| ACYANOTIC TYPE | CYANOTIC TYPE |
| --- | --- |
| Normal color | Cyanosis usually from birth; clubbing of fingers |
| Normal CNS function | May have seizures due to hypoxia; fainting; confusion |
| Possible exercise intolerance | Marked exercise intolerance; may have hypoxic spells following exercise; squats to decrease respiratory distress |
| Possible weight loss or gain (with fluid retention) | Difficulty eating because of inability to breathe at the same time |
| Small stature; failure to thrive | Small stature; failure to thrive |
| Characteristic murmur; increased frequency of respiratory infections | Characteristic murmur; frequent and severe respiratory infections |

3. General effects of heart malformation

a. Increased workload—overloading of chambers resulting in hypertrophy and tachycardia

b. Pulmonary hypertension (increased vascular resistance) resulting in dyspnea, tachypnea, and recurrent respiratory infections

c. Inadequate systemic cardiac output, resulting in exercise intolerance and growth failure

      d. Arterial desaturation from shunting of deoxygenated blood directly into the systemic circulation, resulting in polycythemia, cyanosis, cerebral changes, clubbing, squatting, and metabolic acidemia

      e. Murmurs due to abnormal shunting of blood between two heart chambers or between vessels

    4. Types of defects

      a. Increased pulmonary blood flow (acyanotic)

        1) Ventricular septal defect (VSD)—abnormal opening between right and left ventricles; may vary in size from pinhole to absence of septum

          a) Characterized by loud, harsh murmur

          b) May close spontaneously by age 3—surgery may be indicated (purse-string closure of defect or pulmonary artery banding)

        2) Atrial septal defect (ASD)—abnormal opening between the two atria; severity depends on the size and location

          a) Small defects high on the septum may result in no apparent clinical symptoms

          b) Murmur audible and distinct for defect

          c) Unless defect is severe, prophylactic closure is done in later childhood

        3) Patent ductus arteriosus (PDA)—failure of that fetal structure to close after birth (in fetus, ductus arteriosus connects the pulmonary artery to the aorta to shunt oxygenated blood from placenta directly into systemic circulation, bypassing the lungs)

          a) PDA allows blood to be shunted from aorta (high pressure) to pulmonary artery (low pressure), causing additional blood to be reoxygenated in the lungs; result is increased pulmonary vascular congestion and right ventricular hypertrophy

          b) Characteristic murmur, widened pulse pressure, bounding pulse, and tachycardia

          c) Treatment is surgical intervention to divide or ligate the patent vessel

      b. Obstruction to blood flow from ventricle (acyanotic)

        1) Coarctation of the aorta—narrowing of the aorta

          a) High blood pressure and bounding pulses in areas receiving blood from vessels proximal to the defect; weak or absent pulses distal to defect, cool extremities, and muscle cramps

          b) Murmur may or may not be present

          c) Surgical treatment involves resection of the coarcted portion and end-to-end anastomosis or replacement of the constricted section using a graft

          d) High incidence of complications if left untreated

        2) Pulmonary stenosis—narrowing at the entrance to the pulmonary artery

          a) Resistance to blood flow causes right ventricular hypertrophy

          b) Commonly seen with PDA

      c)    Severity depends on degree of defect

      d)    Surgery recommended for severe defect (pulmonary valvotomy)

    3)   Aortic stenosis—narrowing of aortic valve causes decreased cardiac output

        i)    Murmur usually heard

       ii)    Surgery recommended

c.   Cyanotic—poorly oxygenated venous blood enters systemic circulation; compensatory mechanisms observed in cyanotic heart disease: tachycardia, polycythemia, and posturing (squatting, knee-chest position)—decreased pulmonary blood flow

    1)   Tetralogy of Fallot—four defects: ventricular septal defect, pulmonic stenosis, overriding aorta, right ventricular hypertrophy (first three are congenital, fourth is acquired due to increased pressure within the right ventricle)

      a)    Cyanosis, clubbing of fingers, delayed physical growth and development

      b)    Child often squats or assumes knee-chest position

      c)    Treatment is surgical correction

d.   Mixed blood flow (cyanotic)

    1)   Transposition of the great vessels—pulmonary artery leaves from the left ventricle, and the aorta leaves from the right ventricle

      a)    Unless there is an associated defect to compensate, this condition is incompatible with life

      b)    Depending on severity of condition—severely cyanotic to mild heart failure

      c)    Treatment is surgical correction

    2)   Truncus arteriosus—failure of normal septation and embryonic division of pulmonary artery and aorta, resulting in a single vessel that overrides both ventricles, giving rise directly to the pulmonary and systemic circulations

      a)    Blood from both ventricles enters the common artery and flows either to the lungs or to the aortic arch and body

      b)    Cyanosis, left ventricular hypertrophy, dyspnea, marked activity intolerance, and growth restriction

      c)    Harsh murmur audible; congestive heart failure usually develops

      d)    Palliative treatment—banding both pulmonary arteries to decrease the amount of blood going to lungs

      e)    Corrective treatment—closing ventricular septal defect so truncus originates from left ventricle and creating pathway from right ventricle

    3)   Total anomalous venous return—absence of direct communication between pulmonary veins and left atrium; pulmonary veins attach directly to the right atrium or to various veins draining toward the right atrium

      a)    Cyanosis, pulmonary congestion, and heart failure

      b)    Murmur audible

      c)    Surgical correction involves restoring the normal pulmonary venous circulation

5. Nursing management

    a. Prevent congenital heart disease

        1) Optimal nutrition, prenatal care, and avoidance of drugs and alcohol

        2) Immunization against rubella in females of childbearing age

    b. Recognize early symptoms—cyanosis, poor weight gain, poor feeding habits, exercise intolerance, unusual posturing; carefully evaluate heart murmurs

    c. Help parents adjust to defect

        1) Monitor vital signs and heart rhythm

        2) Prepare client for invasive procedures

        3) Monitor intake and output

        4) Provide calm environment and promote rest

6. Medications

    a. Digoxin

    b. Iron preparations

    c. Diuretics

    d. Potassium

7. Change in feeding pattern for infant

    a. Small amounts every 2 h

    b. Enlarged nipple hole

    c. Diet—low sodium, high potassium

**H.** Sudden infant death syndrome (SIDS)—unexplained sudden death during sleep of a child under 1-year-old

1. Assessment

    a. Occurs during first year of life, peaks at 2–4 mo

    b. Occurs between midnight and 9 A.M.

    c. Increased incidence in winter, peaks in January

2. Analysis

    a. Thought to be brain stem abnormality in neurological regulation of cardiorespiratory control

    b. Third leading cause of death in children from 1 wk to 1 y of age

    c. Higher incidence of SIDS

        1) Infants with documented apparent life-threatening events (ALTEs)

        2) Siblings of infant with SIDS

        3) Preterm infants who have pathological apnea

        4) Preterm infants, especially with low birth weight

        5) Infants of African descent

        6) Multiple births

        7) Infants of addicted mothers

8) Infants who sleep on abdomen

9) Maternal smoking

10) Co-sleeping with parent(s) or multiple family members

11) Soft bedding

3. Nursing management

a. Home apnea monitor

b. Place all healthy infants in supine position to sleep

c. Support parents, family

d. Referral to Sudden Infant Death Foundation

# Selected Neuromuscular Disorders

A. Spina bifida/neural tube defects

1. Description—congenital anomaly of the spinal cord characterized by nonunion between the laminae of the vertebrae

2. Types (*see* Figure 14-4)

a. Dimpling at the site (spina bifida occulta)

b. Bulging, saclike lesion filled with spinal fluid and covered with thin, atrophic, bluish, ulcerated skin (meningocele)

c. Bulging, saclike lesion filled with spinal fluid and spinal cord element (myelomeningocele)

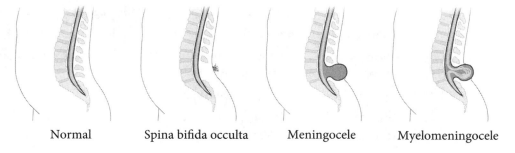

Normal    Spina bifida occulta    Meningocele    Myelomeningocele

**Figure 14-4.** Types of Spina Bifida

3. Risk factors

a. Maternal folic acid deficiency

b. Previous pregnancy affected by neural tubal defect

4. Nursing management

a. Protect lesions from trauma or infection

1) Observe for irritation, CSF leakage, signs of infection, hydrocephalus

2) Maintain optimum asepsis; cover lesion with moist sterile dressings

3) Position client on abdomen or semiprone with sandbags

4) Provide optimum skin care, especially to perineal area

    b.  Identify possible motor and sensory dysfunctions, and report immediately

        1)  Abnormal movement of extremities

        2)  Absent or abnormal reflexes

        3)  Incontinence, fecal impaction

        4)  Flaccid paralysis of lower extremities

    c.  Identify intracranial involvement

        1)  Observe for increased intracranial pressure

            a)  Tense and/or bulging fontanels

            b)  Separated cranial sutures

            c)  Irritability

            d)  High-pitched cry

            e)  Distended scalp veins

            f)  Changes in feeding habits

            g)  Setting-sun sign in the eyes

        2)  Observe for alterations in level of consciousness

            a)  Similar to increased intracranial pressure

            b)  Poor sucking ability

            c)  Poor muscle tone

            d)  Lack of movement

            e)  Weak cry

    d.  Provide frequent sources of stimulation appropriate for child's age level

    e.  Provide postoperative care—vertebral fusion or surgical repair

        1)  Focus observation on detecting signs of meningitis, shock, increased intracranial pressure, and respiratory difficulty

        2)  Family teaching on how to care for child at home

        3)  Referrals for possible physiotherapy, orthopedic procedures, and bowel and bladder management should be discussed with family

**B.**  Cerebral palsy

  1.  Description—a neuromuscular disability in which the voluntary muscles are poorly controlled because of brain damage

  2.  History

    a.  Heredity

    b.  Maternal diabetes, rubella, toxemia during pregnancy

    c.  Rh incompatibility

    d.  Birth injuries

    e.  Infections

3. Assessment

    a. Neonate—cannot hold up head, feeble cry, weakness, inability to feed, body noticeably arched

    b. Infants—failure-to-thrive syndrome present

    c. Toddlers and preschoolers—signs of intellectual delay; distorted physical development pattern, especially walking; spasticity of muscles is a dominant characteristic

4. Nursing management

    a. Preserve physical and mental capacity of the child

        1) Assist with early diagnosis

        2) Assist with physical and occupational therapy

        3) Give referrals to appropriate agencies

    b. Provide emotional support to parents and client

    c. Encourage measures to allow for normal growth

    d. Provide adequate nutrition

        1) Assist with feeding, e.g., place food at back of mouth or on either side of tongue toward cheek with slight downward pressure of the spoon on the tongue

        2) Never tilt head backward when feeding—leads to choking

        3) Set aside ample time for meals

        4) Administer high-calorie diet

**C.** Muscular dystrophy

1. Description—progressive hereditary muscle disorder characterized by muscular weakness

2. Assessment

    a. Leg weakness, flat feet, stumbling and falling, pelvic muscle weakness

    b. Pseudohypertrophy of muscles

    c. Lordosis, scoliosis

    d. Waddling gait, walking on toes

    e. Contractures of elbows, feet, knees, hips

3. Diagnostic tests

    a. Creatinine phosphokinase (CPK) elevated

    b. Abnormal electromyogram

    c. Abnormal muscle biopsy

4. Nursing management

    a. Promote safety due to gait and movement disturbances, use of braces or wheelchair

    b. Assist with diagnostic tests

    c. Client/parent education on nature of the disease

    d. Provide emotional support to child and family

    e. Discuss balance between activity and rest for the child

f. Promote and support growth and development as appropriate

g. Prevent complications of contractures

h. Referrals to appropriate agencies

## Selected Musculoskeletal Disorders

A. Developmental dysplasia of the hip (DDH)
1. Description—inability of the acetabulum to hold the head of the femur
2. Characteristic manifestations
   a. Uneven gluteal folds and thigh creases (more and deeper on involved side)
   b. Limited abduction of hip
   c. Pain on abduction of involved hip
   d. Prominent trochanter
   e. Short limb on affected side
   f. Waddling gait with bilateral dislocation
   g. Limping gait with unilateral dislocation
3. Diagnosis
   a. X-ray evaluations
   b. Clinical signs (*see* Figure 14-5)

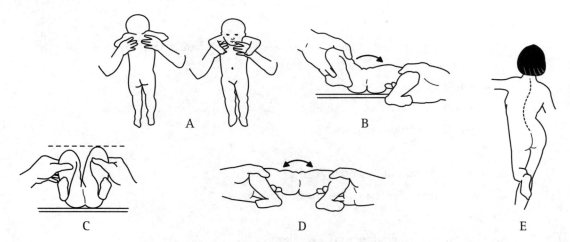

**Figure 14-5.** Developmental Dysplasia of the Hip (DDH)

Signs of congenital dislocation of hip: (A) asymmetry of gluteal and thigh folds; (B) limited hip abduction as seen in flexion; (C) apparent shortening of femur as indicated by knees in flexion; (D) Ortolani sign if infant is under 4 wk of age; (E) Trendelenburg on weight bearing. NOTE: Ortolani sign—palpable click with reduction in abduction and dislocation in adduction; positive sign. Trendelenburg sign—when standing on dislocated side, unable to elevate pelvis of opposite side.

4. Predisposition

   a. Intrauterine position (breech)

   b. Hormonal imbalance

   c. Cultural and environmental influences, e.g., certain groups of people that tightly wrap infants in blankets or strap infant to cradleboard

5. Treatment and nursing management—depends on type of dislocation

   a. Splinting for partial dislocation by use of abduction splints (*see* Figure 14-6)

   b. Hip spica cast after closed reduction for subluxation and complete dislocation (*see* Figure 14-7)

   c. Open reduction if above measures are unsuccessful, i.e., surgical incision is made to directly visualize and reduce the deformity

   d. Provide for safety, mobility

   e. Prevent deformities

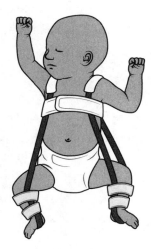

**Figure 14-6.** Pavlik Harness

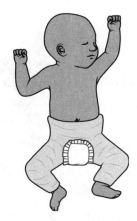

**Figure 14-7.** Hip Spica Cast

B. Fractures

1. Common fractures in children

    a. Bend

        1) Occurs when the bone is bent but not broken

        2) Associated with the flexibility of the bones in young children

        3) Bones can bend 45° or more before breaking

        4) Occur most often in the ulna and fibula, in association with fractures of the radius and tibia, respectively

    b. Buckle fracture

        1) Produced by compression of a porous bone

        2) Appears as a raised or bulging projection at the fracture site

        3) Common in young children

    c. Greenstick fracture

        1) Occurs when a bone bends beyond its limits

        2) Fracture on one side of bone and a bend on the other

2. Traction

    a. 90°-90° traction

        1) Common skeletal traction in children

        2) Affected hip and knee are flexed at 90° angles

        3) Affected lower leg in boot cast or supported in a sling; Steinmann pin or Kirschner wire placed in distal fragment of femur

    b. Buck extension traction

    c. Russell traction

    d. Balanced suspension traction

3. Nursing management

    a. Provide care to child with splint

        1) Encourage normal growth and development by allowing child to perform appropriate activities

        2) Teach parents to reapply splints and explain rationale for maintaining abduction

        3) Tell parents to move child from one room to another for environmental change

        4) Discuss with parents modifications in bathing, dressing, and diapering

        5) Tell parents to touch and hold child to express affection and reinforce security

    b. Provide care to child in cast

        1) Apply principles of cast care

        2) Teach parents cast care if child is being discharged with cast

**C.** Club foot (talipes equinovarus)

   1. Description—rigid abnormality of talus bone at birth; does not involve muscles, tendons, nerves, or blood vessels

   2. Assessment

      a. Adduction and inversion of hind and forward part of the foot (*see* Figure 14-8)

   3. Predisposing factors

      a. Genetics

      b. Environmental

   4. Treatment and management

      a. Foot exercises—manipulation of foot to correct position every 4 h regularly

      b. Casts and splints correct the deformity in most cases if applied early

      c. Surgery is usually required for older child

   5. Nursing management

      a. Early referral

      b. Care of the child in Denis Browne splint

      c. Care of the child with cast

      d. Support normal growth and development

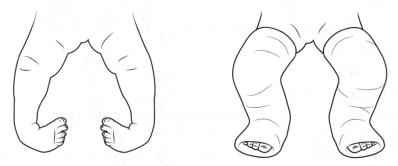

**Figure 14-8.** Casting for Talipes Equinovarus

**D.** Scoliosis

   1. Description—lateral deviation of one or more vertebrae commonly accompanied by rotary motion

   2. Assessment (*see* Figure 14-9)

      a. Poor posture

      b. Unevenness of hips or scapulae

   3. Types

      a. Functional—flexible deviation that corrects by bending

      b. Structural—permanent, hereditary deviation

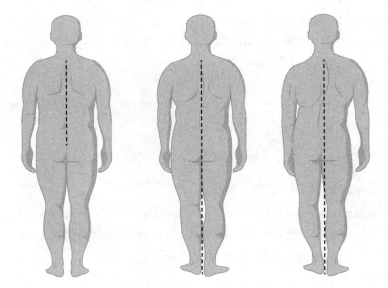

**Figure 14-9.** Scoliosis

4. Treatment and nursing management

   a. Exercise for functional type

   b. Electrostimulation

   c. Braces

      1) Boston brace and thoracolumbosacral (TLSO) brace

      2) Milwaukee brace

   d. Risser-turnbuckle cast

   e. Halo traction

   f. Surgery—spinal fusion with Harrington rod insertion; Dwyer instrumentation with anterior spinal fusion; screw and wire (Luque) instrumentation

   g. Assist in prevention of progression of abnormality—teach isometric exercises to strengthen the abdominal muscles

      1) Sit-ups

      2) Pelvic tilt

      3) Push-up with pelvic tilt

   h. Care for client with brace

      1) Skin care on pressure areas

      2) Wear T-shirt under brace to minimize skin irritation

      3) Provide activities consistent with limitations, yet allow positive peer relationships to promote healthy self-concept

   i. Care for client with cast

   j. Care for client in traction

   k. Provide operative care for client undergoing spinal fusion; apply principles of laminectomy care

## End-of-Chapter Thinking Exercise

The nurse in a pediatric office conducts an assessment on a 20-month-old toddler new to the practice. Upon entering the room, the nurse notes that the client is sitting in the parent's lap. The client weighs 17 pounds (7.7 kg), but the nurse is unable to measure height because even with the parent's assistance, the client begins screaming, clinging to the parent, and will not lie back on the exam table. The nurse asks the parent about eating, sleeping, and playing patterns. The parent states, "I don't understand why my child doesn't talk or walk. My older children were doing those things by this age. She also sleeps much more than my other kids." Upon further assessment, the nurse discovers that the family moved to the area nearly 1 year ago. The parent states, "We are renovating an old farmhouse built in 1924. We have never done anything like this; it needs so much work. We don't have insurance, so I wasn't able to get my child in sooner. But now we are really worried something is wrong with her!"

1. Which assessment findings cause the nurse to be concerned? (Recognize Cues)

2. Which assessment findings lead the nurse to suspect the developmental delays may be related to lead toxicity? (Analyze Cues)

3. What does the nurse anticipate the pediatrician will order next? (Generate Solutions)

# Thinking Exercise Explanations

1. Which assessment findings cause the nurse to be concerned? (Recognize Cues)
   - Irritability
   - Fear
   - Parent reports the child does not walk or talk
   - Child has not received routine well-child checks by a pediatrician
   - Living environment
   - Sleep pattern
   - Less than normal body weight

   New situations, such as an unfamiliar health care provider's office/staff, may cause the toddler to be frightened and uncooperative; however, when there are other indicators, such as the child not walking or talking, the nurse should be concerned. Safety of the living environment will need additional assessment. The average weight of a 20-month-old is 24–25 pounds (10.9–11.4 kg), so the nurse will be concerned about the client's development.

2. Which assessment findings lead the nurse to suspect the developmental delays may be related to lead toxicity? (Analyze Cues)
   - Delays in speech and motor development
   - Irritability
   - Increased somnolence
   - Family is living in an environment that may have lead-based paint and/or lead pipes
   - Less than normal body weight

   The nurse should recognize these indicators as signs of possible lead toxicity.

3. What does the nurse anticipate the pediatrician will order next? (Generate Solutions)
   - Laboratory testing: blood lead level, erythrocyte protoporphyrin (EP) level, and complete blood count (CBC)
   - Long-bone x-rays, such as bilateral femur films
   - Based on laboratory results, a referral to the local health department for a home inspection
   - In-depth assessment of eating, sleeping, play, and motor development patterns by a pediatric occupational therapist or other qualified health care provider
   - Medical records from previous pediatrician (the nurse may ask the parent to sign a release of information form)

   There should be no detectable serum lead level present. Levels of > 5 mcg/dL (0.24 mcmol/L) warrant a referral to the local health department/public health agency to inspect the home. Determining the extent of the developmental delays, by reviewing lab and x-ray results, will help guide the health care team's plan of care.

[ CHAPTER 15 ]

# PSYCHOSOCIAL INTEGRITY

**SECTIONS**

**CONCEPTS COVERED**

1.  Basic Concepts

Table 15-1. Psychosocial Development
Table 15-2. Therapeutic Responses
Table 15-3. Responses to Avoid in Therapeutic Communication
Table 15-4. Treatment Modalities for Mental Illness

2.  Anxiety

Table 15-5. Anxiety Disorders
Table 15-6. Defense Mechanisms
Table 15-7. Nursing Interventions in Anxiety
Table 15-8. Antianxiety Medications

3.  Situational Crises

Table 15-9. Situational/Traumatic Crises
Table 15-10. Nursing Management of Dying Client

4.  Depressive Disorders

Table 15-11. Behavioral Clues of Impending Suicide
Table 15-12. Nursing Management of Depression
Table 15-13. Nursing Considerations for Electroconvulsive Therapy (ECT)
Table 15-14. Antidepressant Medications Overview

5.  Bipolar Disorder

Table 15-15. Bipolar Disorder Medications

6.  Altered Thought Processes

Table 15-16. Schizophrenia
Table 15-17. Antipsychotic Medications
Table 15-18. Nursing Care of a Client Who Acts Withdrawn
Table 15-19. Nursing Care of a Client Who Acts Suspiciously
Table 15-20. Nursing Care of a Client Who Acts Violently

# BASIC CONCEPTS

## Ego Integrity/Self-Concept

## Psychosocial Processes

**A.** Psychosocial well-being

    1. Appearance, behavior, or mood

        a. Well-groomed, relaxed

        b. Self-confident, self-accepting

    2. Speech, thought content, and thought processes

        a. Clear, coherent

        b. Reality based

    3. Sensorium

        a. Oriented to person, place, and time

        b. Good memory

        c. Ability to abstract

    4. Insight and judgment—accurate self-perception and awareness

    5. Family relationships and work habits

        a. Satisfying interpersonal relationships

        b. Ability to trust

        c. Ability to cope effectively with stress

        d. Environmental mastery

**B.** History

    1. Potential support systems or stressors

        a. Religious organization or community support

        b. Family

        c. Socioeconomic resources

        d. Education

        e. Cultural norms

2. Potential risk factors

   a. Family history of mental illness

   b. Medical history—imbalances can cause symptoms resembling emotional illness

   c. Lack of environmental/social support

3. Theorists

   a. Freud—defined parts of the psyche and stages of psychosocial development (*see* Table 15-1)

      1) Id—unconscious, immediate, pleasure principle

      2) Ego—conscious, compromising, based in reality

      3) Superego—both unconscious and conscious, uncompromising, basis of shame and guilt

   b. Erikson—defined stages of psychosocial development throughout life (*see* Table 15-1)

      1) Each stage represents developmental milestones

      2) Completion of one stage is necessary for next stage

   c. Sullivan—theory includes the impact of social environment on interpersonal relationships

      1) Provides basis for many community health models

      2) Hildegard Peplau (nurse theorist) developed Sullivan's theory into a model of the nurse-client relationship

C. Requirements for health maintenance

   1. Satisfaction of basic human needs in order of importance (Maslow)

      a. Physical—oxygen, water, food, sleep, sex

      b. Safety—physical, security, order

      c. Love and belonging—affection, companionship, identification

      d. Esteem and recognition—status, success, prestige

      e. Self-actualization—self-fulfillment, creativity

      f. Aesthetic—harmony, spirituality

   2. Potential nursing diagnoses

      a. Impaired social interactions

      b. Anxiety

      c. Ineffective coping

      d. Self-esteem disturbance

**Table 15-1** Psychosocial Development

| AGE | STAGE OF DEVELOPMENT | | | NORMAL FINDINGS |
|---|---|---|---|---|
| | **Erikson** | **Freud** | **Piaget** | |
| Birth– 1 year | Trust vs. mistrust | Oral stage or infancy | Sensorimotor | Recognizes and attaches to primary caretaker, develops simple motor skills, moves from instant gratification to coping with anxiety<br><br>Learns about self through the environment |
| 1–3 y | Autonomy vs. shame and doubt | Anal stage or toddler-hood | Preoperational | Learns to manipulate environment, learns self-control in toilet training, parallel play<br><br>Develops expressive language and symbolic play |
| 3–6 y | Initiative vs. guilt | Phallic stage or preschool | Preoperational intuitive | Learns symbols and concepts, assertiveness against environment; learns sex role identity |
| 6–12 y | Industry vs. inferiority | Latency stage or school-age | Concrete operational | Sees cause and effect and draws conclusions, develops allegiance to friends, uses energy to industriously create and perform tasks, shows competency in school and with friends |
| 12–20 y | Identity vs. role diffusion | Genital stage or adoles-cence | Formal operational | Thinks abstractly, uses logic and scientific reason, masters independence through rebellion, develops firm sense of self, is strongly influenced by peers, develops sexual maturity, explores sexual relationships |
| 20–45 y | Intimacy vs. isolation | | | Develops lasting intimate relationships and good work relationships |
| 45–65 y | Generativity vs. stagnation | | | Establishes a family and oversees next generation, is productive, shows concern for others |
| 65 y–death | Integrity vs. despair | | | Sees own life as meaningful, is productive, accepts physical changes |

## Communication Skills of the Nurse

A. Therapeutic communication—listening to and understanding client while promoting clarification and insight

1. Goals

   a. To understand client's message (verbal and nonverbal)

   b. To facilitate verbalization of feelings

   c. To communicate understanding and acceptance

   d. To identify problems, goals, and objectives

2. Guidelines

   a. Nonverbal communication constitutes two-thirds of all communication and gives the most accurate reflection of attitude

      1) Physical appearance, body movement, posture, gesture, facial expression

      2) Contact—eye contact, physical distance maintained, ability to touch and be touched

   b. The person's feelings and what is verbalized may be incongruent, e.g., client denies feeling sad but appears morose

   c. Implied messages are as important to understand as overt behavior, e.g., continual interruptions may represent loneliness or fear

3. Phases of a therapeutic relationship

   a. Initiating phase—boundaries of relationship determined

   b. Working phase—client develops insights and learns coping

   c. Terminating phase—work of relationship is summarized

4. Therapeutic responses—techniques that are the main tools to promote therapeutic exchange between nurse and client (*see* Table 15-2)

5. Nontherapeutic responses—responses to avoid (*see* Table 15-3)

**Table 15-2** Therapeutic Responses

| RESPONSE | GOAL/PURPOSE | EXAMPLES |
|---|---|---|
| Using silence (nonverbal) | Allows client time to think and reflect; conveys acceptance<br><br>Allows client to take lead in conversation | Use proper nonverbal communication, remain seated, maintain eye contact, sit quietly and wait |
| Using general leads or broad openings | Encourages client to talk<br><br>Indicates interest in client<br><br>Allows client to choose subject<br><br>Sets tone for depressed client | "What would you like to talk about? Then what? Go on...."<br><br>"What brought you to the hospital?"<br><br>"What can you tell me about your family?" |

*(Continued)*

**Table 15-2** Therapeutic Responses (*Continued*)

| RESPONSE | GOAL/PURPOSE | EXAMPLES |
|---|---|---|
| Clarification | Encourages recall and details of particular experience<br><br>Encourages description of feelings<br><br>Seeks clarification, pinpoints specifics<br><br>Makes sure nurse understands client | "Give me an example."<br><br>"Tell me more."<br><br>"And how do you feel when you're angry?"<br><br>"Who are 'they'?" |
| Reflecting | Paraphrases what client says<br><br>Reflects what client says, especially feelings conveyed | "It sounds like you're feeling angry."<br><br>"In other words, you really felt abandoned."<br><br>"I hear you saying that it was hard to come to the hospital." |

**Table 15-3** Responses to Avoid in Therapeutic Communication

| RESPONSE | EXAMPLES |
|---|---|
| Close-ended questions that can be answered by a "yes" or "no" or other monosyllabic responses; prevents sharing; puts pressure on client | "How many children do you have?"<br><br>"With whom do you live?"<br><br>"Are you feeling better today?" |
| Advice giving encourages dependency; may not be right for a particular client | "Why don't you . . . ?"<br><br>"You really should cut your hair and wear makeup." |
| Responding to questions that are related to one's qualifications or personal life in an embarrassed or concrete way; keep conversation client centered | "Yes, I am highly qualified."<br><br>"You know nurses are not permitted to go out with their clients." |
| Arguing or responding in a hostile way | "If you do not take your medication, there is really nothing we can do to help you." |
| Reassuring; client benefits more by exploring own ideas and feelings | "You will start feeling much better any day."<br><br>"Don't worry; your health care providers will do everything necessary for your care." |
| "Why" questions can imply disapproval; client may become defensive | "Why didn't you take your medication?" |
| Judgmental responses evaluate client using nurse's values | "You were wrong to do that."<br><br>"Don't you think your unfaithfulness has destroyed your marriage?" |

# Treatment Modalities

Techniques that are used to care for the client with psychosocial problems (*see* Table 15-4)

**Table 15-4** Treatment Modalities for Mental Illness

| TYPE | ASSUMPTIONS | FOCUS OF TREATMENT |
|---|---|---|
| Biological | Emotional problem is an illness<br><br>Cause may be inherited or chemical in origin | Medications, electroconvulsive therapy (ECT) |
| Psychoanalytical (individual) | Anxiety results when there is conflict between the id, ego, and superego parts of the personality<br><br>Defense mechanisms form to ward off anxiety | The therapist helps the client to become aware of unconscious thoughts and feelings; understand anxiety and defenses |
| Milieu therapy | Providing a therapeutic environment will help increase client's awareness of feelings, increase sense of responsibility, and help return to community | Positive physical and social environment<br><br>Structured groups and activities<br><br>One-on-one intervention<br><br>May be token program, open wards, self-medication |
| Group therapy | Relationship with others will be re-created among group members and can be worked through; members can also directly help one another | Members meet regularly with a leader to form a stable group<br><br>Members learn new ways to cope with stress and develop insight into their behavior with others |
| Family therapy | The problem is a family problem, not an individual one<br><br>Sick families lack a sense of "I" in each member<br><br>The tendency is to focus on sick member's behavior as the source of trouble<br><br>The sick member's symptom serves a function in the family | Therapist treats the whole family<br><br>Helps members to each develop their own sense of identity<br><br>Points out function of sick member for the rest of the family |
| Activity therapy | Important group interactions occur when group members work on a task together or share in recreation | Organized group activities created to promote socialization, increase self-esteem |

*(Continued)*

**Table 15-4** Treatment Modalities for Mental Illness (*Continued*)

| TYPE | ASSUMPTIONS | FOCUS OF TREATMENT |
|---|---|---|
| Play therapy | Children express themselves more easily in play than in verbal communication<br><br>Choice of colors, toys, and interaction with toys is revealing as reflection of child's situation in the family | Provide materials and toys to facilitate interaction with child, observe play, and help child to resolve problems through play |
| Behavioral therapy and behavior modification | Psychological problems are the result of learning<br><br>Deficiencies can be corrected through learning | Operant conditioning—use of rewards to reinforce positive behavior; perceived and self-reinforcement become more important than the negative behavior |

# ANXIETY

## Cognition, Emotional Process

### Anxiety

An uncomfortable feeling of apprehension or dread that occurs in response to internal or external stimuli

A. Assessment (*see* Table 15-5)

1. Definition: feeling of dread or fear in the absence of an external threat or disproportionate to the nature of the threat

2. Levels of anxiety

   a. Mild—high degree of alertness, mild uneasiness, "butterflies in stomach"

   b. Moderate—increased perspiration, light-headedness, muscle tension, urinary frequency, nausea, anorexia, diarrhea, heart pounding, increased BP, dry mouth, cold, clammy and pale skin, selective inattention, poor comprehension

   c. Severe—most symptoms of moderate anxiety intensified, hyperventilation, dizziness, vomiting, tachycardia, panic, inability to hear or speak, further decreased perception, hallucinations, delusions

   d. Panic—symptoms of severe anxiety and inability to function, dread, terror, personality disorganization

**Table 15-5** Anxiety Disorders

| TYPE | ASSESSMENTS | NURSING CONSIDERATIONS |
|------|-------------|------------------------|
| Phobia | Apprehension, anxiety, helplessness when confronted with phobic situation or feared object<br><br>Examples of specific fears:<br><br>Acrophobia—heights<br><br>Claustrophobia—closed areas<br><br>Agoraphobia—open spaces | Avoid confrontation and humiliation<br><br>Do not focus on getting client to stop being afraid<br><br>Systematic desensitization<br><br>Relaxation techniques<br><br>General anxiety measures<br><br>May be managed with antidepressants |

*(Continued)*

**Table 15-5** Anxiety Disorders (*Continued*)

| TYPE | ASSESSMENTS | NURSING CONSIDERATIONS |
|------|-------------|------------------------|
| Panic disorder | Extreme, overwhelming form of anxiety | Teach, encourage, and support relaxation |
| | Experienced when client has a real or perceived threat | Teach and support self-evaluation scales |
| | Palpitations | Educate and assess medication use and knowledge |
| | Tachycardia | Support use of distraction and positive self-talk |
| | Seating, shaking, nausea | Support participation in therapy treatment |
| | Paresthesia | |
| | Feelings of unreality | |
| Acute stress disorder/ post-traumatic stress disorder | Develops after a traumatic event | Teach, encourage, and support stress management techniques |
| | Determine timing of event | Educate and assess medication use and knowledge |
| | Determine occurrence and timing of symptoms | Support participation in therapy treatment |
| | Assess for history of with 9 or more symptoms from the 5 categories of intrusion, negative mood, dissociation, avoidance and arousal | Perform passive listening to recount of event |
| Obsessive-compulsive disorder (OCD) | Obsession—repetitive, uncontrollable thoughts | Accept ritualistic behavior |
| | Compulsion—repetitive, uncontrollable acts, e.g., rituals, rigidity, inflexibility | Structure environment |
| | | Provide for physical needs |
| | | Offer alternative activities, especially ones using hands |
| | | Guide decisions, minimize choices |
| | | Encourage socialization |
| | | Group therapy |
| | | Managed with clomipramine (tricyclic antidepressant) and selective serotonin reuptake inhibitors (SSRIs) |
| | | Stimulus-response prevention |
| Functional neurologic symptom disorder | Physical symptoms with no organic basis, unconscious behavior—could include blindness, paralysis, convulsions without loss of consciousness, stocking and glove anesthesia; lack of concern about symptoms (la belle indifference) | Diagnostic evaluation |
| | | Discuss feelings rather than symptoms |
| | | Promote therapeutic relationship with client |
| | | Avoid secondary gain |

3. Characteristic findings

   a. Cardiovascular

      1) Increased pulse, blood pressure, and respiration

      2) Palpitations

      3) Chest discomfort/pain

      4) Perspiration

      5) Flushing and heat sensations

      6) Cold hands and feet

      7) Headache

   b. Gastrointestinal

      1) Nausea, vomiting, and diarrhea

      2) Belching

      3) Heartburn

      4) Cramps

   c. Musculoskeletal

      1) Increased muscle tension and tendon reflexes

      2) Increased generalized fatigue

      3) Tremors, jerking of limbs

      4) Unsteady voice

   d. Intellectual

      1) Poor comprehension—may be unable to follow directions

      2) Poor concentration

      3) Selective inattention

      4) Focus on detail

      5) Impaired problem solving

      6) Unable to communicate

         a) Thoughts may become random, distorted, disconnected with impaired logic

         b) Rapid, high-pitched speech

   e. Social and emotional

      1) Feelings of helplessness and hopelessness

      2) Feelings of increased threat, dread, horror, anger, and rage

      3) Use of defense mechanisms and more primitive coping behaviors

         a) Denial

         b) Crying, rocking, shouting, curling up, withdrawal

    4. Predisposing conditions

        a. Prolonged unmet needs of dependency, security, love, and attention

        b. Stress threatening security or self-esteem

        c. Unacceptable thoughts or feelings surfacing to consciousness, e.g., rage, erotic impulses, flashbacks

        d. Older adults—coping mechanisms not as effective when faced with loss of physical or mental function, financial concerns; may report increased physical issues

**B.** Ego defense mechanisms (*see* Table 15-6); used to cope with anxiety and painful feelings

**C.** Nursing management (*see* Table 15-7)

    1. Institute measures to decrease anxiety

    2. Administer medications (*see* Table 15-8)

    3. Goals

        a. To understand client's message (verbal and nonverbal)

        b. To facilitate verbalization of feelings

        c. To communicate understanding and acceptance

        d. To identify problems, goals, and objectives

        e. Follow guidelines regarding communication skills of the nurse (*see* Communication Skills of the Nurse in Section 1 of this chapter)

**Table 15-6** Defense Mechanisms

| MECHANISM | DEFINITION | EXAMPLES |
|---|---|---|
| Denial | Failure to acknowledge an intolerable thought, feeling, experience, reality | Alcoholic says his drinking is not a problem; terminally ill client makes long-range plans |
| Displacement | Redirection of feelings to subject that is acceptable or less threatening | Kicking the dog or yelling at one's spouse after a bad day at work |
| Projection | Attribution to others of one's own unacceptable thoughts, feelings, qualities | Saying someone you are angry with dislikes you; staff nurse complains about the head nurse's poor skills after receiving an unfavorable evaluation |
| Undoing | An attempt to erase an unacceptable act or thought | Excessively apologizing; buying extravagant gifts for one's spouse while having an affair |
| Compensation | An attempt to overcome a real or an imagined shortcoming | A sickly child becoming an athlete |

*(Continued)*

**Table 15-6** Defense Mechanisms (*Continued*)

| MECHANISM | DEFINITION | EXAMPLES |
|---|---|---|
| Substitution | Replacing desired, impractical, or unobtainable object with one that is attainable | Marrying someone who looks like a former fiancée |
| Introjection | Characteristic of another incorporated into oneself | Partner dies and spouse develops symptoms of their illness |
| Repression | Unacceptable thoughts kept from awareness | Forgetting painful experience |
| Reaction formation | Expressing attitude directly opposite to unconscious one | Someone with strong dependency needs chooses a "helping" profession |
| Regression | Returning to an earlier stage of development | Temper tantrums, baby talk, bed-wetting |
| Dissociation | Detachment of painful emotional experience from consciousness | Amnesia |
| Rationalization | Attempts to justify, via logical or acceptable explanations, acts or feelings that are not logical or acceptable | A student who is sexually attracted to her teacher tells herself she needs to stay after class for help with a project |
| Idealization | Glorifying another's characteristics | Only noticing another's positive qualities |
| Identification | Incorporating certain attributes of another into one's own thoughts or behavior | A person dresses like someone she admires |
| Acting out | Using action rather than reflection or feelings during emotional conflict | Client gets mad and stays out late |

**Table 15-7** Nursing Interventions in Anxiety

| GENERAL PRINCIPLES | EXAMPLES |
|---|---|
| Assess level of anxiety | Look at body language, speech patterns, facial expressions, defense mechanisms, and behavior used |
| | Distinguish levels of anxiety (symptoms of sympathetic nervous system stimulation) |
| Keep environmental stresses/stimulation low when anxiety is high | Brief orientation to unit or procedures |
| | Written information to read later when anxiety is lower |
| | Pleasant, attractive, uncluttered environment |
| | Provide privacy if presence of other clients is overstimulating |
| | Provide physical care if necessary |
| | Avoid offering many alternatives or decisions when anxiety is high |
| Assist client to cope with anxiety more effectively | Acknowledge anxious behavior |
| | Always remain with extremely anxious client |
| | Assist client in clarifying own thoughts and feelings |
| | Encourage measures to reduce anxiety, e.g., exercise, activities, talking with friends, hobbies |
| | Assist client in realistically recognizing strengths and capabilities |
| | Provide therapy to develop more effective coping and interpersonal skills, e.g., individual, group |
| | May need to administer antianxiety medications |
| Maintain accepting and helpful attitude toward client | Use unhurried speech |
| | Acknowledge client's distress and concerns about problem |
| | Encourage clarification of feelings and thoughts |
| | Evaluate and manage own anxiety while working with client |
| | Recognize the value of defense mechanisms and realize that client is attempting to make the anxiety tolerable in the best possible way |
| | Do not attempt to remove a defense mechanism at any time |

**Table 15-8** Antianxiety Medications

| MEDICATION | ADVERSE EFFECTS | NURSING CONSIDERATIONS |
|---|---|---|
| **Benzodiazepine Derivatives** | | |
| Chlordiazepox-ide Diazepam | Lethargy, hangover<br><br>Respiratory depression<br><br>Hypotension | CNS depressant<br><br>Use—anxiety, sedation, alcohol withdrawal, seizures<br><br>May result in toxic buildup in older adults<br><br>Potential for physiological addiction/overdose<br><br>Can develop tolerance and cross-tolerance<br><br>Cigarette smoking increases clearance of medication<br><br>Alcohol increases CNS depression<br><br>Increased sedation, fall risk, and confusion in older adults |
| Alprazolam<br><br>Lorazepam<br><br>Oxazepam | Drowsiness, light-headed-ness, hypotension, hepatic dysfunction<br><br>Increased salivation<br><br>Orthostatic hypotension<br><br>Memory impairment and confusion | CNS depressant<br><br>Safer for older adults<br><br>Don't combine with alcohol or other depressants<br><br>Check renal and hepatic function<br><br>Don't discontinue abruptly (true for all antianxiety agents)<br><br>Teach addictive potential |
| Midazolam | Retrograde amnesia, euphoria, hypotension, dysrhythmia, cardiac arrest, respiratory depression | CNS depressant<br><br>Use—preoperative sedation, conscious sedation for endoscopic procedures and diagnostic tests |
| **Anxiolytics Antianxiety Medications** | | |
| Buspirone | Light-headedness<br><br>Confusion<br><br>Hypotension, palpitations | Little sedation<br><br>Requires $\geq$3 weeks to be effective<br><br>Cannot be given as a PRN medication<br><br>Particularly useful for generalized anxiety disorder (GAD)<br><br>No abuse potential<br><br>Used for clients with previous addiction<br><br>Avoid alcohol and grapefruit juice<br><br>Monitor for worsening depression or suicidal tendencies |

*(Continued)*

**Table 15-8** Antianxiety Medications (*Continued*)

| MEDICATION | ADVERSE EFFECTS | NURSING CONSIDERATIONS |
|---|---|---|
| Hydroxyzine | Drowsiness, ataxia | Produces no dependence, tolerance, or intoxication |
| | Leukopenia, hypotension | Can be used for anxiety relief for indefinite periods |
| **Herbals** | | |
| Kava | Impaired thinking, judgment, motor reflexes, vision | Similar activity to benzodiazepines |
| | | Suppresses emotional excitability and produces mild euphoria |
| | Decreased plasma proteins | Do not take with CNS depressants |
| | Thrombocytopenia, leukocytopenia, dyspnea, pulmonary hypertension | Should not be taken by women who are pregnant or lactating or by children under the age of 12 |
| Melatonin | Sedation, confusion, headache, tachycardia | Influences sleep-wake cycles (levels are high during sleep) |
| | | Used for prevention and treatment of jet lag and insomnia |
| | | Use cautiously if given with benzodiazepines and CNS depressants |
| | | Contraindicated in hepatic insufficiency, history of cerebrovascular disease, depression, neurologic disorders |
| Action | Affects neurotransmitters | |
| Indications | Anxiety disorders, insomnia, petit mal seizures, panic attacks, acute manic episodes | |
| Adverse effects | Sedation | |
| | Depression, confusion | |
| | Anger, hostility | |
| | Headache | |
| | Dry mouth, constipation | |
| | Bradycardia | |
| | Elevations in LDH, AST, ALT | |
| | Urinary retention | |
| Nursing considerations | Monitor liver function | |
| | Monitor for therapeutic blood levels | |
| | Avoid alcohol | |
| | Caution when performing tasks requiring alertness (e.g., driving car) | |
| | Benzodiazepines are also used as muscle relaxants, sedatives, hypnotics, anticonvulsants | |

# SITUATIONAL CRISES

## Intracranial Regulation, Emotional Processes

## Crisis

Period in which there is a major change in a person's life, either from an event or a perceived threat

**A.** Characteristics

1. Temporary state of disequilibrium precipitated by an event or a threat

2. Short duration; self-limiting, usually 4–6 wk

3. May offer opportunity to develop new coping abilities; promote growth and new behaviors

4. Typical precipitating factors—developmental stages, situational factors, threats to self-concept

**B.** Assessment of crisis (*see* Table 15-9)

**Table 15-9** Situational/Traumatic Crises

|  | GRIEVING CLIENT | DYING CLIENT | RAPE TRAUMA |
|---|---|---|---|
| **Assessment** | Stages of grief<br><br>  a. Shock and disbelief<br>  b. Awareness of the pain of loss<br>  c. Restitution<br>Acute grief period 4–8 wk<br>Usual resolution within 1 y<br>Long-term resolution over time | Stages of dying<br><br>  a. Denial<br>  b. Anger<br>  c. Bargaining<br>  d. Depression<br>  e. Acceptance | Stages of crisis<br><br>  a. Acute reaction lasts 3-4 wk<br>  b. Reorganization is long-term<br>Common responses to rape<br><br>  a. Self-blame, embarrassment<br>  b. Phobias, fear of violence, death, injury<br>  c. Anxiety, insomnia<br>  d. Wish to escape, move, relocate<br>  e. Psychosomatic disturbances |

(Continued)

**Table 15-9** Situational/Traumatic Crises (*Continued*)

| | GRIEVING CLIENT | DYING CLIENT | RAPE TRAUMA |
|---|---|---|---|
| **Analysis** | Potential problems<br><br>a. Family of deceased or separated<br>   — Guilt<br>   — Anger<br>   — Anxiety<br><br>b. Client undergoing surgery or loss of body part<br>   — Anger<br>   — Withdrawal<br>   — Guilt<br>   — Anxiety<br>   — Loss of role | Potential problems<br><br>a. Avoidance behavior<br>b. Inability to express feelings when in denial<br>c. Feelings of guilt<br>d. Withdrawal<br>e. Lonely, frightened<br>f. Anxiety of client and family | Potential problems<br><br>a. Fears, panic reactions, generalized anxiety<br>b. Guilt<br>c. Inability to cope<br><br>Current crisis may reactivate old, unresolved trauma<br><br>Follow emergency department protocol: may include clothing, hair samples, NPO<br><br>Be alert for potential internal injuries, e.g., hemorrhage |
| **Intervention** | Apply crisis theory<br><br>Focus on the here and now<br><br>Provide support to family when loved one dies<br><br>Provide family privacy<br><br>Encourage verbalization of feelings<br><br>Facilitate expressions of anger and rage<br><br>Emphasize strengths<br><br>Increase ability to cope<br><br>Support adjustment to illness, loss of body part | Apply crisis theory<br><br>Support staff having feelings of loss<br><br>Keep communication open<br><br>Allow expression of feelings<br><br>Focus on the here and now<br><br>Let client know they are not alone<br><br>Provide comforting environment<br><br>Be attentive to need for privacy<br><br>Provide physically comforting care, e.g., back rubs<br><br>Give sense of control and dignity<br><br>Respect client's wishes (cultural and religious beliefs) | Apply crisis theory<br><br>Focus on the here and now<br><br>Write out treatments and appointments for client as anxiety causes forgetfulness<br><br>Record all information in health record<br><br>Give client referrals for legal assistance, supportive psychotherapy, and rape crisis center<br><br>Follow up regularly until client is improved |

1. Stages of crisis

   a. Denial

   b. Increased tension/anxiety

   c. Disorganization—inability to function

   d. Attempts to escape the problem—pretends problem does not exist; blames others

   e. Attempts to reorganize

   f. General reorganization

2. Precipitating factors

   a. Developmental stages

      1) Birth

      2) Adolescence

      3) Midlife

      4) Retirement

   b. Situational factors

      1) Natural disasters

      2) Financial loss

   c. Threats to self-concept

      1) Loss of job

      2) Failure at school

      3) Onset of serious illness

C. Crisis intervention process

   1. Assessment

      a. Explore problem with client

      b. Define the event

      c. Identify client's strengths, previous coping methods used in crisis

      d. Identify client's support system

   2. Planning

      a. Evaluate client's abilities realistically

      b. With client, identify potential solutions to the situation

      c. Encourage exploration of all alternatives, using supports and developing new skills

   3. Intervention

      a. Focus and clarify problem with client

      b. Assist client in identifying feelings and thoughts

      c. Specific discussion of new strategies and ways to solve problem

      d. Rehearsing and evaluating strategies proposed

4. Evaluation and resolution

   a. Review of the event and changes made to cope with situation

   b. Anticipatory guidance to apply learning to future potential situations

   c. Possible referral for long-term assistance if necessary

**D.** Nursing management

1. Goal-directed, focus on the here and now

2. Focus on client's immediate problems

3. Explore nurse's and client's understanding of the problem

   a. Define the event (client may truly not know what has precipitated the crisis)

   b. Confirm nurse's perception by reviewing with client

   c. Identify the factors affecting problem solving

   d. Evaluate how realistically client sees the problems or concerns

4. Help client become aware of feelings and validate them

   a. Acknowledge feelings, e.g., "This must be a painful situation for you."

   b. Avoid blaming client for problems and concerns

   c. Avoid blaming others as this prevents insight

   d. Encourage ventilation with nurse to relieve anxiety

   e. Tell client they will feel better, but it may take 1–2 mo

5. Develop a plan

   a. Encourage client to make as many arrangements as possible (avoid dependence)

   b. Write out information because comprehension is impaired, e.g., referrals

   c. Maximize client's situational supports

6. Find new coping skills and manage feelings

   a. Focus on strengths and current coping skills

   b. Encourage client to form new coping skills and social outlets—reaching out to others

   c. Facilitate future planning

      1) Ask client, "What would you like to do?" and "Where would you like to go from here?"

      2) Give referrals when needed—family counseling, vocational counseling, etc.

E. Grief—self-limiting, normal response to loss (*see* Table 15-9)

1. Examples of precipitating events

   a. Separation, divorce, death

   b. Chronic disease

   c. Trauma, surgery

   d. Newborn with defects or illness

   e. Altered body image

2. Expect a more intense reaction if:

   a. Loss of a child

   b. Unresolved conflict with deceased

   c. Few situational, interpersonal supports

   d. Sudden loss

   e. Poor coping in past with losses

   f. Surgery results in loss of visible body part or one that has special significance, e.g., breast and sexuality, or if procedure is palliative rather than curative

3. Management of grief

   a. Encourage expression of memories, feelings

   b. Accept initial dependency of client

   c. Reassure client of normalcy of reaction—pain, crying, anger, guilt

   d. Recognize importance of event for client and need to mourn

   e. Recognize client's potential need for denial, and support client when beginning to integrate truth

F. Death and dying—stages of dying are not necessarily an orderly progression; may have various feelings within one period, may skip stage or stay with one or two stages (*see* Table 15-10 for nursing management)

1. Denial

2. Anger

3. Bargaining

4. Depression

5. Acceptance

**Table 15-10** Nursing Management of Dying Client

| PROBLEM | INTERVENTION |
|---|---|
| Caregivers have feelings about dying and dying clients, e.g., need to deny, worries about own mortality, anger, feelings of helplessness | Recognize own thoughts and feelings about death and dying |
| | Respect client as having own needs, values, and way of handling situation |
| | Clarify situation |
| | Focus on positive aspects of care given, e.g., less pain, less anxiety |
| Need to maintain open communication with client | Explore client's understanding of problem and prognosis |
| | Clarify misconceptions, e.g., if client feels they will die tomorrow and there is no indication of terminal phase |
| | Use client's questions and statements as guide and focus on feelings |
| | Respect denial rather than give excess information |
| | Respect client's wish for more information re: prognosis, treatment |
| Need for support and hope | Make client aware of what treatment will be provided |
| | Explore fears and reassure client that all modalities possible to relieve pain and suffering will be used |
| | Emphasize that client will not be abandoned no matter how client's illness progresses |
| | Convey idea that day-to-day survival is important and that nurse is interested in client's responses |
| | Plan with client to make the most of each day—e.g., visitors, physical comfort, relief of pain, favorite foods brought in by relatives, taking care of personal and business affairs, pleasurable activities |
| | Explore possibility of hospice care |

# [ SECTION 4 ]

# DEPRESSIVE DISORDERS

## Cellular Regulation, Intracranial Regulation, Behavior

## Depressive Disorders

An overwhelming state of sadness, loss of interest or pleasure, feelings of guilt, disturbed sleep and appetite, low energy, and an inability to concentrate

A. Depression—can be manifested as a single episode or recurrent pattern, varies according to age, race, sex; mood disorder

1. Major depressive disorder (MDD)

   a. Types—melancholia, postpartum, psychotic, agitated, seasonal affective disorder (SAD)

   b. Characterized by symptoms that persist over a minimum 2-week period

   c. MDD involves psychological, biological, and social factors

2. Dysthymic disorder

3. Depressive disorder, not otherwise specified (NOS)

4. Gerontologic considerations

   a. High risk of suicide

   b. Depression underdiagnosed and undertreated

   c. Contributing factors—illness, decreased physical and mental function

B. Assessment

1. Possible changes in self-esteem/self-confidence

   a. Low self-esteem

   b. Self-deprecation

   c. Feelings of helplessness/hopelessness

   d. Obsessive thoughts and fears

   e. Rumination and worries

   f. Sense of doom, failure

   g. Regressed behavior—immature, demanding

2. Possible changes in self-care

    a. Unkempt, depressed appearance

    b. Multiple physical issues reported

    c. Prone to injury, accidents, and infections

    d. Lack of energy; fatigue

    e. Changes in usual sleep pattern

        1) Insomnia or hypersomnia

        2) Feels unrested after night's sleep

    f. Weight loss, poor appetite, or weight gain

    g. Constipation

    h. Amenorrhea

    i. Lack of sexual desire

3. Possible changes in cognitive/mental functioning

    a. Decreased attention span

    b. Decreased concentration

    c. Slowed speech and thought processes

    d. Slowed motor activity

    e. Impaired reality testing (psychotic depression)

    f. Withdrawn

    g. Ambivalent and indecisive behavior

    h. Agitation and psychomotor restlessness

    i. Suicidal ideation (*see* Table 15-11)

**Table 15-11** Behavioral Clues of Impending Suicide

| |
|---|
| 1. Any sudden change in client's behavior |
| 2. Becomes energetic after period of severe depression |
| 3. Improved mood 10–14 d after taking antidepressant may mean suicidal plans made |
| 4. Finalizes business or personal affairs |
| 5. Gives away valuable possessions or pets |
| 6. Withdraws from social activities and plans |
| 7. Appears emotionally upset |
| 8. Presence of weapons, razors, pills (means) |
| 9. Has death plan |
| 10. Leaves a note |
| 11. Makes direct or indirect statements (e.g., "I may not be around then.") |

4. Nursing management (*see* Table 15-12)

    1)  Maintain therapeutic environment Supportive, professional attitude toward client

    2)  Continue ongoing assessment

  a.  Electroconvulsive therapy (ECT) as ordered (*see* Table 15-13)

  b.  Administer medications as ordered (*see* Table 15-14)

**Table 15-12** Nursing Management of Depression

| PROBLEM | INTERVENTION |
|---|---|
| Low self-esteem | Calm, accepting attitude; touch when appropriate (not with psychotic clients); sit with client even if silent; encourage client in an unpressured manner; reassure client that depression generally lifts; avoid cheery attitude or pep talks; note improvements and discuss with client; provide tasks client can accomplish to increase sense of mastery |
| Dependency | Show confidence in client's realistic ability to improve; work with client—avoid doing everything for client or giving advice |
| Anger | Physical activity to channel psychic energy; encourage expressions of anger when appropriate |
| Physical needs | Promote eating; offer small, frequent feedings and favorite foods; offer companionship during meals |
|  | Promote rest; provide quiet sleeping arrangement; stay with client if necessary; offer PRN medication for insomnia; watch client swallow pill |
| Risk of suicide | Monitor for signs of suicidal behavior; remove any potentially dangerous items such as pills, sharp objects, ropelike clothing items, e.g., neckties, pantyhose, belts; close observation—one-to-one; provide concrete assistance, e.g., evaluate resources; give clear explanations and convey sincere desire to help; avoid embarrassment to client by treating client in a dignified, matter-of-fact manner |

**Table 15-13** Nursing Considerations for Electroconvulsive Therapy (ECT)

1. Prepare client by explaining procedure and telling client about potential temporary memory loss and confusion

2. Informed consent, physical exam, labwork

3. NPO after midnight for an early-morning procedure

4. Have client void before ECT

5. Remove dentures, glasses, jewelry

6. Give muscle relaxant to prevent fractures and short-acting barbiturate anesthetic to induce brief general anesthesia

7. Given atropine 30 min before treatment to decrease secretions

8. Have oxygen and suction on hand

9. After procedure, take vital signs, orient client

10. Observe client's reaction and stay with client

11. Observe for sudden improvement and indications of suicidal threats after ECT treatment

**Table 15-14** Antidepressant Medications Overview

| MEDICATION | ADVERSE EFFECTS | NURSING CONSIDERATIONS |
|---|---|---|
| **Monoamine Oxidase Inhibitors (MAOIs)** | | |
| Isocarboxazid<br><br>Tranylcypromine sulfate<br><br>Phenelzine sulfate | Postural hypotension<br><br>If foods with tyramine ingested, can have hypertensive crisis: headache, sweating, palpitations, stiff neck, intracranial hemorrhage<br><br>Potentiates alcohol and other medications | Inhibits monoamine oxidase enzyme, preventing destruction of norepinephrine, epinephrine, and serotonin<br><br>Avoid foods with tyramine—aged cheese, liver, herring, yeast, beer, wine, sour cream, pickled products<br><br>Avoid caffeine, antihistamines, amphetamines<br><br>Takes 3-4 weeks to work<br><br>Avoid tricyclics until 3 weeks after stopping MAOIs<br><br>Monitor vital signs<br><br>Sunblock required |

*(Continued)*

**Table 15-14** Antidepressant Medications Overview (*Continued*)

| MEDICATION | ADVERSE EFFECTS | NURSING CONSIDERATIONS |
|---|---|---|
| **Tricyclics** | | |
| Amitriptyline hydrochloride<br><br>Imipramine<br><br>Desipramine hydrochloride<br><br>Doxepin<br><br>Nortriptyline | Sedation/drowsiness, especially with amitriptyline<br><br>Blurred vision, dry mouth, diaphoresis<br><br>Postural hypotension, palpitations<br><br>Nausea, vomiting<br><br>Constipation, urinary retention<br><br>Increased appetite | Increases brain amine levels<br><br>Suicide risk high after 10–14 days because of increased energy<br><br>Monitor vital signs<br><br>Sunblock required<br><br>Increase fluid intake<br><br>Take dose at bedtime (sedative effect)<br><br>Use sugarless candy or gum for dry mouth<br><br>Delay of 2-6 weeks before noticeable effects |
| **Selective Serotonin Reuptake Inhibitors (SSRI)** | | |
| Fluoxetine<br><br>Paroxetine<br><br>Sertraline hydrochloride | Palpitations, bradycardia<br><br>Nausea, vomiting, diarrhea or constipation, increased or decreased appetite<br><br>Urinary retention<br><br>Nervousness, insomnia | Decreases neuronal uptake of serotonin<br><br>Take in A.M. to avoid insomnia<br><br>Takes at least 4 weeks to work<br><br>Can potentiate effects of digoxin, warfarin, and diazepam<br><br>Used for anorexia |
| **Selective Serotonin-Norepinephrine Reuptake Inhibitors (SSNRI)** | | |
| Venlafaxine Duloxetine | See SSRI above | |
| **Heterocyclics/Atypical** | | |
| Bupropion<br><br>Trazodone | Dry mouth<br><br>Nausea | May require gradual reduction before stopping<br><br>Avoid use with alcohol, other CNS depressants for up to 1 week after end of therapy |
| **Herbals** | | |
| St. John's wort | Dizziness, hypertension, allergic skin reaction, phototoxicity | Avoid use of St. John's wort and MAOI within 2 weeks of each other<br><br>Do not use alcohol<br><br>Contraindicated in pregnancy<br><br>Avoid exposure to sun and use sunscreen<br><br>Discontinue 1 to 2 weeks before surgery |

(*Continued*)

**Table 15-14** Antidepressant Medications Overview (*Continued*)

| MEDICATION | ADVERSE EFFECTS | NURSING CONSIDERATIONS |
|---|---|---|
| Herbal interactions | St. John's wort—interacts with SSRIs; do not take within 2 weeks of MAOI | |
| | Ginseng may potentiate MAOIs | |
| | Avoid ma huang or ephedra with MAOIs | |
| | Kava kava should not be combined with benzodiazepines or opioids due to increased sedation | |
| | Increased use of brewer's yeast with MAOIs can increase blood pressure | |

# [ SECTION 5 ]

# BIPOLAR DISORDER

## Cellular Regulation, Intracranial Regulation, Behavior

## Bipolar Disorder

A. Types
 1. Bipolar I and II, cyclothymic disorder
 2. Mood disorder in which individuals experience the extremes of mood—depression or euphoria

B. Assessment of mania—lasts from a few days to several months
 1. Disoriented, incoherent
 2. Euphoria
 3. Delusions of grandeur
 4. Flight of ideas, impulsive, eccentric
 5. Inappropriate dress, excessive makeup and jewelry
 6. Lacks inhibition; social blunders
 7. Uses sarcastic, profane, and abusive language
 8. Quick-tempered, agitated; impaired judgment
 9. Talks excessively, jokes, dances, sings; hyperactive
 10. Can't stop moving to eat, easily stimulated by environment
 11. Happy/festive or angry/hostile
 12. Weight loss, decreased appetite
 13. Insomnia
 14. Regressed behavior
 15. Sexually indiscreet, hypersexual

C. Characteristics of depression
 1. Weight gain or loss, anorexia
 2. Insomnia or hypersomnia
 3. Decreased sexual desire
 4. Fatigue, decreased activity
 5. May feel hopeless, unhappy, helpless, miserable, guilty

6. Regressive thinking—passive, dependent, decreased motivation, concerned with bodily functions, impaired memory, distorted thought content, slow and diminished speech

7. Delusions possible

8. Socially withdrawn

9. Poor self-esteem

**D.** Etiology

1. Psychodynamics

   a. Bipolar disorder is an affective disorder

   b. Reality contact is less disturbed than in schizophrenia

   c. Elation or grandiosity can be a defense against underlying depression or feelings of low self-esteem

   d. Testing, manipulative behavior results from poor self-esteem

   e. Hypomania (less extreme form)

2. Predisposing factors

   a. Hereditary—genetic

   b. Biochemical

   c. Involvement with alcohol/drugs common (self-medication)

3. Problems

   a. Easily stimulated by surroundings

      1) Hyperactive and anxious

      2) Unable to meet physical needs

   b. Disruptive and intrusive

   c. Denial

   d. Testing, manipulative, demanding behavior

   e. Superficial social relationships

**E.** Nursing management

1. Institute measures to deal with hyperactivity/agitation

   a. Simplify the environment and decrease environmental stimuli

      1) Assign to a single room away from activity

      2) Keep noise level low

      3) Soft lighting

   b. Limit people

      1) Anticipate situations that will provoke or overstimulate client, e.g., activities, competitive situations

      2) Remove to quiet areas

   c.  Distract and redirect energy

      1)  Choose activities for brief attention span, e.g., chores, walks

      2)  Choose physical activities using large movements until acute mania subsides, e.g., dance

      3)  Provide writing materials for busy work when acute mania subsides, e.g., political suggestions, plans

2.  Provide external controls

   a.  Assign one staff person to provide controls

   b.  Do not encourage client when telling jokes or performing, e.g., avoid laughing

   c.  Accompany client to room when hyperactivity is escalating

   d.  Guard vigilantly against suicide as elation subsides and mood evens out

3.  Institute measures to deal with manipulativeness

   a.  Set limits, e.g., limit phone calls when excessive

      1)  Set firm, consistent times for meetings—client often late and unaware of time

      2)  Refuse unreasonable demands

      3)  Explain restrictions on behavior and reasons so client does not feel rejected

   b.  Communicate using a firm, unambivalent, consistent approach

      1)  Use staff consistency in enforcing rules

      2)  Remain nonjudgmental, e.g., when client disrobes say, "I will not allow you to undress here."

      3)  Never threaten or make comparisons with others as it increases hostility and poor coping

   c.  Avoid long, complicated discussions

      1)  Use short sentences with specific, straightforward responses

      2)  Avoid giving advice when solicited, e.g., "I notice you want me to take responsibility for your life."

4.  Meet physical needs

   a.  Meet nutritional needs

      1)  Encourage fluids; offer water every hour because client will not take the time to drink

      2)  Give high-calorie finger foods and drinks to be carried while moving, e.g., cupcakes, sandwiches

      3)  Serve meals on tray in client's room when too stimulated

   b.  Encourage rest

      1)  Sedate PRN

      2)  Encourage short naps

5.  Supervise bathing routines when client plays with water or is too distracted to clean self

6.  Administer medications (*see* Table 15-15)

**Table 15-15** Bipolar Disorder Medications

| MEDICATION | ADVERSE EFFECTS | NURSING CONSIDERATIONS |
|---|---|---|
| Lithium carbonate | Dizziness | Use for control of manic episodes; mood stabilizer |
| | Headache | Blood levels must be monitored frequently |
| | Impaired vision | GI symptoms can be reduced if taken with meals |
| | Fine hand tremors | Therapeutic effects preceded by lag of 1-2 wk |
| | Reversible leukocytosis | Signs of intoxication—vomiting, diarrhea, drowsiness, muscular weakness, ataxia |
| | | Dosage is usually halved during depressive stages of illness |
| | | Initial blood target level = 1-1.5 mEq/L (1-1.5 mmol/L) |
| | | Maintenance blood target level = 0.8-1.2 mEq/L (0.8-1.2 mmol/L) |
| | | Check serum levels 2-3 times weekly when started and monthly while on maintenance; serum levels should be drawn in A.M. prior to dose |
| | | Should have fluid intake of 2,500-3,000 mL/day and adequate salt intake |
| Carbamazepine | Dizziness, vertigo | Mood stabilizer used with bipolar disorder |
| | Drowsiness | Traditionally used for seizures and trigeminal neuralgia |
| | Ataxia | Obtain baseline urinalysis, BUN, liver function tests, CBC |
| | CHF | Shake oral suspension well before measuring dose |
| | Aplastic anemia, thrombocytopenia | When giving by NG tube, mix with equal volume of water, 0.9% NaCl or D5W, then flush with 100 mL after dose |
| | | Take with food |
| | | Drowsiness usually disappears in 3-4 d |
| Divalproex sodium | Sedation | Mood stabilizer used with bipolar disorder |
| | Pancreatitis | Traditionally used for seizures |
| | Indigestion | Monitor liver function tests, platelet count before starting medication and periodically after medication |
| | Thrombocytopenia | Teach client symptoms of liver dysfunction (e.g., malaise, fever, lethargy) |
| | Toxic hepatitis | Monitor blood levels |
| | | Take with food or milk |
| | | Avoid hazardous activities |

7. Help decrease denial and increase client's awareness of feelings

   a. Encourage expression of real feelings through reflecting

   b. Help client acknowledge the need for help when denying it, e.g., "You say you don't need love, but most people need love. It's OK to feel that."

   c. Function as a role model for client by communicating feelings openly

   d. Help client recognize demanding behavior, e.g., "You seem to want others to notice you."

   e. Encourage client to recognize needs of others

   f. Have client verbalize needs directly, e.g., wishes for attention

8. Administer lithium for mania

   a. Physical exam and blood must be done before starting

      1) Contraindications to lithium

         a) Cardiovascular disease

         b) Renal disease

         c) Decreased sodium intake (e.g., in hypertensive clients)

   b. Teach client signs of lithium toxicity

      1) Nausea, vomiting, anorexia

      2) Tremors, ataxia

   c. Do not administer medication with diuretics or if toxicity is suspected

   d. Check serum lithium levels, 2–3 times weekly when beginning and monthly on maintenance

      1) Initial level should be between 1–1.5 mEq/L (1–1.5 mmol/L)

      2) Maintenance level should be between 0.8–1.2 mEq/L (0.8–1.2 mmol/L)

      3) Serum levels should be drawn in the A.M. prior to A.M. dose

# ALTERED THOUGHT PROCESSES

## Cellular Regulation, Cognition, Intracranial Regulation

## Manifestations of Altered Thought Processes

A. Characteristic findings

 1. Withdrawal from relationships and from the world

   a. Neologisms, rhyming

   b. Magical thinking

   c. Social ineptitude—aloof and fails to encourage interpersonal relationships

 2. Inappropriate or no display of feelings

 3. Hypochondriasis, depersonalization

 4. Suspiciousness—sees world as a hostile, threatening place

 5. Poor reality testing

   a. Hallucinations

   b. Delusions—persistent false beliefs

    1) Grandeur—belief that one is special, e.g., a monarch

    2) Persecutory—belief that one is a victim of a plot

    3) Ideas of reference—belief that environmental events are directed toward the self, e.g., client sees people talking and believes they are discussing the client

   c. Illusions—misperceptions of reality

 6. Loose associations

 7. Short attention span, decreased ability to comprehend stimuli

 8. Psychomotor alteration—slow moving, slow speaking

 9. Hyperactivity

   a. Loud, rapid talking

   b. Inability to sit still (akathisia)

 10. Regression

 11. Inability to meet basic survival needs

   a. Unable to feed self properly (poor nutritional habits)

   b. Poor personal hygiene

   c. Inappropriate dress for the weather/environment

**B.** Definitions of characteristic findings

1. Hallucinations—perceptual dysfunction in which false sensory perceptions are experienced in the absence of an external stimulus; visual and auditory hallucinations most common

2. Delusions—persistent false beliefs, rigidly held, that do not stand the test of reality; common types include:

   a. Delusions of grandeur—that one is special in a way that has no basis in reality, e.g., president of the United States

   b. Persecutory—that one is being threatened, e.g., a victim of a plot

   c. Ideas of reference—that situations or events involve them, e.g., thinks people are talking about client; misconstruing trivial remarks

   d. Somatic—that one's body is reacting in a particular way without a basis in reality

3. Illusion—misperception of reality

4. Neologisms—privately invented words that people do not understand

5. Magical thinking—primitive thought process in which one believes thoughts alone can change events

6. Looseness of associations—incoherent, illogical flow of thoughts and ideas producing confusing language

7. Autistic thinking—regressive thought process in which subjective, personal interpretations are not validated with objective reality

8. Word salad—words combined with no logical sequence

**C.** Types

1. Conditions predisposing to withdrawal from reality

   a. Senile dementia

   b. Acute medication psychosis

   c. Biochemical interaction

   d. Ineffective family interaction

   e. Schizophrenia (*see* Table 15-16)

**Table 15-16** Schizophrenia

| SUBTYPES | PRESENTING SYMPTOMS |
|---|---|
| Disorganized | Inappropriate behavior such as silly laughing and regression; transient hallucinations; disorganized behavior and speech |
| Catatonic | Sudden onset of mutism, bizarre mannerisms; remains in stereotyped position with waxy flexibility; may have dangerous periods of agitation and explosivity |
| Paranoid | Late onset in life; characterized by suspicion, ideas of persecution and delusions, and hallucinations; may be angry or hostile |
| Undifferentiated | General symptoms of schizophrenia<br><br>Symptoms of more than one type of schizophrenia |
| Residual | No longer exhibits overt symptoms |

D. Subtypes of schizophrenia

1. Disorganized—type of schizophrenia characterized by inappropriate or flat affect; social withdrawal extreme; disorganized speech and behavior; silliness, inappropriate laughter, grimacing, and regression common

2. Catatonic—stuporous condition associated with rigidity, posturing, waxy flexibility (when limb positioned, stays in that position); may alternate with overactivity and agitation; insidious onset

3. Paranoid—mainly features suspiciousness, distortion, and projection; delusions of grandeur, persecution, or hallucinations may be prominent; if onset occurs later in life, client tends to be less withdrawn from daily activities

4. Undifferentiated—characterized by general symptoms of schizophrenia but does not meet criteria for a particular type (poor overall functioning)

5. Residual—history of at least one psychotic episode but currently without overt psychotic behavior; may be withdrawn but is able to function

E. Nursing management

1. Maintain client safety

   a. Protect from altered thought processes

      1) Decrease sensory stimuli

      2) Remove from areas of tension

      3) Validate reality

      4) Recognize that client is experiencing a hallucination

      5) Do not argue with client

      6) Respond to feeling or tone of hallucination or delusion

      7) Do not reinforce the hallucination

      8) Be alert to any hallucination that commands the client to harm self or others or to do destructive acts

b. Protect from erratic and inappropriate behavior

   1) Communicate in calm, authoritative tone

   2) Address client by name

   3) Observe client for early signs of escalating behavior

c. Administer antipsychotic medications as indicated (*see* Table 15-17)

**Table 15-17** Antipsychotic Medications

| MEDICATION | ADVERSE EFFECTS | NURSING CONSIDERATIONS |
|---|---|---|
| **Conventional High Potency** | | |
| Haloperidol<br>Haloperidol decanoate<br>Fluphenazine<br>Fluphenazine decanoate | Low sedative effect<br>Low incidence of hypotension<br>High incidence of extrapyramidal adverse effects | Used in large doses for assaultive clients<br>Used with older adults (risk of falling reduced)<br>Decanoate: long-acting form given every 2–4 wk;<br>IM into deep muscle Z-track |
| **Conventional Medium Potency** | | |
| Perphenazine | Orthostatic hypotension<br>Dry mouth Constipation | Can help control severe vomiting<br>Medication is available PO, IM, and IV |
| **Conventional Low Potency** | | |
| Chlorpromazine | High sedative effect<br>High incidence of hypotension<br>Irreversible retinitis pigmentosa at 800 mg/day | Educate client about increased sensitivity to sun (as with other phenothiazines)<br>No tolerance or potential for abuse |
| **Atypical** | | |
| Risperidone<br>Quetiapine<br>Ziprasidone<br>Aripiprazole<br>Clozapine<br>Olanzapine | Moderate orthostatic hypotension<br>Moderate sedation<br>Significant weight gain<br>Doses over 6 mg can cause tardive dyskinesia<br>Moderate orthostatic hypotension<br>Moderate sedation<br>Very low risk of tardive dyskinesia and neuroleptic malignant syndrome<br>ECG changes—QT prolongation | Chosen as first-line antipsychotic due to mild extrapyramidal side effects (EPS) and very low anticholinergic adverse effects<br>Chosen as first-line antipsychotic due to mild EPS and very low anticholinergic adverse effects<br>Effective with depressive symptoms of schizophrenia<br>Low propensity for weight gain |

(Continued)

**Table 15-17** Antipsychotic Medications (*Continued*)

| MEDICATION | ADVERSE EFFECTS | NURSING CONSIDERATIONS |
|---|---|---|
| Action | Blocks dopamine receptors in basal ganglia of brain, inhibiting transmission of nerve impulses | |
| Indications | Acute and chronic psychosis | |
| Adverse effects | Akathisia (motor restlessness) | |
| | Dyskinesia (abnormal voluntary movements) | |
| | Dystonias (abnormal muscle tone producing spasms of tongue, face, neck) | |
| | Parkinson syndrome (shuffling gait, rigid muscles, excessive salivation, tremors, masklike face, motor deceleration) | |
| | Tardive dyskinesia (involuntary movements of mouth, tongue, trunk, extremities; chewing motions, sucking, tongue thrusting) | |
| | Photosensitivity | |
| | Orthostatic hypotension | |
| | Neuroleptic malignant syndrome | |
| Nursing considerations | Lowers seizure threshold | |
| | May slow growth rate in children | |
| | Monitor for urinary retention and decreased GI motility | |
| | Avoid alcohol | |
| | May cause hypotension if taken with antihypertensives, nitrates | |
| | Phenothiazines also used | |

2. Establish a therapeutic relationship—engage in individual therapy

   a. Institute measures to promote trust

      1) Same as general withdrawal from reality (*see* Table 15-18)

      2) Be consistent and reliable in keeping all scheduled appointments

      3) Avoid direct questions (client may feel threatened)

      4) Accept client's indifference (e.g., failure to smile or greet nurse) and avoidance behavior (e.g., hostility or sarcasm)

      5) Explain staff changes, especially vacations and absences

   b. Encourage client's affect by verbalizing what you observe, e.g., "You seem to think that I don't want to stay."

   c. Tolerate silences—may have to sit through long silences with client who is too withdrawn to speak (catatonic)

**Table 15-18** Nursing Care of a Client Who Acts Withdrawn

| PROBLEM | INTERVENTIONS |
|---|---|
| Lack of trust and feeling of safety and security | Keep interactions brief, especially orientation |
| | Structure environment |
| | Be consistent and reliable; notify client of anticipated schedule changes |
| | Decrease physical contact |
| | Eye contact during greeting |
| | Maintain attentiveness with head slightly leaning toward client and nonintrusive attitude |
| | Allow physical distance |
| | Accept client's behavior, e.g., silence; maintain matter-of-fact attitude toward behavior |
| Hallucinations | Maintain accepting attitude |
| | Do not argue with client about reality of hallucinations |
| | Comment on feeling, tone of hallucination, e.g., "That must be frightening to you." |
| | Encourage diversional activities, e.g., playing cards, especially activities in which client can gain a sense of mastery, e.g., artwork |
| | Encourage discussions of reality-based interests |
| Lack of attention to personal needs, e.g., nutrition, hygiene | Assess adequacy of hydration, nutrition |
| | Structure routine for bathing, mealtime |
| | Offer encouragement or assistance if necessary, e.g., sit with client or feed client if appropriate |
| | Decrease environmental stimuli at mealtime, e.g., suggest early dinner before dining room crowds |
| | Positioning and skin care for catatonic client |

    d. Accept regression as a normal part of treatment when new stresses are encountered

       1) With delusional regression, respond to associated feeling, not to the delusion, e.g., client claims they have no heart; nursing response, "You must feel empty."

       2) Help pinpoint source of regression, e.g., anxiety about discharge

3. Meet physical needs of severely regressed clients, e.g., catatonic

    a. Poor basic hygiene—may have to be washed initially

    b. Poor nutritional habits—may have to be fed

       1) Ask client to pick up fork; if unable, then feeding is necessary

       2) When ready, encourage client to eat in dining room with others

4. Engage in family therapy—especially when client is returning to family

    a. Understand the problem involves the family—establish a "family client" in need of support

       1) Family helps maintain pathology

       2) Client is often the scapegoat for family problems

    b. All members must be involved to effect change in client

    c. Decrease fusion—give all members a sense of self and independence

5. Engage in socialization or activity group therapy according to client's ability

    a. Accept nonverbal behavior initially

    b. If client cannot tolerate group, do not force or embarrass

    c. Act as a social role model for client

6. Provide simple activities or tasks to promote positive self-esteem and success

    a. Finger painting and clay are good choices for regressed catatonic client

    b. Encourage attendance at occupational, vocational, and art therapy

    c. Avoid competitive situations with paranoid client; solitary activities are better

**F.** Managing withdrawn behavior (*see* Table 15-18)

**G.** Managing suspicious behavior (*see* Table 15-19)

**H.** Managing aggressive/violent behavior (*see* Table 15-20)

**Table 15-19** Nursing Care of a Client Who Acts Suspiciously

| PROBLEM | INTERVENTIONS |
|---|---|
| Mistrust and feeling of rejection | Keep appointments with clients |
| | Clear, consistent communication |
| | Allow client physical distance and keep door open when interviewing |
| | Genuineness and honesty in interactions |
| | Recognize testing behavior and show persistence of interest in client |
| Delusions | Allow client to verbalize the delusion in a limited manner |
| | Do not argue with client or try to convince that delusions are not real |
| | Point out feeling tone of delusion |
| | Provide activities to divert attention from delusions |
| | Solitary activities best at first and then may progress to noncompetitive games or activities |
| | Do not reinforce delusions by validating them |
| | Focus on potential real concerns of client |

**Table 15-20** Nursing Care of a Client Who Acts Violently

| PROBLEM | INTERVENTIONS |
|---|---|
| Increased agitation/ anxiety | Recognize signs of impending violence, e.g., increased motor activity, pacing, or sudden stop—"calm before the storm" |
| | Identify yourself; speak calmly but firmly in normal tone of voice |
| | Help verbalize feelings |
| | Use nonthreatening body language, e.g., arms to side, palm outward, keep distance, avoid blocking exit, avoid body contact |
| | Avoid disagreeing with client or threatening client |
| | Decrease stimuli—remove threatening objects or people |
| Violence | Intercede early |
| | Continue nonthreatening behavior |
| | If client needs to be restrained to protect self or others, get help (at least four people) |
| | Move in organized, calm manner, stating that you want to help and that you will not permit client to harm self or others |
| | Use restraints correctly, e.g., never tie to bedside rail, check circulation frequently |

## [ SECTION 7 ]

# SOCIAL INTERACTIONS

## Interpersonal Relationships

## Manipulative Behavior

A. Assessment

1. Characteristic findings

a. Makes unreasonable requests for time, attention, and favors

b. Divides staff against each other—attempts to undermine nurse's role

c. Intimidates others

1) Uses others' faults to own advantage, e.g., naivete

2) Tries to make others feel guilty

d. Uses seductive and disingenuous approach

1) Make personal approach to staff, e.g., acts more like friend than client

2) Takes advantage of others for own gain

3) Frequently lies and rationalizes

e. May malinger or behave in helpless manner, e.g., feigns illness to avoid task

2. Predisposing conditions

a. Substance abuse, alcoholism

b. Antisocial disorders

c. Bipolar disorders

3. Goals

a. Help client set limits on behavior

b. Help client learn to see the consequences of behavior

c. Help family members understand and deal with client

d. Promote staff cooperation and consistency in caring for client

B. Nursing management

1. Use consistent, undivided staff approach

a. Clearly define expectations of client

b. Adhere to hospital regulations

c. Hold frequent staff conferences to increase staff communication and avoid conflict

2. Set limits

   a. Do not allow behaviors that interfere with the physical and psychological safety of others

   b. Carry out limit setting, avoid threats and promises

   c. Offer alternatives when possible

   d. Remain nonjudgmental

   e. Avoid arguing or allowing client to rationalize behavior

   f. Be brief in discussion

3. Be constantly alert for potential manipulation

   a. Favors, compliments

   b. Attempts to be personal

   c. Malingering, helplessness

4. Be alert for signs of destructive behavior

   a. Suicide

   b. Homicide

## Alcohol Abuse

A. Intoxication (*see* Table 15-21)

   1. Mild—blood alcohol 0.05–0.15%

   2. Moderate—blood alcohol 0.15–0.3%

   3. Severe—blood alcohol 0.3–0.5%

**Table 15-21** Potential Alcohol Intoxication

| ASSESSMENT | NURSING CONSIDERATIONS |
| --- | --- |
| Drowsiness | Monitor vital signs frequently |
| Slurred speech | Allow client to "sleep it off" |
| Tremors | Protect airway from aspiration |
| Impaired thinking/memory loss | Assess need for IV glucose |
| Nystagmus | Assess for injuries |
| Diminished reflexes | Assess for signs of withdrawal and chronic alcohol dependence |
| Nausea/vomiting | Counsel about alcohol use |
| Possible hypoglycemia | Be alert for potential problems of alcohol poisoning and CNS depression |
| Increased respiration | |
| Belligerence/grandiosity | |
| Loss of inhibitions | |
| Depression | |

**B.** Nursing management

1. Counseling the alcoholic

   a. Identify problems related to drinking—in family relationships, work, health, and other areas of life

   b. Help client to see/admit problem

      1) Confront denial with slow persistence

      2) Maintain relationship with client

2. Establishing control of problem drinking

   a. Identify potential problematic settings that trigger drinking behavior

   b. Alcoholics Anonymous—valuable mutual support group

      1) Peers share experiences

      2) Learn to substitute contact with humans for alcohol

      3) Stress living in the present; stop drinking "one day at a time"

   c. Disulfiram—medication used to maintain sobriety; based on behavioral therapy

      1) Once sufficient blood level reached, disulfiram interacts with alcohol to provide severe reaction

      2) Symptoms of disulfiram—alcohol reaction includes flushing, coughing, difficulty breathing, nausea, vomiting, pallor, anxiety

      3) Contraindicated in diabetes mellitus, atherosclerotic heart disease, cirrhosis, kidney disease, psychosis

   d. Assessment of alcohol withdrawal (*see* Table 15-22)

**Table 15-22** Alcohol Withdrawal

| WITHDRAWAL | DELIRIUM TREMENS | NURSING CONSIDERATIONS |
|---|---|---|
| Tremors | Tremors | Administer benzodiazepines, chlordiazepoxide, diazepam |
| Easily startled | Anxiety | |
| Insomnia | Panic | Monitor vital signs, particularly pulse, BP, temperature |
| Anxiety | Disorientation, confusion | Seizure precautions |
| Anorexia | Hallucinations | Provide quiet, well-lit environment |
| Alcoholic hallucinations | Vomiting | Orient client frequently |
| | Diarrhea Paranoia | Don't leave hallucinating, confused client alone |
| | Delusional symptoms | Administer anticonvulsants as needed |
| | Ideas of reference | Administer thiamine IV or IM as needed |
| | Suicide attempts | Administer IV glucose as needed |
| | Grand mal convulsions (especially first 48 h after client stops drinking) | 10% mortality rate |
| | Potential coma/death | |

3. Counseling the spouse of the alcoholic

   a. Initial goal is to help spouse focus on self

   b. Explore life problems from spouse's point of view

   c. Spouse can attempt to help alcoholic once strong enough

   d. Al-Anon—self-help group for spouses and relatives

      1) Learn "loving detachment" from alcoholic

      2) Goal is to try to make one's own life better and not to blame the alcoholic

      3) Provides safe, helpful environment

4. Counseling children of alcoholic parents

   a. Overcome denial of problem

   b. Establish trusting relationship

   c. Work with parents as well; avoid negative reactions to parents

   d. Referral to Alateen—organization for teenagers of alcoholic parent; self-help, similar to Al-Anon

C. Chronic CNS disorders associated with alcoholism (*see* Table 15-23)

**Table 15-23** Chronic CNS Disorders Associated with Alcoholism

| | ALCOHOLIC CHRONIC BRAIN SYNDROME (DEMENTIA) | WERNICKE SYNDROME | KORSAKOFF PSYCHOSIS |
|---|---|---|---|
| **Symptoms** | Fatigue, anxiety, personality changes, depression, confusion<br><br>Loss of memory of recent events<br><br>Can progress to dependent, bedridden state | Confusion, diplopia, nystagmus, ataxia<br><br>Disorientation, apathy | Memory disturbance with confabulation, loss of memory of recent events, learning problems<br><br>Possible problem with taste and smell, loss of reality testing |
| **Nursing considerations** | Balanced diet, abstinence from alcohol | IV or IM thiamin, abstinence from alcohol | Balanced diet, thiamin, abstinence from alcohol |

# Drug Abuse

A. Definition—a physiological and psychological dependence; increasing doses needed creates tolerance for those drugs

B. Substance abusers—have a low frustration tolerance and need for immediate gratification to escape anxiety (*see* Table 15-24)

**Table 15-24** Nonalcohol Substance Abuse

| MEDICATION/DRUG ("STREET NAME") | SYMPTOMS OF ABUSE | SYMPTOMS OF WITHDRAWAL | NURSING CONSIDERATIONS |
|---|---|---|---|
| **Barbiturates** | | | |
| Phenobarbital<br><br>Nembutal<br><br>("downers," "barbs," "pink ladies," "rainbows," "yellow jackets") | Respiratory depression<br><br>Decreased BP and pulse<br><br>Coma, ataxia, seizures<br><br>Increasing nystagmus<br><br>Poor muscle coordination<br><br>Decreased mental alertness | Anxiety, insomnia<br><br>Tremors, delirium<br><br>Convulsions | Maintain airway (intubate, suction)<br><br>Check LOC and vital signs<br><br>Start IV with large-gauge needle<br><br>Give sodium bicarbonate to promote excretion<br><br>Give activated charcoal, use gastric lavage<br><br>Hemodialysis |
| **Narcotics** | | | |
| Morphine<br><br>Heroin ("horse," "junk," "smack")<br><br>Codeine<br><br>Hydromorphone<br><br>Meperidine Methadone—for detoxification and maintenance | Hyperpyrexia<br><br>Seizures, ventricular dysrhythmias<br><br>Euphoria, then anxiety, sadness, insomnia, sexual indifference<br><br>Overdose—severe respiratory depression, pinpoint pupils, coma | Watery eyes, runny nose<br><br>Loss of appetite<br><br>Irritability, tremors, panic<br><br>Cramps, nausea<br><br>Chills and sweating<br><br>Elevated BP<br><br>Hallucinations, delusions | Maintain airway (intubate, suction)<br><br>Control seizures<br><br>Check LOC and vital signs<br><br>Start IV, may be given bolus of glucose<br><br>Have lidocaine and defibrillator available<br><br>Treat for hyperthermia<br><br>Give naloxone to reverse respiratory depression<br><br>Hemodialysis |

*(Continued)*

**Table 15-24** Nonalcohol Substance Abuse (*Continued*)

| MEDICATION/DRUG ("STREET NAME") | SYMPTOMS OF ABUSE | SYMPTOMS OF WITHDRAWAL | NURSING CONSIDERATIONS |
|---|---|---|---|
| **Stimulants** | | | |
| Cocaine ("crack") Amphetamine Benzedrine Dexedrine ("uppers," "pep pills," "speed," "crystal meth") | Tachycardia, increased BP, tachypnea, anxiety Irritability, insomnia, agitation Seizures, coma, hyperpyrexia, euphoria Nausea, vomiting Hyperactivity, rapid speech Hallucinations Nasal septum perforation (cocaine) | Apathy Long periods of sleep Irritability Depression, disorientation | Maintain airway (intubate, suction) Start IV Use cardiac monitoring Check LOC and vital signs Give activated charcoal, use gastric lavage Monitor for suicidal ideation Keep in calm, quiet environment |
| ***Cannabis* Derivatives** | | | |
| Marijuana Hashish ("pot," "weed," "grass," "reefer," "joint," "Mary Jane") | Fatigue Paranoia, psychosis Euphoria, relaxed inhibitions Increased appetite Disoriented behavior | Insomnia, hyperactivity Decreased appetite | Most effects disappear in 5–8 hours as drug wears off May cause psychosis |
| **Hallucinogens** | | | |
| Lysergic acid diethylamide (LSD) Phencyclidine (PCP) ("angel dust," "rocket fuel") Mescaline ("buttons," "cactus") | Nystagmus, marked confusion, hyperactivity Incoherence, hallucinations, distorted body image Delirium, mania, self-injury Hypertension, hyperthermia Flashbacks, convulsions, coma | None | Maintain airway (intubate, suction) Control seizures Check LOC and vital signs "Talk down" client Reduce sensory stimuli Small doses of diazepam Check for trauma, protect from self-injury |

**C.** Addiction—may result from prolonged use of medication for physical or psychological pain

**D.** Nursing management

    1. Observe for signs and symptoms of intoxication or drug use

        a. Examine skin for cuts, needle marks, abscesses, or bruises

        b. Recognize symptoms of individual drug overdose

            1) Hypotension, decreased respirations, constriction (pinpoint) of pupils with narcotics and sedatives

            2) Agitation with amphetamines and hallucinogens

    2. Treat symptoms of overdose

        a. Maintain respiration—airway when needed

        b. IV therapy as necessary

        c. Administer naloxone

            1) Antagonist to narcotics—induces withdrawal, stimulates respirations

            2) Short acting—symptoms of respiratory depression may return; additional doses may be necessary

        d. Gastric lavage for overdose of sedatives taken orally

        e. Dialysis to eliminate barbiturates from system

    3. Observe for signs of withdrawal, e.g., sweating, agitation, panic, hallucinations

        a. Identify drug type

        b. Seizure precautions

        c. Keep airway on hand

        d. Detoxify gradually

            1) Methadone used for long-term maintenance and acute withdrawal (narcotic)

            2) Decreasing doses of methadone used after initial withdrawal until stabilization is achieved

    4. Treat panic from acute withdrawal and/or marked depression

        a. Hospitalize temporarily for psychotic response

        b. Decrease stimuli, provide calm environment

        c. Protect client from self-destructive behavior

        d. Stay with client to reduce anxiety, panic, and confusion

        e. Assure client that hallucinations are from drugs and will subside

        f. Administer medications as indicated to manage symptoms of withdrawal and panic

        g. Monitor vital signs

5. Promote physical health

   a. Identify physical health needs

      1) Rest

      2) Nutrition

      3) Shelter

   b. Complete physical workup

      1) Heroin addicts need to be followed for liver and cardiac complications, sexually transmitted infections (STIs), AIDS

      2) Dental care

6. Administer methadone for maintenance when indicated

   a. Synthetic narcotic—blocks euphoric effects of narcotics

   b. Eliminates cravings and withdrawal symptoms

   c. Daily urine collected to monitor for other drug abuse while on methadone

7. Implement measures for antisocial personality disorders/manipulative behaviors

   a. Structured, nonpermissive environment

   b. Milieu therapy—peer pressure to conform

   c. Set limits but remain nonjudgmental

   d. Refer to drug-free programs (Synanon, Phoenix House, Odyssey House) for confrontation and support to remain drug-free

8. Treat underlying emotional problems

   a. Individual therapy—give support and acceptance

   b. Group therapy—to learn new ways of interacting

   c. Promote use of self-help groups

9. Assist client with rehabilitation, e.g., work programs, vocational counseling, completion of schooling

# ABUSE

## Interpersonal Relationship

## Child Abuse

A. Definition

1. Intentional physical, emotional, and/or sexual misuse/trauma or intentional omission of basic needs (neglect); usually related to diminished/limited ability of parent(s) to cope with, provide for, and/or relate to child

2. Those at high risk include children born prematurely and/or of low birth weight, children under 3 years, and children with physical and/or mental disabilities

B. Assessment

1. Inconsistency between type/location of injury (bruises, burns, fractures, especially chip/spiral) and the history of the incident(s)

2. Unexplained physical or thermal injuries

3. Withdraws or is fearful of parents

4. Sexual abuse—genital lacerations, sexually transmitted diseases

5. Emotional neglect, failure to thrive; disturbed sleep; change in behavior in school

C. Nursing management

1. Provide for physical needs first

2. Mandatory reporting of identified/suspected cases to appropriate agency

3. Nonjudgmental treatment of parents; encourage expression of feelings

4. Provide role modeling to parents

5. Teach growth and development concepts, especially safety, discipline, age-appropriate activities, and human nutrition

6. Provide emotional support for child; play therapy (dolls, drawings, making up stories) may be more appropriate way for child to express feelings

7. Initiate protective placement and/or appropriate referrals for long-term follow-up

8. Documentation should reflect only what nurse saw or was told, not nurse's interpretation or opinion

# Elder Abuse

A. Assessment

1. Battering, fractures, bruises

2. Over/undermedicated

3. Absence of needed dentures, glasses

4. Poor nutritional status, dehydration

5. Physical evidence of sexual abuse

6. Urine burns, excoriations, pressure injuries

B. Analysis

1. Older adults with chronic illness and depletion of financial resources who are dependent on children and grandchildren are particularly at risk

2. Current population trends indicate a decline in amount of people available to care for older adults

C. Nursing management

1. Provide for safety

2. Provide for physical needs first

3. Report to appropriate agencies (state laws vary)

4. Initiate protective placement and/or appropriate referrals

5. Consider client's right of self-determination

# Sexual Abuse

A. Assessment

1. Sexually abused child

   a. Disturbed growth and development

   b. Child becomes protective of others (parents)

   c. Uses defense mechanisms (e.g., denial, dissociation)

   d. Sleep and eating disturbances

   e. Depression and aggression, emotional deadening, amnesia

   f. Poor impulse control

   g. Somatic symptoms (e.g., chronic pain, GI disturbances)

   h. Truancy and running away

   i. Self-destructiveness

2. Adult victims of childhood sexual abuse

    a. Response is similar to delayed post-traumatic stress disorder (PTSD)

    b. Nightmares

    c. Unwanted, intrusive memories

    d. Kinesthetic sensations

    e. Flashbacks

    f. Relationship issues, fear of intimacy, fear of abandonment

3. Sexually abused adult

    a. Uses defense mechanisms (e.g., denial, dissociation)

    b. Relationship issues, abusive relationships, fear of intimacy, fear of abandonment

    c. Somatic issues reported

    d. Homicidal thoughts, violence

    e. Hypervigilance, panic attacks, phobias/agoraphobia

    f. Suicidal thoughts/attempts

    g. Self-mutilation

    h. Compulsive eating/dieting, binging/purging

**B.** Background

1. Victims from every sociocultural, ethnic, and economic group

2. Within the family (incest) and outside the family

3. Usually involves younger, weaker victim

4. Victim is usually urged and coerced, manipulated through fear

5. Difficult to expose abuse; common for child not to be believed

**C.** Nursing management

1. Establish trusting relationship

2. Use empathy, active support, compassion, warmth

3. Nonjudgmental approach

4. Report to appropriate agencies (state laws vary)

5. Group and individual therapy; appropriate referrals (e.g., legal, shelters)

6. Medications as needed (e.g., antianxiety)

# Domestic Violence

**A.** Assessment

1. Frequent visits to health care provider's office or emergency department for unexplained trauma

2. Client being cued, silenced, or threatened by an accompanying family member

3. Evidence of multiple old injuries, scars, healed fractures seen on x-ray

4. Fearful, evasive, or inconsistent replies and nonverbal behaviors, such as flinching when approached or touched

**B.** Background

1. Family violence is usually accompanied by brainwashing (e.g., victims blame themselves, feel unworthy, and fear that they won't be believed)

2. Long-term results of family violence are depression, suicidal ideation, low self-esteem, and impaired relationships outside the family

3. Women, children, and female adolescents are the most common victims

4. Cycle of abuse

   a. Tension building; verbal abuse

   b. Eruption into violent act/behavior

   c. Period of remorse; offering of gifts, thoughtful behaviors, asking forgiveness

   d. Tension builds again

**C.** Nursing management

1. Provide privacy during initial interview to ensure that the perpetrator of violence does not remain with client; make a statement, e.g., "This part of the exam is always done in private."

2. Carefully document all injuries using body maps or photographs (with consent)

3. Determine the safety of client by specific questions about weapons in the home, substance abuse, extreme jealousy

4. Develop a safety or an escape plan with client

5. Refer the client to community resources such as shelters, hotlines, and support groups

# End-of-Chapter Thinking Exercise

(0800) The nurse on the psychiatric unit is assessing a client with a diagnosis of paranoid schizophrenia who was admitted two days ago. At the beginning of the shift, the client was alert but was not oriented to person, place, time, or situation. The client stated, "I don't know you. You came in with them, didn't you? Make them stop yelling at me!" The client proceeded to back up against the wall and would not make eye contact.

(0820) The nurse is unable to locate the client. After the staff searched the unit, the client was found sitting on the floor in the stairway. When approached by hospital security, the client stated, "I am not going to jail. I don't know how to swim."

The nurse reviews the electronic medical record below.

| MEDICATION | DAY 1 | DAY 2 | DAY 3 (TODAY) |
|---|---|---|---|
| Risperidone 1 mg PO daily on days 1 & 2 | 1400 G* (RP)† | 0800 G (SR) | – |
| Risperidone 2 mg PO daily | – | – | 0800 |
| Haloperidol 5 mg PO every 6 hours as needed for mild to moderate agitation | 1600 G (RP) 2315 G (VT) | 0930 G (SR) 1705 G (SR) | 0015 G (VT) |
| Haloperidol 5 mg IM every 6 hours as needed for severe agitation | – | – | – |

*Key: G = given, H = held, R = refused
†Nurse administering the medication placed initials inside ( )

1.  How does the nurse handle this situation? (Generate Solutions)

2.  Which action does the nurse take? (Take Actions)

3.  How does the nurse evaluate the plan of care? (Evaluate Outcomes)

# Thinking Exercise Explanations

1. How does the nurse handle this situation? (Generate Solutions)

   - Recognize that the client is experiencing hallucinations
   - Maintain client safety
   - Establish a therapeutic relationship by responding with a feeling tone (e.g., "You must be scared. You are safe here in the hospital.")
   - Administer antipsychotic medications

   During a crisis situation, the nurse's priority is to ensure that the client and others are physically safe. The nurse should consider the best way to administer an antipsychotic medication during this acute situation.

2. Which action does the nurse take? (Take Actions)

   - Do not argue with or threaten the client
   - Remain at a distance appropriate to ensure safety
   - Speak softly to the client, addressing the client by name
   - Provide gentle reorientation to reality
   - If necessary, administer haloperidol via the IM route

   The nurse will recognize that the client is experiencing an acute episode of hallucinations in which the client believes that the nurse and security team may harm the client or place the client in an unsafe situation. The nurse should speak in a calm voice and reorient the client without arguing. If attempts to de-escalate the situation are unsuccessful, the nurse should administer the medication ordered for severe agitation.

3. How does the nurse evaluate the plan of care? (Evaluate Outcomes)

   - Reassess the client's level of agitation
   - Consider whether the situation was effectively de-escalated
   - Client safety

   Following the acute situation, the nurse should reassess the client's level of agitation and report to the physician for adjustments in medication if needed. Consider whether the approach used to de-escalate the situation worked or whether changes need to be made to the plan of care in the event of another episode. Be alert to any future hallucination that commands the client to harm self or others or to do destructive acts.

# [ CHAPTER 16 ]

# PHARMACOLOGY

## SECTION

# LISTING OF MEDICATIONS

The best way to learn medication information is to use the classification and subclassification systems which group and organize the medications.

Step 1: This section is organized by the most common classifications and subclassifications of medications.

Step 2: Identify the medications included in the classification and subclassification. NCLEX will identify the generic name of the medication.

Step 3: Identify the action or effect of the classification or subclassification.

Step 4: Based on the action of the classification or subclassification, identify the therapeutic use for the medications.

Step 5: Based on the action of the classification or subclassification, identify precautions or contraindications for use of that classification.

Step 6: Adverse effects are more intense effects of the action of the medications included in the classification or subclassification. Knowledge about management of adverse effects is critical when answering questions on NCLEX.

Step 7: Adverse reactions include potentially dangerous consequences related to the action of the medications in the classification or subclassification. The health care provider should be notified when adverse reactions occur.

Step 8: How do you evaluate the effect of the medications in the classification or subclassification? Is it a therapeutic or desired effect? Is it a nontherapeutic or undesired effect?

Emergency Medications for Shock, Cardiac Arrest, and Anaphylaxis

| MEDICATION | ADVERSE EFFECTS | NURSING CONSIDERATIONS |
|---|---|---|
| Norepinephrine | Headache<br><br>Palpitations<br><br>Nervousness<br><br>Epigastric distress<br><br>Angina, hypertension<br>**tissue necrosis with extravasation** | Vasoconstrictor to increase blood pressure and cardiac output<br><br>Reflex bradycardia may occur with rise in BP<br><br>Client should be attended at all times<br><br>Monitor urinary output<br><br>Infuse with dextrose solution, not saline<br><br>Monitor blood pressure<br><br>Protect medication from light |
| Dopamine | Increased ocular pressure<br><br>Ectopic beats<br><br>Nausea<br><br>Tachycardia, chest pain, dysrhythmias | Low-dose–dilates renal and coronary arteries<br><br>High-dose–vasoconstrictor, increases myocardial oxygen consumption<br><br>Headache is an early symptom of medication excess<br><br>Monitor blood pressure, peripheral pulses, urinary output<br><br>Use infusion pump |
| Epinephrine | Nervousness<br><br>Restlessness<br><br>Dizziness<br><br>Local necrosis of skin | Stimulates alpha and beta adrenergic receptors<br><br>Monitor BP<br><br>Carefully aspirate syringe before IM and subcutaneous doses; inadvertent IV administration can be harmful<br><br>Always check strength:<br><br>    1:100 only for inhalation, 1:1,000 for parenteral administration (SC or IM)<br><br>Ensure adequate hydration |
| Isoproterenol | Headache<br><br>Palpitations<br><br>Tachycardia<br><br>Changes in BP<br><br>Angina, bronchial asthma<br><br>Pulmonary edema | Stimulates beta 1 and beta 2 adrenergic receptors<br><br>Used for heart block, ventricular arrhythmias, and bradycardia<br><br>Bronchodilator used for asthma and bronchospasms<br><br>Don't give at bedtime—interrupts sleep patterns<br><br>Monitor BP, pulse |

*(Continued)*

Emergency Medications for Shock, Cardiac Arrest, and Anaphylaxis (*Continued*)

| MEDICATION | ADVERSE EFFECTS | NURSING CONSIDERATIONS |
|---|---|---|
| Phenylephrine | Palpations<br>Tachycardia<br>Hypertension<br>Dysrhythmia<br>Angina<br>Tissue necrosis with extravasation | Potent alpha 1 agonist<br>Used to treat hypotension |
| Dobutamine hydrochloride | Hypertension<br>PVCs<br>Asthmatic episodes<br>Headache | Stimulates beta 1 receptors<br>Incompatible with alkaline solutions (sodium bicarbonate)<br>Administer through central venous catheter or large peripheral vein using an infusion pump<br>Don't infuse through line with other meds (incompatible)<br>Monitor EKG, BP, I and O, serum potassium |
| Milrinone | Dysrhythmia<br>Thrombocytopenia<br>Jaundice | Positive inotropic agent<br>Smooth muscle relaxant used to treat severe heart failure |
| Nitroprusside sodium | Hypotension<br>Increased intracranial pressure | Dilates cardiac veins and arteries<br>Decreases preload and afterload<br>Increases myocardial perfusion<br>Keep in dark place after mixing<br>Use an infusion pump |
| Diphenhydramine HCl | Drowsiness<br>Confusion<br>Insomnia<br>Headache<br>Vertigo<br>Photosensitivity | Blocks effects of histamine on bronchioles, GI tract, and blood vessels |

(*Continued*)

Emergency Medications for Shock, Cardiac Arrest, and Anaphylaxis (*Continued*)

| MEDICATION | ADVERSE EFFECTS | NURSING CONSIDERATIONS |
|---|---|---|
| **Actions** | Varies with med | |
| **Indications** | Hypovolemic shock | |
| | Cardiac arrest | |
| | Anaphylaxis | |
| **Adverse effects** | Serious rebound effect may occur | |
| | Balance between underdosing and overdosing | |
| **Nursing considerations** | Monitor vital signs | |
| | Measure urine output | |
| | Assess for extravasation | |
| | Observe extremities for color and perfusion | |

Adrenocortical Medications: Glucocorticoid

| MEDICATION | ADVERSE EFFECTS | NURSING CONSIDERATIONS |
|---|---|---|
| Cortisone acetate<br><br>Hydrocortisone<br><br>Dexamethasone<br><br>Methylprednisolone<br><br>Prednisone<br><br>Beclomethasone<br><br>Betamethasone<br><br>Budesonide | Increases susceptibility to infection<br><br>May mask symptoms of infection<br><br>Edema, changes in appetite<br><br>Euphoria, insomnia<br><br>Delayed wound healing<br><br>Hypokalemia, hypocalcemia<br><br>Hyperglycemia<br><br>Osteoporosis, fractures<br><br>Peptic ulcer, gastric hemorrhage<br><br>Psychosis | Prevents/suppresses cell-mediated immune reactors<br><br>Used for adrenal insufficiency<br><br>Overdosage produces Cushing's syndrome<br><br>Abrupt withdrawal of medication may cause headache, nausea and vomiting, and papilledema (Addisonian crisis)<br><br>Give single dose before 9 AM<br><br>Give multiple doses at evenly spaced intervals<br><br>Infection may produce few symptoms due to anti-inflammatory action<br><br>Stress (surgery, illness, psychic) may lead to increased need for steroids<br><br>Nightmares are often the first indication of the onset of steroid psychosis<br><br>Check weight, BP, electrolytes, I and O, weight<br><br>Used cautiously with history of TB (may reactivate disease)<br><br>May decrease effects of oral hypoglycemics, insulin, diuretics, $K^+$ supplements<br><br>Assess children for growth restriction<br><br>Protect from pathological fractures<br><br>Administer with antacids<br><br>**Do not stop abruptly**<br><br>Methylprednisolone also used for arthritis, asthma, allergic reactions, cerebral edema<br><br>Dexamethasone also used for allergic disorders, cerebral edema, asthma attack, shock |
| **Action** | Stimulates formation of glucose (gluconeogenesis) and decreases use of glucose by body cells; increases formation and storage of fat in muscle tissue; alters normal immune response | |
| **Indications** | Addison's disease, Crohn's disease, COPD, lupus erythematosus, leukemias, lymphomas, myelomas, head trauma, tumor, to prevent/treat cerebral edema | |
| **Adverse effects** | Psychoses, depression, weight gain, hypokalemia, hypocalcemia, stunted growth in children, petechiae, buffalo hump | |

*(Continued)*

Adrenocortical Medications: Glucocorticoid (*Continued*)

| MEDICATION | ADVERSE EFFECTS | NURSING CONSIDERATIONS |
|---|---|---|
| **Nursing considerations** | Monitor fluid and electrolyte balance<br><br>**Don't discontinue abruptly**<br><br>Monitor for signs of infection | |
| **Herbal interactions** | Senna, celery seed, juniper may decrease serum potassium; when taken with corticosteroids may increase hypoglycemia<br><br>Ginseng taken with corticosteroids may cause insomnia<br><br>Echinacea may counteract effects of corticosteroids<br><br>Licorice potentiates effect of corticosteroids | |

Adrenocortical Medications: Mineralocorticoid

| MEDICATION | ADVERSE EFFECTS | NURSING CONSIDERATIONS |
|---|---|---|
| Fludrocortisone acetate | Hypertension, edema due to sodium retention<br><br>Muscle weakness and dysrhythmia due to hypokalemia | Give PO dose with food<br><br>Check BP, electrolytes, I and O, weight<br><br>Give low-sodium, high-protein, high-potassium diet<br><br>May decrease effects of oral hypoglycemics, insulin, diuretics, $K^+$ supplements |
| **Action** | Increases sodium reabsorption, potassium and hydrogen excretion in the distal convoluted tubules of the nephron | |
| **Indications** | Adrenal insufficiency | |
| **Adverse effects** | Sodium and water retention<br><br>Hypokalemia | |
| **Nursing considerations** | Monitor BP and serum electrolytes<br><br>Daily weight, report sudden weight gain to health care provider<br><br>Used with cortisone or hydrocortisone in adrenal insufficiency | |

Antacid Medications

| MEDICATION | ADVERSE EFFECTS | NURSING CONSIDERATIONS |
|---|---|---|
| Aluminum hydroxide gel<br><br>Calcium carbonate<br><br>Aluminum hydroxide and magnesium trisilicate | Constipation that may lead to impaction, phosphate depletion | Monitor bowel pattern<br><br>Compounds contains sodium; check if client is on sodium-restricted diet<br><br>Aluminum and magnesium antacid compounds interfere with tetracycline absorption<br><br>Encourage fluids<br><br>Monitor for signs of phosphate deficiency—malaise, weakness, tremors, bone pain<br><br>Shake well<br><br>Careful use advised for kidney dysfunction |
| Magnesium hydroxide | Excessive dose can produce nausea, vomiting, and diarrhea | Store at room temperature with tight lid to prevent absorption of $CO_2$<br><br>Prolonged and frequent use of cathartic dose can lead to dependence<br><br>Administer with caution to clients with renal disease |
| Aluminum hydroxide and magnesium hydroxide | Slight laxative effect | Encourage fluid intake<br><br>Administer with caution to clients with renal disease |
| **Action** | Neutralizes gastric acids; raises gastric pH; inactivates pepsin | |
| **Indications** | Peptic ulcer<br><br>Indigestion<br><br>Reflux esophagitis<br><br>Prevent stress ulcers | |
| **Adverse effects** | Constipation, diarrhea<br><br>Acid rebound between doses<br><br>Acid/base Imbalances | |
| **Nursing considerations** | Use medications with sodium content cautiously for clients with cardiac and renal disease<br><br>Absorption of tetracyclines, quinolones, phenothiazines, iron preparations, isoniazid reduced when given with antacids<br><br>Effectiveness of oral contraceptives and salicylates may decrease when given with antacids | |

Anti-Anxiety Medications

| MEDICATION | ADVERSE EFFECTS | NURSING CONSIDERATIONS |
|---|---|---|
| **Benzodiazepine Derivatives** | | |
| Chlordiazepoxide Diazepam | Lethargy, hangover Respiratory depression Hypotension | CNS depressant Use–anxiety, sedation, alcohol withdrawal, seizures May result in toxic build-up in older adults Potential for physiological addiction/overdose Can develop tolerance and cross-tolerance Cigarette smoking increases clearance of medication Alcohol increases CNS depression |
| Alprazolam Lorazepam Oxazepam | Drowsiness, light-headedness, hypotension, hepatic dysfunction Increased salivation Orthostatic hypotension Memory impairment and confusion | CNS depressant Safer for older adults Don't combine with alcohol or other depressants Check renal and hepatic function **Don't discontinue abruptly (true for all antianxiety agents)** Teach addictive potential |
| Midazolam | Retrograde amnesia Euphoria Hypotension Dysrhythmia Cardiac arrest Respiratory depression | CNS depressant Use–preoperative sedation, conscious sedation for endoscopic procedures and diagnostic tests |
| **Anxiolytics Antianxiety Medications** | | |
| Buspirone | Light-headedness Confusion Hypotension, palpitations | Little sedation Requires ≥3 weeks to be effective Cannot be given as a PRN medication Particularly useful for generalized anxiety disorder (GAD) No abuse potential Used for clients with previous addiction Avoid alcohol and grapefruit juice Monitor for worsening depression or suicidal tendencies |

(*Continued*)

Anti-Anxiety Medications (*Continued*)

| MEDICATION | ADVERSE EFFECTS | NURSING CONSIDERATIONS |
|---|---|---|
| Hydroxyzine | Drowsiness, ataxia | Produces no dependence, tolerance, or intoxication |
| | Leukopenia, hypotension | Can be used for anxiety relief for indefinite periods |
| **Herbals** | | |
| Kava | Impaired thinking, judgment, motor reflexes, vision, decreased plasma proteins, thrombocytopenia, leukocytopenia, dyspnea, and pulmonary hypertension | Similar activity to benzodiazepines |
| | | Suppresses emotional excitability and produces mild euphoria |
| | | Do not take with CNS depressants |
| | | Should not be taken by women who are pregnant or lactating or by children under the age of 12 |
| Melatonin | Sedation, confusion, headache, and tachycardia | Influences sleep-wake cycles (levels are high during sleep) |
| | | Used for prevention and treatment of "jet lag" and insomnia |
| | | Use cautiously if given with benzodiazepines and CNS depressants |
| | | Contraindicated in hepatic insufficiency, history of cerebrovascular disease, depression, and neurologic disorders |
| **Action** | Affects neurotransmitters | |
| **Indications** | Anxiety disorders, insomnia, seizures, panic attacks, acute manic episodes | |
| **Adverse effects** | Sedation | |
| | Depression, confusion | |
| | Anger, hostility | |
| | Headache | |
| | Dry mouth, constipation | |
| | Bradycardia | |
| | Elevations in LDH, AST, ALT | |
| | Urinary retention | |
| **Nursing considerations** | Monitor liver function | |
| | Monitor for therapeutic blood levels | |
| | Avoid alcohol | |
| | Caution when performing tasks requiring alertness (e.g., driving car) | |
| | Benzodiazepines are also used as muscles relaxants, sedatives, hypnotics, anticonvulsants | |

Anticholinergic Medications

| MEDICATION | ADVERSE EFFECTS | NURSING CONSIDERATIONS |
|---|---|---|
| Atropine sulfate | Tachycardia<br><br>Headache, blurred vision<br><br>Insomnia, dry mouth<br><br>Dizziness<br><br>Urinary retention<br><br>Angina, mydriasis | Used for bradycardia<br><br>When given PO give 30 minutes before meals<br><br>Check for history of glaucoma, asthma, hypertension<br><br>Monitor I and O, orientation<br><br>When given in nonemergency situations make certain client voids before taking medication<br><br>Educate client to expect dry mouth, increased respiration and heart rate<br><br>Client should avoid heat (perspiration is decreased) |
| Aclidinium<br><br>Tiotropium<br><br>Ipratropium plus albuterol | Dry mouth<br><br>Irritation of pharynx | Used for bronchospasm and long-term treatment of asthma<br><br>Ipratropium administered as aerosol or in nebulizer<br><br>Tiotropium administered in powder form by HandiHaler |
| Benztropine<br><br>Trihexyphenidyl | Urinary retention<br><br>Blurred vision<br><br>Dry mouth<br><br>Constipation | Used for Parkinson's Disease<br><br>Increase fluids, bulk foods and exercise<br><br>Taper before discontinuation<br><br>Orthostatic hypotension precautions |
| Scopolamine | Urinary retention<br><br>Blurred vision<br><br>Dry mouth<br><br>Constipation<br><br>Confusion and sedation | Used for motion sickness<br><br>Transdermal patch<br><br>Contraindicated in acute angle glaucoma |
| **Actions** | Competes with acetylcholine at receptor sites in autonomic nervous system; causes relaxation of ciliary muscles (cycloplegia) and dilation of pupil (mydriasis); causes bronchodilation and decreases bronchial secretions; decreases mobility and GI secretions | |
| **Indications** | Atropine—bradycardia, mydriasis for ophthalmic exam, preoperatively to dry secretions<br><br>Scopolamine—motion sickness, vertigo, mydriasis for ophthalmic exam, preoperative to dry secretions | |

*(Continued)*

Anticholinergic Medications (*Continued*)

| MEDICATION | ADVERSE EFFECTS | NURSING CONSIDERATIONS |
|---|---|---|
| **Adverse effects** | Blurred vision | |
| | Dry mouth | |
| | Urinary retention | |
| | Changes in heart rate | |
| **Nursing considerations** | Monitor for urinary retention | |
| | Contraindicated for clients with glaucoma | |

Anticoagulant Medications

| MEDICATION | ADVERSE EFFECTS | NURSING CONSIDERATIONS |
|---|---|---|
| **Action: Inhibits synthesis of clotting factors** | | |
| Heparin | Can produce hemorrhage from any body site (10%) | Monitor therapeutic partial thromboplastin time (PTT) at 1.5–2.5 times the control without signs of hemorrhage |
| | Tissue irritation/pain at injection site | Lower limit of normal 20–25 sec; upper limit of normal 32–39 sec |
| | Anemia | For IV administration: use infusion pump, peak 5 minutes, duration 2–6 hours |
| | Thrombocytopenia | For injection: give deep SQ; never IM (danger of hematoma), onset 20–60 minutes, duration 8–12 hours |
| | Fever | |
| | Dose-dependent on a PTT | **Antidote: protamine sulfate within 30 minutes** |
| | | Can be allergenic |
| Low-molecular-weight heparin: enoxaparin | Bleeding | Less allergenic than heparin |
| | Minimal widespread effect | Must be given deep SQ, never IV or IM |
| | Fixed dose | Does not require lab test monitoring |

(*Continued*)

Anticoagulant Medications (*Continued*)

| MEDICATION | | ADVERSE EFFECTS | NURSING CONSIDERATIONS |
|---|---|---|---|
| Warfarin | | Hemorrhage<br><br>Diarrhea<br><br>Rash<br><br>Fever | Monitor therapeutic prothrombin time (PT) at 1.3–1.5 times the control, or monitor international normalized ratio (INR)<br><br>Normal PT 9.5–12 sec; normal INR 2–3<br><br>Onset: 36-72 hours, peak 5-7 days, duration: 2–5 days after discontinuation<br><br>**Antidotes: vitamin K, whole blood, plasma**<br><br>Teach measures to avoid venous stasis<br><br>Emphasize importance of regular lab testing<br><br>Client should keep intake of vitamin K consistent: Foods that contain vitamin K include many green vegetables, pork, rice, yogurt, cheeses, fish, milk |
| Fondaparinux | | Hemorrhage<br><br>Thrombocytopenia | SQ only<br><br>PT and aPTT aren't suitable monitoring tests<br><br>Used to treat DVT and acute PE |
| **Action: Inhibits activity of clotting** | | | |
| Dabigatran | Directly inhibits thrombin | PO only<br><br>Used for stroke, DVT, and PE prophylaxis when nonvalvular atrial fibrillation is present<br><br>Age greater than 75, kidney disease, gastrointestinal bleeding, use of NSAIDs increase the risk of bleeding | |
| **Indications** | | For heparin: prophylaxis and treatment of thromboembolic disorders; in very low doses (10–100 units) to maintain patency of IV catheters (heparin flush)<br><br>For warfarin: management of pulmonary emboli, venous thromboembolism, MI, atrial dysrhythmias, post cardiac valve replacement | |
| **Adverse effects** | | Nausea<br><br>Alopecia<br><br>Urticaria<br><br>Hemorrhage<br><br>Bleeding/heparin-induced thrombocytopenia (HIT) | |

(*Continued*)

Anticoagulant Medications (*Continued*)

| MEDICATION | ADVERSE EFFECTS | NURSING CONSIDERATIONS |
|---|---|---|
| **Nursing Considerations** | Check for signs of hemorrhage: bleeding gums, nosebleed, unusual bleeding, black/tarry stools, hematuria, fall in hematocrit or blood pressure, guaiac-positive stools | |
| | Client should avoid IM injections, ASA-containing products, and NSAIDs | |
| | Client should wear medical information tag | |
| | Instruct client to use soft toothbrush, electric razor, to report bleeding gums, petechiae or bruising, epistaxis, black tarry stools | |
| | Monitor platelet counts and signs and symptoms of thrombosis during heparin therapy; if HIT suspected, heparin discontinued and non-heparin anticoagulant given | |
| **Herbal interactions** | Garlic, ginger, ginkgo may increase bleeding when taken with warfarin | |
| | Large doses of anise may interfere with anticoagulants | |
| | Ginseng and alfalfa my decrease anticoagulant activity | |
| | Black haw increases action of anticoagulant | |
| | Chamomile may interfere with anticoagulants | |
| **Vitamin interaction** | Vitamin C may slightly prolong PT | |
| | Vitamin E will increase warfarin's effect | |

Anticonvulsant Medications

| MEDICATION | ADVERSE EFFECTS | NURSING CONSIDERATIONS |
|---|---|---|
| Clonazepam | Drowsiness | Benzodiazepine |
| | Dizziness | **Do not discontinue suddenly** |
| | Confusion | Avoid activities that require alertness |
| | Respiratory depression | |
| Diazepam | Drowsiness, ataxia | IV push doses shouldn't exceed 2 mg/minute |
| | Hypotension | Monitor vital signs–resuscitation equipment available if given IV |
| | Tachycardia | Alcohol increases CNS depression |
| | Respiratory depression | After long-term use, withdrawal leads to symptoms such as vomiting, sweating, cramps, tremors, and possibly convulsions |

(*Continued*)

Anticonvulsant Medications (*Continued*)

| MEDICATION | ADVERSE EFFECTS | NURSING CONSIDERATIONS |
|---|---|---|
| Fosphenytoin | Drowsiness<br><br>Dizziness<br><br>Confusion<br><br>Leukopenia<br><br>Anemia | Used for tonic–clonic seizures, status epilepticus<br><br>Highly protein-bound<br><br>Contact health care provider if rash develops |
| Levetiracetam | Dizziness<br><br>Suicidal ideation | Avoid alcohol<br><br>Avoid driving and activities that require alertness |
| Phenytoin sodium | Drowsiness, ataxia<br><br>Nystagmus<br><br>Blurred vision<br><br>Hirsutism<br><br>Lethargy<br><br>GI upset<br><br>Gingival hypertrophy | Give oral medication with at least 1/2 glass of water, or with meals to minimize GI irritation<br><br>Inform client that red-brown or pink discoloration of sweat and urine may occur<br><br>IV administration may lead to cardiac arrest—have resuscitation equipment at hand<br><br>Never mix with any other medication or dextrose IV<br><br>Instruct in oral hygiene<br><br>Increase vitamin D intake and exposure to sunlight may be necessary with long-term use<br><br>Alcohol increases serum levels<br><br>Increased risk toxicity older adults |
| Primidone | Drowsiness<br><br>Ataxia, diplopia<br><br>Nausea and vomiting | **Don't discontinue use abruptly**<br><br>Full therapeutic response may take 2 weeks<br><br>Shake liquid suspension well<br><br>Take with food if experiencing GI distress<br><br>Decreased cognitive function older adults |
| Magnesium sulfate | Flushing<br><br>Sweating<br><br>Extreme thirst<br><br>Hypotension<br><br>Sedation, confusion | Monitor intake and output<br><br>Monitor magnesium levels<br><br>Before each dose, deep tendon reflexes should be tested<br><br>Vital signs should be monitored often during parenteral administration<br><br>Used for pregnancy-induced hypertension |

(Continued)

Anticonvulsant Medications (*Continued*)

| MEDICATION | ADVERSE EFFECTS | NURSING CONSIDERATIONS |
|---|---|---|
| Valproic acid | Sedation<br><br>Tremor, ataxia<br><br>Nausea, vomiting<br><br>Prolonged bleeding time | Agent of choice in many seizure disorders of young children<br><br>Do not take with carbonated beverage<br><br>Take with food<br><br>Monitor platelets, bleeding time, and liver function tests |
| Carbamazepine | Myelosuppression<br><br>Dizziness, drowsiness<br><br>Ataxia<br><br>Diplopia, rash | Monitor intake and output<br><br>Supervise ambulation<br><br>Monitor CBC<br><br>Take with meals<br><br>Wear protective clothing due to photosensitivity<br><br>Multiple medication interactions |
| Ethosuximide | GI symptoms<br><br>Drowsiness<br><br>Ataxia, dizziness | Monitor for behavioral changes<br><br>Monitor weight weekly |
| Gabapentin | Increased appetite<br><br>Ataxia<br><br>Irritability<br><br>Dizziness<br><br>Fatigue | Monitor weight and behavioral changes.<br><br>Can also be used to treat postherpetic neuralgia, other neuropathic pain, fibromyalgia, prophylaxis of migraine |
| Lamotrigine | Diplopia<br><br>Headaches<br><br>Dizziness<br><br>Drowsiness<br><br>Ataxia<br><br>Nausea, vomiting<br><br>Life-threatening rash when given with valproic acid | Take divided doses with meals or just afterward to decrease adverse effects |

(*Continued*)

Anticonvulsant Medications (*Continued*)

| MEDICATION | ADVERSE EFFECTS | NURSING CONSIDERATIONS |
|---|---|---|
| Topiramate | Ataxia<br><br>Confusion<br><br>Dizziness<br><br>Fatigue<br><br>Vision problems | Adjunct therapy for intractable partial seizures<br><br>Increased risk for renal calculi<br><br>Stop medication immediately if eye problems—could lead to permanent damage |
| **Action** | Decreases flow of calcium and sodium across neuronal membranes | |
| **Indications** | Seizures<br><br>Status epilepticus: diazepam, lorazepam, phenytoin | |
| **Adverse effects** | Cardiovascular depression<br><br>Respiratory depression<br><br>Agranulocytosis<br><br>Aplastic anemia | |
| **Nursing considerations** | Tolerance develops with long-term use<br><br>Don't discontinue abruptly<br><br>Caution with use of medications that lower seizure threshold (MAO inhibitors)<br><br>Barbiturates and benzodiazepines also used as anticonvulsants<br><br>Increased risk adverse reactions older adults | |

Antidepressant Medications: Heterocyclics

| | |
|---|---|
| **Examples** | Bupropion<br><br>Trazodone |
| **Actions** | Does not inhibit MAO; has some anticholinergic and sedative effects; alters effects of serotonin on CNS |
| **Indications** | Treatment of depression and smoking cessation |
| **Adverse effects** | Dry mouth<br><br>Nausea<br><br>Bupropion-insomnia and agitation<br><br>Trazodone-sedation, orthostatic hypotension |
| **Nursing considerations** | **May require gradual reduction before stopping**<br><br>Avoid use with alcohol, other CNS depressants for up to 1 week after end of therapy |

Antidepressant Medications: Monoamine Oxidase (MAO) Inhibitors

| Examples | Phenelzine sulfate, isocarboxazid, tranylcypromine |
|---|---|
| Actions | Interferes with monoamine oxidase, allowing for increased concentration of neurotransmitters (epinephrine, norepinephrine, serotonin) in synaptic space, causing stabilization of mood |
| Indications | Depression |
| | Chronic pain syndromes |
| Adverse effects | Hypertensive crisis when taken with foods containing tyramine (aged cheese, bologna, pepperoni, salami, figs, bananas, raisins, beer, Chianti red wine) or OTC medications containing ephedrine, pseudoephedrine |
| | Photosensitivity |
| | Weight gain |
| | Sexual dysfunction |
| | Orthostatic hypotension |
| Nursing considerations | Not first-line medications for depression |
| | Should not be taken with SSRIs |
| | Administer antihypertensive medications with caution |
| | Avoid use of other CNS depressants, including alcohol |
| | **Discontinue 10 days before general anesthesia** |
| | Medications lower seizure threshold |
| | Monitor for urinary retention |

Antidepressant Medications: Selective Serotonin Reuptake Inhibitors

| Examples | SSRIs: Fluoxetine, Citalopram, Escitalopram, Fluvoxamine, Paroxetine, Sertraline | |
|---|---|---|
| | SNRIs: Venlafaxine, Duloxetine | |
| Actions | Inhibits CNS neuronal uptake of serotonin; acts as stimulant counteracting depression and increasing motivation | |
| Indications | Depression | |
| | Obsessive-compulsive disorders | |
| | Obesity | |
| | Bulimia | |
| Adverse effects | Headache, dizziness | Taste changes |
| | Nervousness | Sweating |
| | Insomnia, drowsiness | Rash |
| | Anxiety | URI |
| | Tremor | Painful menstruation |
| | Dry mouth | Sexual dysfunction |
| | GI upset | Weight gain |
| Nursing considerations | Take in AM | |
| | Takes 4 weeks for full effect | |
| | Monitor weight | |
| | Good mouth care | |
| | Do not administer with MAOIs–risk of serotonin syndrome | |
| | Monitor for thrombocytopenia, leukopenia, and anemia | |

Antidepressant Medications: Tricyclics

| Examples | Amitriptyline |
|---|---|
| | Imipramine |
| **Actions** | Inhibits presynaptic reuptake of neurotransmitters norepinephrine and serotonin; anticholinergic action at CNS and peripheral receptors |
| **Indications** | Depression |
| | Obstructive sleep apnea |
| **Adverse effects** | Sedation |
| | Anticholinergic effects (dry mouth, blurred vision) |
| | Confusion (especially in older adults) |
| | Photosensitivity |
| | Disturbed concentration |
| | Orthostatic hypotension |
| | Bone marrow depression |
| | Urinary retention |
| **Nursing considerations** | Therapeutic effect in 1–3 weeks; maximum response in 6–9 weeks |
| | May be administered in daily dose at night to promote sleep and decrease adverse effects during the day |
| | Orthostatic hypotension precautions |
| | Instruct client that adverse effects will decrease over time |
| | Sugarless lozenges for dry mouth |
| | Do not abruptly stop taking medication (headache, vertigo, nightmares, malaise, weight change) |
| | Avoid alcohol, sleep-inducing medications, OTC medications |
| | Avoid exposure to sunlight, wear sunscreen |
| | Older adults: strong anticholinergic and sedation effects |

Antidepressant Medications: Overview

| MEDICATION | ADVERSE EFFECTS | NURSING CONSIDERATIONS |
|---|---|---|
| **Monoamine oxidase inhibitors (MAOIs)** | | |
| Isocarboxazid<br><br>Tranylcypromine sulfate<br><br>Phenelzine sulfate | Postural hypotension<br><br>If foods with tyramine ingested, can have hypertensive crisis: headache, sweating, palpitations, stiff neck, intracranial hemorrhage<br><br>Potentiates alcohol and other medications | Inhibits monoamine oxidase enzyme, preventing destruction of norepinephrine, epinephrine, and serotonin<br><br>Avoid foods with tyramine—aged cheese, liver, herring, yeast, beer, wine, sour cream, pickled products<br><br>Avoid caffeine, antihistamines, amphetamines<br><br>Takes 3-4 weeks to work<br><br>Avoid tricyclics until 3 weeks after stopping MAO inhibitors<br><br>Monitor vital signs<br><br>Sunblock required |
| **Tricyclics** | | |
| Amitriptyline hydrochloride<br><br>Imipramine<br><br>Desipramine hydrochloride<br><br>Doxepin<br><br>Nortriptyline | Sedation/drowsiness, especially with amitriptyline<br><br>Blurred vision, dry mouth, diaphoresis<br><br>Postural hypotension, palpitations<br><br>Nausea, vomiting<br><br>Constipation, urinary retention<br><br>Increased appetite | Increases brain amine levels<br><br>Suicide risk high after 10-14 days because of increased energy<br><br>Monitor vital signs<br><br>Sunblock required<br><br>Increase fluid intake<br><br>Take dose at bedtime (sedative effect)<br><br>Use sugarless candy or gum for dry mouth<br><br>Delay of 2-6 weeks before noticeable effects |
| **Selective serotonin reuptake inhibitors (SSRIs)** | | |
| Fluoxetine<br><br>Paroxetine<br><br>Sertraline hydrochloride<br><br>Citalopram<br><br>Venlafaxine | Palpitations, bradycardia<br><br>Nausea, vomiting, diarrhea or constipation, increased or decreased appetite, urinary retention<br><br>Nervousness, insomnia | Decreases neuronal uptake of serotonin<br><br>Take in AM to avoid insomnia<br><br>Takes at least 4 weeks to work<br><br>Can potentiate effect of digoxin, warfarin, and diazepam<br><br>Used for anorexia |

(Continued)

Antidepressant Medications: Overview (*Continued*)

| MEDICATION | ADVERSE EFFECTS | NURSING CONSIDERATIONS |
|---|---|---|
| **Serotonin/norepinephrine reuptake inhibitors (SNRIs)** | | |
| Duloxetine | Palpitations, bradycardia<br><br>Nausea, vomiting, diarrhea or constipation, increased or decreased appetite, urinary retention<br><br>Nervousness, insomnia | Decreases neuronal uptake of serotonin<br><br>Take in AM to avoid insomnia<br><br>Takes at least 4 weeks to work<br><br>Can potentiate effect of digoxin, warfarin, and diazepam<br><br>Used for anorexia |
| **Heterocyclics** | | |
| Bupropion<br><br>Trazodone | Dry mouth<br><br>Nausea | May require gradual reduction before stopping<br><br>Avoid use with alcohol, other CNS depressants for up to 1 week after end of therapy |
| **Herbals** | | |
| St. John's wort | Dizziness, hypertension, allergic skin reaction, phototoxicity | Avoid use of St. John's wort and MAOI within 2 weeks of each other<br><br>Do not use alcohol<br><br>Contraindicated in pregnancy<br><br>Avoid exposure to sun and use sunscreen<br><br>Discontinue 1 to 2 weeks before surgery |
| **Herbal interactions** | St. John's wort—interacts with SSRIs; do not take within 2 weeks of MAOI<br><br>Ginseng may potentiate MAOIs<br><br>Avoid Ma huang or ephedra with MAOIs<br><br>Kava kava should not be combined with benzodiazepines or opioids due to increased sedation<br><br>Increase use of Brewer's yeast with MAOIs can increase blood pressure | |

Antidiabetic Medications: Insulin

| INSULIN TYPES | ONSET OF ACTION | PEAK ACTION | DURATION OF ACTION | TIME OF ADVERSE REACTION | CHARACTERISTICS |
|---|---|---|---|---|---|
| **Rapid-acting** | | | | | |
| Lispro | 15-30 min | 0.5-1.5 h | 3-5 h | Midmorning: trembling, weakness | Client should eat within 5-15 min after injection; also used in insulin pumps |
| Aspart | | 1-3 h | 3-5 h | | |
| Glulisine | 15-30 min | 1-1.5 h | 3-5 h | | |
| | 10-15 min | | | | |
| **Short-acting** | | | | | |
| Regular insulin | 30-60 min | 1-5 h | 6-10 h | Midmorning, midafternoon: weakness, fatigue | Clear solution; given 20-30 min before meal; can be alone or with other insulins |
| **Intermediate-acting** | | | | | |
| Isophane (NPH) | 1-2 h | 4-12 h | 16 h | Early evening: weakness, fatigue | White and cloudy solution; can be given after meals |
| **Very long-acting** | | | | | |
| Glargine | 3-4 h | Continuous (no peak) | 24 h | none | Maintains blood glucose levels regardless of meals; cannot be mixed with other insulins; given at bedtime |
| Determir | unknown | Continuous (no peak) | 24 h (varies) | | |
| Degludec | 1 h | 9 h | 24 h | | |

| | |
|---|---|
| **Action** | Reduces blood glucose levels by increasing glucose transport across cell membranes; enhances conversion of glucose to glycogen |
| **Indications** | Type 1 diabetes; type 2 diabetes not responding to oral hypoglycemic agents; gestational diabetes not responding to diet |
| **Adverse effects** | Hypoglycemia |
| **Nursing considerations** | Teach client to rotate sites to prevent lipohypertrophy, fibrofatty masses at injection sites; do not inject into these masses |
| | Only regular insulin can be given IV; all can be given SQ |
| **Herbal interactions** | Bee pollen, ginkgo biloba, glucosamine may increase blood glucose |
| | Basil, bay leaf, chromium, echinacea, garlic, ginseng may decrease blood glucose |

Antidiabetic Medications: Oral

| MEDICATION | ADVERSE EFFECTS | NURSING CONSIDERATIONS |
|---|---|---|
| **Sulfonylureas** | | |
| Glimepiride Glipizide Glyburide | GI symptoms and dermatologic reactions | Only used if some pancreas beta-cell function Stimulates release of insulin from pancreas Many medications can potentiate or interfere with actions Take with food if GI upset occurs |
| **Biguanides** | | |
| Metformin | Nausea Diarrhea Abdominal discomfort | No effect on pancreatic beta cells; decreases glucose production by liver Not given if renal impairment Can cause lactic acidosis Avoid alcohol Do not give with alpha-glucosidase inhibitors |
| **Alpha glucosidase inhibitors** | | |
| Acarbose Miglitol | Abdominal discomfort Diarrhea Flatulence | Delays digestion of carbohydrates Must be taken immediately before a meal Can be taken alone or with other agents |
| **Thiazolidinediones** | | |
| Rosiglitazone Pioglitazone | Infection Headache Pain Rare cases of liver failure | Decreases insulin resistance and inhibits gluconeogenesis Regularly scheduled liver-function studies Can cause resumption of ovulation in perimenopause |
| **Meglitinides** | | |
| Repaglinide | Hypoglycemia GI disturbances URIs Back pain Headache | Increases pancreatic insulin release Medication should not be taken if meal skipped |

(*Continued*)

Antidiabetic Medications: Oral (*Continued*)

| MEDICATION | ADVERSE EFFECTS | NURSING CONSIDERATIONS |
|---|---|---|
| **Gliptins** | | |
| Sitagliptin | Upper respiratory infections<br><br>Hypoglycemia | Enhances action of incretin hormones |
| **Incretin mimetics** | | |
| Exenatide | GI upset<br><br>Hypoglycemia<br><br>Pancreatitis | Interacts with many medications<br><br>Administer 1 hour before meals |
| **Indications** | Type 2 diabetes | |
| **Adverse effects** | Hypoglycemia | |
| **Nursing considerations** | Monitor serum glucose levels<br><br>Avoid alcohol<br><br>Teaching for disease: dietary control, symptoms of hypoglycemia and hyperglycemia<br><br>Good skin care | |
| **Herbal interactions** | Bee pollen, ginkgo biloba, glucosamine may increase blood glucose<br><br>Basil, bay leaf, chromium, echinacea, garlic, ginseng may decrease blood glucose | |

Hypoglycemia Medications

| MEDICATION | ADVERSE EFFECTS | NURSING CONSIDERATIONS |
|---|---|---|
| Glucagon | Nausea, vomiting | Given SQ or IM, onset is 8–10 min with duration of 12–27 min<br><br>Should be part of emergency supplies for diabetics<br><br>May repeat in 15 min if needed |
| **Action** | Hormone produced by alpha cells of the pancreas to simulate the liver to change glycogen to glucose | |
| **Indications** | Acute management of severe hypoglycemia | |
| **Adverse effects** | Hypotension<br><br>Bronchospasm<br><br>Dizziness | |
| **Nursing considerations** | May repeat in 15 minutes if needed<br><br>IV glucose must be given if client fails to respond<br><br>Arouse clients from coma as quickly as possible and give carbohydrates orally to prevent secondary hypoglycemic reactions | |

Antidiarrheal Medications

| MEDICATION | ADVERSE EFFECTS | NURSING CONSIDERATIONS |
|---|---|---|
| Bismuth subsalicylate | Darkening of stools and tongue<br><br>Constipation | Give 2 hours before or 3 hours after other meds to prevent impaired absorption<br><br>Encourage fluids<br><br>Take after each loose stool until diarrhea controlled<br><br>Notify health care provider if diarrhea not controlled in 48 hours<br><br>Absorbs irritants and soothes intestinal muscle<br><br>Do not administer for more than 2 days in presence of fever or in clients less than 3 years of age<br><br>Monitor for salicylate toxicity<br><br>Use cautiously if already taking aspirin<br><br>Avoid use before x-rays (is radiopaque) |
| Diphenoxylate hydrochloride and atropine sulfate | Sedation<br><br>Dizziness<br><br>Tachycardia<br><br>Dry mouth<br><br>Paralytic ileus | Onset 45-60 min<br><br>Monitor fluid and electrolytes<br><br>Increases intestinal tone and decreases peristalsis<br><br>May potentiate action of barbiturates, depressants |
| Loperamide | Drowsiness<br><br>Constipation | Monitor children closely for CNS effects |
| Opium alkaloids | Narcotic dependence, nausea | Acts on smooth muscle to increase tone<br><br>Administer with glass of water<br><br>Discontinue as soon as stools are controlled |
| **Action** | Absorbs water, gas, toxins, irritants, and nutrients in bowel; slows peristalsis; increases tone of smooth muscles and sphincters | |
| **Indications** | Diarrhea | |
| **Adverse effects** | Constipation, fecal impaction<br><br>Anticholinergic effects | |
| **Nursing considerations** | Not used with abdominal pain of unknown origin<br><br>Monitor for urinary retention | |

Antidysrhythmic Medications

| MEDICATION | ADVERSE EFFECTS | NURSING CONSIDERATIONS |
|---|---|---|
| **CLASS IA TYPE** | | |
| Quinidine<br>Procainamide | Hypotension<br>Heart failure | Monitor blood pressure<br>Monitor for widening of the PR, QRS or QT intervals<br>Toxic adverse effects have limited use |
| **CLASS IB** | | |
| Lidocaine | CNS: slurred speech, confusion, drowsiness, confusion, seizures<br>Hypotension and bradycardia | Monitor for CNS adverse effects<br>Monitor BP and heart rate and cardiac rhythm |
| **CLASS IC** | | |
| Flecainide<br>Propafenone HCL | Bradycardia, Hypotension<br>Dysrhythmias<br>CNS: anxiety, insomnia, confusion, seizures | Monitor for increasing dysrhythmias<br>Monitor heart rate and blood pressure<br>Monitor for CNS effects |
| **CLASS II** | | |
| Propranolol<br>Esmolol hydrochloride<br>Acebutolol | Bradycardia and hypotension<br>Bronchospasm<br>Increase in heart failure<br>Fatigue and sleep disturbances | Monitor apical heart rate, cardiac rhythm and blood pressure<br>Assess for shortness of breath and wheezing<br>Assess for fatigue, sleep disturbances<br>Assess apical heart rate for 1 minute before administration |
| **CLASS III** | | |
| Amiodarone hydrochloride,<br>Ibutilide fumarate | Hypotension<br>Bradycardia and atrioventricular block<br>Muscle weakness, tremors<br>Photosensitivity and photophobia<br>Liver toxicity | Continuous monitoring of cardiac rhythm during IV administration<br>Monitor QT interval during IV administration<br>Monitor heart rate, blood pressure during initiation of therapy<br>Instruct client to wear sunglasses and sunscreen |

(*Continued*)

Antidysrhythmic Medications (*Continued*)

| MEDICATION | ADVERSE EFFECTS | NURSING CONSIDERATIONS |
|---|---|---|
| **CLASS IV** | | |
| Verapamil<br>Diltiazem hydrochloride | Bradycardia<br>Hypotension<br>Dizziness and orthostatic hypotension<br>Heart failure | Monitor apical heart rate and blood pressure<br>Instruct clients about orthostatic precautions<br>Instruct clients to report signs of heart failure to health care provider |

Antiemetic Medications

| MEDICATION | ADVERSE EFFECTS | NURSING CONSIDERATIONS |
|---|---|---|
| Prochlorperazine dimaleate | Drowsiness<br>Orthostatic hypotension<br>Diplopia, photosensitivity | Check CBC and liver function with prolonged use<br>Wear protective clothing when exposed to sunlight |
| Ondansetron | Headache, sedation<br>Diarrhea, constipation<br>Transient elevations in liver enzymes | New class of antiemetics—serotonin receptor antagonist<br>Administer 30 min prior to chemotherapy |
| Metoclopramide | Restlessness, anxiety, drowsiness<br>Extrapyramidal symptoms<br>Dystonic reactions | Monitor BP<br>Avoid activities requiring mental alertness<br>Take before meals<br>Used with tube feeding to decrease residual and risk of aspiration<br>Administer 30 min prior to chemotherapy |
| Meclizine | Drowsiness, dry mouth<br>Blurred vision<br>Excitation, restlessness | Contraindicated with glaucoma<br>Avoid activities requiring mental alertness |
| Dimenhydrinate | Drowsiness<br>Palpitations, hypotension<br>Blurred vision | Avoid activities requiring mental alertness |

(*Continued*)

Antiemetic Medications (*Continued*)

| MEDICATION | ADVERSE EFFECTS | NURSING CONSIDERATIONS |
|---|---|---|
| Promethazine | Drowsiness<br>Dizziness<br>Constipation<br>Urinary retention<br>Dry mouth | If used for motion sickness, take 1/2 to 1 hour before traveling; avoid activities requiring alertness; avoid alcohol, other CNS depressants<br>Contraindicated in children less than 2 years old |
| Droperidol | Seizures<br>Arrhythmias<br>Hypotension<br>Tachycardia | Often used either IV or IM in ambulatory care settings; observe for extrapyramidal symptoms (dystonia, extended neck, flexed arms, tremor, restlessness, hyperactivity, anxiety), which can be reversed with anticholinergics |
| **Action** | Blocks effect of dopamine in chemoreceptor trigger zone; increases GI motility | |
| **Indications** | Nausea and vomiting caused by surgery, chemotherapy, radiation sickness, uremia | |
| **Adverse effects** | Drowsiness, sedation<br>Anticholinergic effects | |
| **Nursing considerations** | When used for viral infections may cause Reye's syndrome in clients less than 21 years old<br>Phenothiazine medications are also used as antiemetics | |
| **Herbals** | Ginger—used to treat minor heartburn, nausea, vomiting; may increase risk of bleeding if taken with anticoagulants, antiplatelets, thrombolytic medication; instruct to stop medication if easily bruised or other signs of bleeding noted, report to health care provider; not approved for morning sickness during pregnancy | |

Antifungal Medications

| MEDICATION | ADVERSE EFFECTS | NURSING CONSIDERATIONS |
|---|---|---|
| Amphotericin B | IV: nicknamed "amphoterrible"<br><br>GI upset<br><br>Hypokalemia-induced muscle pain<br><br>CNS disturbances in vision, hearing Peripheral neuritis<br><br>Seizures<br><br>Hematological, renal, cardiac, hepatic abnormalities<br><br>Skin irritation and thrombosis if infiltration of IV occurs | Refrigerate medication and protect from sunlight<br><br>Monitor vital signs; report febrile reaction or any change in function, especially nervous system dysfunction<br><br>Check for hypokalemia<br><br>Meticulous care and observation of injection site |
| Nystatin | Mild GI distress<br><br>Hypersensitivity | Discontinue if redness, swelling, irritation occurs<br><br>Instruct client in good oral, vaginal, skin hygiene |
| Fluconazole | Nausea, vomiting<br><br>Diarrhea<br><br>Elevated liver enzymes | Medication excreted unchanged by kidneys; dosage reduced if creatine clearance is altered due to renal failure<br><br>Administer after hemodialysis |
| Ketoconazole | Headaches, vaginitis, nausea, flu-like symptoms (systemic use) | Reduce dosage hepatic disease<br><br>Monitor CBC, LFTs, cultures<br><br>Give tablet with food or milk |
| **Action** | Impairs cell membrane of fungus, causing increased permeability | |
| **Indications** | Systemic fungal infections (e.g., candidiasis, oral thrush, histoplasmosis) | |
| **Adverse effects** | Hepatotoxicity<br><br>Thrombocytopenia<br><br>Leukopenia<br><br>Pruritus | |
| **Nursing considerations** | Administer with food to decrease GI upset<br><br>Small, frequent meals<br><br>Check hepatic function<br><br>Teach client to take full course of medication, may be prescribed for prolonged period | |

Antigout Medications

| MEDICATION | ADVERSE EFFECTS | NURSING CONSIDERATIONS |
|---|---|---|
| Colchicine | GI upset<br>Agranulocytosis<br>Peripheral neuritis | Anti-inflammatory<br>Give with meals<br>Check CBC, I and O<br>For acute gout in combination with NSAIDs |
| Probenecid | Nausea, constipation<br>Skin rash | For chronic gout<br>Reduces uric acid<br>Check BUN, renal function tests<br>Encourage fluids<br>Give with milk, food, antacids<br>Alkaline urine helps prevent kidney calculi |
| Allopurinol | GI upset<br>Headache, dizziness, drowsiness | Blocks formation of uric acid<br>Encourage fluids<br>Check I and O<br>Check CBC and renal function tests<br>Give with meals<br>Alkaline urine helps prevent kidney calculi<br>Avoid ASA because it inactivates medication |
| **Action** | Decreases production and reabsorption of uric acid | |
| **Indications** | Gout<br>Uric acid stone formation | |
| **Adverse effects** | Aplastic anemia<br>Agranulocytosis<br>Renal calculi<br>GI irritation | |
| **Nursing considerations** | Monitor for renal calculi | |

Antihistamine Medications

| MEDICATION | ADVERSE EFFECTS | NURSING CONSIDERATIONS |
|---|---|---|
| Chlorpheniramine maleate | Drowsiness, dry mouth | Most effective if taken before onset of symptoms |
| Diphenhydramine HCl | Drowsiness<br><br>Nausea, dry mouth<br><br>Photosensitivity | Don't combine with alcoholic beverages<br><br>Give with food<br><br>Use sunscreen<br><br>Older adults: greater risk of confusion and sedation |
| Promethazine HCl | Agranulocytosis<br><br>Drowsiness, dry mouth<br><br>Photosensitivity | Give with food<br><br>Use sunscreen |
| Loratadine<br><br>Cetirizine<br><br>Fexofenadine | Drowsiness | Reduce dose or give every other day for clients with renal or hepatic dysfunction |
| **Action** | Blocks the effects of histamine at peripheral H1 receptor sites; anticholinergic, antipruritic effects | |
| **Indications** | Allergic rhinitis<br><br>Allergic reactions<br><br>Chronic idiopathic urticaria | |
| **Adverse effects** | Depression<br><br>Nightmares<br><br>Sedation | Dry mouth<br><br>GI upset<br><br>Bronchospasm<br><br>Alopecia |
| **Nursing considerations** | Administer with food<br><br>Good mouth care, sugarless lozenges for dry mouth<br><br>Good skin care<br><br>Use caution when performing tasks requiring alertness (e.g., driving car)<br><br>Avoid alcohol | |

Anti-Infective Medications: Aminoglycosides

| **Examples** | Gentamicin |
|---|---|
| | Neomycin |
| | Tobramycin |
| | Amikacin |
| **Actions** | Bacteriocidal |
| | Inhibits protein synthesis of many Gram-negative bacteria |
| **Indications** | Treatment of severe systemic infections of CNS, respiratory, GI, urinary tract, bone, skin, soft tissues, acute pelvic inflammatory disease (PID), tuberculosis (streptomycin) |
| **Adverse effects** | Ototoxicity, Nephrotoxicity |
| | Anorexia, nausea, vomiting, diarrhea |
| **Nursing considerations** | Check eighth cranial nerve function (hearing) |
| | Check renal function (BUN, creatinine) |
| | Usually prescribed for 7–10 days |
| | Encourage fluids |
| | Small, frequent meals |

Anti-Infective Medications: Cephalosporins

| **Examples** | Multiple preparations: |
|---|---|
| | 1st generation example: cephalexin |
| | 2nd generation example: cefoxitin sodium |
| | 3rd generation example: ceftriaxone sodium |
| | 4th generation example: cefepime HCL |
| | 5th generation example: ceftaroline fosamil |
| **Actions** | Bacteriocidal |
| | Inhibits synthesis of bacterial cell wall |

(Continued)

Anti-Infective Medications: Cephalosporins (*Continued*)

| Indications | Pharyngitis |
|---|---|
| | Tonsillitis |
| | Otitis media |
| | Upper and lower respiratory tract infections |
| | Dermatological infections |
| | Gonorrhea |
| | Septicemia |
| | Meningitis |
| | Perioperative prophylaxis |
| | Urinary tract infections |
| **Adverse effects** | Abdominal pain, nausea, vomiting, diarrhea |
| | Increased risk bleeding |
| | Hypoprothrombinemia |
| | Rash |
| | Superinfections |
| | Thrombophlebitis (IV), abscess formation (IM, IV) |
| **Nursing considerations** | Take with food |
| | Administer liquid form to children, don't crush tablets |
| | Have vitamin K available for hypoprothrombinemia |
| | Avoid alcohol while taking medication and for 3 days after finishing course of medication |
| | **Cross allergy with penicillins (cephalosporins should not be given to clients with a severe penicillin allergy)** |
| | Monitor renal and hepatic function |
| | Monitor for Thrombophlebitis |

Anti-Infective Medications: Fluoroquinolones

| | |
|---|---|
| **Examples** | Ciprofloxacin, Levofloxacin |
| **Actions** | Broad-spectrum bactericidal; interferes with DNA replication in Gram-negative bacteria |
| **Indications** | Treatment of infection caused *by E.coli* and other bacteria, chronic bacterial prostatitis, acute sinusitis, postexposure inhalation anthrax |
| **Adverse effects** | Headache<br><br>Nausea<br><br>Diarrhea<br><br>Elevated BUN, AST , ALT, serum creatinine, alkaline phosphatase<br><br>Decreased WBC and hematocrit<br><br>Rash<br><br>Photosensitivity<br><br>Achilles tendon rupture |
| **Nursing considerations** | Culture and sensitivity before starting therapy<br><br>Take 1 h before or 2 h after meals with glass of water<br><br>Encourage fluids<br><br>If needed administer antacids 2 h after medication<br><br>Take full course of therapy<br><br>WARNING: Fluoroquinolones can lead to hypoglycemia and possibly hypoglycemic coma, as well as acute psychosis (e.g., agitation, delirium, disorientation, disturbance in attention, memory impairment, and nervousness). |

Anti-Infective Medications: Lincosamides

| | |
|---|---|
| **Examples** | Clindamycin HCl Phosphate |
| **Action** | Both bacteriostatic and bactericidal, it suppresses protein synthesis by preventing peptide bond formation |
| **Indications** | Staph, strep, and other infections |
| **Adverse effects** | Diarrhea<br><br>Rash<br><br>Liver toxicity |
| **Nursing considerations** | Administer oral med with a full glass of water to prevent esophageal ulcers<br><br>Monitor for persistent vomiting, diarrhea, fever, or abdominal pain and cramping, superinfections |

Anti-Infective Medications: Macrolides

| Examples | Erythromycin |
|---|---|
| | Azithromycin |
| **Actions** | Bacteriostatic; bactericidal; binds to cell membrane and causes changes in protein function |
| **Indications** | Acute infections |
| | Acne and skin infections |
| | Upper respiratory tract infections |
| | Prophylaxis before dental procedures for clients allergic to PCN with valvular heart disease |
| **Adverse effects** | Abdominal cramps, diarrhea |
| | Confusion, uncontrollable emotions |
| | Hepatotoxicity |
| | Superinfections |
| **Nursing considerations** | Take oral med 1 h before or 2–3 h after meals with full glass of water |
| | Take around the clock to maximize effectiveness |
| | Monitor liver function |
| | Take full course of therapy |

Anti-Infective Medications: Penicillins

| Examples | Amoxicillin |
|---|---|
| | Ampicillin |
| | Methicillin |
| | Nafcillin |
| | Penicillin G |
| | Penicillin V |
| **Actions** | Bactericidal; inhibit synthesis of cell wall of sensitive organisms |
| **Indications** | Effective against Gram-positive organisms |
| | Moderate to severe infections |
| | Syphilis |
| | Gonococcal infections |
| | Lyme disease |
| **Adverse effects** | Glossitis, stomatitis |
| | Gastritis |
| | Diarrhea |
| | Superinfections |
| | Hypersensitivity reactions |
| **Nursing considerations** | Culture and sensitivity before treatment |
| | Monitor serum electrolytes and cardiac status if given IV |
| | Monitor and rotate injection sites |
| | Good mouth care |
| | Yogurt or buttermilk if diarrhea develops |
| | Instruct client to take missed medications as soon as possible; do not double dose |

Anti-Infective Medications: Sulfonamides

| Examples | Sulfasalazine |
|---|---|
| | Trimethoprim/Sulfamethoxazole |
| **Actions** | Bacteriostatic; competitively antagonize para-aminobenzoic acid, essential component of folic acid synthesis, causing cell death |
| **Indications** | Ulcerative colitis, Crohn disease |
| | Otitis media |
| | Conjunctivitis |
| | Meningitis |
| | Toxoplasmosis |
| | UTIs |
| | Rheumatoid arthritis |
| **Adverse effects** | Peripheral neuropathy |
| | Crystalluria, proteinuria |
| | Photosensitivity |
| | GI upset |
| | Stomatitis |
| | Hypersensitivity reactions |
| **Nursing considerations** | Culture and sensitivity before therapy |
| | Take with a full glass of water |
| | Take around the clock |
| | Encourage fluid intake (8 glasses of water/day) |
| | Protect from exposure to light (sunscreen, protective clothing) |
| | Good mouth care |

Anti-Infective Medications: Tetracyclines

| | |
|---|---|
| **Examples** | Doxycycline |
| | Minocycline |
| | Tetracycline HCl |
| **Actions** | Bacteriostatic; inhibits protein synthesis of susceptible bacteria |
| **Indications** | Treatment of syphilis, chlamydia, gonorrhea, malaria prophylaxis, chronic periodontitis, acne; treatment of anthrax (doxycycline); as part of combination therapy to eliminate *H. pylori* infections; medication of choice for stage 1 Lyme disease (tetracycline HCl) |
| **Adverse effects** | Discoloration and inadequate calcification of primary teeth of fetus if taken during pregnancy |
| | Glossitis |
| | Dysphagia |
| | Diarrhea |
| | Phototoxic reactions |
| | Rash |
| | Superinfections |
| **Nursing considerations** | Take 1 h before or 2–3 h after meals |
| | Do not take with antacids, milk, iron preparations (give 3 h after medication) |
| | Note expiration date (becomes highly nephrotoxic) |
| | Protect from sunlight |
| | Monitor renal function |
| | Topical applications may stain clothing |
| | Use contraceptive method in addition to oral contraceptives |

Anti-Infective Medications: Vancomycin

| Examples | Vancomycin |
|---|---|
| Action | Bacteriocidal |
| | Binds to bacterial cell wall, stopping its synthesis |
| Indications | Treatment of resistant staph infections, pseudomembranous enterocolitis due to *C. difficile* infection |
| Adverse effects | Thrombophlebitis |
| | Abscess formation |
| | Nephrotoxicity |
| | Ototoxicity |
| Nursing considerations | Monitor renal function and hearing |
| | Poor absorption orally; administer IV: peak 5 minutes, duration 12–24 hours |
| | Avoid extravasation during therapy; it may cause necrosis |
| | Give antihistamine if "red man syndrome": decreased blood pressure, flushing of face and neck |
| | Contact health care provider if signs of superinfection: sore throat, fever, fatigue |

Anti-Infective Medications: Overview

| MEDICATION | ADVERSE EFFECTS | NURSING CONSIDERATIONS |
|---|---|---|
| **Penicillins** | | |
| Ampicillin | Skin rashes, diarrhea | Obtain C and S before first dose |
| Penicillin G potassium | Allergic reactions | Take careful history of penicillin reaction |
| Penicillin G sodium | Renal, hepatic, hematological abnormalities | Observe for 20 minutes post IM injection |
| | Nausea, vomiting | Give 1–2 hours ac or 2–3 hours pc to reduce gastric acid destruction of medication |
| | | Monitor for loose, foul-smelling stool and change in tongue |
| | | Teach to continue medication for entire time prescribed, even if symptoms resolve |
| | | Check for hypersensitivity to other medications, especially cephalosporins |

*(Continued)*

Anti-Infective Medications: Overview (*Continued*)

| MEDICATION | ADVERSE EFFECTS | NURSING CONSIDERATIONS |
|---|---|---|
| **Sulfonamides** | | |
| Sulfasalazine | Nausea, vomiting<br><br>Skin eruption<br><br>Agranulocytosis | Advise client to avoid exposure to sunlight<br><br>Maintain fluid intake at 3,000 mL/day to avoid crystal formation |
| Trimethoprim/<br>Sulfamethoxazole | Hypersensitivity reaction<br><br>Blood dyscrasias<br><br>Rash | Obtain C and S before first dose<br><br>IV solution must be given slowly over 60–90 minutes<br><br>Never administer IM<br><br>Encourage fluids to 3,000 mL/day |
| **Tetracyclines** | Photosensitivity<br><br>GI upset, renal, hepatic, hematological abnormalities<br><br>Dental discoloration of deciduous ("baby") teeth, enamel hypoplasia | Give between meals<br><br>If GI symptoms occur, administer with food EXCEPT milk products or other foods high in calcium (interferes with absorption)<br><br>Assess for change in bowel habits, perineal rash, black "hairy" tongue<br><br>Good oral hygiene<br><br>Avoid during tooth and early development periods (fourth month prenatal to 8 years of age)<br><br>Monitor I and O<br><br>Caution client to avoid sun exposure<br><br>Decomposes to toxic substance with age and exposure to light |
| Doxycycline | Photosensitivity | Check client's tongue for *Monilia* infection |
| **Aminoglycosides** | Ototoxicity cranial nerve VIII<br><br>Nephrotoxicity | Check creatinine and BUN<br><br>Check peak—2 h after med given<br><br>Check trough—at time of dose/prior to med<br><br>Monitor for symptoms of bacterial overgrowth, photosensitivity<br><br>Teach to immediately report tinnitus, vertigo, nystagmus, ataxia<br><br>Monitor I and O<br><br>Audiograms if given long-term |

(*Continued*)

Anti-Infective Medications: Overview (*Continued*)

| MEDICATION | ADVERSE EFFECTS | NURSING CONSIDERATIONS |
|---|---|---|
| Neomycin sulfate | Hypersensitivity reactions | Ophthalmic—remove infective exudate around eyes before administration of ointment |
| **Fluoroquinolones** | | |
| Ciprofloxacin | Seizures<br>GI upset<br>Rash | Contraindicated in children less than 18 years of age<br>Give 2 hours pc or 2 hours before an antacid or iron preparation<br>Avoid caffeine<br>Encourage fluids |
| **Macrolides** | | |
| Azithromycin<br>Erythromycin | Pain at injection site<br>Nausea, diarrhea | Can be used in clients with compromised renal function because excretion is primarily through the bile |
| **Cephalosporins** | | |
| 1st generation example:<br>  Cephalexin<br>2nd generation example:<br>  Cefoxitin sodium<br>3rd generation example:<br>  Ceftriaxone sodium<br>4th generation example:<br>  Cefepime HCL<br>5th generation example:<br>  Ceftaroline fosamil | Diarrhea, nausea<br>Dizziness, abdominal pain<br>Eosinophilia, superinfections<br>Allergic reactions | Can cause false-positive Coombs test (which will complicate transfusion cross-matching procedure)<br>Cross-sensitivity with penicillins<br>Take careful history of penicillin reactions |
| **Glycopeptides** | | |
| Vancomycin | Liver damage | Poor absorption orally, but IV peak 5 minutes, duration 12–24 hours<br>Avoid extravasation during therapy—may cause necrosis<br>Give antihistamine if "red man syndrome": decreased blood pressure, flushing of face and neck<br>Contact health care provider if signs of superinfection: sore throat, fever, fatigue |

(*Continued*)

Anti-Infective Medications: Overview (*Continued*)

| MEDICATION | ADVERSE EFFECTS | NURSING CONSIDERATIONS |
|---|---|---|
| **Lincosamides** | | |
| Clindamycin HCl phosphate | Nausea<br><br>Vaginitis<br><br>Colitis may occur 2–9 days or several weeks after starting meds | Administer oral med with a full glass of water to prevent esophageal ulcers<br><br>Monitor for persistent vomiting, diarrhea, fever, or abdominal pain and cramping |

Anti-Infective Medications: Topical

| MEDICATION | ADVERSE EFFECTS | NURSING CONSIDERATIONS |
|---|---|---|
| Bacitracin ointment | Nephrotoxicity<br>Ototoxicity | Overgrowth of nonsusceptible organisms can occur |
| Neosporin cream | Nephrotoxicity<br>Ototoxicity | Allergic dermatitis may occur |
| Povidone-iodine solution | Irritation | Don't use around eyes<br>May stain skin<br>Don't use full-strength on mucous membranes |
| Silver sulfadiazine cream | Neutropenia<br>Burning | Use cautiously if sensitive to sulfonamides |
| Tolnaftate cream | Irritation | Use small amount of medication<br>Use medication for duration prescribed |
| Nystatin cream | Contact dermatitis | Do not use occlusive dressings |

Antihypertensive Medications: Angiotensin II Receptor Blocker

| Examples | "-sartan" |
|---|---|
| | Candesartan |
| | Eprosartan |
| | Irbesartan |
| | Losartan |
| **Indications** | Hypertension |
| | Heart failure |
| | Diabetic nephropathy |
| | Myocardial infarction |
| | Stroke prevention |
| **Adverse effects** | Angioedema |
| | Renal failure |
| | Orthostatic hypotension |
| **Nursing considerations** | Instruct client about position changes |
| | Monitor for edema |
| | Instruct client to notify health care provider if edema occurs |

Antihypertensive Medications: Angiotensin-Converting Enzyme (ACE) Inhibitor

| Examples | "-pril" |
|---|---|
| | Captopril |
| | Enalapril |
| | Lisinopril |
| | Benazepril |
| | Fosinopril |
| | Quinapril |
| | Ramipril |
| **Actions** | Blocks ACE in lungs from converting angiotensin I to angiotensin II (powerful vasoconstrictor); causes decreased BP, decreased aldosterone secretion, sodium and fluid loss |
| **Indications** | Hypertension |
| | HF |

(*Continued*)

Antihypertensive Medications: Angiotensin-Converting Enzyme (ACE) Inhibitor (*Continued*)

| Adverse effects | Gastric irritation, peptic ulcer, orthostatic hypotension |
|---|---|
| | Tachycardia |
| | Myocardial infarction |
| | Proteinuria |
| | Rash, pruritis |
| | Persistent dry nonproductive cough |
| | Peripheral edema |
| Nursing considerations | Decreased absorption if taken with food—give 1 hour ac or 2 hours pc |
| | Small, frequent meals |
| | Frequent mouth care |
| | Change position slowly |
| | Can be used with thiazide diuretics |

Antihypertensive Medications: Alpha-1 Adrenergic Blocker

| Examples | Doxazosin |
|---|---|
| | Prazosin |
| | Terazosin |
| Actions | Selective blockade of alpha-1 adrenergic receptors in peripheral blood vessels |
| Indications | Hypertension |
| | Benign prostatic hyperplasia |
| | Pheochromocytoma |
| | Raynaud's disease |
| Adverse effects | Orthostatic hypotension |
| | Reflex tachycardia |
| | Nasal congestion |
| | Impotence |
| Nursing considerations | Administer first dose at bedtime to avoid fainting |
| | Change positions slowly to prevent orthostatic hypotension |
| | Monitor BP, weight, BUN/creatinine, edema |

Antihypertensive Medications: Beta-Adrenergic Blocker

| Examples | "-lol" |
|---|---|
| | Atenolol |
| | Nadolol |
| | Propranolol |
| | Metoprolol |
| | Acebutolol |
| | Carvedilol |
| | Pindolol |
| **Actions** | Blocks beta-adrenergic receptors in heart; decreases excitability of heart; reduces cardiac workload and oxygen consumption; decreases release of renin; lowers blood pressure by reducing CNS stimuli |
| **Indications** | Hypertension (used with diuretics) |
| | Angina |
| | Supraventricular tachycardia |
| | Prevent recurrent MI |
| | Migraine headache (propranolol) |
| | Stage fright (propranolol) |
| | Heart failure |
| **Adverse effects** | Gastric pain |
| | Bradycardia/tachycardia |
| | Acute severe heart failure |
| | Cardiac dysrhythmias |
| | Impotence |
| | Decreased exercise tolerance |
| | Nightmares, depression |
| | Dizziness |
| | Bronchospasm (nonselective beta blockers) |
| **Nursing considerations** | **Do not discontinue abruptly, taper gradually over 2 weeks** |
| | Take with meals |
| | Provide rest periods |
| | For diabetic clients, blocks normal signs of hypoglycemia (sweating, tachycardia); monitor blood glucose |
| | Medications have antianginal and antiarrhythmic actions |

Antihypertensive Medication: Calcium Channel Blocker

| Examples | Nifedipine |
|---|---|
| | Verapamil |
| | Diltiazem |
| | Amlodipine |
| | Felodipine |
| **Actions** | Inhibits movement of calcium ions across membrane of cardiac and arterial muscle cells; results in slowed impulse conduction, depression of myocardial contractility, dilation of coronary arteries; decreases cardiac workload and energy consumption, increases oxygenation of myocardial cells |
| **Indications** | Angina |
| | Hypertension |
| | Dysrhythmias |
| | Interstitial cystitis |
| | Migraines |
| **Adverse effects** | Dizziness |
| | Headache |
| | Nervousness |
| | Peripheral edema |
| | Angina |
| | Bradycardia |
| | AV block |
| | Flushing, rash |
| | Impotence |
| **Nursing considerations** | Monitor vital signs |
| | Do not chew or divide sustained-release tablets |
| | Medications also have antianginal actions |
| | Contraindicated in heart block |
| | Contact health care provider if blood pressure less than 90/60 |
| | Instruct client to avoid grapefruit juice |
| | Monitor for signs of heart failure |

Hypertensive Medications: Centrally Acting Alpha-Adrenergic

| | |
|---|---|
| **Examples** | Clonidine<br><br>Methyldopa |
| **Actions** | Stimulates alpha receptors in medulla, causing reduction in sympathetic action in heart; decreases rate and force of contraction, decreasing cardiac output |
| **Indications** | Hypertension |
| **Adverse effects** | Drowsiness, sedation<br><br>Orthostatic hypotension<br><br>CHF |
| **Nursing considerations** | Don't discontinue abruptly<br><br>Monitor for fluid retention<br><br>Older adults: potential for orthostatic hypotension and CNS adverse effects |

Hypertensive Medications: Direct-Acting Vasodilator

| | |
|---|---|
| **Examples** | Hydralazine<br><br>Minoxidil |
| **Actions** | Relaxes smooth muscle of blood vessels, lowering peripheral resistance |
| **Indications** | Hypertension |
| **Adverse effects** | Same as centrally acting alpha adrenergics |
| **Nursing considerations** | Same as centrally acting alpha adrenergics |

Antihypertensive Medications: Overview

| MEDICATION | ADVERSE EFFECTS | NURSING CONSIDERATIONS |
|---|---|---|
| Methyldopa | Drowsiness, dizziness, brady-cardia, hemolytic anemia, fever, orthostatic hypotension | Monitor CBC<br>Monitor liver function<br>Take at bedtime to minimize daytime drowsiness<br>Change position slowly |
| Clonidine | Drowsiness, dizziness<br>Dry mouth, headache<br>Dermatitis<br>Severe rebound hypertension | **Do not discontinue abruptly**<br>Apply patch to nonhairy area (upper outer arm, anterior chest) |

*(Continued)*

Antihypertensive Medications: Overview (*Continued*)

| MEDICATION | ADVERSE EFFECTS | NURSING CONSIDERATIONS |
|---|---|---|
| Atenolol | Bradycardia<br><br>Hypotension<br><br>Bronchospasm | Once-a-day dose increases compliance<br><br>Check apical pulse; if less than 60 bpm hold medication and call health care provider<br><br>**Do not discontinue abruptly**<br><br>Masks signs of shock and hypoglycemia |
| Metoprolol | Bradycardia, hypotension, heart failure, depression | Give with meals<br><br>Teach client to check pulse before each dose; take apical pulse before administration<br><br>Withhold if pulse less than 60 bpm |
| Nadolol | Bradycardia, hypotension, heart failure | Teach client to check pulse before each dose; check apical pulse before administering<br><br>Withhold if pulse less than 60 bpm<br><br>**Do not discontinue abruptly** |
| Hydralazine | Headache, palpitations, edema, tachycardia, lupus erythematosus-like syndrome | Give with meals<br><br>Observe mental status<br><br>Check for weight gain, edema |
| Minoxidil | Tachycardia, angina pectoris, edema, increase in body hair | Teach client to check pulse; check apical pulse before administration<br><br>Monitor I and O, weight |
| Captopril<br>Enalapril<br>Lisinopril | Dizziness<br><br>Orthostatic hypotension | Report swelling of face, lightheadedness<br><br>ACE-inhibitor medication |
| Propranolol | Weakness<br><br>Hypotension<br><br>Bronchospasm<br><br>Bradycardia<br><br>Depression | Beta blocker: blocks sympathetic impulses to heart<br><br>Client takes pulse at home before each dose<br><br>**Dosage should be reduced gradually before discontinued** |
| Nifedipine<br>Verapamil<br>Diltiazem | Hypotension<br><br>Dizziness<br><br>GI distress<br><br>Liver dysfunction<br><br>Jitteriness | Calcium-channel blocker: reduces workload of left ventricle<br><br>Coronary vasodilator; monitor blood pressure during dosage adjustments<br><br>Assist with ambulation at start of therapy<br><br>Avoid grapefruit juice |

(*Continued*)

Antihypertensive Medications: Overview (*Continued*)

| MEDICATION | ADVERSE EFFECTS | NURSING CONSIDERATIONS |
|---|---|---|
| **Herbal interaction** | Ma-huang (ephedra) decreases effect of antihypertensive medications | |
| | Ephedra increases hypertension when taken with beta blockers | |
| | Black cohosh increases hypotensive effects of antihypertensives | |
| | Goldenseal counteracts effects of antihypertensives | |

Antilipemic Medications

| MEDICATION | ADVERSE EFFECTS | NURSING CONSIDERATIONS |
|---|---|---|
| **Bile acid sequestrants** | | |
| Cholestyramine | Constipation | Increases loss of bile acid in feces; decreases cholesterol |
| Colestipol | Rash | Sprinkle powder on noncarbonated beverage or wet food, let stand 2 min, then stir slowly |
| Nicotinic acid | Fat-soluble vitamin deficiency | Administer 1 hour before or 4–6 hours after other meds to avoid blocking absorption |
| | Abdominal pain and bloating | Instruct client to report constipation immediately |
| **HMG-CoA reductase inhibitors (statins)** | | |
| Lovastatin | Myopathy | Decreases LDL cholesterol levels; causes peripheral vasodilation |
| Pravastatin | Increased liver enzyme levels | Take with food; absorption is reduced by 30% on an empty stomach; avoid alcohol |
| Simvastatin | | Contact health care provider if unexplained muscle pain, especially with fever or malaise |
| Atorvastatin | | Take at night |
| Fluvastatin | | Give with caution with ↓ liver function |
| Rosuvastatin | | Avoid grapefruit juice |

(*Continued*)

Antilipemic Medications (*Continued*)

| MEDICATION | ADVERSE EFFECTS | NURSING CONSIDERATIONS |
|---|---|---|
| | | **Nicotinic acid** |
| Niacin | Flushing<br><br>Hyperglycemia<br><br>Gout<br><br>Upper GI distress<br><br>Liver damage | Decreases total cholesterol, LDL, triglycerides, increases HDL<br><br>Flushing will occur several hours after med is taken, will decrease over 2 wk<br><br>Also used for pellagra and peripheral vascular disease<br><br>Avoid alcohol |
| Folic acid derivatives<br><br>Fenofibrate<br><br>Gemfibrozil | Abdominal pain<br><br>Increased risk gall-bladder disease<br><br>Myalgia and swollen joints | Decreases total cholesterol, VLDL, and triglycerides<br><br>Administer before meals<br><br>Instruct clients to notify health care provider if muscle pain occurs |
| **Action** | Inhibits cholesterol and triglyceride synthesis; decreases serum cholesterol and LDLs | |
| **Indications** | Elevated total and LDL cholesterol<br><br>Primary hypercholesterolemia<br><br>Reduce incidence of cardiovascular disease | |
| **Adverse effects** | Varies with medication | |
| **Nursing considerations** | Medication should be used with dietary measures, physical activity, and cessation of tobacco use<br><br>Lipids should be monitored every 6 wk until normal, then every 4–6 months | |
| **Herbals used to lower cholesterol** | Flax or flax seed—decreases the absorption of other medications<br><br>Garlic—increases the effects of anticoagulants; increases the hypoglycemic effects of insulin<br><br>Green tea—produces a stimulant effect with the tea contains caffeine<br><br>Soy | |

Antineoplastic Medications: Antimetabolites

| Examples | Fluorouracil |
|---|---|
| | Mercaptopurine |
| | Methotrexate |
| **Actions** | Closely resembles normal metabolites, "counterfeits" fool cells; cell division halted |
| **Indications** | Acute lymphatic leukemia |
| | Rheumatoid arthritis |
| | Psoriasis |
| | Cancer of colon, breast, stomach, pancreas |
| | Sickle cell anemia |
| **Adverse effects** | Nausea, vomiting |
| | Diarrhea |
| | Stomatitis and oral ulceration |
| | Hepatic dysfunction |
| | Bone marrow suppression |
| | Renal dysfunction |
| | Alopecia |
| **Nursing considerations** | Monitor hematopoietic function |
| | Good mouth care |
| | Small frequent feedings |
| | Counsel about body image changes (alopecia); provide wig |
| | Good skin care |
| | Photosensitivity precautions |
| | Infection control precautions |

Antineoplastic: Antibiotics

| Examples | Dactinomycin |
|---|---|
| | Doxorubicin |
| **Actions** | Interferes with DNA and RNA synthesis |
| **Indications** | Hodgkin's disease |
| | Non-Hodgkin's lymphoma |
| | Leukemia |
| | Many cancers |

*(Continued)*

Antineoplastic: Antibiotics (*Continued*)

| Adverse effects | Bone marrow depression |
|---|---|
| | Nausea, vomiting |
| | Alopecia |
| | Stomatitis |
| | Heart damage |
| | Septic shock |
| **Nursing considerations** | Monitor closely for septicemic reactions |
| | Monitor for manifestations of extravasation at injection site (severe pain or burning that lasts minutes to hours, redness after injection is completed, ulceration after 48 hours) |
| | Instruct client urine and tears may be red in color |
| | Monitor for signs of heart failure |

Antineoplastic Medications: Cytotoxic Agents

| Examples | Busulfan |
|---|---|
| | Chlorambucil |
| | Cisplatin |
| | Cyclophosphamide |
| **Actions** | Interferes with rapidly reproducing cell DNA |
| **Indications** | Leukemia |
| | Multiple myeloma |
| **Adverse effects** | Bone marrow suppression |
| | Nausea, vomiting |
| | Stomatitis |
| | Alopecia |
| | Gonadal suppression |
| | Renal toxicity (cisplatin) |
| | Ototoxicity |
| **Nursing considerations** | Used with other chemotherapeutic agents |
| | Check hematopoietic function weekly |
| | Encourage fluids (10-12 glasses/day) |

Antineoplastics Medication: Hormonal

| Examples | Antiestrogens: Tamoxifen |
|---|---|
| | Aromatase Inhibitors: Anastrozole, Letrozole, Exemestane |
| | Gonadotropin-Releasing Hormone Agonist: Leuprolide |
| | Gonadotropin-Releasing Hormone Antagonists: Degarelix |
| Actions | Tamoxifen–antiestrogen (competes with estrogen to bind at estrogen receptor sites on malignant cells) |
| | Leuprolide–progestin (causes tumor cell regression by unknown mechanism) |
| | Testolactone–androgen (used for palliation in advanced breast cancer) |
| Indications | Breast cancer |
| Adverse effects | Hypercalcemia |
| | Jaundice |
| | Increased appetite |
| | Masculinization or feminization |
| | Sodium and fluid retention |
| | Nausea, vomiting |
| | Hot flashes |
| | Vaginal dryness |
| Nursing considerations | Baseline and periodic gyn exams recommended |
| | Not given IV |
| | Discuss pregnancy prevention |

Antineoplastic Medications: Topoisomerase

| Examples | Irinotecan |
|---|---|
| | Topotecan |
| Actions | Binds to enzyme that breaks the DNA strands |
| Indications | Ovary, lung, colon, and rectal cancers |
| Adverse effects | Bone marrow suppression |
| | Diarrhea |
| | Nausea, vomiting |
| | Hepatotoxicity |

Antineoplastic Medications: Vinca Alkaloids

| Examples | Vinblastine |
| --- | --- |
| | Vincristine |
| **Actions** | Interferes with cell division |
| **Indications** | Hodgkin's disease |
| | Lymphoma |
| | Cancers |
| **Adverse effects** | Bone marrow suppression (mild with VCR) |
| | Neuropathies (VCR) |
| | Stomatitis |
| **Nursing considerations** | Same as antitumor antibiotics |

Antineoplastic Medications: Overview (also see each individual table)

| MEDICATION | ADVERSE EFFECTS | NURSING CONSIDERATIONS |
| --- | --- | --- |
| **Alkylating Medications** | | |
| Busulfan | Bone marrow depression | Check CBC (applies to all medications in this table) |
| | | Most chemotherapy causes stomatitis and requires extra fluids to flush system |
| Chlorambucil | Nausea, vomiting, bone marrow depression, sterility | Monitor for infection |
| | | Avoid IM injections when platelet count is low to minimize bleeding |
| Cyclophosphamide | Alopecia, bone marrow depression, hemorrhagic cystitis, dermatitis, hyperkalemia, hypoglycemia, amenorrhea | Report hematuria, force fluids |
| | | Monitor for infection |
| | | Give antiemetics |
| **Antimetabolites** | | |
| Fluorouracil | Nausea, stomatitis, GI ulceration, diarrhea, bone marrow depression, liver dysfunction, alopecia | Monitor for infection |
| | | Avoid extravasation |
| Methotrexate | Oral and GI ulceration, liver damage, bone marrow depression, stomatitis, alopecia, bloody diarrhea, fatigue | Good mouth care, avoid alcohol |
| | | Monitor hepatic and renal function tests |

(Continued)

Antineoplastic Medications: Overview (also see each individual table) (*Continued*)

| MEDICATION | ADVERSE EFFECTS | NURSING CONSIDERATIONS |
|---|---|---|
| Mercaptopurine | Liver damage, bone marrow depression, infection, alopecia, abdominal bleeding | Check liver function tests |
| Cytarabine | Hematologic abnormalities, nausea, vomiting, rash, weight loss | Force fluids<br><br>Good oral hygiene |
| Hydroxyurea | Bone marrow depression, GI symptoms, rash | Teach client to report toxic GI symptoms promptly |
| **Antibiotic Antineoplastics** | | |
| Doxorubicin | Red urine, nausea, vomiting, stomatitis, alopecia, cardiotoxicity, blisters, bone marrow depression | Check EKG, avoid IV infiltration<br><br>Monitor vital signs closely<br><br>Good mouth care |
| Bleomycin | Nausea, vomiting, alopecia, edema of hands, pulmonary fibrosis, fever, bone marrow depression | Observe for pulmonary complications, treat fever with acetaminophen<br><br>Check breath sounds frequently |
| Dactinomycin | Nausea, bone marrow depression | Give antiemetic before administration |
| **Vinca Alkaloids** | | |
| Vinblastine | Nausea, vomiting, stomatitis, alopecia, loss of reflexes, bone marrow depression | Avoid IV infiltration and extravasation<br><br>Give antiemetic before administration<br><br>Acute bronchospasm can occur if given IV<br><br>Allopurinol given to increase excretion and decrease buildup of urates (uric acid) |
| Vincristine | Peripheral neuritis, loss of reflexes, bone marrow depression, alopecia, GI symptoms | Avoid IV infiltration and extravasation<br><br>Check reflexes, motor and sensory function<br><br>Allopurinol given to increase excretion and decrease buildup of urates (uric acid) |
| **Hormonal Medications** | | |
| Tamoxifen | Transient fall in WBC or platelets Hypercalcemia, bone pain | Check CBC<br><br>Monitor serum calcium<br><br>Nonsteroidal antiestrogen |

Antineoplastic Medications: Nursing Implications for Adverse Effects

| | |
|---|---|
| Bone marrow suppression | Monitor bleeding: bleeding gums, bruising, petechiae, guaiac stools, urine and emesis |
| | Avoid IM injections and rectal temperatures |
| | Apply pressure to venipuncture sites |
| Nausea, vomiting | Monitor intake and output ratios, appetite and nutritional intake |
| | Prophylactic antiemetics may be used |
| | Smaller, more frequent meals |
| Altered immunologic response | Prevent infection by handwashing |
| | Timely reporting of alterations in vital signs or symptoms indicating possible infection |
| Impaired oral mucous membrane; stomatitis | Oral hygiene measures |
| Fatigue | Encourage rest and discuss measures to conserve energy |
| | Use relaxation techniques, mental imagery |

Antiparkinson Medications

| MEDICATION | ADVERSE EFFECTS | NURSING CONSIDERATIONS |
|---|---|---|
| Trihexyphenidyl | Dry mouth | Acts by blocking acetylcholine at cerebral synaptic sites |
| | Blurred vision | |
| | Constipation, urinary hesitancy | Intraocular pressure should be monitored |
| | Decreased mental acuity, difficulty concentrating, confusion, hallucination | Supervise ambulation |
| | | Causes nausea if given before meals |
| | | Suck on hard candy for dry mouth |
| Benztropine mesylate | Drowsiness, nausea, vomiting | Acts by lessening cholinergic effect of dopamine deficiency |
| | Atropine-like effects—blurred vision, mydriasis | Suppresses tremor of Parkinsonism |
| | Antihistaminic effects—sedation, dizziness | Most adverse effects are reversed by changes in dosage |
| | | Additional drowsiness can occur with other CNS depressants |

Antiparkinson Medications (*Continued*)

| MEDICATION | ADVERSE EFFECTS | NURSING CONSIDERATIONS |
|---|---|---|
| Levodopa | Nausea and vomiting, anorexia<br><br>Postural hypotension<br><br>Mental changes: confusion, agitation, mood alterations<br><br>Cardiac arrhythmias<br><br>Twitching | Precursor of dopamine<br><br>Thought to restore dopamine levels in extrapyramidal centers<br><br>Administered in large prolonged doses<br><br>Contraindicated in glaucoma, hemolytic anemia<br><br>Give with food<br><br>Monitor for postural hypotension<br><br>Avoid OTC meds and foods that contain vitamin $B_6$ (pyridoxine); reverses effects |
| Bromocriptine mesylate<br><br>Pergolide | Dizziness, headache, hypotension<br><br>Tinnitus<br><br>Nausea, abdominal cramps<br><br>Pleural effusion<br><br>Orthostatic hypotension | Give with meals<br><br>May lead to early postpartum conception<br><br>Monitor cardiac, hepatic, renal, hematopoietic function |
| Carbidopa–Levodopa | Hemolytic anemia<br><br>Dystonic movements, ataxia<br><br>Orthostatic hypotension<br><br>Dysrhythmias<br><br>GI upset, dry mouth | Stimulates dopamine receptors<br><br>Don't use with MAO inhibitors<br><br>Advise to change positions slowly<br><br>Take with food |
| Amantadine | CNS disturbances, hyperexcitability<br><br>Insomnia, vertigo, ataxia<br><br>Slurred speech, convulsions | Enhances effect of L-Dopa<br><br>Contraindicated in epilepsy, arteriosclerosis<br><br>Antiviral |
| **Action** | Levodopa—precursor to dopamine that is converted to dopamine in the brain<br><br>Bromocriptine—stimulates postsynaptic dopamine receptors | |
| **Indications** | Parkinson's disease | |
| **Adverse effects** | Dizziness<br><br>Ataxia<br><br>Confusion<br><br>Psychosis<br><br>Hemolytic anemia | |

(*Continued*)

Antiparkinson Medications (*Continued*)

| MEDICATION | ADVERSE EFFECTS | NURSING CONSIDERATIONS |
|---|---|---|
| **Nursing considerations** | Monitor for urinary retention<br><br>Large doses of pyridoxine (vitamin B$_6$) decrease or reverse effects of medication<br><br>Avoid use of other CNS depressants (alcohol, narcotics, sedatives)<br><br>Anticholinergics, dopamine agonists, MAO inhibitors, catechol-*O*-methyltransferase (COMT) inhibitors, and antidepressants may also be used | |

Antiplatelet Medications

| MEDICATION | ADVERSE EFFECTS | NURSING CONSIDERATIONS |
|---|---|---|
| Adenosine diphosphate (ADP) receptor antagonists<br><br>Ticlopidine<br><br>Clopidogrel | Thrombocytopenic purpura<br><br>GI upset | Prevents platelet aggregation<br><br>Higher risk of hemorrhage with ticlopidine |
| Dipyridamole<br><br>Dipyridamole plus aspirin | Headache<br><br>Dizziness<br><br>EKG changes<br><br>Hypertension, hypotension | Administer 1 h ac or with meals<br><br>Monitor BP<br><br>Check for signs of bleeding |
| Glycoprotein IIb and IIIa receptor antagonists<br><br>Eptifibatide<br><br>Abciximab | GI, retroperitoneal, and urogenital bleeding | Does not increase risk of fatal hemorrhage or hemorrhagic stroke |
| Salicylates | Short-term use—GI bleeding, heartburn, occasional nausea<br><br>Prolonged high dosage—salicylism: metabolic acidosis, respiratory alkalosis, dehydration, fluid and electrolyte imbalance, tinnitus | Observe for bleeding gums, bloody or black stools, bruises<br><br>Give with milk, water, or food, or use enteric-coated tablets to minimize gastric distress<br><br>Contraindications—GI disorders, severe anemia, vitamin K deficiency<br><br>Anti-inflammatory, analgesic, antipyretic |
| **Action** | Interferes with platelet aggregation | |

(*Continued*)

Antiplatelet Medications (*Continued*)

| MEDICATION | ADVERSE EFFECTS | NURSING CONSIDERATIONS |
|---|---|---|
| **Indications** | Venous thrombosis | |
| | Pulmonary embolism | |
| | CVA and acute coronary prevention | |
| | Post cardiac surgery; post percutaneous coronary interventions | |
| | Acute coronary syndrome | |
| **Adverse effects** | Hemorrhage, bleeding | |
| | Thrombocytopenia | |
| | Hematuria | |
| | Hemoptysis | |
| **Nursing considerations** | Teach client to check for signs of bleeding | |
| | Inform health care provider or dentist before procedures | |
| | Older adults at higher risk for ototoxicity | |
| | Instruct client to contact health care provider before taking any over-the-counter medications | |
| | Instruct client to avoid ginkgo, garlic and ginger herbal preparations | |
| **Gerontologic considerations** | Dipyridamole causes orthostatic hypotension in older adults | |
| | Ticlopidine–greater risk of toxicity with older adults | |

Antipsychotic Medications

| MEDICATION | ADVERSE EFFECTS | NURSING CONSIDERATIONS |
|---|---|---|
| **Conventional high potency** | | |
| Haloperidol | Low sedative effect | Used in large doses for assaultive clients |
| Fluphenazine | Low incidence of hypotension | Used with older adults (risk of falling reduced) |
| | High incidence of extrapyramidal adverse effects | Decanoate: long-acting form given every 2–4 wk; |
| | | IM into deep muscle Z-track |

(*Continued*)

Antipsychotic Medications (*Continued*)

| MEDICATION | ADVERSE EFFECTS | NURSING CONSIDERATIONS |
|---|---|---|
| **Conventional medium potency** | | |
| Perphenazine | Orthostatic hypotension<br><br>Dry mouth Constipation | Can help control severe vomiting<br><br>Medication is available PO, IM, and IV |
| **Conventional low potency** | | |
| Chlorpromazine | High sedative effect<br><br>High incidence of hypotension<br><br>Irreversible retinitis pigmentosus at 800 mg/day | Educate client about increased sensitivity to sun (as with other phenothiazines)<br><br>No tolerance or potential for abuse |
| **Atypical** | | |
| Risperidone | Moderate orthostatic hypotension<br><br>Moderate sedation<br><br>Significant weight gain<br><br>Doses over 6 mg can cause tardive dyskinesia | Chosen as first-line antipsychotic due to mild EPS and very low anticholinergic adverse effects |
| Quetiapine | Moderate orthostatic hypotension<br><br>Moderate sedation<br><br>Very low risk of tardive dyskinesia and neuroleptic malignant syndrome | Chosen as first-line antipsychotic due to mild EPS and very low anticholinergic adverse effects |
| Ziprasidone<br>Aripiprazole<br>Clozapine<br>Olanzapine | ECG changes—QT prolongation | Effective with depressive symptoms of schizophrenia<br><br>Low propensity for weight gain |
| **Action** | Blocks dopamine receptors in basal ganglia of brain, inhibiting transmission of nerve impulses | |
| **Indications** | Acute and chronic psychosis | |

*(Continued)*

Antipsychotic Medications (*Continued*)

| MEDICATION | ADVERSE EFFECTS | NURSING CONSIDERATIONS |
|---|---|---|
| **Adverse effects** | Akathisia (motor restlessness) | |
| | Dyskinesia (abnormal voluntary movements) | |
| | Dystonias (abnormal muscle tone producing spasms of tongue, face, neck) | |
| | Parkinson syndrome (shuffling gait, rigid muscles, excessive salivation, tremors, mask-like face, motor deceleration) | |
| | Tardive dyskinesia (involuntary movements of mouth, tongue, trunk, extremities; chewing motions, sucking, tongue thrusting) | |
| | Photosensitivity | |
| | Orthostatic hypotension | |
| | Neuroleptic malignant syndrome | |
| **Nursing considerations** | Lowers seizure threshold | |
| | May slow growth rate in children | |
| | Monitor for urinary retention and decreased GI motility | |
| | Avoid alcohol | |
| | May cause hypotension if taken with antihypertensives, nitrates | |
| | Phenothiazines also used | |

Antipsychotic Medications: Adverse Effects

| MEDICATION | ADVERSE EFFECTS | NURSING CONSIDERATIONS |
|---|---|---|
| Extrapyramidal | Pseudoparkinsonism | Pharmacologic management of Parkinsonian adverse effects: benztropine or trihexyphenidyl |
| | Dystonia (muscle spasm) | |
| | Acute dystonic reaction | Recognize early symptoms of acute dystonic reaction |
| | Early signs: tightening of jaw, stiff neck, swollen tongue | |
| | Late signs: swollen airway, oculogyric crisis | Notify health care provider for IM diphenhydramine protocol |
| | Akathisia (inability to sit or stand still, foot tap, pace) | |
| | Tardive dyskinesia (abnormal, involuntary movements); may be irreversible | |

(*Continued*)

Antipsychotic Medications: Adverse Effects (*Continued*)

| MEDICATION | ADVERSE EFFECTS | NURSING CONSIDERATIONS |
|---|---|---|
| Anticholinergic | Blurred vision<br><br>Dry mouth<br><br>Nasal congestion<br><br>Constipation<br><br>Acute urinary retention | Educate client that some anticholinergic adverse effects often diminish over time<br><br>Maintain adequate fluid intake and monitor I and O |
| Sedative | Sleepiness<br><br>Possible danger if driving or operating machinery | Monitor sedative effects and maintain client safety |
| Hypotensive | Orthostatic hypotension is common | Frequent monitoring of BP and advise client to rise slowly |
| Other | Phototoxicity | Educate client regarding need for sunscreen |
| Neuroleptic malignant syndrome | Rigidity<br><br>Fever<br><br>Sweating<br><br>Autonomic dysfunction (dysrhythmias, fluctuations in BP)<br><br>Confusion<br><br>Seizures, coma | Immediately withdraw antipsychotics<br><br>Control hyperthermia<br><br>Hydration<br><br>Dantrolene (muscle relaxant) used for rigidity and severe reactions<br><br>Bromocriptine (dopamine receptor antagonist) used for CNS toxicity and mild reactions |
| Atropine psychosis | Skin hot to touch without fever–"red as a beet" (flushed face)<br><br>Dehydration–"dry as a bone"<br><br>Altered mental status–"mad as a hatter" | Reduce or discontinue medication<br><br>Hydration<br><br>Stay with client while confused, for safety |

Antipsychotic Medications: Degree of Adverse Effects

| ACTION | BLOCKS POSTSYNAPTIC DOPAMINE RECEPTORS IN BRAIN |
|---|---|
| **Indications** | Psychotic disorders |
| | Severe nausea and vomiting |
| **Adverse effects** | Drowsiness |
| | Pseudoparkinsonism |
| | Dystonia |
| | Akathisia |
| | Tardive dyskinesia |
| | Neuroleptic malignant syndrome |
| | Dysrhythmias |
| | Photophobia |
| | Blurred vision |
| | Photosensitivity |
| | Lactation |
| | Discolors urine pink to red-brown |
| **Nursing considerations** | May cause false-positive pregnancy tests |
| | Dilute oral concentrate with water, saline, 7-Up, homogenized milk, carbonated orange drink, fruit juices (pineapple, orange, apricot, prune, V-8, tomato, use 60 mL for each 5 mL of medication |
| | Do not mix with beverages that contain caffeine (coffee, tea, cola) or apple juice; incompatible |
| | Monitor vital signs |
| | Takes 4–6 weeks to achieve steady plasma levels |
| | Monitor bowel function |
| | Monitor older adults for dehydration (sedation and decreased thirst sensation) |
| | Avoid activities requiring mental alertness |
| | Avoid exposure to sun |
| | Maintain fluid intake |
| | May have anticholinergic and antihistamine actions |

Antipsychotic Medications: Degree of Adverse Effects for Selected Antipsychotics

| MEDICATION | EXTRA PYRAMIDAL | ANTI CHOLINERGIC | SEDATIVE | HYPOTENSIVE |
|---|---|---|---|---|
| Chlorpromazine | ↑ | ↑↑ | ↑↑↑ | ↑↑↑ |
| Thioridazine | ↑ | ↑↑↑ | ↑↑↑ | ↑↑ |
| Trifluoperazine | ↑↑↑ | ↑ | ↑ | ↑ |
| Fluphenazine | ↑↑↑ | ↑ | ↑ | ↑ |
| Perphenazine | ↑↑↑ | ↑ | ↑↑ | ↑ |
| Haloperidol | ↑↑↑ | ↑ | ↑ | ↑ |
| Thiothixene | ↑↑ | ↑ | ↑ | ↑↑ |

KEY: ↑ mild; ↑↑ moderate; ↑↑↑ severe

Antipyretic Medications

| MEDICATION | ADVERSE EFFECTS | NURSING CONSIDERATIONS |
|---|---|---|
| Acetaminophen | Overdosage may be fatal<br>GI adverse effects are not common | Do not exceed recommended dose |
| Salicylates | Short-term use—GI bleeding, heartburn, occasional nausea<br><br>Prolonged high dosage—salicylism: metabolic acidosis, respiratory alkalosis, dehydration, fluid and electrolyte imbalance, tinnitus | Observe for bleeding gums, bloody or black stools, bruises<br><br>Give with milk, water, or food, or use enteric-coated tablets to minimize gastric distress<br><br>Contraindications—GI disorders, severe anemia, vitamin K deficiency<br><br>Anti-inflammatory, analgesic, antipyretic |
| **Action** | Antiprostaglandin activity in hypothalamus reduces fever; causes peripheral vasodilation; anti-inflammatory actions | |
| **Indications** | Fever | |

*(Continued)*

Antipyretic Medications (*Continued*)

| MEDICATION | ADVERSE EFFECTS | NURSING CONSIDERATIONS |
|---|---|---|
| **Adverse effects** | GI irritation<br><br>Occult bleeding<br><br>Tinnitus<br><br>Dizziness<br><br>Confusion<br><br>Liver dysfunction (acetaminophen) | |
| **Nursing considerations** | Aspirin contraindicated for client less than 21 years old due to risk of Reye syndrome<br><br>Aspirin contraindicated for clients with bleeding disorders due to anticlotting activity<br><br>NSAIDs are also used for fever | |

Antithyroid Medications

| MEDICATION | ADVERSE EFFECTS | NURSING CONSIDERATIONS |
|---|---|---|
| Methimazole<br>Propylthiouracil | Leukopenia, fever<br><br>Rash, sore throat<br><br>Jaundice | Inhibits synthesis of thyroid hormone by thyroid gland<br><br>Check CBC and hepatic function<br><br>Give with meals<br><br>Report fever, sore throat to health care provider |
| Iodine solution<br>Potassium iodide | Nausea, vomiting, metallic taste<br><br>Rash | Iodine preparation<br><br>Used 2 weeks prior to surgery; decreases vascularity, decreases hormone release<br><br>Only effective for a short period<br><br>Give after meals<br><br>Dilute in water, milk, or fruit juice<br><br>Stains teeth<br><br>Give through straw |
| Radioactive iodine ($^{131}$I) | Feeling of fullness in neck<br><br>Metallic taste<br><br>Leukemia | Destroys thyroid tissue<br><br>Contraindicated for women of childbearing age<br><br>Fast overnight before administration<br><br>Urine, saliva, vomit radioactive 3 days<br><br>Use full radiation precautions<br><br>Encourage fluids |

(*Continued*)

Antithyroid Medications (*Continued*)

| MEDICATION | ADVERSE EFFECTS | NURSING CONSIDERATIONS |
|---|---|---|
| **Action** | Antithyroid medications—inhibit oxidation of iodine | |
| | Iodines—reduce vascularity of thyroid gland; increases amount of inactive (bound) hormone; inhibits release of thyroid hormones into circulation | |
| **Indications** | Hyperthyroidism | |
| | Thyrotoxic crisis | |
| **Adverse effects** | Nausea, vomiting | |
| | Diarrhea | |
| | Rashes | |
| | Thrombocytopenia | |
| | Leukopenia | |
| **Nursing considerations** | Changes in vital signs or weight and appearance may indicate adverse reactions, which should lead to evaluation of continued medication use | |

Thyroid Replacement Medications

| MEDICATION | ADVERSE EFFECTS | NURSING CONSIDERATIONS |
|---|---|---|
| Levothyroxine | Nervousness, tremors | Tell client to report chest pain, palpitations, sweating, nervousness, shortness of breath to health care provider |
| | Insomnia | |
| | Tachycardia, palpitations | |
| | Dysrhythmias, angina | |
| Liothyronine sodium | Excessive dosages produce symptoms of hyperthyroidism | Take at same time each day |
| | | Take in AM |
| | | Monitor pulse and BP |
| **Action** | Increases metabolic rate of body | |
| **Indications** | Hypothyroidism | |
| **Adverse effects** | Nervousness | |
| | Tachycardia | |
| | Weight loss | |

(*Continued*)

Thyroid Replacement Medications (*Continued*)

| MEDICATION | ADVERSE EFFECTS | NURSING CONSIDERATIONS |
|---|---|---|
| **Nursing considerations** | Obtain history of client's medications | |
| | Enhances action of oral anticoagulants, antidepressants | |
| | Decreases action of insulin, digitalis | |
| | Obtain baseline vital signs | |
| | Monitor weight | |
| | Avoid OTC medications | |

Antituberculotic Medications

| MEDICATION | ADVERSE EFFECTS | NURSING CONSIDERATIONS |
|---|---|---|
| | | **First-line medications** |
| Isoniazid | Hepatitis | Pyridoxine ($B_6$): 10–50 mg as prophylaxis for neuritis; 50–100 mg as treatment |
| | Peripheral neuritis | Teach signs of hepatitis |
| | Rash | Check liver function tests |
| | Fever | Alcohol increases risk of hepatic complications |
| | | Therapeutic effects can be expected after 2–3 weeks of therapy |
| | | Monitor for resolution of symptoms (fever, night sweats, weight loss); hypotension (orthostatic) may occur initially, then resolve; caution client to change position slowly |
| | | Give before meals |
| | | Do not combine with phenytoin, causes phenytoin toxicity |
| Ethambutol | Optic neuritis | Use cautiously with renal disease |
| | | Check visual acuity |
| Rifampin | Hepatitis | Orange urine, tears, saliva |
| | Fever | Check liver function tests |
| | | Can take with food |
| Streptomycin | Nephrotoxicity | Check creatinine and BUN |
| | VIII nerve damage | Audiograms if given long-term |

(*Continued*)

Antituberculotic Medications (*Continued*)

| MEDICATION | ADVERSE EFFECTS | NURSING CONSIDERATIONS |
|---|---|---|
| **Second-line medications** | | |
| Para-amino-salicylic acid | GI disturbances<br>Hepatotoxicity | Check for ongoing GI adverse effects |
| Pyrazinamide | Hyperuricemia<br>Anemia<br>Anorexia | Check liver function tests, uric acid, and hematopoietic studies |
| **Action** | Inhibits cell wall and protein synthesis of *Mycobacterium tuberculosis* | |
| **Indications** | Tuberculosis<br>INH—used to prevent disease in person exposed to organism | |
| **Adverse effects** | Hepatitis<br>Optic neuritis<br>Seizures<br>Peripheral neuritis | |
| **Nursing considerations** | Used in combination (2 medications or more)<br>Monitor for liver damage and hepatitis<br>With active TB, the client should cover mouth and nose when coughing, confine used tissues to plastic bags, and wear a mask with crowds until three sputum cultures are negative (no longer infectious)<br>In health care facilities, client is placed under airborne precautions and workers wear a N95 or high-efficiency particulate air (HEPA) respirator until the client is no longer infectious | |

## Antitussive/Expectorant Medications

| MEDICATION | ADVERSE EFFECTS | NURSING CONSIDERATIONS |
|---|---|---|
| Dextromethorphan hydrobromide | Drowsiness<br><br>Dizziness | Antitussive<br><br>Onset occurs within 30 min, lasts 3-6 hours<br><br>Monitor cough type and frequency |
| Guaifenesin | Dizziness<br><br>Headache<br><br>Nausea, vomiting | Expectorant<br><br>Monitor cough type and frequency<br><br>Take with glass of water |
| **Action** | Antitussives—suppresses cough reflex by inhibiting cough center in medulla<br><br>Expectorants—decreases viscosity of bronchial secretions | |
| **Indications** | Coughs due to URI<br><br>COPD | |
| **Adverse effects** | Respiratory depression<br><br>Hypotension<br><br>Bradycardia<br><br>Anticholinergic effects<br><br>Photosensitivity | |
| **Nursing considerations** | Older adult clients may need reduced dosages<br><br>Avoid alcohol | |

## Antiviral Medications

| MEDICATION | ADVERSE EFFECTS | NURSING CONSIDERATIONS |
|---|---|---|
| Acyclovir | Headaches, dizziness<br><br>Seizures<br><br>Diarrhea | Used for herpes simplex and herpes zoster<br><br>Given PO, IV, topically<br><br>Does not prevent transmission of disease<br><br>Slows progression of symptoms<br><br>Encourage fluids<br><br>Check liver and renal function tests |

(Continued)

Antiviral Medications (*Continued*)

| MEDICATION | ADVERSE EFFECTS | NURSING CONSIDERATIONS |
|---|---|---|
| Ribavirin | Worsening of pulmonary status, bacterial pneumonia<br><br>Hypotension, cardiac arrest | Used for severe lower respiratory tract infections in infants and children<br><br>Must use special aerosol-generating device for administration<br><br>Can precipitate<br><br>Contraindicated in females who may become pregnant during treatment |
| Zidovudine | Anemia<br><br>Headache<br><br>Anorexia, diarrhea, nausea, GI pain<br><br>Paresthesias, dizziness<br><br>Insomnia<br><br>Agranulocytosis | Used for HIV infection<br><br>Teach clients to strictly comply with dosage schedule |
| Zalcitabine | Oral ulcers<br><br>Peripheral neuropathy, headache<br><br>Vomiting, diarrhea<br><br>CHF, cardiomyopathy | Used in combination with zidovudine for advanced HIV |
| Didanosine | Headache<br><br>Rhinitis, cough<br><br>Diarrhea, nausea, vomiting<br><br>Pancreatitis, granulocytopenia<br><br>Peripheral neuropathy<br><br>Seizures<br><br>Hemorrhage | Used for HIV infection<br><br>Monitor liver and renal function studies<br><br>Note baseline vital signs and weight<br><br>Take on empty stomach<br><br>Chew or crush tablets |
| Famciclovir | Fatigue, fever<br><br>Nausea, vomiting, diarrhea, constipation<br><br>Headache, sinusitis | Used for acute herpes zoster (shingles)<br><br>Obtain baseline CBC and renal function studies<br><br>Remind clients they are contagious when lesions are open and draining |

(*Continued*)

Antiviral Medications (*Continued*)

| MEDICATION | ADVERSE EFFECTS | NURSING CONSIDERATIONS |
|---|---|---|
| Ganciclovir | Fever | Used for retinitis caused by cytomegalovirus |
| | Rash | Check level of consciousness |
| | Leukemia | Monitor CBC, I and O |
| | Seizures | Report any dizziness, confusions, seizures immediately |
| | GI hemorrhage | Need regular eye exams |
| | MI, stroke | |
| Amantadine | Dizziness | Used for prophylaxis and treatment of influenza A |
| | Nervousness | Orthostatic hypotension precautions |
| | Insomnia | Instruct clients to avoid hazardous activities |
| | Orthostatic hypotension | |
| Oseltamivir | Nausea, vomiting | Used for the treatment of Types A and B influenza |
| Zanamivir | Cough and throat irritation | Best effect if given within 2 days of infection |
| | | Instruct clients that medication will reduce flu-symptom duration |
| **Action** | Inhibits DNA or RNA replication in virus | |
| **Indications** | Recurrent HSV 1 and 2 in immunocompromised clients | |
| | Encephalitis | |
| | Herpes zoster | |
| | HIV infections | |
| **Adverse effects** | Vertigo | |
| | Depression | |
| | Headache | |
| | Hematuria | |
| **Nursing considerations** | Encourage fluids | |
| | Small, frequent feedings | |
| | Good skin care | |
| | Wear glove when applying topically | |
| | Not a cure, but relieves symptoms | |

Attention-Deficit Hyperactivity Disorder Medications

| MEDICATION | ADVERSE EFFECTS | NURSING CONSIDERATIONS |
|---|---|---|
| Methylphenidate | Nervousness, palpitations<br><br>Insomnia<br><br>Tachycardia<br><br>Weight loss, growth suppression | May precipitate Tourette's syndrome<br><br>Monitor CBC, platelet count<br><br>Has paradoxical calming effect in ADD<br><br>Monitor height/weight in children<br><br>Monitor BP<br><br>Avoid drinks with caffeine<br><br>Give at least 6 hours before bedtime<br><br>Give pc |
| Dextroamphetamine sulfate | Insomnia<br><br>Tachycardia, palpitations | Controlled substance<br><br>May alter insulin needs<br><br>Give in AM to prevent insomnia<br><br>Don't use with MAO inhibitor (possible hypertensive crisis) |
| **Action** | Increases level of catecholamines in cerebral cortex and reticular activating system | |
| **Indications** | Attention-deficit hyperactivity disorder (ADHD)<br><br>Narcolepsy | |
| **Adverse effects** | Restlessness<br><br>Insomnia<br><br>Tremors<br><br>Tachycardia<br><br>Seizures | |
| **Nursing considerations** | Monitor growth rate in children | |

Bipolar Disorder Medications

| MEDICATION | ADVERSE EFFECTS | NURSING CONSIDERATIONS |
|---|---|---|
| Lithium | Dizziness<br><br>Headache<br><br>Impaired vision<br><br>Fine hand tremors<br><br>Reversible leukocytosis | Use for control of manic episodes in the syndrome of manic-depressive psychosis; mood stabilizer<br><br>Blood levels must be monitored frequently<br><br>GI symptoms can be reduced if taken with meals<br><br>Therapeutic effects preceded by lag of 1–2 weeks<br><br>Signs of intoxication—vomiting, diarrhea, drowsiness, muscular weakness, ataxia<br><br>Dosage is usually halved during depressive stages of illness<br><br>Initial blood target level = 1–1.5 mEq/L(1-1.5 mmol/L)<br><br>Maintenance blood target level = 0.8-1.2 mEq/L (0.8-1.2 mmol/L)<br><br>Check serum levels 2-3 times weekly when started and monthly while on maintenance; serum levels should be drawn in AM prior to dose<br><br>Should have fluid intake of 2,500–3,000 mL/day and adequate salt intake |
| Carbamazepine | Dizziness, vertigo<br><br>Drowsiness<br><br>Ataxia<br><br>CHF<br><br>Aplastic anemia, thrombocytopenia | Mood stabilizer used with bipolar disorder<br><br>Traditionally used for seizures and trigeminal neuralgia<br><br>Obtain baseline urinalysis, BUN, liver function tests, CBC<br><br>Shake oral suspension well before measuring dose<br><br>When giving by NG tube, mix with equal volume of water, 0.9% NaCl or $D_5$ W, then flush with 100 mL after dose<br><br>Take with food<br><br>Avoid grapefruit juice<br><br>Drowsiness usually disappears in 3–4 days |
| Divalproex sodium | Sedation<br><br>Pancreatitis<br><br>Indigestion<br><br>Thrombocytopenia<br><br>Toxic hepatitis | Mood stabilizers used with bipolar disorder<br><br>Traditionally used for seizures<br><br>Monitor liver function tests, platelet count before starting med and periodically after med<br><br>Teach client symptoms of liver dysfunction (e.g., malaise, fever, lethargy)<br><br>Monitor blood levels<br><br>Take with food or milk<br><br>Avoid hazardous activities |

*(Continued)*

Bipolar Disorder Medications (*Continued*)

| MEDICATION | ADVERSE EFFECTS | NURSING CONSIDERATIONS |
|---|---|---|
| **Action** | Reduces amount of catecholamines released into synapse and increases reuptake of norepinephrine and serotonin from synaptic space; competes with $Na^+$ and $K^+$ transport in nerve and muscle cells | |
| **Indications** | Manic episodes | |
| **Adverse effects** | GI upset | |
| | Tremors | |
| | Polydipsia, polyuria | |
| **Nursing considerations** | Monitor serum levels carefully | |
| | Severe toxicity: exaggerated reflexes, seizures, coma, death | |

Bone-Resorption Inhibitors (Bisphosphonates) Medications

| MEDICATION | ADVERSE EFFECTS | NURSING CONSIDERATIONS |
|---|---|---|
| Alendronate | Esophagitis | Prevention and treatment of postmenopausal osteoporosis, Paget disease, glucocorticoid-induced osteoporosis |
| Risedronate | Arthralgia | |
| Ibandronate | Nausea, diarrhea | Instruct clients to take medication in the morning with 6–8 ounces of water before eating and to remain in upright position for 30 minutes |
| | | Bone density tests may be monitored |

Bronchodilators/Mucolytic Medications

| MEDICATION | ADVERSE EFFECTS | NURSING CONSIDERATIONS |
|---|---|---|
| Terbutaline sulfate | Nervousness, tremor | Short-acting beta agonist most useful when about to enter environment or begin activity likely to induce asthma attack |
| | Headache | |
| | Tachycardia | Pulse and blood pressure should be checked before each dose |
| | Palpitations | |
| | Fatigue | |

(*Continued*)

Bronchodilators/Mucolytic Medications (*Continued*)

| MEDICATION | ADVERSE EFFECTS | NURSING CONSIDERATIONS |
|---|---|---|
| Ipratropium bromide<br>Tiotropium | Nervousness<br>Tremor<br>Dry mouth<br>Palpitations | Cholinergic antagonist<br>Don't mix in nebulizer with cromolyn sodium<br>Not for acute treatment<br>Teach use of metered dose inhaler: inhale, hold breath, exhale slowly |
| Albuterol | Tremors<br>Headache<br>Hyperactivity<br>Tachycardia | Short-acting beta agonist most useful when about to enter environment or begin activity likely to induce asthma attack<br>Monitor for toxicity if using tablets and aerosol<br>Teach how to correctly use inhaler |
| Epinephrine | Cerebral hemorrhage<br>Hypertension<br>Tachycardia | When administered IV monitor BP, heart rate, EKG<br>If used with steroid inhaler, use bronchodilator first, then wait 5 minutes before using steroid inhaler (opens airway for maximum effectiveness) |
| Salmeterol | Headache<br>Pharyngitis<br>Nervousness<br>Tremors | Dry powder preparation<br>Not for acute bronchospasm or exacerbations |
| Montelukast sodium<br>Zafirlukast<br>Zileuton | Headache<br>GI distress | Used for prophylactic and maintenance therapy of asthma<br>Liver tests may be monitored<br>Interacts with theophylline |
| Acetylcysteine | Bronchospasm<br>Nausea<br>Vomiting | Mucolytic<br>Administered by nebulization into face mask or mouthpiece<br>Bronchospasm most likely to occur in asthmatics<br>Open vials should be refrigerated and used within 90 hours<br>Clients should clear airway by coughing prior to aerosol |

Carbonic Anhydrase Inhibitor Medications

| MEDICATION | ADVERSE EFFECTS | NURSING CONSIDERATIONS |
|---|---|---|
| Acetazolamide | Lethargy, depression<br><br>Anorexia, weakness<br><br>Decreased $K^+$ level, confusion | Used for glaucoma<br><br>Assess client's mental status before repeating dose |
| **Action** | Decreases production of aqueous humor in ciliary body | |
| **Indications** | Open-angle glaucoma | |
| **Adverse effects** | Blurred vision<br><br>Lacrimation<br><br>Pulmonary edema | |
| **Nursing considerations** | Monitor client for systemic effects | |

Cardiac Glycoside (Digitalis) Medications

| MEDICATION | ADVERSE EFFECTS | NURSING CONSIDERATIONS |
|---|---|---|
| Digoxin | Anorexia<br><br>Nausea<br><br>Bradycardia<br><br>Visual disturbances<br><br>Confusion<br><br>Abdominal pain | Administer with caution to older adults or clients with renal insufficiency<br><br>Monitor renal function and electrolytes<br><br>Instruct clients to eat high-potassium foods<br><br>Take apical pulse for 1 full minute before administering<br><br>Notify health care provider if apical pulse less than 60 (adult), less than 90–110 (infants and young children), less than 70 (older children)<br><br>Digitalizing dose (oral) aimed at administering the medication in divided dosages over a period of 24 hours or days until an "optimum" cardiac effect is reached. Not used frequently. –0.5 to 0.75 mg PO, then 0.25 mg PO every 6–8 hrs to a total dose of 1–1.5 mg<br><br>Digitalizing dose (IV)–0.25 to 0.5 mg IV, then 0.25 mg IV to a total dose of 1 mg<br><br>Digoxin immune fab–used for treatment of life-threatening toxicity<br><br>Maintenance dose 0.125–0.5 mg IV or PO (average is 0.25 mg)<br><br>Teach client to check pulse rate and discuss adverse effects<br><br>Low $K^+$ increases risk of digitalis toxicity<br><br>Serum therapeutic blood levels 0.5–2 ng/mL (0.64–2.56 nmol/L)<br><br>Toxic blood levels > 2 ng/mL (2.56 nmol/L) |

*(Continued)*

Cardiac Glycoside (Digitalis) Medications (*Continued*)

| MEDICATION | ADVERSE EFFECTS | NURSING CONSIDERATIONS |
|---|---|---|
| Action | Increases force of myocardial contraction and slows heart rate by stimulating the vagus nerve and blocking the AV node | |
| Indications | Heart failure, dysrhythmias | |
| Adverse effects | Tachycardia, bradycardia, heart block | |
| | Anorexia, nausea, vomiting | |
| | Halos around dark objects, blurred vision, halo vision | |
| | Dysrhythmias, heart block | |
| Nursing considerations | Instruct client to eat high potassium foods | |
| | Monitor for digitalis toxicity | |
| | Risk of digitalis toxicity increases if client is hypokalemic | |
| Herbal interactions | Licorice can potentiate action of digoxin by promoting potassium loss | |
| | Hawthorn may increase effects of digoxin | |
| | Ginseng may falsely elevate digoxin levels | |
| | Ma-huang (ephedra) increases risk of digitalis toxicity | |

Cytoprotective Medications

| MEDICATION | ADVERSE EFFECTS | NURSING CONSIDERATIONS |
|---|---|---|
| Sucralfate | Constipation | Take medication 1 hour ac |
| | Dizziness | Should not be taken with antacids or $H_2$ blockers |
| Action | Adheres to and protects ulcer's surface by forming a barrier | |
| Indications | Duodenal ulcer | |
| Adverse effects | Constipation | |
| | Vertigo | |
| | Flatulence | |
| Nursing considerations | Action lasts up to 6 h | |
| | Give 2 hours before or after most medications to prevent decreased absorption | |

Disease-Modifying Antirheumatic Medications (DMARDS)

| MEDICATION | ADVERSE EFFECTS |
|---|---|
| **Nonbiologic DMARDs** | |
| Methotrexate | Serious infection |
| Hydroxychloroquine sulfate | Cancer |
| | Impaired liver and kidney function |
| Sulfasalazine | |
| Cyclosporine | |
| **Biologic DMARDs** | |
| Etanercept | Bacterial infection |
| Infliximab | Invasive fungal infection |
| Adalimumab | Injection site reaction |
| Anakinra | |
| Rituximab | |
| Abatacept | |
| **Action** | Non-biologic DMARDs: |
| | Interfere with immune system |
| | Indirect and nonspecific effect |
| | Biologic DMARDs: |
| | Interfere with immune system (tumor necrosis factor, interleukins, T- or B-cell lymphocytes) |
| **Indications** | Rheumatoid arthritis |
| | Psoriasis |
| | Inflammatory bowel disease |
| **Adverse effects** | Stomatitis |
| | Liver toxicity |
| | Bleeding |
| | Anemia |
| | Infections Hypersensitivity |
| | Kidney failure |
| **Nursing considerations** | Precautions: infections, bleeding disorders |
| | Monitor liver function tests |
| | Monitor BUN and creatinine |
| | Monitor for signs of infection |
| | Monitor response to medication |
| | Teach client about risk of live vaccines |
| | Teach client to avoid alcohol |
| | Teach client about risk of infection |

Diuretic Medications

| MEDICATION | ADVERSE EFFECTS | NURSING CONSIDERATIONS |
|---|---|---|
| **Thiazide diuretics** | | |
| Hydrochlorothi-azide<br>Chlorothiazide | Hypokalemia<br>Hyperglycemia<br>Blurred vision<br>Loss of $Na^+$<br>Dry mouth<br>Hypotension | Monitor electrolytes, especially potassium<br>I and O<br>Monitor BUN and creatinine<br>Don't give at bedtime<br>Weigh client daily<br>Encourage potassium-containing foods |
| **Potassium–sparing** | | |
| Spironolactone | Hyperkalemia<br>Hyponatremia<br>Hepatic and renal damage<br>Tinnitus<br>Rash | Used with other diuretics<br>Give with meals<br>Avoid salt substitutes<br>containing potassium<br>Monitor I and O |
| **Loop diuretics** | | |
| Furosemide<br>Ethacrynic acid | Hypotension<br>Hypokalemia<br>Hyperglycemia<br>GI upset<br>Weakness | Monitor BP, pulse rate, I and O<br>Monitor potassium<br>Give IV dose over 1–2 minutes → diuresis in 5–10 min<br>After PO dose diuresis in about 30 min<br>Weigh client daily<br>Don't give at bedtime<br>Encourage potassium-containing foods |
| Ethacrynic acid<br>Bumetanide | Potassium depletion<br>Electrolyte imbalance<br>Hypovolemia<br>Ototoxicity | Supervise ambulation<br>Monitor blood pressure and pulse<br>Observe for signs of electrolyte imbalance |
| **Osmotic diuretic** | | |
| Mannitol | Dry mouth<br>Thirst | I and O must be measured<br>Monitor vital signs<br>Monitor for electrolyte imbalance |

*(Continued)*

Diuretic Medications (*Continued*)

| MEDICATION | ADVERSE EFFECTS | NURSING CONSIDERATIONS |
|---|---|---|
| | | **Other** |
| Chlorthalidone | Dizziness<br><br>Aplastic anemia<br><br>Orthostatic hypotension | Acts like a thiazide diuretic<br><br>Acts in 2–3 h, peak 2–6 h, lasts 2–3 days<br><br>Administer in AM<br><br>Monitor output, weight, BP, electrolytes<br><br>Increase $K^+$ in diet<br><br>Monitor glucose levels in diabetic clients<br><br>Change position slowly |
| **Action** | Thiazides—inhibits reabsorption of sodium and chloride in distal renal tubule<br><br>Loop—inhibits reabsorption of sodium and chloride in loop of Henle and distal renal tubules<br><br>Potassium-sparing—blocks effect of aldosterone on renal tubules, causing loss of sodium and water and retention of potassium<br><br>Osmotic—pulls fluid from tissues due to hypertonic effect | |
| **Indications** | Heart failure<br><br>Hypertension<br><br>Renal diseases<br><br>Diabetes insipidus<br><br>Reduction of osteoporosis in postmenopausal women | |
| **Adverse effects** | Dizziness, vertigo<br><br>Dry mouth<br><br>Orthostatic hypotension<br><br>Leukopenia<br><br>Polyuria, nocturia<br><br>Photosensitivity<br><br>Impotence<br><br>Hypokalemia (except for potassium-sparing)<br><br>Hyponatremia | |

(*Continued*)

Diuretic Medications (*Continued*)

| MEDICATION | ADVERSE EFFECTS | NURSING CONSIDERATIONS |
|---|---|---|
| **Nursing considerations** | Take with food or milk | |
| | Take in AM | |
| | Monitor weight and electrolytes | |
| | Protect skin from the sun | |
| | Diet high in potassium for loop and thiazide diuretics | |
| | Limit potassium intake for potassium-sparing diuretics | |
| | Used as first-line medications for hypertension | |
| **Herbal interactions** | Licorice can promote potassium loss, causing hypokalemia | |
| | Aloe can decrease serum potassium level, causing hypokalemia | |
| | Ginkgo may increase blood pressure when taken with thiazide diuretics | |

Electrolytes and Replacement Solutions

| MEDICATION | ADVERSE EFFECTS | NURSING CONSIDERATIONS |
|---|---|---|
| Calcium carbonate<br>Calcium chloride | Dysrhythmias<br>Constipation | Foods containing oxalic acid (rhubarb, spinach), phytic acid (bran, whole cereals), and phosphorus (milk, dairy products) interfere with absorption<br><br>Monitor EKG<br><br>Take 1–1.5 h pc if GI upset occurs |
| Magnesium chloride | Weak or absent deep tendon reflexes<br><br>Hypotension<br><br>Respiratory paralysis | Respirations should be greater than 16/min before medication given IV<br><br>Test deep tendon reflexes before each dose<br><br>Monitor I and O |
| Potassium chloride<br>Potassium gluconate | Dysrhythmias, cardiac arrest<br><br>Abdominal pain<br><br>Respiratory paralysis | Monitor EKG and serum electrolytes<br><br>Take with or after meals with full glass of water or fruit juice |
| Sodium chloride | Pulmonary edema | Monitor serum electrolytes |

Electrolyte Modifier Medication

| Action | Alkalinizing agents—release bicarbonate ions in stomach and secrete bicarbonate ions in kidneys |
|---|---|
| | Calcium salts—provide calcium for bones, teeth, nerve transmission, muscle contraction, normal blood coagulation, cell membrane strength |
| | Hypocalcemic agents—decrease blood levels of calcium |
| | Hypophosphatemic agents—bind phosphates in GI tract lowering blood levels; neutralize gastric acid, inactivate pepsin |
| | Magnesium salts—provide magnesium for nerve conduction and muscle activity and activate enzyme reactions in carbohydrate metabolism |
| | Phosphates—provide body with phosphorus needed for bone, muscle tissue, metabolism of carbohydrates, fats, proteins, and normal CNS function |
| | Potassium exchange resins—exchange $Na^+$ for $K^+$ in intestines, lowering $K^+$ levels |
| | Potassium salts—provide potassium needed for cell growth and normal functioning of cardiac, skeletal, and smooth muscle |
| | Replacement solution—provide water and $Na^+$ to maintain acid-base and water balance, maintain osmotic pressure |
| | Urinary acidifiers—secrete $H^+$ ions in kidneys, making urine acidic |
| | Urinary alkalinizers—convert to sodium bicarbonate, making the urine alkaline |
| **Indications** | Fluid and electrolyte imbalances |
| | Renal calculi |
| | Peptic ulcers |
| | Osteoporosis |
| | Metabolic acidosis or alkalosis |
| **Adverse effects** | See individual medications |
| **Nursing considerations** | Monitor clients with HF, hypertension, renal disease |

Genitourinary Medications

| MEDICATION | ADVERSE EFFECTS | NURSING CONSIDERATIONS |
|---|---|---|
| Nitrofurantoin | Diarrhea | Anti-infective |
| | Nausea, vomiting | Check CBC |
| | Asthma attacks | Give with food or milk |
| | | Avoid acidic foods (cranberry juice, prunes, plums), which increase medication action |
| | | Check I and O |
| | | Monitor pulmonary status |
| Phenazopyridine | Headache | Urinary tract analgesic, spasmolytic |
| | Vertigo | Inform client that urine will be bright orange |
| | | Take with meals |
| **Anticholinergics** | | |
| Oxybutynin | Drowsiness | Used to reduce bladder spasms and treat urinary incontinence |
| Darifenacin | Blurred vision | |
| Solifenacin | Dry mouth | Increase fluids and fiber in diet |
| Tolterodine | Constipation | Oxybutynin-older adults require higher dose and have greater incidence of adverse effects |
| | Urinary retention | |
| **Anti-impotence** | | |
| Sildenafil | Headache | Treatment of erectile dysfunction |
| Vardenafil | Flushing | Take 1 hour before sexual activity |
| Tadalafil | Hypotension | Never use with nitrates—could have fatal hypotension |
| | Priapism | Do not take with alpha blockers, e.g., doxazosin-risk of hypotension |
| | | Do not drink grapefruit juice |
| **Testosterone inhibitors** | | |
| Finasteride | Decreased libido | Treatment of benign prostatic hyperplasia (BPH) by Proscar; male hair loss by finasteride |
| | Impotence | |
| | Breast tenderness | Pregnant women should avoid contact with crushed medication or client's semen—may adversely affect male fetus |

GI Ulcer Disease Medications

| MEDICATION | ADVERSE EFFECTS | NURSING CONSIDERATIONS |
|---|---|---|
| H$_2$-antagonists | | |
| Cimetidine | Diarrhea | Bedtime dose suppresses nocturnal acid production |
| Ranitidine | Confusion and dizziness (esp. in older adults with large doses) | Compliance may increase with single-dose regimen |
| Famotidine | | Avoid antacids within 1 hour of dose |
| Nizatidine | | Dysrhythmias |
| | Headache | Cimetidine–greater incidence of confusion and agitation with older adults |
| Antisecretory agents | | |
| Omeprazole | Dizziness | Typically administered 30 to 60 minutes before breakfast |
| Lansoprazole | Diarrhea | Do not crush sustained-release capsule; contents may be sprinkled on food or instilled with fluid in NG tube |
| Rabeprazole | | |
| Esomeprazole | | |
| Pantoprazole | | |
| Prostaglandin analogs | | |
| Misoprostol | Abdominal pain | Notify health care provider if diarrhea more than 1 week or severe abdominal pain or black, tarry stools |
| | Diarrhea (13%) | |
| | Miscarriage | |
| **Nursing considerations** | Other medications may be prescribed, including antacids (time administration to avoid canceling med effect) and antimicrobials to eradicate *H. pylori* infections | |
| | Client should avoid smoking, alcohol, ASA, and caffeine, all of which increase stomach acid | |

Eye Medications: Overview

| MEDICATION | ADVERSE EFFECTS | NURSING CONSIDERATIONS |
|---|---|---|
| Methylcellulose | Eye irritation if excess is allowed to dry on eyelids | Lubricant<br><br>Use eyewash to rinse eyelids of "sandy" sensation felt after administration |
| Polyvinyl alcohol | Blurred vision<br><br>Burning | Artificial tears<br><br>Applied to contact lenses before insertion |
| Tetrahydrozoline | Cardiac irregularities<br><br>Pupillary dilation, increased intraocular pressure<br><br>Transient stinging | Used for ocular congestion, irritation, allergic conditions<br><br>Rebound congestion may occur with frequent or prolonged use<br><br>Apply light pressure on lacrimal sac for 1 min instillation |
| Timolol maleate<br>Levobunolol | Eye irritation<br><br>Hypotension | Beta-blocking agent<br><br>Reduces intraocular pressure in management of glaucoma<br><br>Apply light pressure on lacrimal sac for 1 min following instillation<br><br>Monitor BP and pulse |
| Proparacaine HCl<br><br>Tetracaine HCl, cocaine | Corneal abrasion | Topical anesthetic<br><br>Remind client not to touch or rub eyes while anesthetized<br><br>Patch the eye to prevent corneal abrasion |
| Prednisolone acetate | Corneal abrasion | Topical steroid<br><br>Steroid use predisposes client to local infection |
| Gentamicin<br>Tobramycin | Eye irritation; itching, redness | Anti-infective agent<br><br>Clean exudate from eyes before use |
| Idoxuridine | Eye irritation<br><br>Itching lids | Topical antiviral agent<br><br>Educate client about possible adverse effects |
| Dipivefrin HCl | Increase in heart rate and blood pressure | Adrenergic<br><br>Monitor vital signs because of systemic absorption |
| Flurbiprofen | Platelet aggregation disorder | Nonsteroidal anti-inflammatory agents<br><br>Monitor client for eye hemorrhage<br><br>Client should not continue wearing contact lens |
| **Nursing considerations** | Place pressure on tear ducts for one minute<br><br>Wash hands before and after installation<br><br>Do not touch tip of dropper to eye or body | |

Eye Medications: Miotic

| MEDICATION | ADVERSE EFFECTS | NURSING CONSIDERATIONS |
|---|---|---|
| Pilocarpine | Painful eye muscle spasm, blurred or poor vision in dim lights<br><br>Photophobia, cataracts, or floaters | Teach to apply pressure on lacrimal sac for 1 min following instillation<br><br>Used for glaucoma<br><br>Caution client to avoid sunlight and night driving |
| Carbachol | Headache<br><br>If absorbed systemically, can cause sweating, abdominal cramps, and decreased blood pressure | Cholinergic (ophthalmic)<br><br>Similar to acetylcholine in action<br><br>Produces pupillary miosis during ocular surgery |
| **Action** | Causes contraction of sphincter muscles of iris, resulting in miosis | |
| **Indications** | Pupillary miosis in ocular surgery<br><br>Primary open-angle glaucoma | |
| **Adverse effects** | Headache<br><br>Hypotension<br><br>Bronchoconstriction | |
| **Nursing considerations** | Teach how to instill eye drops correctly<br><br>Apply light pressure on lacrimal sac for 1 minute after medication instilled<br><br>Avoid hazardous activities until temporary blurring disappears<br><br>Transient brow pain and myopia are common initially, disappear within 10–14 days | |

Eye Medications: Mydriatic and Cycloplegic

| MEDICATION | ADVERSE EFFECTS | NURSING CONSIDERATIONS |
|---|---|---|
| Atropine sulfate | Blurred vision, photophobia<br><br>Flushing, tachycardia<br><br>Dry mouth | Contraindicated with narrow-angle glaucoma<br><br>Suck on hard candy for dry mouth |
| Cyclopentolate | Photophobia, blurred vision<br><br>Seizures<br><br>Tachycardia | Contraindicated in narrow-angle glaucoma<br><br>Burns when instilled |
| **Action** | Anticholinergic action leaves the pupil under unopposed adrenergic influence, causing it to dilate | |

(Continued)

Eye Medications: Mydriatic and Cycloplegic (*Continued*)

| MEDICATION | ADVERSE EFFECTS | NURSING CONSIDERATIONS |
|---|---|---|
| **Indications** | Diagnostic procedures<br>Acute iritis, uveitis | |
| **Adverse effects** | Headache<br>Tachycardia<br>Blurred vision<br>Photophobia<br>Dry mouth | |
| **Nursing considerations** | Mydriatics cause pupil dilation; cycloplegics paralyze the iris sphincter<br>Watch for signs of glaucoma (increased intraocular pressure, headache, progressive blurring of vision)<br>Apply light pressure on lacrimal sac for 1 minute after instilling medication<br>Avoid hazardous activities until blurring of vision subsides<br>Wear dark glasses | |

Heavy Metal Antagonist Medications

| MEDICATION | ADVERSE EFFECTS | NURSING CONSIDERATIONS |
|---|---|---|
| Deferoxamine mesylate | Pain and induration at injection site<br>Urticaria<br>Hypotension<br>Generalized erythema | Used for acute iron intoxication, chronic iron overload |
| Dimercaprol | Hypertension<br>Tachycardia<br>Nausea, vomiting<br>Headache | Used for treatment of arsenic, gold, and mercury poisoning; acute lead poisoning when used with edetate calcium disodium<br>Administered as initial dose because of its improved efficiency in removing lead from brain tissue |

(*Continued*)

Heavy Metal Antagonist Medications (*Continued*)

| MEDICATION | ADVERSE EFFECTS | NURSING CONSIDERATIONS |
|---|---|---|
| Edetate calcium disodium (EDTA) | | Used for acute and chronic lead poisoning, lead encephalopathy |
| | | Renal tubular necrosis |
| | | Multiple deep IM doses or IV |
| | | Very painful—local anesthetic procaine is injected with the medication (drawn into syringe last, after which the syringe is maintained with needle held slightly down so that it is administered first); rotate sites; provide emotional support and play therapy as outlet for frustration |
| | | Ensure adequate hydration and monitor I and O and kidney function—CaNa$_2$, EDTA and lead are toxic to kidneys |
| | | Seizure precautions—initial rapid mobilization of lead may cause an increase in brain lead levels, exacerbating symptoms |
| **Action** | Forms stable complexes with metals | |
| **Indications** | Poisoning (gold, arsenic) | |
| | Acute lead encephalopathy | |
| **Adverse effects** | Tachycardia | |
| | Burning sensation in lips, mouth, throat | |
| | Abdominal pain | |
| **Nursing considerations** | Monitor I and O, BUN, EKG | |
| | Encourage fluids | |

Immunosuppressant Medications

| MEDICATION | INDICATIONS FOR USE |
|---|---|
| Azathioprine | Prevent renal transplant rejection |
| | Treat severe rheumatoid arthritis not responsive to other treatments |
| Cyclosporine | Prevent rejection of solid organ (heart, kidney, liver) transplants |
| | Prevent graft-versus-host disease in bone marrow transplant |
| Tacrolimus | Prevent liver, kidney, and heart transplant rejection |
| Etanercept | Rheumatoid arthritis treatment (acts to reduce the immune response resulting in inflammation and pain) |
| Infliximab | Treatment of Crohn's disease (inflammatory bowel disease thought to have autoimmune origins) |
| | Treatment of rheumatoid arthritis |
| Methotrexate | Treatment of severe rheumatoid arthritis unresponsive to other treatments |
| Prednisone | Autoimmune disease |
| Prednisolone | |
| Basiliximab | Post transplant surgery |
| Daclizumab | |

Immunomodulator Medications

| MEDICATION | ADVERSE EFFECTS |
|---|---|
| Beta interferons | "Flu-like" symptoms |
| Interferon beta-1a | Liver dysfunction |
| Interferon beta-1b | Bone marrow depression |
| | Injection site reactions |
| | Photosensitivity |
| Glatiramer acetate | Central nervous system infection (natalizumab) |
| Natalizumab | |
| **Action** | Modify the immune response |
| | Decrease the movement of leukocytes into the central nervous system neurons |
| **Indications** | Multiple sclerosis |

(Continued)

Immunomodulator Medications (*Continued*)

| MEDICATION | ADVERSE EFFECTS |
|---|---|
| **Adverse effects** | "Flu-like" symptoms |
| | Liver dysfunction |
| | Bone marrow depression |
| | Injection site reactions |
| | Photosensitivity |
| | Central nervous system infection (natalizumab) |
| **Nursing considerations** | Monitor liver function tests |
| | Monitor complete blood count |
| | Subcutaneous injection: rotate injection sites, apply ice, and then use warm compresses, analgesics for discomfort |
| | Photosensitivity precautions |
| | Monitor for signs of depression |

Iron Preparation Medication

| MEDICATION | ADVERSE EFFECTS | NURSING CONSIDERATIONS |
|---|---|---|
| Ferrous sulfate | Nausea Constipation Black stools | Food decreases absorption but may be necessary to reduce GI effects Monitor Hgb, Hct Dilute liquid preparations in juice, but not milk or antacids Use straw for liquid to avoid staining teeth |
| Iron dextran | Nausea Constipation Black stools | IM injections cause pain and skin staining; use the Z-track technique to put med deep into buttock; IV administration is preferred |
| **Action** | Iron salts increase availability of iron for hemoglobin | |
| **Indications** | Iron-deficiency anemia | |
| **Adverse effects** | Constipation, diarrhea | |
| | Dark stools | |
| | Tooth enamel stains | |
| | Seizures | |
| | Flushing, hypotension | |
| | Tachycardia | |

(Continued)

Iron Preparation Medication (*Continued*)

| MEDICATION | ADVERSE EFFECTS | NURSING CONSIDERATIONS |
|---|---|---|
| **Nursing considerations** | Take iron salts on empty stomach (absorption is reduced by one-third when taken with food) | |
| | Absorption of iron decreased when administered with tetracyclines, antacids, coffee, tea, milk, eggs (bind to iron) | |
| | Concurrent use of iron decreases effectiveness of tetracyclines and quinolone antibiotics | |
| | Vitamin C increases absorption of iron salts | |
| | Vitamin E delays therapeutic responses to iron salts | |

Laxatives and Stool Softener Medications

| MEDICATION | ADVERSE EFFECTS | NURSING CONSIDERATIONS |
|---|---|---|
| Bisacodyl | Mild cramps, rash, nausea, diarrhea | Stimulant<br>Tablets should not be taken with milk or antacids (causes dissolution of enteric coating and loss of cathartic action)<br>Can cause gastric irritation<br>Effects in 6–12 hours |
| Mineral oil | Pruritus ani, anorexia, nausea | Lubricant<br>Administer in upright position<br>Prolonged use can cause fat-soluble vitamin malabsorption |
| Docusate | Few adverse effects<br>Abdominal cramps | Stool softener<br>Contraindicated in atonic bowel, nausea, vomiting, GI pain<br>Effects in 1-3 days |
| Milk of Magnesia | Hypermagnesemia, dehydration | Saline agent<br>$Na^+$ salts can exacerbate heart failure |
| Psyllium hydrophilic mucilloid | Obstruction of GI tract | Take with a full glass of water; do not take dry<br>Report abdominal distention or unusual amount of flatulence |
| Polyethylene glycol and electrolytes | Nausea and bloating | Large-volume product—allow time to consume it safely |

*(Continued)*

Laxatives and Stool Softener Medications (*Continued*)

| MEDICATION | ADVERSE EFFECTS | NURSING CONSIDERATIONS |
|---|---|---|
| **Action** | Bulk-forming—absorbs water into stool mass, making stool bulky, thus stimulating peristalsis | |
| | Lubricants—coat surface of stool and soften fecal mass, allowing for easier passage | |
| | Osmotic agents and saline laxatives—draw water from plasma by osmosis, increasing bulk of fecal mass, thus promoting peristalsis | |
| | Stimulants—stimulate peristalsis when they come in contact with intestinal mucosa | |
| | Stool softeners—soften fecal mass | |
| **Indications** | Constipation | |
| | Preparation for procedures or surgery | |
| **Adverse effects** | Diarrhea | |
| | Dependence | |
| **Nursing considerations** | Contraindicated for clients with abdominal pain, nausea and vomiting, fever (acute abdomen) | |
| | Chronic use may cause hypokalemia | |

Minerals

| MEDICATION | ADVERSE EFFECTS | NURSING CONSIDERATIONS |
|---|---|---|
| Calcium | Cardiac dysrhythmias | Give 1 hour before meals |
| | Constipation | Give 1/3 dose at bedtime |
| | Hypercalcemia | Monitor for urinary stones |
| | Renal calculi | |
| Vitamin D | Seizures | Treatment of vitamin D deficiency, rickets, psoriasis, rheumatoid arthritis |
| | Impaired renal function | |
| | Hypercalcemia | Check electrolytes |
| | Renal calculi | Restrict use of antacids containing Mg |
| Sodium fluoride | Bad taste | Observe for synovitis |
| | Staining of teeth | |
| | Nausea, vomiting | |
| Potassium | Nausea, vomiting | Prevention and treatment of hypokalemia |
| | Cramps, diarrhea | Report hyperkalemia: lethargy, confusion, fainting, decreased urine output |
| | | Report continued hypokalemia: fatigue, weakness, polyuria, polydipsia, cardiac changes |

Musculoskeletal Medications

| MEDICATION | ADVERSE EFFECTS | NURSING CONSIDERATIONS |
|---|---|---|
| Neostigmine | Nausea, vomiting | Monitor vital signs frequently |
| | Abdominal cramps | Have atropine injection available |
| | Respiratory depression | Observe for improvement in strength, vision, ptosis 45 min after each dose |
| | Bronchoconstriction | |
| | Hypotension | Schedule dose before periods of fatigue (e.g., ac) |
| | Bradycardia | Take with milk or food |
| | | Potentiates action of morphine |
| | | Diagnostic test for myasthenia gravis |
| Pyridostigmine bromide | Seizures | Monitor vital signs frequently |
| | Bradycardia | Have atropine injection available |
| | Hypotension | Take extended-release tablets same time each day at least 6 hours apart |
| | Bronchoconstriction | |
| | | Medication of choice for myasthenia gravis to improve muscle strength |
| Alendronate sodium | Vitamin D deficiency | Prevents and treats osteoporosis |
| | Osteomalacia | Longer-lasting treatment for Paget's disease |
| | | Take in AM at least 30 min before other medication, food, water, or other liquids |
| | | Should sit up for 30 min after taking medication |
| | | Use sunscreen and wear protective clothing |
| Glucosamine | Nausea, heartburn, diarrhea | Antirheumatic |
| | | Contraindicated with shellfish allergy, pregnancy, and lactation |
| | | May worsen glycemic control |
| | | Must be taken on regular basis to be effective |
| **Action** | Inhibits destruction of acetylcholine released from parasympathetic and somatic efferent nerves | |
| **Indications** | Myasthenia gravis | |
| | Postoperative and postpartum functional urinary retention | |

(*Continued*)

Musculoskeletal Medications (*Continued*)

| MEDICATION | ADVERSE EFFECTS | NURSING CONSIDERATIONS |
|---|---|---|
| **Adverse effects** | Bronchoconstriction | |
| | Diarrhea | |
| | Respiratory paralysis | |
| | Muscle cramps | |
| **Nursing considerations** | Give with milk or food | |
| | Administer exactly as ordered and on time | |
| | Doses vary with client's activity level | |
| | Monitor vital signs, especially respirations | |

Nitrates/Antianginal Medications

| MEDICATION | ADVERSE EFFECTS | NURSING CONSIDERATIONS |
|---|---|---|
| Nitroglycerin | Flushing | Renew supply every 3 months |
| | Hypotension | Avoid alcoholic beverages |
| | Headache | Sublingual dose may be repeated every 5 minutes for 3 doses |
| | Tachycardia | |
| | Dizziness | Protect medication from light |
| | Blurred vision | Should wet tablet with saliva and place under tongue |
| Isosorbide | Headache | Change position slowly |
| | Orthostatic | Take between meals |
| | Hypotension | Don't discontinue abruptly |
| **Action** | Relaxes vascular smooth muscle; decreases venous return; decreases arterial blood pressure; reduces myocardial oxygen consumption | |
| **Indications** | Angina | |
| | Perioperative hypertension | |
| | CHF associated with MI | |
| | Raynaud's disease (topical) | |

*(Continued)*

Nitrates/Antianginal Medications (*Continued*)

| MEDICATION | ADVERSE EFFECTS | NURSING CONSIDERATIONS |
|---|---|---|
| **Adverse effects** | Hypotension | |
| | Tachycardia | |
| | Headache | |
| | Dizziness | |
| | Syncope | |
| | Rash | |
| **Nursing considerations** | Take sublingual tablets under tongue or in buccal pouch; tablet may sting | |
| | Check expiration date on bottle | |
| | Discard unused med after 6 months. Take sustained-release tablets with water, don't chew them | |
| | Administer topically over 6 × 6 inch area using applicator, cover with plastic wrap, rotate sites | |
| | Administer transdermal to skin free of hair; do not apply to distal extremities; remove before defibrillation or cardioversion | |
| | Administer transmucosal tablets between lip and gum above the incisors or between cheek and gum; do not swallow or chew | |
| | Administer translingual spray into oral mucosa; do not inhale | |
| | Withdraw medication gradually over 4-6 wks | |
| | Provide rest periods | |
| | Teach to take medication when chest pain anticipated | |
| | May take q 5 min × 3 doses | |
| | Beta-adrenergic blockers and calcium-channel blockers also used for angina | |

Nonsteroidal Anti-Inflammatory Medications (NSAIDs)

| MEDICATION | ADVERSE EFFECTS | NURSING CONSIDERATIONS |
|---|---|---|
| Ibuprofen | GI upset—nausea, vomiting, diarrhea, constipation | Use cautiously with aspirin allergy, asthma or nasal polyps |
| | Skin eruption, dizziness, headache, fluid retention | Give with milk |
| | GI bleeding, prolonged bleeding | Observe for bleeding |
| | Stevens-Johnson syndrome | Observe for skin rash |

(*Continued*)

Nonsteroidal Anti-Inflammatory Medications (NSAIDs) (*Continued*)

| MEDICATION | ADVERSE EFFECTS | NURSING CONSIDERATIONS |
|---|---|---|
| Indomethacin | Peptic ulcer, ulcerative colitis<br><br>Headache, dizziness<br><br>Bone marrow depression | Observe for bleeding tendencies<br><br>Monitor I and O |
| Naproxen | Headache, dizziness, epigastric distress | Administer with food<br><br>Optimal therapeutic response is seen after 2 weeks of treatment<br><br>Use cautiously in client with history of aspirin allergy, asthma or nasal polyps |
| Celecoxib | Fatigue<br><br>Anxiety, depression, nervousness<br><br>Nausea, vomiting, anorexia<br><br>Dry mouth, constipation | COX-2 inhibitor<br><br>Increasing doses do not appear to increase effectiveness<br><br>Do not take if allergic to sulfonamides, ASA, or NSAIDs |
| Ketorolac | Peptic ulcer disease<br><br>GI bleeding, prolonged bleeding<br><br>Renal impairment | Dosage is decreased in clients greater than 65 years or with impaired renal function<br><br>Duration of treatment is less than 5 days |
| **Actions** | NSAIDs inhibit prostaglandins<br><br>COX-2 inhibitors block the enzyme responsible for inflammation without blocking the COX-1 enzyme<br><br>ASA has antiplatelet activity | |
| **Indications** | Pain, fever, arthritis, dysmenorrhea<br><br>ASA: transient ischemic attacks, prophylaxis of MI, ischemic stroke, angina<br><br>Ibuprofen: gout, dental pain, musculoskeletal disorders | |
| **Adverse effects** | Headache<br><br>Eye changes<br><br>Dizziness<br><br>Somnolence<br><br>GI disturbances<br><br>Constipation<br><br>Bleeding<br><br>Rash | |

*(Continued)*

Nonsteroidal Anti-Inflammatory Medications (NSAIDs) (*Continued*)

| MEDICATION | ADVERSE EFFECTS | NURSING CONSIDERATIONS |
|---|---|---|
| **Nursing considerations** | Take with food or after meals | |
| | Periodic ophthalmologic exam | |
| | Monitor liver and renal function | |
| | Avoid OTC medications; may contain similar medications | |
| | Also have analgesic and antipyretic actions | |
| | Post op clients with adequate pain relief have fewer complications and a shorter recovery | |
| | Pain is the fifth vital sign and needs to be assessed with others | |

Opioid Analgesic Medications

| MEDICATION | ADVERSE EFFECTS | NURSING CONSIDERATIONS |
|---|---|---|
| Morphine sulfate | Dizziness, weakness | Give in smallest effective dose |
| | Sedation or paradoxical excitement | Observe for development of dependence |
| | Nausea, flushing, and sweating | Encourage respiratory exercises |
| | Respiratory depression, decreased cough reflex | Use cautiously to prevent respiratory depression |
| | Constipation, miosis, hypotension | Monitor vital signs |
| | | Monitor I and O, bowel patterns |
| | | Used for cardiac clients—reduces preload and afterload pressures, decreasing cardiac workload |
| Codeine | Same as morphine | Less potent and less dependence potential compared with morphine |
| | High dose may cause restlessness and excitement | |
| | Constipation | |
| Methadone | Same as morphine | Observe for dependence, respiratory depression |
| | | Encourage fluids and high-bulk foods |
| Hydromorphone | Sedation, hypotension | Keep narcotic antagonist (naloxone) available |
| | Urine retention | Monitor bowel function |
| Oxycodone and acetaminophen | Lightheadedness, dizziness, sedation, nausea | Administer with milk after meals |
| Oxycodone and aspirin | Constipation, pruritus | |
| | Increased risk bleeding (oxy and ASA) | |

Opioid Analgesic Medications (*Continued*)

| MEDICATION | ADVERSE EFFECTS | NURSING CONSIDERATIONS |
|---|---|---|
| Hydrocodone/ acetaminophen | Confusion<br>Sedation<br>Hypotension<br>Constipation | Use with extreme caution with MAO inhibitors<br>Additive CNS depression with alcohol, antihistamines, and sedative/hypnotics |
| **Action** | Produces analgesia, euphoria, sedation; acts on CNS receptor cells | |
| **Indications** | Moderate-to-severe pain<br>Chronic pain<br>Preoperative medication | |
| **Adverse effects** | Dizziness<br>Sedation<br>Respiratory depression<br>Cardiac arrest<br>Hypotension | |
| **Nursing considerations** | Provide narcotic antagonist if needed<br>Turn, cough, deep breathe<br>Safety precautions (side rails, assist when walking)<br>Avoid alcohol, antihistamines, sedative, tranquilizers, OTC medications<br>Avoid activities requiring mental alertness | |

Paget Disease Medications

| MEDICATION | ADVERSE EFFECTS | NURSING CONSIDERATIONS |
|---|---|---|
| Calcitonin | Nausea, vomiting, flushing of face<br>Increased urinary frequency | Retards bone resorption<br>Decreases release of calcium from bone<br>Relieves pain<br>Observe for symptoms of tetany<br>Give at bedtime |
| Etidronate disodium | Diarrhea | Prevents rapid bone turnover<br>Don't give with food, milk, or antacids (reduces absorption)<br>Monitor renal function |

(*Continued*)

Paget Disease Medications (*Continued*)

| MEDICATION | ADVERSE EFFECTS | NURSING CONSIDERATIONS |
|---|---|---|
| Alendronate | Esophagitis | Suppress bone reabsorption |
| | | Give in morning on an empty stomach, with a full glass of water |
| | | Remain upright for 30 minutes |
| **Action** | Inhibits osteocytic activity | |
| **Indications** | Paget disease | |
| **Adverse effects** | Decreased serum calcium | |
| | Facial flushing | |
| **Nursing considerations** | Monitor serum calcium levels | |
| | Facial flushing and warmth last 1 h | |

Thrombolytic Medications

| MEDICATION | ADVERSE EFFECTS | NURSING CONSIDERATIONS (SPECIFIC) |
|---|---|---|
| Reteplase Alteplase Tissue plasminogen activator | Bleeding | Tissue plasminogen activator is a naturally occurring enzyme |
| | | Low allergenic risk but high cost |
| | | Administered as initial bolus followed by 90 minute IV infusion |
| Tenecteplase | Bleeding | Single IV bolus |
| **Action** | Break down plasminogen into plasmin, which dissolves the fibrin network of a clot | |
| **Indications** | MIs within the first 6 hours after symptoms, limited arterial thrombosis, thrombotic strokes, occluded shunts, PE (alteplase) | |
| | MIs (Reteplase and Tenecteplase) | |
| **Nursing considerations (general)** | Check for signs of bleeding; minimize number of punctures for inserting IVs; avoid IM injections; apply pressure at least twice as long as usual after any puncture; avoid high dose therapy with anticoagulants and antiplatelet medications until thrombolytic action has subsided | |

Vitamins

| MEDICATION | ADVERSE EFFECTS | NURSING CONSIDERATIONS |
|---|---|---|
| Cyanocobalamin (Vitamin $B_{12}$) | Anaphylaxis<br><br>Urticaria | Treatment of vitamin $B_{12}$ deficiency, pernicious anemia, hemorrhage, renal and hepatic diseases<br><br>Monitor reticulocyte count, iron, and folate levels<br><br>Don't mix with other solutions in syringe<br><br>Monitor $K^+$ levels<br><br>Clients with pernicious anemia need monthly injections |
| Folic acid | Bronchospasm<br><br>Malaise | Treatment of anemia, liver disease, alcoholism, intestinal obstruction, pregnancy<br><br>Don't mix with other meds in syringe |
| **Action** | Coenzymes that speed up metabolic processes | |
| **Indications** | Vitamin deficiencies | |
| **Adverse effects** | Some vitamins are toxic at high levels | |
| **Nursing considerations** | Avoid exceeding RDA (recommended daily allowance) | |

Men's Health Medications

| MEDICATION | ADVERSE EFFECTS | NURSING CONSIDERATIONS |
|---|---|---|
| **Alpha$_1$-adrenergic blockers** | | |
| Terazosin | Dizziness<br><br>Headache<br><br>Weakness<br><br>Nasal congestion<br><br>Orthostatic hypotension | Used to decrease urinary urgency, hesitancy, nocturia in prostatic hyperplasia<br><br>Caution to change position slowly<br><br>Avoid alcohol, CNS depressant, hot showers due to orthostatic hypotension<br><br>Requires titration<br><br>Administer at bedtime due to risk orthostatic hypotension<br><br>Effects may not be noted for 4 weeks |
| Tamsulosin | Dizziness<br><br>Headache | Used to decrease urinary urgency, hesitancy, nocturia in prostatic hyperplasia<br><br>Caution to change position slowly<br><br>Administer 30 min. after same meal each day |

*(Continued)*

Men's Health Medications (*Continued*)

| MEDICATION | ADVERSE EFFECTS | NURSING CONSIDERATIONS |
|---|---|---|
| **5-alpha-reductase inhibitor** | | |
| Finasteride | Decreased libido<br><br>Impotence | Used to treat benign prostatic hyperplasia by slowing prostatic growth<br><br>May decrease serum PSA levels<br><br>6-12 months therapy required to determine if medication effective<br><br>May cause harm to male fetus. Pregnant women should not be exposed to semen of partner taking finasteride or they should not handle crushed medication<br><br>Monitor liver function tests |
| Dutasteride | Decreased libido<br><br>Impotence | Used to treat benign prostatic hyperplasia by slowing prostatic growth<br><br>May cause harm to male fetus. Pregnant women should not be exposed to semen of partner taking finasteride or they should not handle crushed medication<br><br>Monitor liver function |
| **Anti-impotence agents** | | |
| Sildenafil<br><br>Vardenafil<br><br>Tadalafil | Headache<br><br>Flushing<br><br>Dyspepsia<br><br>Nasal congestion<br><br>Mild visual disturbance | Enhances blood flow to the corpus cavernosum to ensure erection to allow sexual intercourse<br><br>Should not take with nitrates in any form due to dramatic decrease in blood pressure<br><br>Usually taken 1 hour before sexual activity (sildenafil, vardenafil)<br><br>Tadalafil has longer duration of action (up to 36 hours)<br><br>Should not take more than one time per day<br><br>Notify health care provider if erection lasts longer than 4 hours<br><br>Avoid grapefruit juice |
| Saw palmetto | Urinary antiseptic used to treat PBH; may cause false-negative PSA test result | |

Women's Health Medications

| MEDICATION | ADVERSE EFFECTS | NURSING CONSIDERATIONS |
|---|---|---|
| **Contraceptives, systemic** | | |
| Example: Ethinyl Estradiol/ norgestrel | Headache<br>Dizziness<br>Nausea<br>Breakthrough bleeding, spotting | Used to prevent pregnancy<br>Use condoms against sexually transmitted diseases<br>Take pill at same time every day<br>No smoking |
| **Contraceptives, systemic** | | |
| Levonorgestrel | Breakthrough bleeding, spotting | Prevention of pregnancy for 5 years as a contraceptive implant; emergency contraceptive in oral form when given within 72 hours of unprotected intercourse |
| **Estrogens** | | |
| Estradiol<br>Estrogens conjugated | Nausea<br>Gynecomastia<br>Contact lens intolerance | Treatment of menopausal symptoms, some cancers<br>Prevention of osteoporosis<br>Client should contact health care provider if there are breast lumps, vaginal bleeding, edema, jaundice, dark urine, clay-colored stools, dyspnea, blurred vision, numbness or stiffness in leg, chest pain |
| **Progestins** | | |
| Medroxyprogesterone acetate | Nausea<br>Contact lens intolerance | Management of abnormal uterine bleeding; prevent endometrial changes of estrogen replacement therapy, some cancers |
| **Actions** | Female hormones | |
| **Indications** | Contraceptives<br>Treatment of menopausal symptoms<br>Prevention of osteoporosis | |
| **Adverse effects** | Nausea<br>Breakthrough bleeding<br>Headache | |

*(Continued)*

Women's Health Medications (*Continued*)

| MEDICATION | ADVERSE EFFECTS | NURSING CONSIDERATIONS |
|---|---|---|
| **Nursing considerations** | Client should know when to take medication and what to do for skipped doses | |
| | Client should know when to contact prescribing health care provider (signs of thrombosis/thromboembolism) | |
| | Contraindications: smoking, thrombophlebitis, cerebrovascular disease | |
| | Some oral contraceptives can elevated blood glucose, so monitor, especially in prediabetic or already diagnosed diabetics | |
| **Herbal** | Black cohosh—relieves hot flashes; may increase hypotensive effect of antihypertensives; do not take for more than 6 months | |

Herbal Supplements

| SUPPLEMENT | ADVERSE EFFECTS/ CONTRAINDICATIONS | NURSING CONSIDERATIONS |
|---|---|---|
| IMMUNE SYSTEM | | |
| **Echinacea** | | |
| Immunostimulant, anti-inflammatory, antiviral, antibacterial<br><br>Used to prevent and treat colds, flu, wound healing, urinary tract infections | Immune suppression, tingling sensation and/or unpleasant taste on tongue, nausea, vomiting, allergic reactions | Decreases effectiveness of immunosuppressants<br><br>Contraindicated in autoimmune diseases<br><br>Avoid if allergic to ragweed, members of daisy family of plants |
| **Garlic** | | |
| Antimicrobial, antilipidemic, antithrombotic, antitumor, anti-inflammatory<br><br>Used to reduce cholesterol, prevent atherosclerosis, cancer, stroke, and MI; decrease blood pressure, prevent and treat colds and flu | Flatulence, heartburn, halitosis, irritation of mouth, esophagus, stomach, allergic reaction<br><br>Contraindicated with peptic ulcer, reflux | May potentiate anticoagulant and antiplatelets, antihyperlipidemics, antihypertensives, antidiabetic agents, and herbs with these effects<br><br>May decrease efficacy of cyclosporine, hormonal contraceptives<br><br>Avoid if allergic to members of the lily family of plants |

(*Continued*)

Herbal Supplements (*Continued*)

| SUPPLEMENT | ADVERSE EFFECTS/ CONTRAINDICATIONS | NURSING CONSIDERATIONS |
|---|---|---|
| **Ginseng** | | |
| Stimulant and tonic to immune and nervous systems<br><br>Used to increase stamina, as aphrodisiac, adjunct chemotherapy and radiation therapy | Headache, insomnia, nervousness, palpitations, excitation, diarrhea, vaginal bleeding<br><br>May cause headache, tremors, irritability, manic episodes if combined with MAOIs or caffeine | May falsely elevate digoxin levels; observe for signs usually associated with high digoxin levels<br><br>May antagonize warfarin<br><br>Potentiates antidiabetic agents, steroids, estrogens<br><br>Caution with cardiovascular disease, hypotension, hypertension, steroid therapy |
| FEMALE REPRODUCTIVE SYSTEM | | |
| **Evening Primrose Oil** | | |
| Anti-inflammatory, sedative, astringent<br><br>Used for premenstrual and menopausal problems, rheumatoid arthritis, elevated serum cholesterol, hypertension, eczema, diabetic neuropathy | Headache, rash, nausea, seizures, inflammation<br><br>Contraindicated for clients with epilepsy, schizophrenia | May potentiate antiplatelet and anticoagulant meds<br><br>Increases risk for seizures when taken with phenothiazines, antidepressants |
| MUSCULOSKELETAL SYSTEM | | |
| **Chondroitin** | | |
| Collagen synthesis<br><br>Used for arthritis for cartilage synthesis (with glucosamine) | Dyspepsia, nausea | May potentiate effects of anticoagulants |
| **Glucosamine** | | |
| Collagen synthesis<br><br>Used for arthritis for cartilage synthesis (with chondroitin) | Dyspepsia, nausea | May impede insulin secretion or increase resistance |

(*Continued*)

Herbal Supplements (*Continued*)

| SUPPLEMENT | ADVERSE EFFECTS/ CONTRAINDICATIONS | NURSING CONSIDERATIONS |
|---|---|---|
| **NEUROLOGICAL SYSTEM** | | |
| **Capsicum/Cayenne Pepper** | | |
| Analgesia, improves blood circulation<br><br>Used for arthritis, bowel disorders, nerve pain, PAD, chronic laryngitis, personal self-defense spray | GI discomfort, burning pain in eyes, nose, mouth, blepharospasm and swelling in eyes, skin tissue irritation, cough, bronchospasm<br><br>Avoid if allergic to ragweed or to chili pepper | May decrease effectiveness of antihypertensives, increases risk of cough with ACE inhibitors<br><br>May potentiate antiplatelet and anticoagulant meds and herbs<br><br>May cause hypertensive crisis with MAOIs<br><br>Increases theophylline absorption |
| **Feverfew** | | |
| Analgesic, antipyretic<br><br>Used for migraine prophylaxis, fever, menstrual problems, arthritis | Mouth ulcers, heartburn, indigestion, dizziness, tachycardia, allergic reactions | Potentiates antiplatelet and anticoagulant meds<br><br>Do not stop abruptly—causes moderate-to-severe pain with joint and muscle stiffness<br><br>Caution if allergic to daisy family of plants |
| **GASTROINTESTINAL SYSTEM** | | |
| **Flaxseed** | | |
| Laxative, anticholesteremic<br><br>Used for constipation, decrease cholesterol, prevent atherosclerosis, colon disorders | Diarrhea, flatulence, nausea<br><br>Contraindicated if client has strictures or acute GI inflammation | May decrease absorption of oral meds—do not take within 2 hrs<br><br>Immature flax seeds can be very toxic<br><br>Increase fluids to minimize flatulence |
| **Ginger** | | |
| Antiemetic, antioxidant, digestive aid, anti-inflammatory<br><br>Used for nausea, vomiting, indigestion, gas, lack of appetite | Minor heartburn, dermatitis<br><br>Contraindicated with gallstones | May potentiate antiplatelet and anticoagulant meds, antidiabetic meds, herbs that increase bleeding times |

(*Continued*)

Herbal Supplements (*Continued*)

| SUPPLEMENT | ADVERSE EFFECTS/ CONTRAINDICATIONS | NURSING CONSIDERATIONS |
| --- | --- | --- |
| **Licorice** | | |
| Demulcent (soothes), expectorant, anti-inflammatory <br><br> Used for coughs, colds, stomach pains, ulcers | Hypokalemia, headache, edema, lethargy, hypertension, heart failure (with overdose), cardiac arrest <br><br> Contraindicated in renal or liver disease, heart disease, hypertension; caution with hormonal contraceptives | Decreases effect of spironolactone <br><br> Avoid use with digoxin, loop diuretics, corticosteroids |
| GENITOURINARY SYSTEM | | |
| **Saw Palmetto** | | |
| Mild diuretic, urinary antiseptic <br><br> Used for BPH, increasing sexual vigor, cystitis | Constipation, diarrhea, nausea, decreased libido, back pain | May interact with hormonal meds such as HRT and oral contraceptives <br><br> May cause a false-negative PSA test result |
| PSYCHIATRIC | | |
| **Chamomile** | | |
| Sedative/hypnotic, anti-inflammatory, antispasmodic, anti-infective <br><br> Used for stress, anxiety, insomnia, GI disorders | Allergic reactions, contact dermatitis, vomiting, depression | May potentiate sedatives and anticoagulants <br><br> Avoid if allergic to ragweed, members of daisy family of plants |
| **Kava** | | |
| Anti-anxiety, sedative/hypnotic, muscle relaxant <br><br> Used for anxiety, insomnia, seizure disorders | Hepatotoxicity, psychological dependence, mild euphoria, fatigue, sedation, suicidal thoughts, visual problems, scaly skin reaction <br><br> Contraindicated in Parkinson's, history of stroke, endogenous depression | May potentiate sedative effects of other sedating meds (benzodiazepines, barbiturates), anticonvulsants, and herbs (chamomile, valerian) |
| **Melatonin** | | |
| Hormone from pineal gland <br><br> Used for insomnia, jet lag | Headache, confusion, sedation, tachycardia | Potentiates CNS depressants <br><br> May decrease effectiveness of immunosuppressants, Procardia |

(Continued)

Herbal Supplements (*Continued*)

| SUPPLEMENT | ADVERSE EFFECTS/ CONTRAINDICATIONS | NURSING CONSIDERATIONS |
|---|---|---|
| **St. John's wort** | | |
| Antidepressant, sedative effects, antiviral, antimicrobial<br><br>Used for mild to moderate depression, sleep disorders, skin and wound healing | Photosensitivity, fatigue, allergic reactions, dry mouth, dizziness, restlessness, nausea<br><br>Contraindicated for major depression, transplant recipients, clients taking SSRIs (increases risk of serotonin syndrome), MAOIs (increases risk of hypertensive crisis), hormonal contraceptives | Usually decreases effectiveness of (digoxin, antineoplastics, antiviral AIDS medications, anti-rejection medications, theophylline, warfarin, hormonal contraceptives<br><br>May potentiate medications and herbs with sedative effects<br><br>Should avoid tyramine in diet, OTC meds |
| **Valerian** | | |
| Sedative/hypnotic, antispasmodic<br><br>Used for insomnia, restlessness, anxiety | Headache, blurred vision, nausea, excitability<br><br>Contraindicated in liver disease may be hepatotoxic | May potentiate other CNS depressant meds, antihistamines, and sedating herbs |
| CARDIOVASCULAR SYSTEM | | |
| **Ginkgo** | | |
| Enhances cerebral and peripheral blood circulation; antidepressive<br><br>Used for dementia, short-term memory loss, vertigo, PADs, depression, sexual dysfunction (including from SSRIs) | Headache, GI upset, contact dermatitis, dizziness | May potentiate antiplatelet and anticoagulant meds, ASA, NSAIDs, and herbs, which increase bleeding time<br><br>May potentiate MAOIs<br><br>May decrease effectiveness of anticonvulsants |
| **Hawthorn** | | |
| Antianginal, antiarrhythmic, vasodilator, antihypertensive, antilipidemic<br><br>Used for mild to moderate heart failure, hypertension, cholesterol reduction | Nausea, fatigue, sweating | May potentiate or interfere with wide range of cardiovascular meds used for CHF, angina, arrhythmias, hypertension, vasodilation<br><br>Potentiates digoxin<br><br>Potentiates CNS depressants<br><br>Avoid if allergic to members of the rose family of plants |

(Continued)

Herbal Supplements (*Continued*)

| SUPPLEMENT | ADVERSE EFFECTS/ CONTRAINDICATIONS | NURSING CONSIDERATIONS |
|---|---|---|
| RESPIRATORY SYSTEM | | |
| **Eucalyptus** | | |
| Decongestant, anti-inflammatory, antimicrobial, antifungal<br><br>Used for coughs, bronchitis, nasal congestion, sore muscles, wounds | Nausea, vomiting, epigastric burning, dizziness, muscle weakness, seizures<br><br>Contraindicated with liver disease, inflammation of intestinal tract | Potentiates antidiabetic meds and possibly other herbs that cause hypoglycemia<br><br>May increase metabolism of any medications metabolized in liver |

Medication Interactions with Grapefruit Juice (Increased Serum Medication Levels)

Anti-anxiety: buspirone, midazolam, triazolam

Anti-dysrhythmic: amiodarone

Anti-seizure: carbamazepine

Calcium channel blockers: amlodipine, diltiazem, felodipine, nicardipine, nifedipine, nimodipine, nisoldipine, verapamil

Erectile dysfunction: sildenafil, tadalafil

Immunosuppressants to prevent organ transplant rejection: cyclosporine, sirolimus, tacrolimus

SSRIs: fluoxetine, fluvoxamine, sertraline

Statins: lovastatin, simvastatin

Caffeine (stimulant)

Dextromethorphan(cough suppressant)

Pimozide (Tourette)

Praziquantel (schistosomiasis)

# End-of-Chapter Thinking Exercise

The nurse receives report on an older adult client being discharged from the hospital tomorrow morning. The client was admitted 6 days ago with a right leg deep vein thrombosis extending from the ankle to the hip that required treatment with an intravenous heparin drip. The heparin has been discontinued and replaced with warfarin 5 mg PO daily to begin tomorrow. Past medical history (PMH) includes two admissions last year for pneumonia, anemia (iron deficiency), and a gastrointestinal (GI) bleed that required cautery 6 months ago. The client lives alone and has the assistance of a neighbor to pick up groceries, prescriptions, and take the client to health care provider appointments. The nurse is asked to conduct client teaching about warfarin.

1.  What resources does the nurse use when providing teaching on warfarin? (Generate Solutions)

2.  What does the nurse teach about warfarin therapy? (Take Action)

3.  How does the nurse evaluate the client's understanding of the teaching? (Evaluate Outcomes)

# Thinking Exercise Explanations

1. What resources does the nurse use when providing teaching on warfarin? (Generate Solutions)

   - Agency-generated client education materials
   - The health care provider's order for warfarin, including dosage and frequency
   - Protocol for follow-up lab testing

   Most hospitals have a database of educational materials for use in teaching clients. The nurse should review these materials, the health care provider's order, and the protocol for follow-up lab testing as warfarin therapy requires frequent blood draws to monitor international normalized ratio (INR) levels.

2. What does the nurse teach about warfarin therapy? (Take Action)

   - Measures to avoid venous stasis
   - Emphasize the need for frequent lab monitoring
   - Maintain consistent intake of foods that contain vitamin K
   - Use a soft toothbrush and electric razor
   - Report bleeding gums, bruising, epistaxis, and black tarry stools
   - Report other adverse effects such as diarrhea, rash, or fever
   - Do not take any new medications without consulting the health care provider

   The nurse will teach the client to avoid venous stasis by getting up and walking every 1–2 hours during the day, avoid lengthy travel in cars or planes, and avoid sitting or standing still for long periods of time. The client will need to understand there will be frequent visits to the lab (2–3 times/week initially until INR is regulated), adverse effects to report, and to use a soft toothbrush and electric razor to avoid bleeding. The nurse will need to review dietary considerations, such as maintaining a consistent intake of foods that contain vitamin K (e.g., dark leafy greens, pork, rice, yogurt, cheese, fish, milk). Because vitamin K reverses the effects of warfarin, consistency of intake is important once levels become therapeutic. This consistency will allow the client to continue eating foods they like while remaining therapeutic with the INR levels. Finally, instruct the client not to add any over-the-counter or herbal medications (e.g., garlic, ginkgo) to the medication regimen without first checking with the health care provider as many of these interact with warfarin and may alter coagulation times.

3. How does the nurse evaluate the client's understanding of the teaching? (Evaluate Outcomes)

   - Ask the client to repeat back information regarding lab monitoring, examples of how to avoid venous stasis and bleeding, and adverse effects that should be reported
   - Ask about the client's plan for getting to lab appointments
   - Ask the client to describe foods that will be eaten for breakfast, lunch, and dinner

   To ensure the client understands the teaching, the nurse should ask the client to repeat key points back to the nurse and have the client describe who will bring the client to lab appointments. Dietary considerations are extremely important in maintaining a therapeutic INR while taking warfarin. The nurse should review menu options for each meal (breakfasts, lunches, etc.) and allow the client to select foods that are appropriate while taking warfarin.

[ CHAPTER 17 ]

# TERMINOLOGY

## SECTIONS

1. Nursing Abbreviations
2. Medication Terminology
3. Terminology Used for Documentation

# NURSING ABBREVIATIONS

| | |
|---|---|
| A and P | anterior and posterior |
| ABC | airway, breathing, circulation |
| abd | abdomen |
| ABG | arterial blood gas |
| ABO | system of classifying blood groups |
| ac | before meals |
| ACE | angiotensin-converting enzyme |
| ACS | acute compartment syndrome |
| ACTH | adrenocorticotrophic hormone |
| ad lib | freely, as desired |
| ADH | antidiuretic hormone |
| ADL | activities of daily living |
| AFP | alpha-fetoprotein |
| AIDS | acquired immunodeficiency syndrome |
| AKA | above-knee amputation |
| ALL | acute lymphocytic leukemia |
| ALP | alkaline phosphatase (formerly SGPT) |
| ALS | amyotrophic lateral sclerosis |
| ALT | alanine aminotransferase |
| AMI | antibody-mediated immunity |
| AML | acute myelogenous leukemia |
| amt | amount |
| ANA | antinuclear antibody |
| ANS | autonomic nervous system |
| AP | anteroposterior |

*(Continued)*

| APC | atrial premature contraction |
|-----|------------------------------|
| aq | water |
| ARDS | adult respiratory distress syndrome |
| ASD | atrial septal defect |
| ASHD | atherosclerotic heart disease |
| AST | aspartate aminotransferase (formerly SGOT) |
| ATP | adenosine triphosphate |
| AV | atrioventricular |
| BCG | bacille Calmette-Guerin |
| bid | two times a day |
| BKA | below-knee amputation |
| BLS | basic life support |
| BMR | basal metabolic rate |
| BP | blood pressure |
| BPH | benign prostatic hyperplasia |
| bpm | beats per minute |
| BPR | bathroom privileges |
| BSA | body surface area |
| BUN | blood, urea, nitrogen |
| C | centigrade, Celsius |
| $\overline{c}$ | with |
| C and S | culture and sensitivity |
| Ca | calcium |
| CA | cancer |
| cal | calorie(s) |
| CABG | coronary artery bypass graft |
| CAD | coronary artery disease |
| caps | capsules |
| CAPD | continuous ambulatory peritoneal dialysis |
| CBC | complete blood count |
| CBI | continuous bladder irrigation |

*(Continued)*

| CC | chief complaint |
|----|----|
| CCU | coronary care unit, critical care unit |
| CDC | Centers for Disease Control and Prevention |
| CHF | congestive heart failure |
| CK | creatine kinase |
| Cl | chloride |
| CLL | chronic lymphocytic leukemia |
| cm | centimeter |
| CMV | cytomegalovirus infection |
| CNS | central nervous system |
| CO | carbon monoxide, cardiac output |
| $CO_2$ | carbon dioxide |
| comp | compound |
| cont | continuous |
| COPD | chronic obstructive pulmonary disease |
| CP | cerebral palsy |
| CPAP | continuous positive airway pressure |
| CPK | creatine phosphokinase |
| CPR | cardiopulmonary resuscitation |
| CRP | C-reactive protein |
| CSF | cerebrospinal fluid |
| CT | computerized tomography |
| CTD | connective tissue disease |
| CTS | carpal tunnel syndrome |
| cu | cubic |
| CVA | costovertebral angle |
| CVC | central venous catheter |
| CVP | central venous pressure |
| D and C | dilation and curettage |
| DIC | disseminated intravascular coagulation |
| DIFF | differential blood count |

*(Continued)*

| dil | dilute |
|-----|--------|
| DJD | degenerative joint disease |
| DKA | diabetic ketoacidosis |
| dL | deciliter (100 mL) |
| DM | diabetes mellitus |
| DNA | deoxyribonucleic acid |
| DNR | do not resuscitate |
| DOE | dyspnea on exertion |
| DTaP | vaccine for diphtheria, pertussis, tetanus |
| D/W | dextrose in water |
| Dx | diagnosis |
| ECF | extracellular fluid |
| ECG or EKG | electrocardiogram |
| ECT | electroconvulsive therapy |
| ED | emergency department |
| EDD | estimated date of delivery |
| EEG | electroencephalogram |
| EMD | electromechanical dissociation |
| EMG | electromyography |
| ENT | ear, nose, and throat |
| ESR | erythrocyte sedimentation rate |
| ESRD | end-stage renal disease |
| ET | endotracheal tube |
| 4 × 4 | piece of gauze 4 inches by 4 inches used for dressings |
| F | Fahrenheit |
| FBD | fibrocystic breast disease |
| FBS | fasting blood sugar |
| FDA | Food and Drug Administration |
| FFP | fresh frozen plasma |
| FHR | fetal heart rate |
| fl | fluid |

*(Continued)*

| FM | fetal movement |
|---|---|
| FSH | follicle-stimulating hormone |
| ft | foot, feet (unit of measure) |
| FUO | fever of undetermined origin |
| g, gm | gram |
| GB | gallbladder |
| GFR | glomerular filtration rate |
| GH | growth hormone |
| GI | gastrointestinal |
| gr | grain |
| GSC | Glasgow coma scale |
| gtts | drops |
| GU | genitourinary |
| GYN | gynecological |
| (H) | hypodermically |
| h or hr | hour(s) |
| Hb or Hgb | hemoglobin |
| hCG | human chorionic gonadotropin |
| $HCO_3$ | bicarbonate |
| Hct | hematocrit |
| HD | hemodialysis |
| HDL | high-density lipoproteins |
| Hg | mercury |
| Hgb | hemoglobin |
| HGH | human growth hormone |
| HHNC | hyperglycemia hyperosmolar nonketotic coma |
| HIV | human immunodeficiency virus |
| HLA | human leukocyte antigen |
| hPL | human placental lactogen |
| HR | heart rate |
| hr | hour |

*(Continued)*

| $H_2O$ | water |
|---|---|
| HSV | herpes simplex virus |
| HTN | hypertension |
| Hx | history |
| Hz | hertz (cycles/second) |
| I and O | intake and output |
| IAPB | intra-aortic balloon pump |
| IBS | irritable bowel syndrome |
| ICF | intracellular fluid |
| ICP | intracranial pressure |
| ICS | intercostal space |
| ICU | intensive care unit |
| ID | intradermal |
| IDDM | insulin-dependent diabetes mellitus |
| IgA | immunoglobulin A |
| IM | intramuscular |
| in | inch(es) |
| IOP | increased intraocular pressure |
| IPG | impedance plethysmogram |
| IPPB | intermittent positive-pressure breathing |
| IU | international unit |
| IUD | intrauterine device |
| IV | intravenous |
| IVC | intraventricular catheter |
| IVP | intravenous pyelogram |
| JRA | juvenile rheumatoid arthritis |
| $K^+$ | potassium |
| kcal | kilocalorie (food calorie) |
| kg | kilogram |
| KO, KVO | keep vein open |
| KS | Kaposi sarcoma |

*(Continued)*

| KUB | kidneys, ureters, bladder |
|---|---|
| L | liter |
| lab | laboratory |
| lb | pound |
| LBBB | left bundle branch block |
| LDH | lactate dehydrogenase |
| LDL | low-density lipoproteins |
| LE | lupus erythematosus |
| LH | luteinizing hormone |
| liq | liquid |
| LLQ | left lower quadrant |
| LOC | level of consciousness |
| LP | lumbar puncture |
| LPN, LVN | licensed practical or vocational nurse |
| Lt | left |
| LTC | long-term care |
| LUQ | left upper quadrant |
| LV | left ventricle |
| m | meter, micron |
| MAO, MAOI | monoamine oxidase inhibitors |
| MAST | military antishock trousers |
| MCH | mean corpuscular hemoglobin |
| MCV | mean corpuscular volume |
| MD | muscular dystrophy |
| MDI | metered dose inhaler |
| mEq | milliequivalent |
| Mg | magnesium |
| mcg | microgram |
| mg | milligram |
| MG | myasthenia gravis |
| MI | myocardial infarction |

*(Continued)*

| min | minute(s) |
|---|---|
| mL | milliliter |
| mm | millimeter |
| MMR | vaccine for measles, mumps, rubella |
| mo | month(s) |
| MRI | magnetic resonance imaging |
| MS | multiple sclerosis |
| MRSA | methicillin-resistant *Staphylococcus aureus* |
| N | nitrogen, normal (strength of solution) |
| $Na^+$ | sodium |
| NaCl | sodium chloride |
| NANDA | North American Nursing Diagnosis Association |
| NG | nasogastric |
| NGT | nasogastric tube |
| NIDDM | non-insulin-dependent diabetes mellitus |
| NLN | National League for Nursing |
| noc | at night |
| NPO | nothing by mouth |
| NS | normal saline |
| NSAIDs | nonsteroidal anti-inflammatory drugs |
| NSNA | National Student Nurses' Association |
| NST | non-stress test |
| $O_2$ | oxygen |
| OB-GYN | obstetrics and gynecology |
| OCT | oxytocin challenge test |
| OD | right eye |
| OOB | out of bed |
| OPC | outpatient clinic |
| OR | operating room |
| OS | left eye |
| OSHA | Occupational Safety and Health Administration |

*(Continued)*

| OT | occupational therapy |
|---|---|
| OTC | over the counter (medication that can be obtained without a prescription) |
| OU | both eyes |
| oz | ounce |
| $\bar{p}$ | after |
| P | pulse, pressure, phosphorus |
| PA Chest | posterior-anterior chest x-ray |
| PAC | premature atrial complexes |
| $PaCO_2$ | partial pressure of carbon dioxide in arterial blood |
| PAD | peripheral artery disease |
| $PaO_2$ | partial pressure of oxygen in arterial blood |
| Pap | Papanicolaou smear |
| PAT | paroxysmal atrial tachycardia |
| pc | after meals |
| PCA | patient-controlled analgesia |
| $PCO_2$ | partial pressure of carbon dioxide |
| PCP | *Pneumocystis carinii* pneumonia |
| PD | peritoneal dialysis |
| PDA | patent ductus arteriosus |
| PE | pulmonary embolism |
| PEEP | positive end-expiratory pressure |
| PERRLA | pupils equal, round, react to light and accommodation |
| PET | postural emission tomography |
| PFT | pulmonary function tests |
| pH | hydrogen ion concentration |
| PICC | peripherally inserted central catheter |
| PID | pelvic inflammatory disease |
| PIH | pregnancy-induced hypertension |
| PKD | polycystic disease |
| PKU | phenylketonuria |
| PMI | point of maximal impulse |

*(Continued)*

| PMS | premenstrual syndrome |
|---|---|
| PN | parenteral nutrition |
| PND | paroxysmal nocturnal dyspnea |
| PO | by mouth |
| PO$_2$ | partial pressure of oxygen |
| PPD | positive purified protein derivative (of tuberculin) |
| PPN | partial parenteral nutrition |
| pro time | prothrombin time |
| PRN, prn | as needed, whenever necessary |
| PSA | prostate-specific antigen |
| psi | pounds per square inch |
| PT | physical therapy, prothrombin time |
| PTCA | percutaneous transluminal coronary angioplasty |
| PTH | parathyroid hormone |
| PTT | partial thromboplastin time |
| PUD | peptic ulcer disease |
| PVC | premature ventricular contraction |
| PSP | phenol-sulfonephthalein |
| q | every |
| q 2 h | every two hours |
| q 4 h | every four hours |
| QA | quality assurance |
| qid | four times a day |
| qs | quantity sufficient |
| R | rectal temperature, respirations, roentgen |
| RA | rheumatoid arthritis |
| RAI | radioactive iodine |
| RAIU | radioactive iodine uptake |
| RAS | reticular activating system |
| RBBB | right bundle branch block |
| RBC | red blood cell or count |

*(Continued)*

| RCA | right coronary artery |
|---|---|
| RDA | recommended dietary allowance |
| resp | respirations |
| RF | rheumatic fever, rheumatoid factor |
| Rh | antigen on blood cell indicated by $+$ or $-$ |
| RIND | reversible ischemic neurologic deficit |
| RLQ | right lower quadrant |
| RN | registered nurse |
| RNA | ribonucleic acid |
| R/O | rule out, to exclude |
| ROM | range of motion (of joint) or rupture of membranes |
| Rt | right |
| RUQ | right upper quadrant |
| Rx | prescription |
| $\bar{s}$ | without |
| s | second(s) (unit of measure) |
| S or Sig | (Signa) to write on label |
| SA | sinoatrial node |
| SaO$_2$ | systemic arterial oxygen saturation (%) |
| sat sol | saturated solution |
| SBE | subacute bacterial endocarditis |
| SDA | same-day admission |
| SDS | same-day surgery |
| sed rate | sedimentation rate |
| SI | International System of Units |
| SIADH | syndrome of inappropriate antidiuretic hormone |
| SIDS | sudden infant death syndrome |
| SL | sublingual |
| SLE | systemic lupus erythematosus |
| SOB | short of breath |
| sol | solution |

(*Continued*)

| SMBG | self-monitoring blood glucose |
|---|---|
| SMR | submucous resection |
| sp gr | specific gravity |
| spec | specimen |
| SS | soap suds |
| SSKI | saturated solution of potassium iodide |
| stat | immediately |
| STI | sexually transmitted infection |
| Syr | syrup |
| T | temperature, thoracic (to be followed by the number designating specific thoracic vertebra) |
| T and A | tonsillectomy and adenoidectomy |
| T and C | type and cross-match |
| tabs | tablets |
| TB | tuberculosis |
| TED | antiembolitic stockings |
| temp | temperature |
| TENS | transcutaneous electrical nerve stimulation |
| TIA | transient ischemic attack |
| TIBC | total iron-binding capacity |
| tid | three times a day |
| tinct | tincture |
| TMJ | temporomandibular joint |
| t-PA | tissue plasminogen activator |
| TPR | temperature, pulse, respiration |
| TQM | total quality management |
| TSE | testicular self-examination |
| TSH | thyroid-stimulating hormone |
| tsp | teaspoon |
| TSS | toxic shock syndrome |

*(Continued)*

| TURP | transurethral prostatectomy |
|------|------------------------------|
| UA | urinalysis |
| ung | ointment |
| URI | upper respiratory tract infection |
| UTI | urinary tract infection |
| VAD | venous access device |
| VDRL | Venereal Disease Research Laboratory (test for syphilis) |
| VF, Vfib | ventricular fibrillation |
| vol | volume |
| VPC | ventricular premature complexes |
| VS | vital signs |
| VSD | ventricular septal defect |
| VTE | venous thromboembolism |
| WBC | white blood cell or count |
| WHO | World Health Organization |
| wk | week(s) |
| wt | weight |
| y | years(s) |

| DO NOT USE | USE INSTEAD |
|------------|-------------|
| U, u | unit |
| Q.D., QD, q.d., qd, | daily |
| Q.O.D., QOD, q.o.d., qod | every other day |
| MS, $MSO_4$, $MgSO_4$ | morphine or magnesium sulfate |
| http://www.jointcommission.org/assets/1/18/Do_Not_Use_List.pdf | |

# MEDICATION TERMINOLOGY

| Action | Description of the method of how a medication works. |
|---|---|
| Adverse effects | Actions of a medication other than that for which it was given. Adverse effects may or may not be harmful to the person and may or may not require a lowering of the dosage or discontinuance of the medication. |
| Ampoule | Sealed, sterile glass container containing one dose of medication. May be in liquid form or a powder that must be diluted. |
| Aqueous solution | One or more substances dissolved in water or alcohol. Solutions are translucent and do not have to be shaken. |
| Aqueous suspension | An insoluble medication in hydrated form. Must be shaken before pouring. |
| Capsules | Gelatin containers for medications and that may be plain or enteric coated. Plain capsules dissolve in the stomach. Enteric capsules dissolve in the small intestine. |
| Disposable plastic syringe | Equipment used for injections consisting of plunger inserted into a barrel, which contains a needle. All parts of the syringe except the outside of the barrel, handle of the plunger, and needle cap are considered sterile. |
| Elixirs | Aromatic, sweetened beverages containing alcohol and used as flavoring vehicles. |
| Emulsion | Suspension of fat or oil in water. |
| Enteric-coated capsules | Capsules that dissolve in the alkaline secretions of the small intestine rather than the acid secretions of the stomach. This prevents gastric irritation and protects the medication from being inactivated by stomach acid. |
| Extracts | Concentrated preparations of vegetable or animal medications that contain the active ingredients of the medication. They can be liquid or pills. |
| Generic name | Official name of the medication that is never changed and is used in all countries. It relates to the chemical formula and is the name under which the medication is listed in official publications. A medication can have several trade names but only one generic name. |

*(Continued)*

| Lotion | Liquid suspension intended for external use on the skin. |
|---|---|
| Nursing implications | Actions of the nurse related to the administration of a medication. |
| Ointment | Semisolid preparation of a medication in a petroleum jelly or lanolin base that is intended for external use but may penetrate the skin. It is used for its soothing, astringent, or bacteriostatic effects. |
| Paste | Ointment-like preparation that tends to absorb secretions. It softens and penetrates the skin less than ointments. |
| Pills | Globular, oval, or flattened materials containing a mixture of a medication with some cohesive material. |
| Powders | Fine particles of solid medications. |
| Route | Method of administration of a medication, i.e., IM (intramuscular), IV (intravenous), SQ or SC (subcutaneous), topical, PO (oral), intradermal, SL (sublingual). |
| Spansule | Timed-release capsule that contains small particles of the medication coated with materials that take varying amounts of time to dissolve. This prolongs action for as long as 24 hours. |
| Spirits | Concentrated, alcoholic solutions of volatile substances. The dissolved substances may be solids, liquids, or gases. |
| Suppository | Mixture of a medication in a firm base that is molded so it can be inserted into a body cavity, i.e., rectum, vagina, urethra. |
| Syrup | Aqueous solution of sucrose or sugar. It is added to a medication to disguise an unpleasant taste or to soothe mucous membranes. |
| Tablets | Powdered medications that are compressed or molded into shape. When they are scored, i.e., have lines drawn in them, they may be broken along the line; otherwise, they must be given whole. |
| Teaching about medications | Clients should be taught how to administer the medication, the proper dosage and frequency of the medication, how the medication works, possible adverse effects, and signs of effectiveness of the medication. |
| Tincture | Alcoholic or hydroalcoholic solutions usually prepared from plants or chemical substances. |
| Toxic effects | Untoward or severe nontherapeutic effects of the medication that are dangerous to the person and require the medication to be discontinued immediately or the dosage lowered. |
| Trade name | Brand name or registered trademark of a medication used by the manufacturer. Medications can have several trade names, depending on which company which manufactures the medication. |

*(Continued)*

| Troches or lozenges | Flat, round, or rectangular mediations that are held in the mouth until they dissolve. They are usually used for their local soothing effect but may cause a systemic effect. |
|---|---|
| Uses | Medical diagnoses for which a medication is administered. |
| Vials | Glass containers with rubber stoppers that contain multiple doses of medication. Powders in vials are diluted with either sterile water or sterile saline. |

# TERMINOLOGY USED FOR DOCUMENTATION

| TERM | DEFINITION |
| --- | --- |
| abduction | to move away from the midline |
| abraded | scraped |
| acetonuria | acetone in the urine |
| adduction | to move toward the midline |
| afebrile | without fever |
| albuminuria | albumin in the urine |
| ambulatory | walking |
| amenorrhea | absence of menstruation |
| amnesia | loss or defective memory |
| ankyloses | stiff joint |
| anorexia | loss of appetite |
| anuria | total suppression of urination |
| apnea | short periods when breathing has ceased |
| arthritis | inflammation of joint |
| asphyxia | suffocation |
| atrophy | wasting |
| auscultation, auscultate | to listen for sounds |
| bradycardia | heartbeat less than 60 beats per minute |
| Cheyenne-Stokes respirations | abnormal breathing pattern: increasing rate and depth of respirations, followed by decreasing depth and rate, followed with periods of apnea |
| choluria | bile in the urine |
| clonic tremor | shaking with intervals of rest |
| conjunctivitis | inflammation of conjunctiva |

*(Continued)*

| TERM | DEFINITION |
|------|-----------|
| coryza | watery drainage from nose |
| cyanotic | bluish in color due to poor oxygenation |
| defecation | bowel movement |
| dental caries | decay of the teeth |
| dentures | false teeth |
| diarrhea | excessive or frequent defecation |
| diplopia | double vision |
| distended | appears swollen |
| diuresis | large amount of urine voided |
| dorsal recumbent | lying on back, knees flexed and apart |
| dysmenorrhea | painful menstruation |
| dyspnea | difficulty breathing |
| dysrhythmia, arrhythmia | abnormal heart rhythm |
| dysuria | painful urination |
| edematous | puffy, swollen |
| emaciated | thin, underweight |
| emetic | agent given to produce vomiting |
| enuresis | bed-wetting |
| epistaxis | nosebleed |
| eructation | belching |
| erythema | redness |
| eupnea | normal breathing |
| excoriation | raw surface |
| exophthalmos | abnormal protrusion of eyeball |
| extension | to straighten |
| fatigued | tired |
| feigned | pretended |
| fetid | foul |
| fixed | motionless |
| flaccid | soft, flabby |

*(Continued)*

| TERM | DEFINITION |
|------|------------|
| flatus, flatulence | gas in the digestive tract |
| flexion | bending |
| flushed | pink or hot |
| Fowler position | semi-erect, knee flexed, head of bed elevated 45-60° |
| gavage | forced feeding through tube passed into stomach |
| glossy | shiny |
| glycosuria | glucose in the urine |
| guaiac | test for occult blood |
| gustatory | dealing with taste |
| heliotherapy | using sunlight as a therapeutic agent |
| hematemesis | blood in vomitus |
| hematuria | blood in the urine |
| hemiplegia | paralysis of one side of the body |
| hemoglobinuria | hemoglobin in the urine |
| hemoptysis | spitting of blood |
| horizontal | flat |
| hydrotherapy | using water as a therapeutic agent |
| hyperpnea | rapid breathing |
| hypertonic | concentration greater than body fluids |
| hypotonic | concentration less than body fluids |
| infrequent | not often |
| insomnia | inability to sleep |
| instillation | pouring into a body cavity |
| intermittent | starting and stopping, not continuous |
| intradermal | within or through the skin |
| intramuscular | within or through the muscle |
| intraspinal | within or through the spinal canal |
| intravenous | within or through the vein |
| involuntary, incontinent | unable to control bladder or bowels |
| isotonic | having the same tonicity or concentration as body fluids |

*(Continued)*

| TERM | DEFINITION |
|---|---|
| jackknife position | prone with hips over break in table and feet below level of head |
| jaundice | yellow color |
| knee-chest position | in face down position resting on knees and chest |
| kyphosis | humpback, concavity of spine |
| labored | difficult, requires an effort |
| lacerated | torn, broken |
| lateral position | on the side, knees flexed |
| lithotomy position | on back, buttocks near edge of table, knees well flexed and separated |
| lochia | drainage from the vagina after delivery |
| lordosis | swayback convexity of spine |
| manipulation, manipulate | to handle |
| menopause | cessation of menstruation |
| menorrhagia | profuse menstruation |
| metrorrhagia | variable amount of uterine bleeding occurring at frequent but irregular intervals |
| miosis | contraction of pupil |
| moist | wet |
| monoplegia | paralysis of one limb |
| mucopurulent | drainage containing mucus and pus |
| mydriasis | dilation of pupil |
| myopia | near-sightedness |
| nausea | desire to vomit |
| necrosis | death of tissue |
| nocturia | frequent voiding at night |
| obese | overweight |
| objective | able to document other than by observation |
| oliguria | scant urination, less than 400 mL in 24 hours |
| orthopnea | inability to breath or difficulty breathing lying down |
| palliative | offering temporary relief |
| pallor | pale |

*(Continued)*

| TERM | DEFINITION |
| --- | --- |
| palpation, palpate | to feel with hands or fingers |
| paraplegia | paralysis of legs |
| paroxysm | spasms or convulsive seizure |
| paroxysmal | coming in seizures |
| pediculi, pediculosis | lice |
| percussion, percuss | to strike |
| persistent | lasting over a long time |
| petechia | small rupture of blood vessels |
| photophobia | sensitive to light |
| photosensitivity | skin reaction caused by exposure to sunlight |
| pigmented | containing color |
| polyuria | increased amount of voiding |
| profuse, copious | large amount |
| projectile | ejected or projected some distance |
| pronation | to turn downward |
| prone | on abdomen, face turned to one side |
| prophylactic | preventative |
| protruding | extends outward |
| pruritus | itching |
| ptosis | drooping eyelid |
| purulent | drainage containing pus |
| pyrexia | elevated temperature |
| pyuria | pus in the urine |
| radiating | spreads to distant areas |
| radiotherapy | using x-ray or radium as a therapeutic agent |
| rales, crackles | abnormal breath sounds; indicate fluid in alveoli |
| rapid | quickly |
| rotation | to move in circular pattern |
| sanguineous | bloody drainage |
| scanty | small amount |

*(Continued)*

| TERM | DEFINITION |
|------|------------|
| semi-Fowler position | semi-erect, head of bed elevated 30–45° |
| serous | drainage of lymphatic fluid |
| Sims position | on left side, left arm behind back, left leg slightly flexed, right leg slightly flexed |
| sprain | wrenching of joint |
| stertorous | snoring |
| stethoscope | instrument used for auscultation |
| strabismus | squinting |
| stuporous | partial unconsciousness |
| subcutaneous | under the skin |
| subjective | observed |
| sudden onset | started all at once |
| superficial | on the surface only |
| supination | to turn upward |
| suppurating | discharging pus |
| syncope | fainting |
| syndrome | group of symptoms |
| tachycardia | fast heartbeat, greater than 100 beats per minute |
| tenacious | tough and sticky |
| thready | barely perceptible |
| tonic tremor | continuous shaking |
| Trendelenburg position | flat on back with pelvis higher than head, foot of bed elevated 6 inches |
| tympanic, tympanites | bell-like, resonant distention of abdomen due to presence of gas or air in intestine or peritoneal cavity |
| urticaria | hives or wheals, eruption on skin or mucous membranes |
| vertigo | dizziness |
| vesicle | fluid-filled blister |
| visual acuity | sharpness of vision |
| void, micturate | to urinate or pass urine |

# INDEX

## A

Abdominal assessment, 17
  liver function testing, 283
  neonates, 555
  preparation, 6
Abdominal hernia, 316
Abdominal respiration, 9, 195
Abdominoperineal resection, 302
Abortion
  history in prenatal assessment, 530
  spontaneous, 559, 560, 560*t*
Abruptio placentae, 561–562
Abuse
  of persons, 685–688
  of substances (*See* Alcohol abuse; Substance abuse)
Accommodation disorders, 458*t*
ACE. *See* Angiotensin-converting enzyme (ACE) inhibitors
Acetaminophen overdose, 610–611
ACLS (advanced cardiac life support), 130–131
Acne vulgaris, 69
Acoustic meatus, 465, 466*f*
Acoustic neuroma, 435–436
Acquired human immunodeficiency syndrome. *See* AIDS
Acromegaly, 328–330, 329*t*
Activities of daily living (ADL), guidelines, 34
Activity, physiological need for, 29
Acute drug psychosis, 670
Acute epiglottitis, 210
Acute kidney injury, 369–370
Acute laryngotracheobronchitis, 210
Acute leukemia, 487
Acute otitis media, 468–469
Acute pancreatitis, 295–296
Acute pulmonary edema, myocardial infarction, 158
Acyanotic heart anomalies, 619*t*, 620–621
ADC (AIDS-dementia complex), 233
Addiction, management of, 681*t*–682*t*, 683–684
Addison's disease, 335–336, 335*t*
Adenoma, pituitary, 328
Adenomastectomy, 515
ADHD. *See* Attention deficit hyperactivity disorder

ADH (antidiuretic hormone) deficiencies, 331, 331*t*–332*t*
ADL (activities of daily living), guidelines, 34
Adolescence
  growth and development in, 593–596, 593*t*–594*t*
  physical examinations, 604
  pregnancy in, 558
  psychosocial issues, 637*t*
  safety issues, 40
Adrenal gland disorders, 335–341
  Addison's disease, 335–336, 335*t*
  Cushing's disease, 335*t*, 339–341
  medications, 337*t*–339*t*, 341*t*
Adrenocortical hypofunction, 335
Adrenocortical medications, 697*t*–698*t*
Adulthood (developmental phase), 596, 597*t*, 598*t*
Advanced cardiac life support (ACLS), 130–131
Adventitious lung sounds, 15, 195
African-American clients, nutritional intake of, 249
Afterload, cardiac output, 127
Afterpains, 551
Agonal respirations, 195
AIDS (acquired human immunodeficiency syndrome), 231–237, 234*t*
  medications, 235*t*
  in pregnancy, 559
AIDS-dementia complex (ADC), 233
Airway resistance, 193
Al-Anon, 680
Alcohol abuse, 678–680
  congenital malformations and, 619
  intoxication, 678, 678*t*
  neonatal complications, 569
  withdrawal, 679, 679*t*
Alcoholics Anonymous, 679
Alimentary canal, 245
Alkylating antineoplastic medications, 477*t*
Allergies, 236
  antihistamine medications, 723*t*
Alpha-1 adrenergic blockers, 376*t*, 736*t*
Alpha radiation, 477
5-Alpha-reductase inhibitor, 376*t*
Altered thought processes, 669–676, 671*t*
  medications, 672*t*–675*t*

Alternative/complementary therapies
  herbal supplements, 406*t*, 661*t*, 713*t*, 795*t*–800*t*
  menopause, 503
  Parkinson's disease, 448
  perioperative care, 74
  radiation therapy, 477
  seizure management, 423
  skin cancer, 490
Alveolar ventilation, 194
Alzheimer's disease, 452–453
Ambulation, rehabilitation for, 31*t*–32*t*, 32–34
Amenorrhea, 503
American Cancer Society warning signs, 475
Amino acids, nutrition and, 251
Aminoglycosides, 724*t*
Amniocentesis, 557
Amnion, 523–524
Amputation, 394, 395*t*
Amylase, 282
Amyotrophic lateral sclerosis, 441–442
Analgesia
  labor and delivery, 541, 542*t*, 543
  opioid analgesics, 789*t*–790*t*
Anal phase of development, 587
Anaphylaxis medications, 178*t*–180*t*, 694*t*–696*t*
Anderson tube, 301
Anemia
  hemolytic, 236, 573
  iron-deficiency anemia, 223–225
  megaloblastic, 226–227
  pernicious anemia, 255, 262
Anesthesia
  intraoperative care, 73*t*–74*t*
  labor and delivery, 542–543, 542*t*
Angina pectoris, 161–162, 161*f*
  medications, 163*t*, 786*t*–787*t*
Angiotensin-converting enzyme (ACE) inhibitors
  heart failure, 156
  table of, 735*t*–736*t*
Angiotensin-receptor blockers (ARBs)
  heart failure management, 156
  table of, 735*t*
Angle of Louis, 15

Anisocytosis, 222

Ankylosing spondylitis, 398–399

Antacids, 699*t*

Antepartal care, 523–534

Anthropoid pelvis, 502

Antianginals, 163*t*, 786*t*–787*t*

Antianxiety medications, 649*t*–650*t*,
700*t*–701*t*

Antibacterials, 734*t*

Antibiotics, 724*t*

   antitumor, 479*t*, 743*t*–744*t*

   *See also* Anti-infective medications

Antibodies, 237

Anticancer medications

   antineoplastic medications, 477*t*–481*t*,
743*t*–748*t*

   chemotherapy, 477, 477*t*, 488, 490

   side effects, 748*t*

Anticholinergic medications, 702*t*–703*t*

Anticoagulant medications, 164*t*–166*t*,
703*t*–705*t*

Anticonvulsant medications, 419*t*–422*t*,
705*t*–708*t*

Antidepressant medications, 660*t*–662*t*,
708*t*–713*t*

Antidiabetic medications, 326, 714*t*–716*t*

Antidiarrheal medications, 309*t*, 717*t*

Antidiuretic hormone (ADH) deficiencies,
331, 331*t*–332*t*

Antidysrhythmics, 142*t*–143*t*

Antiemetic medications, 272*t*, 719*t*–720*t*

Antifungal medications, 721*t*

Antigens, 237

   prostate-specific, 519

Antigout medications, 401*t*, 722*t*

Antihistamine medications, 723*t*

Antihypertensive medications, 170*t*–172*t*,
735*t*–741*t*

Anti-infective medications, 724*t*–734*t*

Antilipemic medications, 741*t*–742*t*

Antimetabolites, antineoplastic medications,
478*t*, 743*t*

Antineoplastic medications, 477*t*–481*t*,
743*t*–748*t*

Antiparkinson medications, 748*t*–750*t*

Antiplatelet medications, 750*t*–751*t*

Antipsychotic medications, 672*t*–673*t*,
751*t*–756*t*

Antipyretic medications, 756*t*–757*t*

Antiretroviral medications, 235, 235*t*

Antirheumatic medications, 770*t*

Antithyroid medications, 757*t*–758*t*

Antituberculotics medications, 213*t*–214*t*,
759*t*–760*t*

Antitumor antibiotics, 479*t*, 743*t*–744*t*

Antitussive/expectorant medications, 761*t*

Antiviral medications, 761*t*–763*t*

Anus

   functional assessment, 299

   physical assessment, 18

Anxiety, 643–650

   assessment of, 643–646

   coping mechanisms for, 646*t*–647*t*

   disorders, 643*t*–644*t*

   medications, 649*t*–650*t*

   nursing interventions in, 646, 648*t*

Aortic stenosis, 621

Apgar score, 546, 546*t*

Apical rate, neonatal assessment, 553

Apnea

   defined, 195

   physical assessment, 10

Appendicitis, 310–311

ARBs. *See* Angiotensin-receptor blockers

Arterial blood pressure, intravenous therapy
and, 106

Arterial peripheral vascular disease,
182–184

Arteries, 125–126

Arthritis

   juvenile rheumatoid, 398

   medications, 770*t*

   osteoarthritis, 383, 399–400

   rheumatoid, 237, 396–397

Ascending colon, 299

Ascending colostomy, 303, 304*f*

ASD (atrial septal defect), 620

Aspirin, poisoning from, 610

Asthma, 203

Athlete's foot, 68

Atria, anatomy, 122

Atrial dysrhythmias, 135*f*

Atrial fibrillation, 137, 137*f*

Atrial flutter, 136–137, 136*f*

Atrial septal defect (ASD), 620

Atrial tachycardia, 135–136, 135*f*

Atrioventricular (AV) node, 124, 125*f*

Atrioventricular valves, 122

Atrophic vaginitis, 509

Atrophy, skin, 66

Attention deficit hyperactivity disorder
(ADHD), 432

   medications, 433*t*, 764*t*

Auditory canal, 465, 466*f*

Auricle, anatomy and physiology, 465, 466*f*

Auscultation

   pediatric assessment, 603

   physical assessment, 7–8

Autistic thinking, 670

Autoimmune diseases, 236

Autonomic dysreflexia, spinal cord
injury, 438

Autonomic nervous system, cardiac function,
126–127

Autosomal defects, 598

AV (atrioventricular) node, 124, 125*f*

Avulsion injuries, 387

## B

Babinski's sign, 555

Balanced suspension, 388, 390*f*

Ballottement, physical assessment, 6

Barium enema, 264, 300

Barium swallow, 263

Basal cell carcinoma, 489

Basal ganglia, 412*f*, 413

Baths, therapeutic, 60, 60*t*

Battle's sign, 36

Bell's palsy, 435

Bend fracture, 628

Benign prostatic hyperplasia/hypertrophy
(BPH), 368, 518–519

Beriberi, 254

Beta-adrenergic blockers, 156, 737*t*

Beta radiation, 477

Biliary atresia, 294

Biliary carcinoma, 294

Biliary tract

   anatomy and function, 282

   disorders of, 292–295

Billroth I and II surgical procedures, 278

Biophysical profile, fetal assessment, 558

Biopsies

   female reproductive system, 507–508

   liver, 283

   testicular, 518

Bipolar disorder, 663–667

   medications, 666*t*, 765*t*–766*t*

Birth asphyxia, 569

Birthmarks, 554

Bisphosphonates, bone-resorption inhibitors,
766*t*

Bladder

   anatomy and physiology, 356

   urinary retention, 359–360

Bleeding, in pregnancy, 560–562

Blindness, 460–461

Blood components, 109*t*, 219

   in pregnancy, 528

   transfusion reactions, 236

Blood disorders, 221–230

Blood group compatibility, 111*t*

Blood pressure, 10
 cardiac function, 127
 intravenous therapy and, 106
 neonatal assessment, 553
 pediatric assessment, 604
Blood tests
 glucose monitoring, 324
 nutritional assessment, 262, 263*t*
Blood transfusions, 108–111, 236
Blood vessels
 congenital malformations, 571, 621
 coronary, 122, 123*f*
 medications affecting, 739*t*–741*t*
 pregnancy, 524
Body structure and function, maintenance
  and promotion, 28–29
Bone
 diseases, 396–406
 fractures, 385–392, 386*f*, 628
 graft, low back pain, 385
Bone resorption inhibitors, 766*t*
Boredom, prevention of, 37
Boston brace, 630
Bowel disorders, 306–316
 abdominal hernia, 316
 appendicitis, 310–311
 celiac disease, 310
 constipation, 306–308, 307*t*
 diarrhea, 308
 diverticular disease, 314–315
 ileitis, 312
 intestinal obstruction, 315
 malabsorption syndrome, 308, 310
 Meckel's diverticulum, 311–312
 necrotizing enterocolitis, 574–575
 neonatal assessment, 555
 peritonitis, 311
 postpartum period, 551
 ulcerative colitis, 314
Bowel surgery, 302–306, 304*f*
BPH (benign prostatic hyperplasia/
  hypertrophy), 368, 518–519
Braces, scoliosis, 630
Brachytherapy, 483
Brain
 abscess, 445–446
 anatomy and function, 411–414, 412*f*
 organic brain syndrome, 429–430
Brain stem, 413
Breastfeeding, 549–550, 550*t*
 breast-milk jaundice, 573
Breasts
 anatomy and function, 502

cancer of, 515
 hypoplasia/hyperplasia, 514
 infections, 514–515
 physical assessment, 16
 postpartum care, 549–550
 in pregnancy, 527
 problems related to, 514–515
Breathing patterns
 alterations, 195–214
 definitions, 195
 normal, 192
 physical assessment, 9–10
 *See also* Respiration
Breath sounds, 196*t*
Breech presentation, 535
Bronchitis, chronic, 203
Bronchodilators, 204*t*, 210, 766*t*–767*t*
Bronchodilators/mucolytic medications, 203
Brudzinski's sign, 444
Buckle fracture, 628
Buck's traction, 389, 389*f*
Bundle branch block, 139–140
Bundle of His, 124
Burn management, 111–115, 113*t*–114*t*
 burn classifications, 112*t*
 eyes, 459*t*
Bursitis, 400

## C

Cajun clients, nutritional intake of, 249
Calcium
 imbalances, 95–97
 preparations, 403*t*–404*t*
Calcium channel blockers, 738*t*
Caloric requirements, adult, 262
Cancer, 475–485
 antineoplastic medications, 477*t*–481*t*,
  743*t*–748*t*
 assessment, 475
 chemotherapy, 477, 477*t*, 744*t*
 classifications, 476–477
 etiology, 475–477
 overview, 475–485
 *See also specific types of cancer,
  e.g.: Leukemia*
Candida albicans
 AIDS clients, 232
 vaginal infection, 509
Cantor tube, 301
Capillaries, 126
Captopril, 156
Caput succedaneum, 554
Carbamazepine, 666*t*
Carbohydrates, 250–251, 262

Carbonic anhydrase inhibitors, 768*t*
Carcinoma, larynx, 495–496
Cardiac arrest, medications for, 178*t*–180*t*,
  694*t*–696*t*
Cardiac conduction system, 123–125
Cardiac cycle, 125
Cardiac decompensation, 151
Cardiac disease, in pregnancy, 566
Cardiac disturbances, 131–133, 131*t*
Cardiac function
 anatomy of cardiovascular system, 121–123,
  121*f*
 angina pectoris, 161–162
 basic principles, 123–125
 heart failure, 147–157
 myocardial infarction, 157–161
Cardiac glycosides, 152, 153*t*, 768*t*–769*t*
Cardiac medications, 160*t*
Cardiac output, 127
 alterations, 129–166
 disturbances, 131–133
 rhythm disturbances, 133–147
Cardiac reserve, 125
Cardiac workload, prevention of increase in,
  37
Cardiogenic shock, 176
Cardiopulmonary arrest, 129–131
Cardiovascular system
 anatomy, 121–123, 121*f*
 cardiac function, 123–125, 125*f*
 postoperative care, 77
 vascular system, 125–127
Cardioversion, 144*t*, 145
Carvedilol, 156
Casting
 club foot, 629*f*
 fractures, 391–392
 hip spica cast, 627, 627*f*
 scoliosis, 630
Cataracts, 462–463
Catatonic schizophrenia, 671, 671*t*
Catheterization
 total parenteral nutrition, 267
 urinary, 361–363, 361*t*
CCT/OCT (contraction/stress test), 558
Cecum, 299
Celiac disease, 310
Cellular differentiation, cancer and, 475
Centrally-acting alpha-adrenergics, 739*t*
Central nervous system (CNS), 411–414,
  412*f*
 alcohol-related disorders, 680*t*
Central venous access devices (CVADs),
  106–108